Intensive Care Nursing

A framework for practice

Third edition

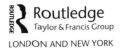 Philip Woodrow

Clinical scenarios by Jane Roe

Routledge
Taylor & Francis Group

LONDON AND NEW YORK

First published 2000
by Routledge

Second edition published 2006
by Routledge

This edition published 2012
by Routledge
2 Park Square, Milton Park, Abingdon, Oxon OX14 4RN

Simultaneously published in the USA and Canada
by Routledge
711 Third Avenue, New York, NY 10017

Routledge is an imprint of the Taylor and Francis Group, an informa business

Main text © 2000, 2006 and 2012 Philip Woodrow

Clinical Scenarios © 2000, 2006 and 2012 Jane Roe

British Library Cataloguing in Publication Data
A catalogue record for this book is available from the British Library

Library of Congress Cataloging in Publication Data
Woodrow, Philip, 1957–
Intensive care nursing : a framework for practice / Philip Woodrow. – 3rd ed.
p. cm.
Includes bibliographical references and index.
1. Intensive care nursing. I. Title.
RT120.I5W66 2011
610.73'6–dc22
2011002387

ISBN: 978–0–415–58451–7 (hbk)
ISBN: 978–0–415–58452–4 (pbk)
ISBN: 978–0–203–80812–2 (ebk)

Typeset in Sabon and Futura
by Florence Production Ltd
Printed in the UK by Ashford Colour Press Ltd

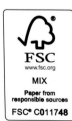

FSC
www.fsc.org
MIX
Paper from
responsible sources
FSC® C011748

To the States or any one of them, or any city of the States,
Resist much, obey little,
Once unquestioning obedience, once fully enslaved,
Once fully enslaved, no nation, state, city, of this earth,
ever afterwards resumes its liberty.

Walt Whitman

Fashion, even in medicine.

Voltaire

Contents

List of illustrations		xi
Preface		xv
Acknowledgements		xvi
List of abbreviations		xvii

Part I

▪ **Contexts of care**   **1**

1	Nursing perspectives	3
2	Humanism	11
3	Psychological care	18

Part II

▪ **Fundamental aspects**   **29**

4	Artificial ventilation	31
5	Airway management	47
6	Sedation	59
7	Acute pain management	68
8	Thermoregulation	79
9	Nutrition and bowel care	86
10	Mouthcare	96
11	Eyecare	103
12	Skincare	109
13	Children in adult ICUs	115
14	Older patients in ICUs	123
15	Infection control	130
16	Pandemic planning	139

Part III

▪ **Monitoring**   **147**

| 17 | Respiratory monitoring | 149 |
| 18 | Gas carriage | 161 |

19 Arterial blood gas analysis and acid/base balance   171
20 Haemodynamic monitoring   184
21 Blood results   198
22 ECGs and dysrhythmias   213
23 Neurological monitoring   234

Part IV

■ **Micropathologies**   **245**

24 Cellular pathology   247
25 Immunity and immunodeficiency   254
26 Disseminated intravascular coagulation (DIC)   260

Part V

■ **Respiratory**   **267**

27 Acute respiratory distress syndrome (ARDS)   269
28 Alternative ventilatory modes   275

Part VI

■ **Cardiovascular**   **283**

29 Acute coronary syndromes   285
30 Cardiac intervention and surgery   292
31 Shock   304
32 Sepsis   317
33 Fluid management   325
34 Inotropes and vasopressors   336
35 Vascular surgery   346

Part VII

■ **Neurological**   **353**

36 Central nervous system injury   355
37 Peripheral neurological pathologies   370

Part VIII

■ **Abdominal**   **377**

38 Acute kidney injury   379
39 Haemofiltration   389
40 Gastrointestinal bleeds   398
41 Liver failure   405
42 Obstetric emergencies   415
43 Transplants   423

Part IX

◼ **Metabolic**   **431**

44   Severe acute pancreatitis   433
45   Diabetic crises   440
46   Self-poisoning   446

Part X

◼ **Professional**   **455**

47   Professional perspectives   457
48   Transferring critically ill patients   463
49   Managing the ICU   469
50   Cost of intensive care   478

Glossary   485
References   493
Index   557

Illustrations

Figures

5.1	ETT just above the carina	49
5.2	High- and low-pressure ETT cuffs	53
5.3	The nasal cavity	54
7.1	Referred pain	71
7.2	Dermatomes	75
9.1	Krebs' (citric acid) cycle	88
9.2	Bristol Stool Form Chart	92
10.1	Oral (buccal) cavity	98
11.1	External structure of the eye	107
17.1	Auscultation sites for breath sounds (anterior chest wall)	152
17.2	Breath waveform	153
17.3	Pressure waveform	154
17.4	Flow waveform	155
17.5	Volume waveform	155
17.6	Pressure:volume loop	155
17.7	Flow:volume loop	157
18.1	Oxygen dissociation curve	165
18.2	Carbon dioxide dissociation curve	167
19.1	Origin of acid/base imbalance	174
20.1	Arterial trace	187
20.2	Main central venous cannulation sites	188
20.3	CVP waveform	190
22.1	Normal sinus rhythm	215
22.2	Chest lead placement	216
22.3	Action potential	218
22.4	Premature atrial ectopic	221
22.5	Multifocal ventricular ectopics	222
22.6	Sinus arrhythmia	222
22.7	Supraventricular tachycardia	223
22.8	Atrial fibrillation	223
22.9	Atrial flutter	225
22.10	Wolff-Parkinson-White syndrome	225
22.11	Junctional (or 'nodal') rhythm	226

22.12	First-degree block	226
22.13	Second-degree block (type 1)	227
22.14	Second-degree block (type 2)	227
22.15	Third-degree block	228
22.16	Bundle branch block	228
22.17	Bigeminy and trigeminy	229
22.18	Ventricular tachycardia	229
22.19	Torsades de pointes	230
22.20	Ventricular fibrillation	230
23.1	Cross-section of the cranium	236
23.2	Pressure:volume curve	236
23.3	Intracranial hypertension and tissue injury: a vicious circle	237
23.4	Normal ICP waveform	241
24.1	Cell structure	248
29.1	Acute coronary syndromes	287
29.2	Coronary arteries, with anterior myocardial infarction	287
31.1	Intra-aortic balloon pump	312
31.2	Arterial pressure trace	313
31.3	Ventricular assist devices	314
33.1	Normal distribution of body water	326
33.2	Perfusion gradients	327
39.1	Ultrafiltration	390
39.2	Convection	391
40.1	Tamponade ('Minnesota') tube	401

Tables

1.1	Levels of care	4
4.1	Commonly used abbreviations and terms	32
6.1	Ramsay scale	63
13.1	Normal cardiovascular vital signs in children	118
17.1	Sputum colour – possible causes	151
18.1	Partial pressures of gases at sea level	162
18.2	Some factors affecting oxygen dissociation	165
19.1	Some abbreviations commonly found on blood gas samples	178
19.2	Normal levels of electrolytes and metabolites	178
20.1	Normal flow monitoring parameters	192
21.1	Erythrocyte results	200
21.2	Normal white cell counts	202
21.3	Main biochemistry results	209
22.1	Framework for ECG interpretation	217
22.2	Likely lead changes with myocardial infarction	219
32.1	Terminology of sepsis	319
32.2	Significance of abnormal procalcitonin (PCT) levels	321
33.1	Summary of fluids (simplified)	328
34.1	Main target receptors for drugs	339

35.1   Common complications of open surgery to the aorta   350
36.1   Possible main aspects of medical management of traumatic
        brain injury   360
36.2   Priorities of care during fitting   362
39.1   Main differences between CVVH and CVVHD   391
41.1   Main liver function tests   408
43.1   Brainstem death: preconditions   425
44.1   Priorities of nursing care for pancreatitis   435

Preface

This book is for ICU nurses. Intensive care is a diverse speciality, with many sub-specialities. Even within a single ICU, the range of pathologies and treatments seen may vary widely. No text can hope to cover every possible condition readers may see, and general texts cannot cover topics comprehensively. My aim for this edition, as in the previous ones, is to offer nurses working in general ICUs an overview of the more commonly encountered pathologies and treatments. This text will probably be most useful about 6–12 months into ICU nursing careers, so assumes that readers are already qualified nurses, with experience of caring for ventilated patients, but wish to develop their knowledge and practice further. Because some knowledge is assumed, 'fundamental knowledge' is listed at the start of many chapters for readers to pursue any assumed aspects of which they are unsure. 'Further reading' at the end of each chapter identifies some useful, and usually relatively easily accessible, resources for readers to pursue. Definitions of some technical terms can be found in the glossary – where these terms appear in the text for the first time they are italicised, although italics are sometimes used for other reasons, for example the standard practice of italicising names of publications and micro-organisms, or for emphasis.

This book focuses on the nursing care of level 3 patients. Level 2 patients are the focus of a companion volume (Moore and Woodrow, 2009). Where reasonably possible, overlap between the two books is avoided, but some overlap is inevitable; some topics that may be relevant to level 3 patients are included in the other text – for example, intrapleural chest drains. The title and terminology 'intensive care unit (ICU)' has been retained, rather than replaced with the often used 'critical care unit (CCU)', largely to avoid confusion with 'coronary care unit' (also CCU).

This third edition has provided the opportunity to update and develop contents. Much more could be covered, but a larger book would be less affordable, more unwieldy and less used. My priority in revising this book has therefore been to identify core issues within a text of similar length. Some links made to incorporate topics into chapters are tenuous, but I hope that their presence justifies this approach.

This decade the volume of journal articles has increased exponentially. While academic rigour and research integrity are probably higher than ever, relevance to nursing practice is arguably lower. Medical literature has produced many meta-analyses, many of which are useful, but some draw on too little and too-dated evidence. Searching literature is therefore necessarily selective, and is heavily reliant on guidelines, meta-analyses and publications from key organisations, as well as being influenced by serendipity.

Many controversies are identified, but all aspects of knowledge and practice should be actively questioned and constantly reassessed. I have tried to minimise errors, but some are almost inevitable in a text this size; like any other source, it should be read critically. If this book encourages further debate among practising nurses it will have achieved its main purpose. References to statute and civil law usually relate to England and Wales, so readers in Scotland, Northern Ireland and outside the United Kingdom should check applicability to local legal systems. My hope remains that this book benefits readers, and so contributes to delivering quality patient care.

Philip Woodrow, 2011

Acknowledgements

As with previous editions, John Albarran has reviewed all chapters of this book, and made many valuable comments. Over the years and editions, the text has also been influenced by input from many other people, including reviewers, colleagues in the British Association of Critical Care Nurses, and East Kent Hospitals University NHS Foundation Trust – especially the staff of its three ICUs at Kent and Canterbury (Canterbury), Queen Elizabeth the Queen Mother (Margate) and William Harvey (Ashford) hospitals. I am especially grateful to the team at Routledge for commissioning this third edition, and supporting it throughout its development.

The second edition scenarios by Jane Roe have been revised by Philip Woodrow, who also wrote the scenarios for Chapters 16 and 48.

Harmony Pathology is in the process of standardising normal references ranges for laboratory results throughout the UK. Most Harmony ranges were issued at a very late stage of production of this book, and so could not be incorporated into the text. Many references ranges given will therefore now differ slightly from those issued by laboratories.

Further information can be found at: www.harmonypathology.org.uk.

Abbreviations

<	less than
>	more than
A	alveolar
a	arterial
AAA	abdominal aortic aneurysm
ABC	actual bicarbonate
ABCDE	airway, breathing, circulation/cardiovascular, disability, exposure
ABGs	arterial blood gases
Acb	*Acinetobacter baumanii*
ACCP	American Society of Critical Care Physicians
ACS	acute coronary syndrome
ACT	activated clotting time
ACTH	adrenocorticotrophic hormone
ADH	antidiuretic hormone
AF	atrial fibrillation
AIDP	acute inflammatory demyelinating polyneuropathy
AIDS	acquired immune deficiency syndrome
AKI	acute kidney injury
ALI	acute lung injury
ALP/alk phos	alkaline phosphatase
ALT	alanine aminotransferase
AMAN	acute motor axonal neuropathy
AMSAN	acute motor sensory axonal neuropathy
AMV	assisted mandatory ventilation
ANP	atrial natriuretic peptide (also called atrial natriuretic factor (ANF))
APACHE	Acute Physiology and Chronic Health Evaluation
APRV	airway pressure release ventilation
APT	activated prothrombin time
APTT	activated partial thromboplastin time
APV	adaptive pressure ventilation
ARC	AIDS-related complex
ARDS	acute respiratory distress syndrome

ARDSNet	Acute Respiratory Distress Syndrome Network
ASB	assisted spontaneous breathing
AST	aspartate aminotransferase
ASV	adaptive support ventilation
ATN	acute tubular necrosis
ATP	adenosine triphosphate
AV	atrioventricular (node)
BACCN	British Association of Critical Care Nurses
BAPEN	British Association of Parenteral and Enteral Nutrition
BE	base excess
BIS	bispectral index
BiVAD	biventricular assist device
BMI	body mass index
BNF	*British National Formulary*
BP	blood pressure
bpm	depending on context, 'beats per minute' (heart rate) or 'breaths per minute' (respiratory rate)
BPS	Behavioral Pain Scale
BTS	British Thoracic Society
c	capillary
CABG	coronary artery bypass graft
CAM-ICU	Confusion Assessment Measurement for ICU
CCU	coronary care unit (also critical care unit)
CD4, CD8	CD = cluster designation, the numbers refer to different types
C. diff	*Clostridium difficile*
CFAM	cerebral function analysing monitor
CFM	cerebral function monitor
CI	cardiac index
CIDP	chronic inflammatory demyelinating polyneuropathy
CK	creatine kinase
CLOD	Clinical Lead Organ Donation
CMV	controlled mandatory ventilation *or* cytomegalovirus (depending on context)
CNS	central nervous system
CNST	Clinical Negligence Scheme for Trusts
CO	cardiac output
COHb	carboxyhaemoglobin
COP	colloid osmotic pressure
COPD	chronic obstructive pulmonary disease
CPAP	continuous positive airway pressure
CPB	cardiopulmonary bypass
CPP	cerebral perfusion pressure
CRP	C-reactive protein
CRRT	continuous renal replacement therapy (blanket term used to describe any mode)
CSF	cerebrospinal fluid

CT	computerised tomography (scan)
CVC	central venous catheter
CVP	central venous pressure; blood volume
CVVH	continuous venovenous haemofiltration
CVVHD	continuous venovenous haemodiafiltration
CXR	chest X-ray
Da	Daltons (molecular weight)
dB	decibels
DCD	donation following cardiac death
DDS	Delirium Detection Score
delta P (ΔP)	amplitude of oscillation
DES	drug-eluding stents
DH	Department of Health
DIC	disseminated intravascular coagulation
DKA	diabetic ketoacidosis
dl	decilitre(s)
DNA	deoxyribonucleic acid
DO_2	delivery of oxygen
DO_2I	delivery of oxygen index
DPG	diphosphoglycerate
DSA	digital subtraction angiography
DSH	deliberate self-harm
DVT	deep vein thrombosis
ECG	electrocardiograph
ECLA	extracorporeal lung assist
ECMO	extracorporeal membrane oxygenation
E. coli	*Escherichia coli*
EEG	electroencephalography
EfCCNa	European federation of Critical Care Nursing associations
eGFR	estimated glomerular filtration rate; normal > 90 ml/minute
EPAP	expired positive airway pressure
ERCP	endoscopic retrograde cholangiopancreatography
ESPEN	European Society of Parenteral and Enteral Nutrition
$etCO_2$	end-tidal carbon dioxide
ETT	endotracheal tube
EVAR	endovascular aneurysm repair
EVLW	extra vascular lung water
F	fractional concentration in dry gas
FADH	flavin adenine dinucleotide
FDP	fibrin degradation product
FFP	fresh frozen plasma
FG	French Gauge
FiO_2	fraction of inspired oxygen (expressed as a decimal fraction, so FiO_2 1.0 = 100 per cent or pure oxygen)
FRC	functional residual capacity
GABA	gamma-aminobutyric acid

GBS	Guillain-Barré syndrome
GCS	Glasgow Coma Scale (assessment of level of consciousness)
G-CSF	granulocyte colony-stimulating factor
GFR	*see* eGFR
GGT	gamma glutamyl transpeptidase
GI	gastrointestinal
GTN	glyceryl trinitrate
GvHD	graft versus host disease
HAART	highly active antiretroviral therapy
HAI	healthcare-associated infection (previously called 'hospital-acquired infection')
HbA	adult haemoglobin
HbF	foetal haemoglobin (abnormal after 3 months of age)
HbS	sickle cell haemoglobin
HBV	hepatitis B virus
HCOOP	Health Care of Older People
HCO_3^-	bicarbonate
Hct	haematocrit (also called 'packed cell volume')
HCV	hepatitis C virus
HDL-C	high-density lipoprotein cholesterol
HDU	high-dependency unit
HELLP	haemolysis, elevated liver enzymes and low platelets
HES	hydroxyethyl starch
HFJV	high-frequency jet ventilation
HFOV	high-frequency oscillatory ventilation
HFV	high-frequency ventilation
HHb	deoxyhaemoglobin
HHS	hyperosmolar hyperglycaemic state (= HONKS)
Hib	*Haemophilus influenza* type b
HIT/HITTS	heparin-induced thrombocytopaenia and thrombosis syndrome
HIV	human immunosuppressive virus
HLA	human leucocyte antigen
HME	heat/moisture exchange(r)
HONKS	hyperosmolar non-ketotic state (= HHS)
HPA	hypothalamic-pituitary-adrenal
HR	heart rate
HRQL	Health-related Quality of Life
HSD	hypertronic saline dextran
HUS	haemolytic uraemic syndrome
Hz	hertz
I	ideal
IABP	intra-aortic balloon pump
IAP	intra-abdominal pressure
ICDSC	International Care Delirium Score Checklist
ICN	International Council of Nurses

ICNARC	Intensive Care National Audit and Research Centre
ICP	intracranial pressure
ICS	Intensive Care Society
ICU	intensive care unit
IDDM	insulin-dependent diabetes mellitus
I:E	inspiratory to expiratory ratio (on ventilator)
Ig	immunoglobulin (e.g. IgA = immunoglobulin A)
iLA	interventional lung assist
IMA	internal mammary artery
INR	international normalised ratio (measures clotting time)
IPAP	inspired positive airway pressure
IRV	inverse ratio ventilation
iu	international units
IVI	intravenous infusion
kcal	kilocalorie(s)
kDa	kiloDaltons (molecular weight) = 1000 daltons (Da)
kPa	kilopascals
LBBB	left bundle branch block
LCW	left cardiac work
LCWI	left cardiac work index
LIMA	left internal mammary artery
LSD	lysergic acid
LVAD	left ventricular assist device
LVSW	left ventricular stroke work
LVSWI	left ventricular stroke work index
MAAS	Motor Activity Assessment Scale
MAP	mean arterial pressure
MARS	Molecular Adsorbent Recirculating System
MC+S	microscopy, culture and sensitivity
MCD	mean cylindrical diameter
MCH	mean corpuscular haemoglobin
MCHC	mean corpuscular haemoglobin concentration
MCV	mean cell volume
MDMA	3–4 methylenedioxymethamphetamine (Ecstasy)
MetHb	methaemoglobin
MEWS	Modified Early Warning Score
MHRA	Medicines and Healthcare products Regulatory Agency
MI	myocardial infarction
mmHg	millimetres of mercury
mmol	millimole(s)
MMV	mandatory minute ventilation
MODS	multi-organ dysfunction syndrome (same as MOF)
MOF	multi-organ failure (same as MODS)
mPaw	mean airway pressure
MRI	magnetic resonance imaging

MRSa	meticillin-resistant *Staphylococcus aureus*, also called multi-resistant *Staphylococcus aureus*; in USA is spelt 'methicillin'
MSSa	meticillin-sensitive *Staphylococcus aureus*
MV	mandatory ventilation
NADH	nicotinamide adenine dinucleotide
NASH	non-alcoholic steatohepatitis
NCEPOD	National Confidential Enquiry into Patient Outcome and Death
ng	nanogram(s)
NGAL	neutrophil gelatinase-associated lipocalin
NHSBT	NHS Blood and Transplant
NICE	National Institute for Health and Clinical Excellence
NIDDM	non-insulin-dependent diabetes mellitus
NIRS	near infrared spectroscopy
NIV	non-invasive ventilation
NJ	nasojejunal
NMC	Nursing and Midwifery Council
nmol	nanomole(s)
NO	nitric oxide
NOS	nitrogen oxygen species (= nitrogen free radicals)
NPSA	National Patient Safety Agency
NSAID	non-steroidal anti-inflammatory drug
NSTE-ACS	non-ST elevation acute coronary syndrome (also called NSTEMI)
NSTEMI	non-ST elevation myocardial infarction (also called NSTE-ACS)
Nu-DESC	Nursing Delirium Screening Scale
O_2Hb	fraction of total haemoglobin combined with oxygen
OI	oxygen index
OPCAB	off-pump coronary artery bypass
P	pressure, or partial pressure
PAC	pulmonary artery catheter
PAF	platelet-activating factor
PAFC	pulmonary artery flotation catheter
$PaCO_2$	arterial carbon dioxide (from blood gas)
PaO_2	partial pressure of arterial oxygen
PAP	pulmonary artery pressure
PAV	proportional assist ventilation
PC	pressure control
PCA	patient-controlled analgesia
PCI	percutaneous coronary intervention
pCO_2	partial pressure of arterial carbon dioxide
PCP	*Pneumocystis jirovici* (formerly called *Pneumocystis carinii* pneumonia)
PCT	procalitonin
PCV	packed cell volume (also called 'haematocrit')

PDI	phosphodiesterase inhibitor
PE	pulmonary embolism
PEA	pulseless electrical activity
PEEP	positive end expiratory pressure
PEG/PEJ	percutaneous endoscopic gastrostomy/jejunostomy
PFC	perfluorocarbon
PGD	patient group direction
PGE_2	prostaglandin E_2
PGI_2	prostaglandin I_2 (also called 'prostacyclin')
pH	acid/base balance
pHi	intramucosal pH
PICC	peripherally inserted central cannula
PICCO	peripherally inserted continuous cardiac output
PICU	paediatric intensive care unit
PJP	*see PCP*
PN	parenteral nutrition
pPCI	primary percutaneous coronary intervention
PPE	personal protective equipment
PPI	proton pump inhibitor
PPV	pulse pressure variation
PR	per rectum (= digital rectal examination)
PRVC	pressure-regulated volume control
PS	pressure support
PSIMV	pressure-synchronised intermittent mandatory ventilation
PSV	pressure support ventilation
PTCA	percutaneous transluminal coronary angioplasty
PTSD	post-traumatic stress disorder
PT	prothrombin time
PTT	partial thromboplastin time
PUFAs	polyunsaturated fatty acids
PVR	pulmonary vascular resistance
PVRI	pulmonary vascular resistance index
Q	volume of blood
QALYs	Quality-adjusted Life Years
QT	interval between the start of the Q wave and the end of the T wave on the ECG complex (= duration of ventricular excitability)
QTc	QT interval corrected to what it would be if heart rate were 60
RASS	Richmond Agitation and Sedation Scale
RBBB	right bundle branch block
RBC	red blood cell
RCN	Royal College of Nursing
RCOG	Royal College of Obstetricians and Gynaecologists
RCP	Royal College of Physicians
RCW	right cardiac work
RCWI	right cardiac work index

REM	rapid eye movement
RHb	reduced or deoxygenated haemoglobin
RNA	ribonucleic acid (part of cells)
ROS	reactive oxygen species (= oxygen free radicals)
RR	respiratory rate
RSBI	rapid shallow breathing index
rt-PA	recombinant tissue plasminogen activator
RVSW	right ventricular stroke work
RVSWI	right ventricular stroke work index
SA	sinoatrial (node)
SaO_2	saturation of arterial oxygen
SAPS	Simplified Acute Physiology Score
SARS	severe acute respiratory syndrome
SAS	Sedation-Agitation Scale (Riker)
SBC	standardised bicarbonate
SBE	standardised base excess
SCBU	special care baby unit
SCI	spinal cord injury
$ScvO_2$	central venous oxygen saturation
SDD	selective digestive decontamination
SI	Système Internationale
SIMV	synchronised intermittent mandatory ventilation
SIRS	systemic inflammatory response syndrome
SjO_2	jugular venous bulb saturation
SNOD	Senior Nurse Organ Donation
SOD	selective oral decontamination
SOIV	swine origin influenza virus
SPC	Summary of Product Characteristics
SpO_2	pulse oximetry
SSI	signs and symptoms of infection
STE-ACS	ST elevation acute coronary syndrome (also called STEMI)
STEMI	ST elevation myocardial infarction (also called STE-ACS)
SV	stroke volume
SVI	stroke volume index
SvO_2	mixed venous oxygen saturation
SVR	systemic vascular resistance
SVRI	systemic vascular resistance index
SVV	stroke volume variation
SVT	supraventricular tachycardia
TB	tuberculosis
TBI	traumatic brain injury
tCO^2	total carbon dioxide
TEB	thoracic electrical bioimpedance
TEDS™	thromboembolism deterrent stockings
TEG	thromboelastography
TENS	transcutaneous electrical nerve stimulation

TIPSS	transjugular intrahepatic portosystemic shunt
TMP	transmembrane pressure
TNFα	tumour necrosis factor alpha
TP	total protein
t-PA, rt-PA	(recombinant) tissue plasminogen activator
TRALI	transfusion-related acute lung injury
TTP	thrombotic thrombocytopaenia purpura
TV	tidal volume (also written at V_t)
UA	unstable angina
UTI	urinary tract infection
v	venous
VAD	ventricular assist device
VALI	ventilator-associated lung injury (see VILI)
VAP	ventilator-associated pneumonia
VILI	ventilator-induced lung injury (see VALI)
VO_2	consumption of oxygen
VO_2I	consumption of oxygen index
V/Q	(alveolar) ventilation to (pulmonary capillary) perfusion ratio; normal V/Q = 0.8
VRE	vancomycin-resistant *Enterococci*
V_t	tidal volume (also written at TV)
VT	ventricular tachycardia
VTE	venous thromboembolism
WBC	white blood cell (count)
WCC	white cell count
WHO	World Health Organization
WPW	Wolff-Parkinson-White syndrome

Part I

Contexts of care

Chapter 1

Nursing perspectives

Contents

Introduction	4
Technology	5
The patient . . .	5
. . . their relatives . . .	5
. . . and the nurse	7
Stress	8
Duty of care	8
Implications for practice	9
Summary	9
Further reading	10
Clinical questions	10

Introduction

This book is about the nursing care of critically ill (level 3 – see Table 1.1) patients; a companion book (Moore and Woodrow, 2009) focuses on level 2 patients.

The fifty years of ICUs have seen various technologies, drugs and protocols launched as panaceas for problems of critical illness. While many have found a valid niche, initial hopes have often been largely disappointed. What has been constant is the contribution of nurses and nursing to outcomes for critically ill patients. So what is the purpose of nurses in ICUs? What does critical illness, and admission to intensive care, cost patients and their families? In the busyness of everyday practice, these fundamental questions can too easily be forgotten. Nursing is expensive, costing more than one-quarter of acute Trust budgets, and although ICU staffing costs vary, high nurse:patient ratios necessitate the need for ICU nurses to clarify their value (Bray *et al.*, 2009). This book explores issues for ICU nursing practice; this section establishes core fundamental aspects of ICU nursing. To help readers articulate the importance of their role, this first chapter explores what nursing means in the context of intensive care, while Chapter 2 outlines two schools of psychology (Humanism and Behaviourism) that have influenced healthcare and society.

A recurring theme of the pathologies described comprises two responses:

- inflammation
- stress.

These are defensive/protective responses. Balanced responses (appropriate to the threat) often help resolve non-critical illness. Critical illness typically occurs with imbalanced responses – insufficient response means disease can cause death, while excessive response becomes pathological. Many critically ill patients suffer systemic inflammatory response syndrome (SIRS), where the main problems are caused by excessive, body-wide inflammatory responses.

Table 1.1 Levels of care

Level 0	Patients whose needs can be met through normal ward care in an acute hospital.
Level 1	Patients at risk of their condition deteriorating, or those recently relocated from higher levels of care, whose needs can be met on an acute ward with additional advice and support from the critical care team.
Level 2	Patients requiring more detailed observation or intervention, including support for a single failing organ system or post-operative care and those 'stepping down' from higher levels of care.
Level 3	Patients requiring advanced respiratory support alone, or basic respiratory support together with support of at least two organ systems. This level includes all complex patients requiring support for multi-organ failure.

Source: DH (2000a)

Technology

Intensive care is a young speciality. The first purpose-built intensive care unit (ICU) in the UK opened in 1964 (Ashworth, personal communication). ICUs offer potentially life-saving intervention during acute physiological crises, with emphasis on medical need and availability of technology.

Technology provides valuable means of monitoring and treatment, but can also be dehumanising (Almerud *et al.*, 2007). To achieve a patient-centred focus, patients, not machines, must remain central to each nurse's role (ICN, 2006). ICU patients, often disempowered by their disease and drugs, are confronted with environments designed for medical and technical use that can create barriers for patients and their care (Eriksson *et al.*, 2010). ICU nurses can valuably use technology to promote physical recovery, but patients, rather than machines, should be the focus of nursing care. Nurses should develop therapeutic and humanistic environments that help the patient as a whole person towards their recovery (Almerud *et al.*, 2007). For patients, caring behaviour and relieving their fear and worries are the most valuable aspects of nursing (Hofhuis *et al.*, 2008a).

The patient . . .

Patients are admitted to intensive care because physiological crises threaten one or more body systems, and ultimately life. Care therefore needs to focus primarily on supporting failed systems. This book discusses various aspects of technological and physiological care, many chapters focusing on specific systems and treatments. But these aspects should be placed in the context of the whole person. People are influenced by, and interact with, their environment. Extrinsic needs for:

- dignity
- privacy
- psychological support and
- spiritual support

define each person as a unique individual, rather than just a biologically functioning organism.

Uniquely among healthcare workers, nurses are with the patient throughout their hospital stay. A fundamental role of nurses is therefore to be with and be for the patient, as a whole person (McGrath, 2008). Person-centred care is widely cited in strategic documents, policy statements and organisational values, but its evaluation tends to be narrow and reductionist (Manley and McCormac, 2008).

. . . their relatives . . .

Although evidence is limited (Prinha and Rowan, 2008), relatives are an important part of each person's life (Burr, 1998), giving patients courage to struggle for survival (Bergbom and Askwall, 2000). So caring for relatives is an important part of patient care (Endacott, 2007; Prinha and Rowan, 2008). In contrast to the often high-tech focus of staff, families of intensive care patients often focus on fundamental aspects of physiological needs, such as shaving (Ryan, 2004), pain relief and communication (Tingle, 2007). Relatives' values and perspectives often differ from those of nurses (Endacott, 2007). Rather than hovering by bedsides, afraid to touch their loved ones in case they interfere with some machine, relatives should be offered opportunities to be actively involved in care (Azoulay *et al.*, 2003), without being made to feel guilty or becoming physically exhausted.

Physiological crises of patients often create psychological crises for their relatives, especially with end-of-life decisions (Azoulay *et al.*, 2005). Holistic patient care should include caring for their families and other significant people in their lives (Greenwood, 1998; Whyte and Robb, 1999). Too often, focus on tasks, however futile, can lead ICU nurses to neglect the support needed by families (Brenner, 2002).

Relatives may be angry. They are usually angry at the disease, but it is difficult to take anger out on a disease. Instead, anger, complaints or passive withdrawal may be directed at those nearby, who are usually nurses (Maunder, 1997). Most relatives display symptoms of anxiety or depression (Jones *et al.*, 2004), yet these symptoms too often remain unnoticed. They may blame themselves, however illogically, for their loved one's illness. Feeling guilty and distressed, they may neglect their own physical needs, such as rest (van Horn and Tesh, 2000) and food. Facilities for relatives should include a waiting room near the unit, somewhere to stay overnight and facilities to make refreshments (NHS Estates, 2003).

Relatives need information, both to cope with their own psychological crises and to make decisions. They often have a psychological need for hope, but with one-fifth of patients dying on the unit, and additional post-discharge mortality and morbidity, there may be little hope to offer. If death seems likely, relatives need to know so they can start grieving (Wright, 2007). Communication by staff is often ineffective (Azoulay *et al.*, 2000). Information given should be consistent, so should be recorded in multidisciplinary notes. Relatives will often anticipate a more positive outcome than physicians (Lee Char *et al.*, 2010), so may be unconvinced when bad news is broken. Of all staff, nurses are best placed to meet relatives' needs, yet needs are not always met (Holden *et al.*, 2002).

Nearly one-fifth of ICU patients die (Vincent *et al.*, 2009). Changes may be rapid and unpredictable. Where possible, both the nurse caring for the patient and a senior doctor should inform the family of anticipated outcomes, away from the patient's bedside, preferably in a room where discussion will not be interrupted by other people or telephones. The door should be closed for privacy, but access to doors should not be obstructed in case distressed relatives need to escape. Everyone should sit down, as family members may faint, and staff should not stand above relatives. Posture, manner and voice should be as open as possible. Tissues should be available. Having witnesses is useful in case relatives later complain. Detailed records of discussions should be recorded.

Relatives should be given time to think about information, express their emotions, ask anything they wish, and offered the opportunity to return if they wish. An information book, including details of who to contact or support groups (such as Cruse), is useful. Further discussion on bereavement can be found in Woodrow (2009).

... and the nurse

Nurses monitor and assess patients. But nurses also provide care. Assessment is fundamental to providing care, but excessive paperwork can be a hindrance. Nursing assessments should therefore remain patient-focused, enabling nurses and others to deliver effective care. Proliferation of policies, protocols and competencies is often intended to ensure quality and parity of care wherever patients are admitted and whoever cares for them. But each patient is an individual and needs individualised nursing care. While guidance and safeguards can be useful, nurses need to maintain and develop knowledge and skills to be able to adapt care to individualised patient needs.

Nurses should collaborate with other professions (NMC, 2008a). Nurse:patient ratios for level 3 patients should be 1:1 (EfCCNa, 2007; Bray et al., 2009). The UK faces specific challenges: UK ICU patients are sicker than in most countries (Mandelstam, 2007; Higgs, 2009a), there are fewer ICU beds per 100 hospital beds (ICS, 2006) and per 100,000 population (Adhikari et al., 2010) than in other developed, and many third world, countries. The Department of Health (DH, 2000a) recommends flexible use of beds for level 2 and level 3 patients. For level 2 patients, nurse:patient ratios should be 1:2 (EfCCNa, 2007; Bray et al., 2009). While this may reflect acuity of disease, it often fails to reflect nursing workload: level 2 patients are usually conscious but may be acutely disorientated/confused, whereas level 3 patients are often unconscious, so more nursing time may be consumed in maintaining safety for level 2 patients. Decreasing staffing levels increases complication rates (EfCCNa, 2007) and mortality (West et al., 2004; Cho et al., 2008).

Nurses and nursing have valuable roles within intensive care. But staff are an expensive commodity. Even if economic pressures are ignored, the global shortage of nurses and an ageing workforce (Buchan, 2002) limit supply. A pragmatic solution to both economic and recruitment limitations has been to develop support worker roles. Most units employing support workers have found they provide valuable contributions to teamwork, provided the skill mix of nurses is not reduced inappropriately (RCN, 2003a). British Association of Critical Care Nurses (BACCN) guidelines should protect patients, nurses and support workers from inappropriate delegation (Bray et al., 2009).

Intensive care can support failing physiological systems, but too often opportunities to prevent physiological deterioration before life-threatening crises are missed. Critical Care Outreach (= Medical Emergency Teams in Australia) aims to enable earlier detection and support of problems to prevent ICU admission becoming necessary, and to follow up patients discharged from

ICUs to help their recovery. Critical Care Outreach is discussed in Higgs (2009b). Similarly, pre-surgical high-dependency units (HDUs) enable optimisation (non-invasive ventilation (NIV), aggressive fluid management, inotropes), and so reduce complications (Wilson *et al.*, 1999). Pre-surgical high dependency has not so far been widely adopted in the UK.

Stress

Stress is frequently experienced by patients in ICUs (Samuelson *et al.*, 2007), but it can also be a problem for relatives and staff. Stress is both a psychological and physiological phenomenon. Psychology and physiology interact. Critically ill patients suffer physiological stress from their illness, and psychological stress from negative emotions, such as fear. The stress response is a primitive defence mechanism, activating the hypothalamic-pituitary-adrenal (HPA) axis (Marik and Zaloga, 2002). The pituitary gland releases adrenocorticotrophic hormone (ACTH), which stimulates adrenal gland production of adrenaline (epinephrine) and noradrenaline (norepinephrine), with increased production of other hormones, including cortisol. This 'fight or flight' response, discussed further in Chapter 31, increases:

- heart rate
- stroke volume
- systemic vascular resistance
- respiration rate
- blood sugar
- fluid retention.

While protective in an acutely life-threatening confrontation, all factors are frequently detrimental with critical illness. Caring for both physical and psychological needs, nurses can add a humane, holistic perspective into patient care, transcending an often hostile environment (McGrath, 2008).

Duty of care

Nurses' primary duty of care should be to their patients. This includes a duty to maintain confidentiality (NMC, 2008a). If patients are unable to express their wishes, and what information they wish shared with others, nurses should be cautious about sharing information even with close relatives and friends. Usually, if patients are unconscious, information will be given to the identified next of kin, who will usually be asked to liaise with other family and friends. Sensitive information should not be disclosed to anyone not directly involved in a patient's care, or if it is unnecessary to do so. Especial care should be taken with telephone conversations, both because the other person may not be who they claim to be, and because reactions are unpredictable. Requirements of the Mental Capacity Act 2005 (see Chapter 3) should be observed. If in doubt, advice should be sought, if necessary from the Trust's legal department.

Implications for practice

- Nurses need technical knowledge and skills, but nursing is more than being a technician.
- ICU nurses have a unique role in providing holistic, patient-centred care that can humanise a hostile environment for their patients.
- Nurses have a professional duty of confidentiality to their patients, which remains after patients die.
- Physiology and psychology interact, so although the physiological crisis necessitating ICU admission is the focus of treatment, holistic care includes meeting physical and psychological needs. Reducing psychological distress reduces the stress reponse, and so promotes physiological recovery.
- Relatives experience psychological distress. Holistic patient care should include care of relatives and significant others.
- Nursing values underpin each nurse's actions; clarifying values and beliefs helps each nurse and each team increase self-awareness.
- Patient experiences are central to ICU nursing, so consider what patients are experiencing.

Summary

Much of this book necessarily focuses on technological/pathological aspects of knowledge needed for ICU nursing, but the busyness of clinical practice brings dangers of paying lip service to psychological needs in care plans and course assignments, while not meeting them in practice. Psychological care is not an abstract nicety; it affects physiology, and so remains fundamental to nursing care. This chapter is placed first to establish fundamental nursing values before considering individual pathologies and treatments; nursing values can (and should) then be applied to all aspects of holistic patient care.

Intensive care is labour intensive; nursing costs consume considerable portions of budgets. ICU nursing therefore needs to assert its value by:

- recognising nursing knowledge;
- valuing nursing skills;
- offering holistic patient/person-centred care.

Person-centred care involves nurses being there for each patient, rather than the institution.

Having recognised the primacy of the patient, nurses can then develop their valuable technological skills, together with other resources, to fulfil their unique role in the multidisciplinary team for the benefit of patients. ICU nurses should value ICU nursing on its own terms, to humanise the environment for their patients. Relatives are an important part of the person's life, and have valuable roles to play in holistic care. But relatives also have needs that are often exacerbated by their loved one's critical illness, and that may remain unmet. The beliefs, attitudes and philosophical values of nurses will ultimately determine nursing's economic value.

Further reading

Patient perspectives, such as Almerud *et al.* (2007) and Crunden (2010) provide valuable, if salutary, reading. Johns (2005) provides a useful reminder of humane perspectives. Work pressure and limited resources can prevent ideals being realised, but Bray *et al.* (2009) offer guidelines for staffing levels.

Clinical questions

Q.1 Identify environmental, cultural, behavioural and physiological factors from your own clinical area that may contribute to the suffering and dehumanisation of patients in the ICU.

Q.2 Outline specific resources and nursing strategies that can minimise the suffering and dehumanisation of patients.

Q.3 Consider the role of a Consultant Nurse within the ICU. What are the responsibilities of a Consultant Nurse and how may their contribution to patient care be evaluated?

Q.4 Reflect on the assessment of patient dependency in your own clinical area. Does this consider:

- patients' need for nursing interventions;
- medical interventions;
- level of technology?

Chapter 2

Humanism

Contents

Introduction   12
Behaviourism   12
Behaviourism in practice   13
Time out   13
Humanism   14
Lifelong learning   14
Evidence   15
Implications for practice   15
Summary   16
Further reading   16
Clinical scenario   17

Introduction

We are products of history. Nursing and healthcare have developed significantly in recent years, and applicability of evidence from a decade or more ago is rightly questioned. But this does risk jettisoning awareness of philosophies that have influenced practice. Passive acceptance of philosophy can be dangerous, as philosophy affects our values – how we approach patients and patient care. Our values may be either explicit or implicit, and influence both individual attitudes and the culture we work in (Sarvimaki and Sanderlin Benko, 2001). Values therefore influence care. Chapter 1 identified the need to explore values and beliefs about ICU nursing. This chapter describes and contrasts two influential philosophies to supply a context for developing individual beliefs and values. This is not a book about philosophy, so descriptions of these movements are brief and simplified; readers are encouraged to pursue their ideas through further reading.

The label 'humanism' has been variously used through human history, probably because its connotations of human welfare and dignity sound attractive. The Renaissance Humanist movement included such influential philosophers as Erasmus and More. In this text, humanism is a specifically twentieth-century movement in philosophy, led primarily by Abraham Maslow (1908–1970) and Carl Rogers (1902–1987).

The Humanist movement, sometimes called the 'third force' (the first being psychoanalysis, the second Behaviourism), was a reaction to Behaviourism. This chapter therefore begins by describing Behaviourism. Two world wars, and other traumatic events of the twentieth century, have however replaced some of Humanism's classical optimism with an emphasis on recovering humane values from the impersonality of bureaucratic and technological systems (Walter, 1997).

Behaviourism

Behaviourist theory was developed largely by Watson (1924/1998), drawing on Pavlov's famous animal experiments: if each stimulus eliciting a specific response could be replaced by another (associated) stimulus, the desired response (behaviour) could still be achieved ('conditioning').

Behaviourism therefore focuses on outward, observable behaviours. Behaviourist theory enabled social control, so became influential when society valued a single, socially desirable, behaviour. For Behaviourists, learning *is* a change in behaviour (Reilly, 1980).

Holloway and Penson (1987) suggested that nurse education contains a 'hidden curriculum' controlling behaviour of students and their socialisation into nursing culture; nearly a quarter of a century later Benner *et al.* (2008) called for nurse education to move from focusing on socialisation and role-taking to formation. Through Gagné's (1975, 1985) influence, many nurses accepted and adopted a Behaviouristic competency-orientated culture, without always being made aware of its philosophical framework. Hendricks-Thomas and Patterson (1995) suggest that Behaviouristic philosophy is often covert, masked under the guise of Humanism. Increasingly, learner-centred teaching (Carter, 2009) and reflection (Gustafsson and Fagerberg, 2004) have replaced didactic education, enabling nurses to respond to individual patients and situations.

Behaviourist theory relies largely on animal experiments, but humans do not always function like animals, especially where cognitive skills are concerned. Focusing on outward behaviour does not necessarily change inner values. People can adopt various behaviours in response to external motivators (e.g. senior nursing/medical staff), but once stimuli are removed, behaviour may revert; when no external motivator exists, people are usually guided by internal motivators, such as their own values. So if internal values remain unaltered, desired behaviour exists only as long as external motivators remain.

Behaviourism relies on rewards and punishments to motivate individuals to conform to desired behaviour. Rewards and punishments used by Behaviourism are public – external to the individual – such as essay grades, job promotion, salary or loss of privileges. Humanism also uses rewards and punishments, but relies on internal ends, such as self-actualisation and individual conscience. Humanism is therefore dependent on the individual valuing a moral code.

Behaviourism in practice

Time out

A patient in the ICU attempts to remove his endotracheal tube. There have been no plans to extubate as yet.

Options:

> explanation (cognitive)
> accepting extubation
> analgesia and sedation (control)
> restraint (e.g. chemical – sedation).

Comment:

Here, 'pure' Behaviourism has already been tempered with humanitarianism: to try to comfort. Nevertheless, description remains deliberately Behaviouristic, seeing the problem as behaviour (extubation). While extubation causes justifiable concern, behaviour is a symptom of more complex psychology. The patient attempts extubation because the tube causes distress. Until underlying problems are resolved, they remain problems; restraint only delays resolution.

No philosophy is ideal for all circumstances, and few are without some merit. In this scenario, Behaviourism may justifiably 'buy time' until the underlying pathophysiology is resolved or reduced, when extubation will be desirable rather than a problem. Behavioural approaches can be useful, but they can also be harmful, dehumanising others to lists of task-orientated responses. Preregistration courses emphasise learning outcomes, creating passive learners (Romyn, 2001). Analysing values and beliefs, understanding the implications they have for practice, and selecting appropriate approaches to each context all enable nurses to give humanistic, individualised care.

Humanism

The Humanist movement was concerned that Behaviourism overemphasised animal instincts and attempted to control outward behaviour. People who are controlled too often learn to become helpless (Seligman, 1975). Humanism emphasises inner values that distinguish people from animals – a 'person-centred' philosophy. Rather than emphasising society's needs, Humanism emphasises the needs of the individual self. Simplistically, Behaviourism can be viewed as attempting to control, whereas Humanism attempts to empower. Seeing patients as human beings, and placing them at the centre of care, is therefore fundamental to nursing (Hofhuis *et al.*, 2008a). Maslow's *Motivation and Personality* (1954/1987) popularised the concept of 'holism' (the whole person). Humanists believe people have a psychological need to (attempt to) achieve and realise their maximum potential. Maslow (1954/1987) described a hierarchy of needs, self-actualisation being the highest. Roper *et al.* (1996) adopted Maslow's hierarchy into their nursing model, although arguably to Behaviouristic ends.

Emphasis on inner values led Humanist educationalists to concentrate on developing and/or attempting to change inner values. Values that are internalised will continue to influence actions after external motivators are removed. Changes in nursing practice made to conform with the desires of one person may not continue after that person has left, or even when they are not present (e.g. days off), but changes made because staff wish change to occur will continue as long as consensus remains.

Concern for inner values and holistic approaches to care makes Humanism compatible with many aspects of healthcare and nursing, although familiarity with terms can reduce them to levels of cliché. Patients believe empowerment helps their recovery (Williams and Irurita, 2004). Humanism has much to offer nurses in analysing their philosophies of care and practice, but no ideas should be accepted uncritically.

Lifelong learning

Where Behaviourist education aimed to achieve conformity, Humanist education sought to promote individuality; this reflects the training versus education debate. Training seeks to equip learners with a repertoire of behavioural responses to specific stimuli, usually with a 'hidden curriculum' of indoctrinating conformity. Such training is often time-limited. In animals, stimulus–response reactions are often simple (as with Pavlov's dogs). Training equips the learner to be reactive to problems (stimuli) rather than proactive (to prevent potential problems occurring). Conditioned responses can be life-saving during a cardiac arrest, but 'training' fails to develop higher skills to work constructively through actual and potential human problems.

Facts and ideas are quickly outdated (Rogers, 1983), so are less valued by Humanists than development of skills to enable personal growth (Maslow, 1971) and learning (Rogers, 1983). Humanism seeks to develop higher cognitive and affective skills to analyse issues according to individual needs, most valuable human interactions occurring above stimulus–response levels. For healthcare, Humanism promotes a person-centred philosophy that enables learning to continue beyond designated courses; each clinical area becomes a place for learning, and nurses should be extending and developing their skills through practice.

Many nursing actions have (literally) vital effects. Professional safety is necessary (Rogers, 1951), and most countries have professional regulatory bodies (e.g. the Nursing and Midwifery Council (NMC)), but emphasis on individualised learning (e.g. learning contracts), reflection and lifelong learning (NMC, 2008a) recognises that learning processes must be meaningful for each individual rather than determined by Behaviourist objectives and outcomes. NMC requirements for pre-registration emphasise that attendance at study days does not ensure learning has taken place.

Evidence

Humanism and person-centred care has a weak research base (Traynor, 2009), so acceptance or rejection of its philosophy remain largely subjective. Arguably, research-based approaches conflict with Humanism's fundamental beliefs in individualism; Rogers' early work did attempt to adapt traditional scientific research processes to Humanism, but his later work adopts more discursive, subjective approaches.

Much learning occurs through making mistakes; individualistic learning necessarily means making mistakes. Accepting the possibility of mistakes involves taking risks. Human fallibility should be recognised – expecting that mistakes will not occur, and so treating them as unacceptable, is unrealistic (DH, 2000b). However, errors with critically ill patients can cause significant, potentially fatal, harm. ICU staff, especially managers, need to achieve the difficult balance between facilitating positive learning environments and maintaining safety for patients and others.

Implications for practice

- Philosophy (beliefs and values) influences practice, so to understand our practice, we need to understand our underlying beliefs and values.
- Changing inner values, rather than just outward behaviour, ensures continuity when external stimuli are removed.

- Healthcare, nursing and ICUs retain Behaviouristic legacies that can undermine individualistic, patient-centred care.
- Humanism emphasises inner values and individualism, so Humanistic nursing helps humanise ICUs for patients by placing them at the centre of care.
- Nurses should seek to humanise the potentially alien environments and practices of the ICU for their patients.
- Humans are fallible, so mistakes will occur. Accepting this fallibility encourages errors to be acknowledged and learnt from, thus limiting future risks.

Summary

Philosophy is not an abstract theoretical discipline, but something underlying and influencing all aspects of practice, so is relevant to each chapter in this book. Our beliefs, even if we are unaware of their source, influence our practice. Nurses can humanise care by (Andrew, 1998):

- being there
- sharing
- supporting
- involving
- interpreting
- advocating.

This chapter has outlined two influential and opposing philosophies; applying these beliefs to nursing values (see Chapter 1) helps clarify our own and others' motivation.

Further reading

Many texts identified in Chapter 1 reflect (often unacknowledged) Humanistic philosophy, but the best resources remain the classic texts that developed Behaviourism and Humanism. Skinner (1971) gives interesting late perspectives on Behaviourism, while Gagné's (1975, 1985) influence entrenched Behaviourism in a generation of nurse education. Maslow (1954/1987) is a classic text of Humanistic philosophy. Rogers is equally valuable, and more approachable; his 1967 text synthesises his ideas, while his 1983 book valuably discusses educational theory. Benner *et al.* (2008) outlines USA proposals for changes to nurse education that largely reject Behaviourism in favour of Humanistic values.

Clinical scenario

James Oliver is a 35-year-old who was admitted to the ICU with a Glasgow Coma Scale (GCS) of 6 following an unsuccessful attempt at suicide. He is invasively ventilated, but without sedation in order to facilitate the weaning process. He continually reaches towards his oral endotracheal tube (ETT). This behaviour causes the nurse to respond.

Q.1 Describe a 'Behaviourist' response by the nurse to Mr Oliver reaching for his ETT.

Q.2 Explain how a 'Humanistic' response would differ from a 'Behaviourist' response in this situation. Consider the values that underpin each response, for example safety, duty of care, autonomy, motivation of Mr Oliver, and also his needs.

Q.3 Review your own practice and evaluate typical responses to this patient's gesture. What are your own and others' motivating values? How might the presence of a nurse with Mr Oliver influence his and the nurse's responses?

Chapter 3

Psychological care

Contents

Fundamental knowledge   18
Introduction   19
Delirium   19
Time out 1   20
Time out 2   21
Sensory input   21
Making sense of environments   23
Noise   24
Circadian rhythm   24
Sleep   24
Post-traumatic stress disorder   25
Safety   25
Recovery   26
Implications for practice   26
Summary   27
Further reading   27
Clinical scenario   27

Fundamental knowledge

Sensory receptors and nervous system
Motor nervous system
Autonomic nervous system
Stress response (see Chapter 1)
Psychological coping mechanisms – e.g. denial

18

Introduction

In the busyness of attempting to resolve acute physiological crises, psychological care can be consigned to afterthoughts. But physiology and psychology interact; psychological stressors cause physiological stress responses (see Chapters 1 and 31):

- *tachypnoea*
- *tachycardia*
- *hypertension*
- *hyperglycaemia*
- *immunocompromise*
- *oedema* formation.

All of these usually complicate critical illness.

Anxiety, delirium and post-traumatic stress disorder (PTSD) are common problems for ICU patients, and adversely affect morbidity and mortality. Since Ashworth's classic 1980 study, ICU nurses have been aware of problems from psychoses, and these have been given many names; but while progress has been made, many challenges remain.

Delirium

Most mechanically ventilated patients suffer delirium (acute confusion) (Jones, 2007; Waters, 2008; Davydow *et al.*, 2009; NICE, 2010a). In addition to psychological stress to patients and families, and other effects of morbidity, such as reduced motivation and prolonged recovery, delirium is associated with mortality rates of 25–33 per cent (Pisani *et al.*, 2009; Heymann *et al.*, 2010; NICE, 2010a).

Delirium may be:

- hyperactive
- hypoactive
- mixed.

Hyperactive and mixed delirium often cause bizarre actions, but hypoactive delirium more often causes withdrawal – remaining quiet, passive and unnoticed. Delirium is usually hypoactive (Pun and Ely, 2007), and so undiagnosed (Page, 2010).

All ICU patients should be assessed for delirium (Page, 2010). Arbour *et al.* (2009) suggest clinical scoring remains the 'gold standard', with assessment tools including:

- Nursing Delirium Screening Scale (Nu-DESC);
- International Care Delirium Score Checklist (ICDSC);
- Delirium Detection Score (DDS);

■ Confusion Assessment Measurement for ICU (CAMICU, available on the Vanderbilt website);
■ sedation assessment.

However, quantifying delirium does not in itself treat problems; assessment tools are only useful if findings influence action.

Delirium is difficult to manage, but can be reduced by (Page, 2010):

■ patient orientation
■ communication
■ mobilisation
■ analgesia
■ rationalising drugs.

Drugs may reduce delirium, haloperidol usually being the most effective (Borthwick *et al.*, 2006; Devlin *et al.*, 2008; Page, 2010). Haloperidol has few side effects (Ely *et al.*, 2004). Alcohol withdrawal can be treated with chlordiazepoxide or benzodiazepines. Sedation may provide *anxiolysis* (see Chapter 6), but is also a chemical restraint, so is not a substitute for nursing care. However, while drugs may change behavioural responses to delirium, they do not change underlying causes. Active observation and proactive nursing can do much to humanise care and environments, removing many factors that contribute to delirium.

Time out 1

ICU environments are abnormal. Using your senses – sight, hearing, touch, taste, smell – take two or three minutes to list your own impressions of your current environment; complete this before reading any further. Repeat this exercise on your ICU.

Review your lists, noting down beside each item whether impressions were perceived through sight, hearing, touch, taste or smell. Some items may be perceived by more than one sense. How often was each sense used?

Most items are probably listed under sight, followed by a significant number under hearing. Touch is probably a poor third, with few (if any) under taste or smell. This reflects usual human use of senses: most input is usually through sight and hearing, with very limited inputs perceived from other senses.

Time out 2

Imagine yourself as a patient in your own ICU. Jot down under each of the five senses any inputs you are likely to receive.

When finished, review your lists, analysing how many of these inputs are 'normal' for you. Remember, most people usually rely on visual and auditory inputs.

Sensory input

Even if eyes are/can open, ICU patients often have distorted *vision* from:

- drugs, e.g. opioids may cause blurred vision;
- absence of glasses, if normally worn;
- restricted visual field from positioning of head or equipment such as ventilator circuits.

Absence of vision may be caused by:

- periorbital oedema (preventing eye opening);
- exposure keratopathy (see Chapter 11).

Walls and ceilings are usually visually unstimulating; overhead equipment may be frightening. Waking to this alien environment, and trying to rationalise it, is likely to cause bizarre interpretation. Watching overhead monitors detracts from eye contact (non-verbal communication) and becomes dehumanising. Nurses should actively develop non-verbal skills (e.g. open body language, quality touch). Windows with views help maintain orientation to normality, so views should not be obscured by blinds, or beds placed so patients are unable to see out of windows.

Hearing is often unaltered by critical illness; over half of ICU patients remember nurses speaking to them (Margarey and McCutcheon, 2005), so staff and visitors should assume patients can hear normally. Communication is fundamental to nursing care, yet aural communication may be impaired because:

- patients are unable to respond to cues;
- hearing aids are missing, faulty or not switched on;
- the cochlear nerve is damaged by *ototoxic* drugs (e.g. gentamicin, furo-semide);
- English is not understood, or is not the person's first language.

Conversation is too often confined to either instructions or others' conversation (e.g. medical/nursing/team discussions, sometimes spoken across patients, often in jargon). Instructions, although valid in themselves, should be supplemented by quality conversation.

Touch is a major means of non-verbal communication, especially with impaired vision. Most touch in ICUs remains task-orientated. Task-orientated touch is necessary, but reduces individuals to commodities, reinforcing their dehumanisation. Caring touch reduces stress responses (Henricson *et al.*, 2008) and is valued by patients (Henricson *et al.*, 2009), yet is frequently underused in ICUs. Overload of abnormal tactile sensations may be caused by:

- unfamiliar bedding (e.g. people used to duvets);
- pulling from tubes/drains/leads;
- oral endotracheal tubes;
- endotracheal suction;
- pressure area care, passive movements and body positioning.

Patients may appreciate their pillow being turned or their hand being held. Human touch is valuable, especially if provided by loved ones.

Various receptors sense information about the body's internal and external environment. Proprioceptors, in the musculoskeletal system, provide information about body movement. Prolonged intervals between movement, common in most unconscious patients, result in lack of signals. Any movement sensed, such as movement in hoists or for procedures, may cause abnormal proprioceptive stimulation.

Barrier nursing, and reverse barrier nursing, can reduce infection. But for most people isolation is stressful and can cause depression (Catalano *et al.*, 2003) and delay weaning (Wenham and Pittard, 2009). Isolation also reduces surveillance by staff and can result in higher rates of falls (Maben, 2009). Social isolation may be overt (e.g. gowns and masks, emphasising subhuman 'untouchable' status, restricting visiting) or covert (e.g. avoidance of patients who have nit infestation, or depriving patients of quality touch and meaningful conversation).

Warm environments (above 24°C) contribute to poor sleep, as probably experienced by readers during warm summer nights. Ambient temperature in most ICUs usually exceeds 24°C.

Few ICU patients receive oral diets, so *taste* is limited to thirst and drugs (e.g. metronidazole causes a metallic taste) and anything remaining in the mouth:

- blood
- vomit
- mucus
- mouthwash/oral drug
- toothpaste
- fungal infections (*Candida albicans* – 'thrush'), stomatitis.

Being thirsty is one of the memories of ICU patients (Margarey and McCutcheon, 2005). Taste relies largely on smell, so reduced olfactory input (from intubation) reduces perception of taste.

Air turbulence over four nasal conchae (or tubinates) exposes *smells* to olfactory chemoreceptors. Intubation bypasses this mechanism, so sense of smell is usually reduced, although not absent. ICU smells are often abnormal:

- 'hospital' smells (disinfectant, diarrhoea, body fluids);
- human smells (perfume, body odours);
- putrefying wounds;
- nasogastric feeds.

Making sense of environments

The reticular activating system, near the medulla, filters information from the senses. Normally nearly all information is blocked, with only the few meaningful (for the individual) stimuli reaching the cerebral cortex, where we make sense of our environment. Removing irrelevant stimuli prevents sensory overload, keeping us sane. Reticular activating system dysfunction may be caused by 'psychedelic' drugs (e.g. ketamine, lysergic acid – LSD, ecstasy – see Chapter 46) or:

- reduced sensory input
- relevance deprivation
- repetitive stimulation
- unconsciousness.

(O'Shea, 1997)

Responses depend on both *reception* (sensory stimuli) and *perception* (sensory transmission to, and interpretation by, higher centres). Hallucinations vary, often being vivid and usually terrifying. Sensory deprivation can cause acute psychoses, delusions, severe depression and PTSD (Egerod *et al.*, 2007; Åkerman *et al.*, 2010), which may persist for many days, months and possibly years.

Intubation prevents ICU patients from speaking, and conscious ICU patients often have psychomotor weakness, which makes writing difficult. Patients find not being able to communicate extremely stressful (Wenham and Pittard, 2009). Gestures, facial expression and physiological signs (e.g. tachycardia) may be attempts to communicate, or indicate comfort, pain or anxiety. Conscious intubated patients often mouth words, but the effectiveness of this varies with their mouthing and others' ability to lip-read. Speaking valves and devices exist for patients with tracheostomies.

Understanding patients' perceptions and interpretations is not always possible, but can make sense of hallucinations and bizarre actions. Reported experiences often suggest profound fear; nurses (and other healthcare professionals) may become devils/tormentors, so nurses attempting to explore fears or reassure patients may meet resistance.

Explanations may reduce anxiety and psychological (and so physical) pain (Hayward, 1975). But, like any physiological intervention, reality orientation is not beneficial for everyone, and quality and quantity affect its effectiveness. Inappropriate reality orientation can provoke aggression.

Noise

ICUs are noisy. Christensen (2007) found that the lowest noise levels measured on ICUs were 50 decibels (dB) (mean 56–42 dB), while Akansel and Kaymakçi (2008) measured 49–89 dB (mean 65). Much noise is unavoidable, inevitably continuing overnight, and this can disturb sleep (Lawson *et al.*, 2010). Nurses should actively reduce unnecessary noise, especially overnight. Physical pain is caused by 130 dB, while prolonged exposure to 85–90 dB causes hearing loss (Stansfeld and Matheson, 2003).

Circadian rhythm

Circadian rhythm (change in body function over a day) is individual to each person, with normal slight variations between each day. Critical illness and abnormal environments (ICUs) can severely disrupt circadian rhythm. Circadian rhythm usually peaks at about 1800 hours and ebbs between 0300 and 0600. Most nurses working night duty experience the ebb stage (Muecke, 2005), so should avoid high-risk actions (e.g. extubation) at this time. During this ebb, reduced peripheral circulation may cause *ischaemia* (e.g. 'night cramps').

Circulating catecholamine and cortisol levels peak at around 0600 hours (Chassard and Bruguerolle, 2004). Sympathetic stimulation makes the cardio-vascular system hyperdynamic – tachycardia, vasoconstriction. Peak time for myocardial infarctions and strokes is 0600–1000 hours (Soo *et al.*, 2000), so early morning stimulation (e.g. washes) are best avoided with vulnerable patients.

Sleep

Sleep is essential to physical and psychological health; sleep deprivation increases mortality (Friese *et al.*, 2009), yet many ICU patients sleep poorly (Tembo and Parker, 2009). Sleep cycles are usually about 90 minutes, with the final stage (*rapid eye movement* – REM) being the most restorative (Wenham and Pittard, 2009). This is the stage most often lost in ICUs (Friese *et al.*, 2007).

ICU nurses should facilitate sleep by:

- ensuring night-time environments are as quiet and dark as reasonably possible;
- minimising interruptions, and allowing 90–120 minutes between interventions likely to disturb sleep;
- providing earplugs/eyeshades if desired;
- assessing effects of any night sedation used;
- individual assessment of sleeping pattern/needs.

Earplugs and eye masks can improve sleep overnight (Richardson *et al.*, 2007), although a small-scale study of noise-reducing earphones found that five of the eleven patients who tried them found them intolerable, while the other six slept better than the control group (Hassall *et al.*, 2010).

Dimming lights mimics day/night cycles, but 'dimmed' lighting often exceeds levels most nurses would choose for their own bedrooms at night. However, some patients may find some light comforting.

Afternoon rest periods of 90–120 minutes provide the opportunity for patients to recuperate from often physically tiring morning activities.

Post-traumatic stress disorder (PTSD)

Like delirium, many ICU patients experience PTSD (Pun and Ely, 2007). Åkerman *et al.* (2010) suggest that one-third of ICU patients have delusional memories; this may be an underestimate. Memories of the ICU are often incomplete and compressed. 'Missing time' can be psychologically traumatic. 'Patient diaries' recording significant events during their illness that patients may want to find out about can be a valuable way to come to terms with 'missing time' (Combe, 2005; Egerod *et al.*, 2007; Åkerman *et al.*, 2010), although evidence for their benefits or potential harm remains weak (Egerod *et al.*, 2007).

Professional duties of confidentiality, other ethical issues and workload (Åkerman *et al.*, 2010) may limit staff keeping patient diaries, but they could usefully be kept by families, who are more likely to record what would interest patients. Where diaries are used, opportunities for follow-up discussion and explanations should be available. Follow-up can be provided through:

- Critical Care Outreach;
- return visits to the unit;
- ICU follow-up clinics.

Some ICUs have developed follow-up clinics. Much initial literature about these was enthusiastic, but Cuthbertson *et al.* (2009) found nurse-led follow-up clinics to be neither effective nor cost-effective.

Safety

Patient safety is central to healthcare, being enshrined in all professional codes, national bodies such as the National Patient Safety Agency (NPSA), and such classic resources as Nightingale (1859/1980) and Roper *et al.* (1996). Confused patients may cause harm to themselves. While the law expects healthcare professionals will act in patients' best interests (Dimond, 2008), how far 'best interests' includes restraining confused patients from harming themselves is ethically and legally debatable. The five key principles of the Mental Capacity Act 2005 identify that:

- staff must presume capacity to make decisions until proved otherwise;
- staff must support people to make their own decisions using 'all practical means';
- staff must not treat people as lacking capacity to make decisions because their decision is unwise;

- patients' best interests are paramount;
- decisions by others must interfere least with rights and freedom of action of those lacking capacity.

Rights of the incapacitated are enforceable through a Court of Protection. However, when a confused patient attempts to self-extubate, there is not time to seek guidance from courts or lawyers.

Restraint is sometimes necessary to prevent patients harming themselves (e.g. self-extubation), but means used must be proportional to the harm (Musters, 2010), and restraint may actually increase self-extubation rates (Chang *et al.*, 2008). Physical restraints are marketed, but ICUs should be cautious about introducing them as they may cause more harm than good (Hine, 2007). Where physical restraints are used, local protocols should be developed (Bray *et al.*, 2004) to protect both staff and patients. Traditionally, the UK has preferred chemical to physical restraint, although ethical and legal differences between the two are also debatable (Bray *et al.*, 2004). Sedatives are discussed further in Chapter 6.

Recovery

Despite complications, most ICU patients survive critical illness. Transfer to wards can cause relocation stress (Strahan and Brown, 2005). Weaning care by reducing:

- time spent with patients
- monitoring (equipment, frequency)

helps adjustment to non-intensive care environments ('de-ICUing').

Implications for practice

- Many ICU patients suffer delirium, PTSD and other psychological problems.
- Psychology affects health; psychological ill-health increases mortality and morbidity.
- Psychological problems are not always obvious, and may remain undetected.
- Haloperidol is generally the first-line drug for delirium in ICUs.
- Good psychological care can prevent problems.
- Sensory imbalance is a symptom of psychological pain, provoking a stress response; alleviating pain provides both humanitarian and physiological benefits, so should be fundamental to nursing assessment and care.
- Sensory imbalance can be reduced by:

  - creating environments that minimise sensory monotony or overload;
  - providing patients with explanations, and helping them to understand what they are experiencing;
  - where patients are able to participate in care, encouraging them to take active roles.

- Monitors should be sited unobtrusively.
- Facilitating sleep is usually the nurse's most important role overnight.
- Patient diaries can be a useful means for patients to come to terms with 'missing time' and PTSD, but there should be opportunities for patients to discuss these after ICU discharge.
- With recovery, care should be weaned to prepare patients for ward environments ('de-ICU').

Summary

The significance of psychology is often acknowledged in academic assignments, but not so often translated into practice. Critical care nurses necessarily prioritise resolving physiological crises. But psychological problems are common, and complicate recovery. Nurses can valuably humanise environments for patients, and help promote psychological well-being.

Further reading

The National Institute for Health and Clinical Excellence (NICE) provides guidance for post-ICU rehabilitation (2009a) and delirium (2010a). The forthcoming Danish guidelines for patient diaries should prove useful; until then Egerod *et al.* (2007) and Åkerman *et al.* (2010) offer different, valuable perspectives. Jones has led aftercare initiatives; her 2007 review provides a useful summary. Nursing articles frequently appear on various aspects; Tembo and Parker's (2009) review of sleep is a recent, valuable example. Borthwick *et al.* (2006) review pharmacology for delirium, while Page (2010) provides a medical review.

Clinical scenario

Robert Duke is 67 years old and was admitted to the ICU 26 days ago following emergency abdominal surgery. His past medical history includes chronic obstructive pulmonary disease (COPD), smoking and heavy alcohol use. Mr Duke has a tracheostomy and his respiratory support has been weaned to bilevel NIV. He continues to have copious secretions requiring clearance, and also has twice-daily 5 mg nicotine patch applications. Mr Duke refuses to cooperate with nursing care and avoids eye contact with everyone except his wife. He appears sleep deprived and, as observations indicate, he takes 15-minute naps at night, with a total of two hours' sleep recorded in 24 hours.

Q.1 Note the best methods to determine Mr Duke's psychological state, for example, mood, anxiety, understanding, consent to treatments, pain, discomfort, etc. How will you assess Mr Duke's communication abilities and understanding of his situation?

Q.2 Identify risk factors associated with development of sensory imbalance and delirium in the ICU for Mr Duke. How can these risks be minimised?

Q.3 Consider strategies to improve his experience of critical care and include specific interventions for psychological and physical comfort.

Part II

Fundamental aspects

Chapter 4

Artificial ventilation

Contents

Fundamental knowledge   31
Introduction   32
Respiratory failure   33
Artificial ventilation   34
Modes of ventilation   34
Settings   37
Independent lung ventilation   39
Care of ventilated patient   40
Safety   40
System complications   41
Ventilator-associated lung injury 42
Weaning   43
Implications for practice   44
Summary   45
Further reading   45
Clinical scenario   46

Fundamental knowledge

Respiratory anatomy and physiology
Normal (negative pressure) breathing and mechanics
  of normal breathing
Dead space and normal lung volumes
Experience of nursing ventilated patients
Local weaning protocols/guidelines

Introduction

Ventilation is the process by which gases move in and out of the lungs. When self-ventilation is, or is likely to be, inadequate due to disease or drugs, artificial ventilation may be required. Artificial ventilation may fully replace patients' own ventilation, or support self-ventilation.

Intensive care units developed from respiratory units. Providing mechanical ventilation, and so caring for ventilated patients, is fundamental to intensive care nursing. Nurses should have a safe working knowledge of whichever machines and modes they use – manufacturers' literature and company representatives are usually good sources for information. This chapter discusses the main components of ventilation, more commonly used modes, and identifies complication of positive pressure ventilation on other body systems. Table 4.1 lists commonly used abbreviations and terms, but terminology of modes varies

Table 4.1 Commonly used abbreviations and terms

Abbreviation	Term
AMV	assisted mandatory ventilation
APRV	airway pressure release ventilation
APV	adaptive pressure ventilation
ASV	adaptive support ventilation
barotrauma	damage to alveoli from excessively high (peak) airway pressure
CMV	controlled mandatory ventilation
FiO_2	fraction of inspired oxygen (expressed as a decimal fraction, so FiO_2 1.0 = 100% or pure oxygen)
I:E	inspiratory to expiratory ratio (on ventilator)
MMV	mandatory minute ventilation
open lung strategies	strategies to keep alveoli constantly open, and so prevent atelectasis
PAV	proportional assist ventilation
permissive hypercapnia	tolerating abnormally high arterial carbon dioxide tensions ($PaCO_2$) to enable smaller tidal volumes
pressure support	self-ventilating (triggered) breaths have volume augmented by the ventilator until preset airway pressure is reached
PRVC	pressure-regulated volume control
PS	pressure support
respiratory failure	Type 1: oxygenation failure – hypoxia ($PaO_2 < 8$ kPa) with normocapnia ($PaCO_2 < 6$ kPa); Type 2: ventilatory failure – hypoxia ($PaO_2 < 8$ kPa) with hypercapnia ($PaCO_2 > 6$ kPa)
SIMV	synchronised intermittent mandatory ventilation
trigger	when patient-initiated breaths generate sufficient negative pressure, trigger initiates inspiratory phases through ventilators
V/Q	(alveolar) ventilation to (pulmonary capillary) perfusion ratio; normal V/Q = 0.8
VALI	ventilator-associated lung injury (see VILI)
VILI	ventilator-induced lung injury (see VALI)
volutrauma	damage from alveolar distension (excessive volume); also called 'volotrauma'

between manufacturers and authors. Additional ventilatory options are discussed in Chapter 28. Negative pressure ventilation is rarely used in ICUs, so is not discussed in this book. Oxygen toxicity is discussed in Chapter 18.

Frequently-used ventilator settings are discussed, but different diseases need different supports, and the variety of adjustments that can be offered means different practitioners will often prefer different options. Anaesthetists normally decide ventilator settings, although experienced nurses often make small adjustments. If in doubt about any settings, nurses should always seek further advice.

Invasive ventilation can be life-saving, but dying sedated and intubated on a busy ICU is not a dignified death. Invasive ventilation should therefore only be used for potentially recoverable conditions. When patients cannot make competent decisions for themselves, nurses (as patients' advocates) should contribute actively to multidisciplinary decisions. A useful ethical maxim is whether proposed interventions are likely to prolong life or prolong death.

Respiratory failure

There are two types of respiratory failure:

- Type 1: oxygenation failure – hypoxia (PaO_2 < 8 kPa) with normocapnia ($PaCO_2$ < 6 kPa);
- Type 2: ventilatory failure – hypoxia (PaO_2 < 8 kPa) with hypercapnia ($PaCO_2$ > 6 kPa).

(British Thoracic Society (BTS), 2002)

Gas exchange in lungs is determined by three factors:

- *ventilation* (V) – breath size;
- *perfusion* (Q) – pulmonary blood flow;
- *diffusion* – movement of gases across tissue between pulmonary blood and alveolar air.

At rest, healthy average-sized adults breathe about four litres each minute, with cardiac output of about five litres. This creates ventilation:perfusion (*V/Q*) ratios of 4:5, or 0.8. Perfusion without ventilation is called a shunt. *Shunting* can also occur at tissue level (reduced oxygen extraction ratio – see Chapter 20).

Carbon dioxide is 20 times more soluble than oxygen. In health, the distance between alveolar air and pulmonary blood is miniscule – 0.2–0.4 micrometers (erythrocyte diameter is about 7 micrometers). So in health, poorer solubility of oxygen is insignificant. However, diseases increasing distance between alveolar air and pulmonary blood (such as pulmonary oedema) inhibit oxygen transfer, causing type 1 respiratory failure.

Air contains virtually no carbon dioxide (0.04 per cent). Carbon dioxide is a waste product of cell metabolism. Provided metabolism and carbon dioxide production remain constant, blood levels depend on removal, which is mainly affected by breath size, flow ('washout') and frequency (rate). Type 2 respiratory failure may be caused by any disease that limits breath size, such as neuro-muscular weakness (e.g. Guillain-Barré syndrome (GBS)), bronchoconstriction (COPD) or extensive alveolar damage (emphysema, acute respiratory distress syndrome (ARDS)). Carbon dioxide production can be affected by nutrition – feeds such as Pulmocare® produce less carbon dioxide than standard feeds.

Artificial ventilation

Artificial ventilation attempts to temporarily replace or support patients' own ventilation. This may be planned as part of post-operative care, or necessitated by existing or potentially imminent severe respiratory failure. If intubation is necessary, delay can be fatal (Esteban *et al.*, 2004).

Ventilators also have various safety features, including apnoea back-up, which changes self-ventilating modes to mandatory ones if apnoea persists beyond preset limits (often 20 seconds).

Oxygenation relies on functional alveolar surface area, so is determined by:

- mean airway pressure
- inspiration time
- positive end expiratory pressure (PEEP)
- FiO_2
- pulmonary blood flow.

Carbon dioxide removal requires active tidal ventilation, so is affected by:

- inspiratory pressure
- tidal volumes
- expiratory time
- frequency and flow of breath.

Manipulating these factors can optimise ventilation while minimising complications.

Modes of ventilation

Ventilators were originally classified by their cycles:

- time (controlled by rate or I:E ratio);
- volume (delivers gas until preset tidal volume is reached);
- pressure (delivers gas until present airway pressure reached);
- flow (rarely used).

Although most modern ventilators mix these cycles in an often bewildering variety of modes and names, historical origins often clarify what they offer.

Dual modes combine advantages of volume-controlled ventilation (constant minute volume) and pressure-controlled ventilation (rapid, variable flow). However, depending on settings, some ventilators may fail to control minute volume. Choice of modes will depend partly on options available, partly on preference and partly on need. For example, effects of sleep were discussed in Chapter 3.

Fully regulated volume ventilation is *controlled mandatory ventilation* (*CMV*). Modern ventilators usually offer various mandatory and self-ventilating modes, many 'dual control' – combining pressure limitation with guaranteed tidal volume. With apnoea, ventilators switch automatically to back-up modes that ensure ventilation. Modes and options used depend largely on patients' needs, but also on available technology, which varies slightly between clinicians' preferences and manufacturers. All settings should be considered in the context of individual patient needs and problems, and other ventilator settings.

Pressure control (*PC*) is a mode usually used with children (up to about 8–12 years) due to the need to avoid cuffed endotracheal tubes. With adult ventilation, pressure control is usually an adjunct to prevent excessive pressure (and so *barotrauma*) in other modes.

Some of the more commonly available modes on ventilators are:

■ pressure-regulated volume control (PRVC), also called adaptive pressure ventilation (APV);
■ synchronised intermittent mandatory ventilation (SIMV);
■ adaptive support ventilation (ASV);

and various 'self-ventilating' modes such as:

■ pressure support ventilation (PSV);
■ continuous positive airway pressure (CPAP);
■ airway pressure release ventilation (APRV);
■ bilevel positive airway pressure;
■ proportional assist ventilation (PAV);
■ non-invasive ventilation (NIV).

PRVC controls volume, so is essentially CMV, but ceases if maximum preset pressure is reached (to prevent barotrauma – see Table 4.1). Self-ventilating breaths are often difficult (but vary between manufacturers), so this mode is not suitable for weaning.

SIMV was an early weaning mode, reducing frequency of ventilator breaths while synchronising with patient-initiated breaths to prevent hyperinflation and barotrauma.

Relatively rarely used now, it is usually combined with pressure regulation (to limit barotrauma) and pressure support (see Table 4.1) – PSIMV. It should not now be used for weaning (Brignall and Davidson, 2009).

ASV adjusts various aspects (mandatory rate, tidal volume, inspiratory pressure, inspiratory time, I:E ratio) to maintain preset minute volume. ASV may be useful for weaning (Petter *et al.*, 2003) or to replace conventional ventilation (Iotti *et al.*, 2010), although its use is limited, and most studies recommend other modes.

PSV is a self-ventilating, flow-cycled, mode. Once a breath is triggered, pressure support delivers gas until preset pressure is reached, adding volume to weak breaths, so compensating for respiratory muscle weakness. Although often available as a mode in its own right, it is also often used as an adjunct with other modes (pressure support – PS). PS is often commenced at 20 cmH$_2$O, then weaned usually by increments of 2; once pressure support is 8–10 cmH$_2$O, extubation is usually possible. PSV is the most widely used weaning mode (Brignall and Davidson, 2009). However, it is less conducive to sleep than assist control ventilation (Figueroaa-Ramos *et al.*, 2009), so is generally not a good choice for night-time.

CPAP is a self-ventilating form of PEEP (see page 38), and is available on many ventilators, although more often bilevel modes (see below) are used. CPAP stabilises and recruits alveoli, enables gas exchange to continue between breaths, and can resolve pulmonary oedema. Expired positive airway pressure (EPAP) of bilevel modes has similar benefits to CPAP.

APRV provides CPAP, with periodic release of pressure to a lower level (Habashi, 2005). This makes it an 'open lung' approach, with ventilation occurring during release rather than inspiratory phases, allowing clearance of carbon dioxide. Reducing the pressure difference encourages spontaneous ventilation, and so can be useful for weaning. Work of breathing on APRV is similar to PSV (Uyar *et al.*, 2005)

Bilevel positive airway pressure is like two alternating levels of CPAP: higher pressure on inspiration (inspired positive airway pressure – IPAP), and lower during expiration (expired positive airway pressure – EPAP). EPAP provides all the benefits of PEEP/CPAP, while higher inspiratory pressures increase tidal volume. Colloquially often called BiPAP®, this is a brand name, so ventilators that include this option often prefix the 'PAP' with another letter – for example, SPAP. Although not strictly NIV, high-flow humidified nasal oxygen (e.g. Vapotherm™, Optiflow™) has also proved an effective support for many patients, and is often tolerated better than CPAP or BiPAP (Turnbull, 2008). NIV is often useful for:

- attempts to avoid intubation (e.g. Guillain-Barré syndrome);
- patients who have been deemed not suitable for invasive ventilation ('ceiling treatment');
- weaning, especially for patients with COPD (Burns *et al.*, 2009; Ferrer *et al.*, 2009).

NIV is discussed further in Moore and Woodrow (2009).

PAV allows ventilators to adjust (proportion) airway pressure according to patients' effort (Hess, 2002), thus compensating for changes in lung compliance and resistance. It is currently not available on many ventilators.

Settings

Within each mode various settings can 'fine-tune' ventilation. Different modes and ventilators offer different options, but core options are:

- tidal volume
- minute volume
- respiratory rate
- oxygen.

Increasing one or more of the first three usually clears more carbon dioxide. Additional options usually include:

- PEEP
- I:E ratio
- trigger.

Tidal volume (V_t) affects gas exchange, but can also cause shearing damage to lungs; settings therefore balance oxygenation and carbon dioxide removal against limiting lung injury. Patients at greatest risk from alveolar trauma usually have poor compliance, low functional lung volumes, and hypoxia. The Acute Respiratory Distress Syndrome Network (ARDSNet, 2008) recommends initial tidal volumes of 8 ml/kg, reducing quickly to 6 ml/kg (420 ml for 70 kg patients), which may necessitate accepting *permissive hypercapnia*. Larger tidal volumes may be used for patient without ARDS, although risks of ventilator-associated lung injury (see page 42) should be considered. Gas exchange may be improved through adjusting other aspects (e.g. inspiratory flow, mean airway pressure, PEEP).

Minute volume is the sum of tidal volume multiplied by respiratory rate (if both are constant):

minute volume = tidal volume × respiratory rate.

Setting two of these components on any ventilator necessarily sets the third. All three are usually monitored.

Respiratory rate is usually set between 8 and 16 breaths per minute if ventilation is fully controlled, but reducing respiratory rate is a useful means of weaning. If treatment is withdrawn, the rate will usually be set at 8.

Oxygen is usually adjusted according to partial pressure of arterial oxygen (PaO_2) and saturation targets, although other aspects (e.g. PEEP) also affect oxygenation. In ICUs, oxygen is usually recorded as FiO_2; this means 'fraction of inspired oxygen', so pure (100 per cent) oxygen is an FiO_2 of 1.0, while 50 per cent oxygen is an FiO_2 of 0.5. Prolonged use of high concentration can cause oxygen toxicity, discussed in Chapter 18.

Positive end expiratory pressure (PEEP)

PEEP:

- prevents *atelectasis*;
- recruits collapsed alveoli;
- facilitates oxygen exchange during expiratory pause, so improving oxygenation.

Increasing PEEP can therefore be an alternative or supplement to increasing inspired oxygen. High PEEP (e.g. 20 cmH$_2$O) is sometimes used for 'open lung strategies' to prevent VALI.

Respiratory muscles normally relax passively with expiration, leaving residual gas within airways, usually exerting 2–2.5 cmH$_2$O pressure and so maintaining alveolar patency. This is variously called 'auto-PEEP', 'intrinsic PEEP', 'natural PEEP', 'air trapping' and 'breath stacking'. Intubation prevents upper (but not lower) airway closure, so measured airway pressure returns to *zero-PEEP* at the end of expiration.

However, increased intrathoracic pressure can:

- cause barotrauma;
- cause gas trapping and hypercapnia;
- reduce venous return (increasing cardiac workload);
- increase work of breathing on self-ventilating modes, by increasing resistance to expiration.

Optimal PEEP is much debated. PEEP of 10 cmH$_2$O may increase extra-vascular lung water (Maybauer *et al.*, 2006), but mortality from ARDS is not significantly affected whether high or low levels of PEEP are used (Briel *et al.*, 2010). ARDSNet (2008) recommends increasing PEEP according to FiO$_2$. With conditions such as asthma, where gas-trapping from bronchospasm is a major problem, minimal or (more often) no PEEP is used (Brenner *et al.*, 2009).

Inspiratory:expiratory (I:E) ratio

Breaths have three active phases:

- inspiration
- pause/plateau/inspiratory pause
- expiration

and a fourth passive phase:

- expiratory pause.

Normal I:E ratios are about 1:2, with plateau usually being adjusted separately. I:E ratio cannot be regulated in self-ventilating modes.

Awake patients are unlikely to tolerate significantly different ratios. However, reduced airflow (poor lung compliance, e.g. ARDS) necessitates relatively longer inspiratory time. Oxygen transfer occurs primarily during inspiration and plateau; incomplete expiration (e.g. short expiratory phase; gas trapping) increases alveolar carbon dioxide concentrations, reducing *diffusion* from blood. Changing the I:E ratio therefore manipulates alveolar gas exchange. Prolonging pause/plateau time has similar effects to PEEP – increasing gas exchange, but also increasing intrathoracic pressure. Bronchospasm (e.g. asthma) reduces expiratory flow, needing longer expiratory time.

Trigger senses patient-initiated breaths. Making trigger levels less negative makes it easier to initiate breaths through the ventilator, so can be useful for weaning. With most modes, triggered breaths are additional to preset volumes.

At rest, self-ventilation negative pressure is approximately –3 mmHg; trigger levels below this can cause discomfort (fighting). Settings close to zero are usually used (e.g. 0.5–2). Settings of zero can cause autocycling, the ventilator triggering itself at the end of each expiratory phase. Trigger/sensitivity settings normally allow for PEEP (but check manufacturers' information), so trigger of –0.5 cmH$_2$O with PEEP of 5 allows triggering at +4.5 cmH$_2$O.

Self-ventilating modes rely on patient-initiated breaths. If patients are gas-trapping (e.g. asthma), they may generate insufficient negative pressure to trigger ventilators.

Pressure limit terminates inspiration once preset limits are reached, even if preset volumes have not been achieved, to prevent barotrauma. Target plateau (peak) pressure should be below 30 cmH$_2$O (ARDSNet, 2008).

Inverse ratio ventilation (IRV) uses ratios of 1:1 or below, making expiratory time abnormally short. Advantages of IRV are:

- alveolar recruitment from prolonged inspiration time;
- alveolar stabilisation from shorter expiratory time (like PEEP);
- increased mean airway pressure (increased ventilation) without raising peak pressure (barotrauma).

However, IRV is physiologically abnormal, so can only be used with mandatory ventilation and usually necessitates additional sedation and often paralysis. IRV further increases intrathoracic pressure, compromising cardiac output.

Independent lung ventilation

With single-lung pathology, patients may benefit from different modes of ventilation being used to each lung. Independent lung ventilation requires double lumen endotracheal tubes, one lumen entering each bronchus. Independent ventilators, each using any available mode, may then be used for each lung.

Independent lung ventilation may be impractical due to:

- insufficient available ventilators;
- increased costs and workload (e.g. ventilator observations are doubled);
- danger to safety (access to patient, consuming more nursing time).

Care of ventilated patient

Ventilators are usually complex machines, and can be a source of fear for many nurses new to ICUs, but while technical skills are essential, the focus of care should remain the individual patient as a person. Care should be patient-centred, holistic, respectful and dignified – themes underlying many chapters in this book. Artificial ventilation causes potential problems with:

- safety;
- replacing normal functions (see Chapter 5);
- system complications.

Safety

Individual patient handover is usually at the bedside. During handover, and frequently during their shift, nurses should observe their patients':

- general appearance (e.g. colour, position, facial expression);
- level of sedation;
- comfort (signs of pain, body position/alignment, coughing/gagging from tube).

Following handover, respiratory observations include:

- chest wall movement (bilateral);
- lung auscultation to identify air entry (see Chapter 17) and lung sounds; if secretions (rattles) are heard, suction is usually needed;
- ETT size and position;
- cuff pressure (see Chapter 5);
- effectiveness of sedation and analgesia (usually through scoring systems).

Additional observations should be individualised to the patient, but may include:

- Glasgow Coma Scale (GCS);
- arterial blood gas analysis.

Following handover, the ventilator should be checked for:

- all settings, and whether they are appropriate for the patient;
- alarm limits;
- what effort/breaths (if any) the patient is making, and size of self-ventilating tidal volumes;
- ventilator waveforms (if available) – see Chapter 17.

Layout of bed areas should minimise nurses having to turn their backs on their patients. Alarms do not replace the need for nursing observation, but are useful adjuncts, so should be set narrowly enough to provide early warning of significant changes, but with sufficient leeway to avoid causing patients or family unnecessary distress.

Safety equipment and back-up facilities in case of ventilator, power or gas failure should include:

■ manual rebreathing bag, with suitable connections;
■ full oxygen cylinders;
■ reintubation and suction equipment (check suction equipment works).

Additional safety equipment may also be needed (e.g. tracheal dilators). Nurses should check all safety equipment at the start of each shift.

System complications

All body systems are affected by artificial ventilation. Managing artificial ventilation focuses on avoiding or limiting ventilator-induced damage rather than achieving 'normal' gases. Generally, higher pressures create more complications, so the ideal pressure is the lowest one that achieves the aims, so it is normally best to start with low pressures and increase according to needs (Royal College of Physicians – RCP, 2008).

Respiratory: The main complication, VALI, is discussed below. Other respiratory complications include:

■ increased work of breathing (in self-ventilating modes/breaths) from narrow, rigid tubes;
■ induced diaphragmatic weakness (from potentially as little as 18 hours' diaphragmatic rest) (Tobin *et al.*, 2010).

Artificial support should therefore be increased if patients show signs of exhaustion or become tachypnoeic with low tidal volumes. Optimal ventilation will however be individual to each patient, with modes and settings varying between clinicians. If severe respiratory failure causes prolonged weaning, patients may benefit by 'resting' overnight on ventilator-initiated modes, to resume weaning the following day.

Cardiovascular: Normal respiration aids cardiac return through negative intrathoracic pressure. Conversely, positive pressure ventilation:

■ impedes venous return;
■ increases right ventricular workload;
■ causes cardiac *tamponade*.

So positive pressure ventilation increases venous, while reducing arterial pressures, potentially causing:

- oedema (including pulmonary);
- hypoperfusion/failure of all organs.

Oedema may be caused by:

- venous congestion;
- renin-angiotensin-aldosterone response;
- antidiuretic hormone secretion;
- atrial natriuretic peptide (ANP).

Liver dysfunction from:

- diaphragmatic compression (raised intrathoracic pressure);
- portal congestion and hypertension (impaired venous return);
- ischaemia (arterial *hypotension*);

reduces:

- *albumin* production;
- drug or toxin metabolism;
- clotting factor production;
- *complement* production (infection control);

so causing:

- reduced *colloid osmotic pressure* (*hypovolaemia*, hypotension, oedema);
- toxicity (e.g. ammonia can cause coma);
- *coagulopathy*;
- opportunistic infection.

Neurological: Reduced cerebral blood flow predisposes to confusion/delirium.

Ventilator-associated lung injury (VALI)

Positive pressure can cause chronic lung damage. Identified or speculated causes of VALI include:

- *barotrauma*, from high airway pressure;
- *volutrauma*, from overdistension, usually caused by large tidal volumes;
- *atelectrauma* – possible damage from continual opening and closure of alveoli;
- *biotrauma* – pro-inflammatory *cytokine* release from alveolar distortion;
- *oxygen toxicity* (see Chapter 18).

(Pinhu *et al.*, 2003; Cooper, S.J., 2004)

Most recent changes in ventilatory practice aim to prevent VALI.

Barotrauma can be reduced by pressure-limiting ventilation, and adjusting ventilatory patterns. Lung function is affected by the way positive pressure is applied, so maximising tidal volume while minimising peak pressures optimises gas exchange while limiting barotrauma (Bigatello *et al.*, 2005), which can be adjusted using pressure:volume waveforms (see Chapter 17).

Cooper (S.J., 2004) recommends that VALI can be minimised through:

- open lung strategies: PEEP + prone position (or continuous lateral rotation therapy if prone contraindicated);
- semi-recumbent position;
- low tidal volumes;
- pressure-limited ventilation.

Weaning

With severe respiratory failure, artificial ventilation may be life-saving. But prolonging ventilation is unnecessarily costly, both to patients (morbidity, risks – especially ventilator-associated pneumonia) and to ICUs (workload, cost). While early extubation is desirable, premature extubation increases morbidity and mortality, often necessitating reintubation (Macnaughton, 2004). Judging the optimal time for weaning is therefore challenging. If weaning is likely to be slow, tracheostomy increases success and survival (Wu *et al.*, 2010). Prolonged (18–69 hours) complete diaphragmatic inactivity damages muscle fibres, so should be avoided if possible (Tobin *et al.*, 2010).

Daily 'sedation holds' (see Chapter 6) help assess the likely success of weaning/extubation.

Debate persists over what are the most reliable weaning criteria, but frequently used ones include:

- underlying pathologies resolving;
- appropriate ventilator settings (e.g. PEEP 5, $FiO_2 < 0.5$);
- measured respiratory function (e.g. blood gases, pH 7.3–7.45, $PaO_2{:}FiO_2$ ratio > 26; rapid shallow breathing index < 100 – see Chapter 17);
- other respiratory assessments (e.g. chest X-ray (CXR), auscultation);
- stability and function of other systems (especially cardiovascular);
- sedation score/status;
- therapeutic drugs – usually sedatives and inotropes are discontinued before weaning; paralysing agents should always be discontinued before weaning;
- any other risk factors (e.g. bleeding).

There is no generally accepted ideal weaning mode. Widely used modes are:

- assisted spontaneous breathing (ASB);
- pressure support (PS) (Koksal *et al.*, 2004);
- non-invasive ventilation (NIV) (Ferrer *et al.*, 2009).

43

Boles *et al.* (2007) recommend a spontaneous breathing trial of initially 30 minutes, using either a T-piece or low-level PS; if the trial fails, PS or assist–control ventilation are recommended modes, with NIV being considered to reduce intubation time. Most now use PS ventilation for weaning (Brignall and Davidson, 2009). Various weaning protocols have been developed and recommended, claiming to reduce both the number of ventilator-dependent days and length of ICU stay. However, weaning requires great skill (Crocker, 2009), and over-rigid use of protocols may delay more proactive, and equally (or more) successful, weaning using skilled clinical judgement (Blackwood *et al.*, 2004; Krishnan *et al.*, 2004). Care given is more important than the weaning mode used (Wu *et al.*, 2010). Psychological factors, such as communication and sleep, significantly influence success (Brignall and Davidson, 2009). Weaning should therefore be individualised to each patient and is best managed by experienced nurses (Crocker, 2009). With the array of weaning options available on most ventilators, locally preferred weaning methods are more likely to succeed (Blackwood *et al.*, 2004), and modes that are effective for one patient are not always effective for another. If initial short-term weaning plans fail, slower weaning plans should be instigated. Occasionally, patients may need referral to centres specialising in long-term ventilation.

Where further aggressive intervention would be inappropriate, teams may plan a 'one-way wean'. This may be part of terminal care or with hope of survival but recognising the futility of reintubation, but raises ethical issues about certainty of prognosis and value of life. Ideally, patients would participate in decision-making, but this is not always possible. Where expected outcome of a one-way wean is rapid death, withdrawal of life-prolonging treatment should not mean withdrawal of all treatment. Terminal care, however brief, should aim to provide patients with the best possible death that can reasonably, and legally, be offered. However, what makes a 'good death' is value-laden, so may vary greatly between patients – some patients might choose to die fully sedated and analgesed, while others might choose consciousness even at the cost of possible pain.

Implication for practice

- Critically ill (level 3) patients usually need mechanical ventilation.
- Nurses have a central role in managing ventilation, so need technical knowledge of equipment to care safely and effectively for their patients.
- Any machine can be inaccurate or fail; nurses should check all alarms and safety equipment at the start of each shift; ventilator function should be checked through recorded observations (at least hourly) and continuously by visual observation and setting appropriate alarm parameters (often within 10 per cent); remember alarms may also fail.

- Check the patient – air entry, appearance, and effectiveness of ventilation (pulse oximetry (SpO$_2$), tidal volume, arterial blood gases (ABGs)).
- Ventilators include default settings – know your machine and check these.
- Check alarm parameters at the start of every shift.
- Positive pressure ventilation affects all body systems; function of other systems should be continuously and holistically assessed.
- Ventilated patients depend on nurses to provide fundamental aspects of care (e.g. mouthcare).
- All intubation/mask equipment can cause damage – ties/tapes can occlude venous flow or cause direct trauma (e.g. tapes across open corneas); CPAP or other close fitting masks and endotracheal cuffs can cause pressure sores.
- In addition to maintaining safe technological environments, nurses should provide psychological care through explanations and reassurance.
- Early weaning reduces morbidity, but premature weaning creates complications. Ability to wean should be assessed. Weaning necessitates close monitoring and observation, revising plans if patients appear unable to cope.

Summary

Breathing is vital to life. Patients rely on nurses and others to maintain safety. When breathing is wholly or partly replaced by mechanical ventilation, maintaining safety includes ensuring adequate ventilation.

Most ICU patients need ventilatory support. Many modes and options are available, although not all modes discussed are available on all machines. Choice should be adapted to individualised patient needs, which relies on nurses to continually monitor and assess their patients. Nurses therefore need a working knowledge of equipment on their unit, and should be familiar with local protocols.

Positive pressure ventilation compromises function of other body systems. Nurses should assess complications from artificial ventilation, preventing risks where possible, minimising risks that cannot be avoided, and replacing lost functions through fundamental care.

Further reading

Manuals/information on machines used on your unit should be read. Most specialist texts include sections on ventilators and ventilation. A two-part article (Couchman *et al.*, 2007 and Coyer *et al.*, 2007) provides a good review of many topics in this and other chapters. Much recent literature debates weaning; Boles *et al.* (2007) and Cocker (2009) are especially useful. Nava and Hill (2009) review non-invasive ventilation.

Clinical scenario

Robert Hook is 32 years old with acute pancreatitis, bilateral pleural effusions, hypoxia, metabolic acidosis, tachypnoea and renal impairment. He was admitted to the ICU for mechanical ventilation following four days of NIV and worsening respiratory function. He is orally intubated, weighs 106 kg, has copious white secretions via his ETT and is draining thick sinus fluid into his oropharynx.

Ventilator settings	Patient-initiated variables
Mode SIMV – pressure cycled	
Respiratory rate 18 bpm	Respiratory rate 26 bpm
Airway pressure 22 cmH$_2$O	Airway pressure 24 cmH$_2$O
PEEP 9 cmH$_2$O	TV 710 to 750 ml
I:E ratio 1:2	MV 18 to 19.5 litres/minute
FiO2 0.6	SpO$_2$ 100%

Arterial blood gas result	Other blood results	Vital observations
pH 7.41	Hb 9.8 g/dl	Temperature 39.6°C
PaO$_2$ 14.5 kPa	WBC 15.5 x 10^{-9}/litre	Heart rate 118 bpm
PaCO$_2$ 6.69 kPa	Platelets 132 x 10^{-9}/litre	BP 140/55 mmHg
HCO$_3^-$ 27.6 mmol/litre	CRP 83 mg/litre	CVP 15 cmH$_2$O
BE 4.5 mmol/litre	Albumin 13 g/litre	
SaO$_2$ 97%	Phosphate 1.23 mmol/litre	
	Magnesium 0.6 mmol/litre	
	Chloride 117 mmol/litre	

Q.1 With this mode of ventilation, list other parameters that may be set, and specify alarm limits. What other observations should be documented?

Q.2 Interpret Mr Hook's results and suggest changes to the ventilator settings. Identify potential complications of mechanical ventilation and strategies to minimise these for Mr Hook.

Q.3 Assess Mr Hook's readiness to wean using evidence-based criteria, estimate PaO$_2$/FiO$_2$ ratio and rapid shallow breathing index (RSBI = f/V$_t$). Devise a weaning plan for him, including modes, parameters and indicators of success.

Chapter 5

Airway management

Contents

Fundamental knowledge   47
Introduction   48
Intubation   48
Extubation   49
Extubation stridor   50
Tracheostomy   50
Problems from intubation   52
Humidification   53
Suction   55
Catheters   56
Implications for practice   57
Summary   57
Further reading   57
Clinical scenario   58

Fundamental knowledge

Glossopharyngeal nerves
Oropharynx, and proximity of oesophagus to trachea
Tracheal anatomy, mucociliary mechanism ('ladder')
Cricoid anatomy
Carina and positions of right and left main bronchi
Differences between paediatric and adult trachea
Alveolar physiology
Dead space

Introduction

Ventilatory support usually necessitates insertion of *endotracheal tubes* (*ETTs*) or formation of a *tracheostomy*. ICU nurses caring for intubated patients are therefore responsible for ensuring patency of, and minimising complications from, artificial airways. This chapter describes types of tubes usually used in ICUs, the main complications of intubation and controversies surrounding endotracheal suction.

Physiological airways:

- warm
- moisten and
- filter

inspired air. Bypassing part of physiological airways necessitates replacing lost functions, as well as minimising complications. Airway management has been much studied, resulting in many changes to technology and practice. Older literature therefore often has limited value for current care. But evidence is often limited or questionable for many aspects, making recommendations necessarily tentative.

Intubation

Traditionally intubation could be:

- oral
- nasal
- tracheostomy.

Oral tubes cause gagging, but are easier to insert. ETTs are rigid, limiting lumen size and increasing airway resistance (especially nasal tubes).

Nasal tubes are narrow, increasing airway resistance, and cause sinusitis, which may increase ventilator-associated pneumonia (VAP) (Dodek *et al.* 2004), so are rarely used unless oral intubation is contraindicated (e.g. dental or head/neck surgery).

Nurses assisting with intubation may be asked to apply cricoid pressure. Cricoid cartilage (C5–C6 – just below the 'Adam's apple') is the only complete ring of cartilage in the trachea, so cricoid pressure (pressing cricoid cartilage down with three fingers towards the patient's head) compresses the pharynx against cervical vertebra, preventing gastric reflux and aspiration. Pressure is maintained until the endotracheal tube cuff is inflated.

To ventilate both lungs, ETTs should end above the carina (see Figure 5.1); this should be checked by:

- auscultating for air entry;
- ensuring chest movement is bilateral;
- X-rays.

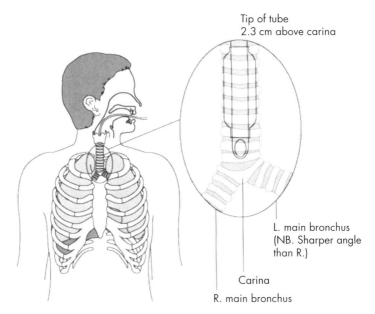

Tip of tube
2.3 cm above carina

L. main bronchus
(NB. Sharper angle
than R.)

Carina

R. main bronchus

Figure 5.1 ETT just above the carina

Accidental single bronchus intubation usually occurs in the right main bronchus, which is more vertical to the trachea than the left main bronchus. Misplaced tubes should be repositioned by anaesthetists and reassessed.

Endotracheal tubes are manufactured in a single (long) length, so almost invariably require cutting to minimise ventilatory *dead space*, usually to 21 cm (female) and 23 cm (male). Children's airways differ from those of adults, and are discussed in Chapter 13.

Most ETTs used in ICUs are bacteriostatic, to reduce VAP (Kollef *et al.*, 2008). Antiseptic-coated tubes hold promise, but currently cannot be recommended (Pneumatikos *et al.*, 2009). Some tubes have subglottic drainage ports, but while this reduces colonisation and VAP, it does not reduce mortality (Pneumatikos *et al.*, 2009).

Extubation

Planned extubation should occur as soon as patients are able to adequately self-ventilate. If not already identified by medical plans, nurses should check that medical staff are satisfied for patients to be extubated.

The usual procedure for extubation is:

1   Inform patient; assemble equipment; hand hygiene.
2   Endotracheal suction, to remove any significant airway secretions.
3   Orotracheal suction, to remove secretions on top of the cuff.
4   Deflation of ETT cuff, cutting tube holder/tapes.

5   Endotracheal suction; remove ETT with suction catheter.
6   Offer the patient mouthwash.
7   Commence oxygen via facemask, usually with slightly more oxygen than used with ventilation.
8   Continuous pulse oximetry, with ABG 20–30 minutes after extubation.

However, during extubation, subglottic secretions may be aspirated, causing pneumonitis, pneumonia, and possibly extubation failure (Hodd *et al.*, 2010). Scales and Pilsworth (2007) describe an alternative 'positive pressure technique', to prevent hypoxia and atelectasis: delivering a positive pressure breath using a rebreathe bag with 100 per cent oxygen. Simultaneously deflate the ETT cuff and immediately withdraw the tube without suction; following extubation, patients should immediately cough. However, this technique requires rapid and complex coordination, and the only support cited is a paediatric study. Hodd *et al.* (2010) identify alternative methods to clear secretions:

- adjusting PEEP on ventilators;
- extubating with cuff inflated;
- asking patients to cough;

but acknowledge that effectiveness remains unproven.

Extubation stridor

If bronchospasm is anticipated, cuffs should be deflated before extubation. Normally, this would create an airleak, usually audible, and cause loss of tidal volume; if bronchospasm is present no airleak will be heard/measured, so extubation should not proceed, and an anaesthetist should review the patient. Laryngeal oedema often causes hoarseness following extubation, making patients temporarily hoarse or speechless. Children, having smaller airways, are especially liable to oedematous obstruction, but 10–15 per cent of intubated patients develop laryngeal oedema (Lermitte and Garfield, 2005), so Fan *et al.* (2008) suggest giving steroids before extubation to reduce incidence of laryngeal oedema and the need for reintubation, although this is not generally routinely practised. Stridor may be treated with:

- nebulised adrenaline (1 mg in 5 ml saline);
- steroids (e.g. dexamethasone);
- Heliox (see Chapter 18).

If stridor cannot be rapidly reversed, reintubation is usually necessary.

Tracheostomy

Tracheostomies avoid many complications of oral and nasal intubation. They halve dead space, making the work of breathing, and so weaning, easier. Debate about optimal timing of tracheostomies persists; Blot *et al.* (2008) found no benefit from early tracheostomy, but Möller *et al.* (2005) found that early tracheostomy reduced VAP, while Wu *et al.* (2010) suggest that tracheostomy may increase survival.

Tracheostomies are usually formed percutaneously rather than surgically (Freeman *et al.*, 2000), as percutaneous insertion has fewer complications (Eggert and Jarwood, 2003). However, surgical tracheostomies may be created if percutaneous approaches are contraindicated; Regan (2009) lists absolute contraindications as:

■ uncorrected coagulopathy;
■ infection over site;
■ extreme ventilator and oxygenation demand;
■ tracheal obstruction;

and relative contraindications as:

■ unfavourable neck anatomy;
■ emergency airway management.

Alternatively, Pratt *et al.* (2008) list relative contraindications as:

■ children < 12;
■ anatomic abnormality of trachea;
■ pulsating palpable blood vessels over site;
■ active infection over site;
■ occluding mass or goitre over site;
■ short or obese neck;
■ PEEP > 15 cm H_2O;
■ platelets < 40;
■ INR > 10;
■ limited ability to extend cervical spine;
■ history of difficult intubation.

Percutaneous stomas take 7–10 days to mature (Broomhead, 2002), so if replaced before this time the stoma may occlude more rapidly than surgical stomas. With early displacement of either surgical or percutaneous tubes it is safer to reintubate (Broomhead, 2002).

Emergency bedside equipment should include:

■ tracheal dilators
■ spare tubes: one the same size and one a size smaller
■ suction
■ syringe.

Tracheostomies are seldom stitched into skin, but if they are a stitch cutter is also needed. Nurses caring for patients with a tracheostomy should check this emergency equipment is easily accessible at the start of their shift.

Frequency of tracheostomy dressing depends on both the wound and the type of dressing used. If the stoma looks infected, it should be redressed. Otherwise, most tracheostomy dressings should be replaced daily or according to local protocols.

Because tracheostomies reduce dead space, decannulation significantly increases the work of breathing, by 30 per cent (Chadda *et al.*, 2002). Weaning from a tracheostomy should therefore be a carefully planned and staged process to minimise need for recannulation:

- remove or minimise CPAP and pressure support (CPAP no more than 5 cmH_2O);
- initially use a T-piece rather than tracheal mask; T-pieces provide some PEEP and a reservoir of oxygen-rich gas.

Minitracheostomies (crichothyroidotomy), initially developed to facilitate removal of secretions, can also be used for high-frequency, but not conventional, ventilation. Non-invasive positive pressure ventilation may avoid the necessity for intubation.

Problems from intubation

Intubation is often a necessary medical solution that creates various nursing problems.

Coughing is a protective mechanism, removing foreign bodies, including respiratory pathogens, from the airway. This reflex can also be triggered by oral endotracheal tubes and suction catheters, causing distress, possibly necessitating sedation.

Artificial airways can *damage tissue*, especially lips, gums, cilia and mucus-producing goblet cells (non-specific immunity). Condition of lips and gums should be assessed, and tissues protected as necessary – various commercial products can cushion pressure from tapes on lips. Tube position on the lips/gums should be changed at least daily.

Cuff pressures of about 20 cmH_2O reduce aspiration, and so VAP (Pneumatikos *et al.*, 2009; Torres *et al.*, 2009). But cuff pressure exceeding *capillary occlusion pressure* can cause *tracheal ulcers*. 'High-volume low-pressure' 'profile' cuffs (see Figure 5.2) reduce cuff pressure by exerting lower pressure over an extended area. Unlike pressure sores on skin, tracheal epithelium is not directly visible. Average capillary occlusion pressure is about 30 cmH_2O, but can be lower (see Chapter 12), especially in hypotensive ICU patients. Cuff pressures should be checked and recorded at least once each shift, and whenever cuff volume is changed. Most cuff pressure manometers display 'safe' ranges of 20–25 cmH_2O.

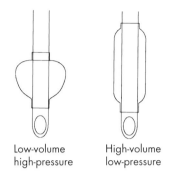

Low-volume   High-volume
high-pressure   low-pressure

Figure 5.2 High- and low-pressure ETT cuffs

Impaired cough and swallowing reflexes may cause *aspiration* of saliva and gastric secretions. Profile cuffs rarely completely seal lower airways, making some aspiration almost inevitable. Risks of aspiration pneumonia can be reduced by nursing patients at 45° (Drakulovic *et al.*, 1999).

Although secured with tapes, ETTs can become displaced, rising up the airway. Therefore, each shift the length of the ETT at the lips should be recorded, and if tube movement is suspected, an anaesthetist informed.

Oral ETTs cause *hypersalivation* and impair swallowing reflexes (see Chapter 10), with drying of mucosa near the lips and saliva accumulation (and potential aspiration) in the throat. 'Bubbling' sounds during inspiratory phases of ventilation indicate the need to remove secretions and check cuff pressure. Nasal intubation and tracheostomy prevent hypersalivation, but tracheal secretions may still accumulate.

Tubes bypass and damage non-specific immune defences (e.g. cilia). Immuno-compromise, together with impaired cough reflex, predisposes patients to infection. Endotracheal intubation displaces the *isothermic saturation boundary* further down the trachea, further impairing mucociliary clearance (Ward and Park, 2000).

Sympathetic nervous stimulation from intubation and suction initiates *stress responses* (see Chapter 1). Direct *vagal* nerve stimulation (anatomically close to the trachea) can cause *bradycardic* dysrhythmias and blocks, especially during intubation.

Oral ETTs cause discomfort and *anxiety*; nasal tubes and tracheostomies are usually tolerated better. Patients' inability to speak due to intubation through their vocal cords should be explained.

Humidification

The upper airway:

- warms
- moistens
- filters

inhaled air (see Figure 5.3). Endotracheal intubation bypasses these normal physiological mechanisms, necessitating artificial replacement. Oxygen is a dry gas, so inadequate humidification dries exposed membranes (below the endotracheal tube), damaging cilia and drying mucus. Stickier, thicker mucus, and impaired cilial clearance, reduce airflow and increase infection risks.

During inspiration, airways warm air to body temperature. This is normally reached just below the carina, sometimes called the 'isothermic saturation boundary' (Dutta *et al.*, 2006). Warm air transports more water vapour than cold air, so fully saturated room air/gas (100 per cent relative humidity) will not be fully saturated once warmed to body temperature. Ideally, tracheal gas temperature should be 32–36°C.

Humidification may be achieved by:

- heat/moisture exchange (HME) filters;
- hot-water humidifiers;
- large-volume nebulisers ('cold-water humidifiers');
- nebulisers (e.g. saline).

Instilling bolus saline is not recommended (Blackwood, 1999).

Heat/moisture exchangers (HMEs) use hydrophobic membranes to repel airway moisture, are very efficient bacterial filters (95–100 per cent efficacy (Lawes, 2003)), and reflect heat. They cause less infection risk than heated humidifiers (Torres *et al.*, 2009), but should be changed daily (or more frequently if soiled).

HMEs increase dead space (Morán *et al.*, 2006), so are usually best avoided in children (Ward and Park, 2000) and patients with COPD (Girault *et al.*, 2003) or asthma (Oddo *et al.*, 2006).

Hot-water humidifiers warm inspired air to preset temperatures, usually 37°C. Most systems are self-filling, avoiding the need to break circuits. As with HMEs, significant technological improvements invalidate many early studies. Nurses should monitor and record humidifier temperature, keep fluid bags easily

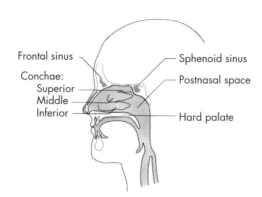

Figure 5.3 The nasal cavity

visible and replace them when empty. Circuits should be changed according to manufacturers' instructions.

Large-volume nebulisers (usually called 'cold-water humidifiers') provide less efficient humidification (BTS, 2008), but carry fewer risks from infection and tracheal burns. Water bottles should be replaced when empty, and circuits changed according to manufacturers' instructions.

Nebulisation delivers particles initially into airways, so where drug effects are desired primarily within airways, such as bronchodilators (e.g. salbutamol) or pulmonary vasodilators (*prostacyclin*), nebulisation is often the best route, although it may create the paradox that drugs mainly reach open parts of lungs, whereas effects may be needed most in collapsed airways. This makes nebulisation a poor choice for antibiotics. Nebulising saline (2–5 ml) delivers droplets directly to airway epithelium, is an efficient means of humidification (BTS, 2008) and may help mobilise secretions.

Different types of nebulisers create different-sized droplets. Droplets of 5 microns are deposited in the trachea, whereas droplets of 2–5 microns will reach the bronchi, and droplets below 2 microns reach alveoli. Most nebulisers deliver 2–5 micron droplets, but ultrasonic nebulisers deliver smaller droplets (below 1 micron).

Nebulisers should ideally be placed near the patient, just before the Y connection, with no HME between the nebuliser and the ETT. Some ventilators include nebuliser circuits, but if using oxygen/air flow meters, 6–8 litre flow is needed to generate effective droplets. HMEs should be placed on return circuits to protect ventilators. Nebulisers should be cleaned or replaced after use, as static fluid is a medium for bacterial growth. Nebulisers should be cleaned and dried after each use (Medicines and Healthcare products Regulatory Agency (MHRA), 2004).

Suction

Endotracheal suction is usually necessary to remove accumulated secretions, but can cause:

- distress
- infection
- trauma
- hypoxia
- atelectasis

so should be performed when needed, not routinely. Indications include:

- rattling/bubbling on auscultation;
- sudden increases in airway pressure;
- audible 'bubbling';
- sudden hypoxia (e.g. in SpO_2).

Suction is painful (Arroyo-Novoa *et al.*, 2009), so warn patients before suctioning, and pass tubes steadily, but not aggressively.

Negative (suction) pressure damages delicate tracheal epithelium (Maggiore *et al.*, 2003), causing possible:

- haemorrhage
- oedema
- stenosis
- metaplasia.

Negative pressure should be sufficient to clear secretions, but low enough to minimise trauma. Suction pressures, usually measured in kilopascals (kPa) but sometimes in millimetres of mercury (mmHg), should be displayed on equipment. Many ICU nurses limit negative pressure to 20 kPa, although the Intensive Care Society (ICS, 2008) recommends 13–16 kPa when suctioning through tracheostomies.

Suction removes oxygen from airways and can cause atelectasis. Suction should therefore be as brief as possible (maximum 10 seconds). Nurses are recommended to hold their own breath during each pass: when they need oxygen, so will their patient.

Endotracheal suction can cause bronchoconstriction (sympathetic stress response), and possible hypoxia. It is common practice to preoxygenate prior to suction, although evidence is sparse; Demir and Dramali (2005) found no benefits from routine preoxygenation, but failure to preoxygenate is probably more dangerous than routine preoxygenation, so preoxygenating all patients (100 per cent oxygen for 3–5 minutes) is recommended. Most ventilators include time-limited control for delivery of 100 per cent oxygen.

Care, and problems, should be fully recorded, to help later staff decide how and when to suction.

Catheters

Oral secretions are often best removed with Yankauer catheters (Dean, 1997). Closed-circuit suction is almost always used with intubated ICU patients, 'open' suction largely being limited to self-ventilating patients who have a tracheostomy but whose cough reflex is too weak to effectively clear secretions. Open suction is discussed further in Moore and Woodrow (2009). Closed-circuit systems maintain ventilation and PEEP when passing catheters, enabling slower (less traumatic) catheter introduction. In-line circuits should be changed according to manufacturers' instructions.

Many texts (usually anecdotally) recommend that catheters should not exceed half to two-thirds ETT diameter, although it is probably better to individualise selection to patient need – using the smallest size that will remove secretions. Smaller catheters cause less trauma, but remove fewer secretions. For adults, standard catheter sizes are French Gauge (FG) 10 (black), 12 (white) and sometimes FG 14 (green). Watery secretions can usually be easily removed with FG 10, but thicker secretions usually need larger sizes; it is usually best to commence with FG 12, and change size as necessary. Smaller sizes will be needed for children (note that some colours are similar to those of adult sizes).

Implications for practice

- Nurses assisting with intubation may have to perform cricoid pressure, so should be familiar with how to perform it.
- ETT cuff pressures should be checked each shift, and whenever any change in pressure is suspected. Pressures should not exceed 25 cmH$_2$O (3.3 kPa).
- Unless other positions are specifically indicated, patients should be nursed semi-recumbent.
- Airway humidification is essential to maintain effective mucociliary clearance.
- Suction should never be 'routine', but performed when indicated.
- Negative pressure during suction should not exceed 20 kPa.

Summary

Intubation remains a medical intervention, but nurses monitor and manage artificial airways, so should:

- maintain safe environments, including ensuring safety equipment;
- replace lost/impaired physiological functions, including humidification and clearing secretions;
- individually assess each patient for risk factors caused by intubation.

They should also plan individualised care accordingly. No aspect of airway management is routine. Respiratory assessment, including breath sounds, is discussed in Chapter 17.

Further reading

Tracheostomy care is discussed in greater detail in Moore and Woodrow (2009), and the ICS (2008) provides guidelines for care. Arroyo-Novoa *et al.* (2008) researched patient experiences of being suctioned. Although not designed for ICUs, BTS (2008) guidelines for acute oxygen therapy provide valuable evidence. Scales and Pilsworth (2007) provide a nursing guide to extubation.

Clinical scenario

Tony Richards is 45 years old, very hirsute with a thick bushy beard and weighs 160 kg. He was admitted to the ICU following elective surgery for closer airway management. He was a difficult intubation (Grade 3) and mechanically ventilated via a size 9 ETT, with length 21 cm marking at his lips and cuff pressures of 35cmH$_2$O. Mr Richards is ready for extubation and biting on his ETT.

Q.1 List the equipment and process used to prepare Mr Richards for extubation. Identify the most suitable type of respiratory support for him. Provide a rationale for your suggestion.

Fifteen minutes after extubation Mr Richards develops an audible stridor with intermittent gurgling noises from his throat. His respiratory rate changes from 18 to 28 bpm.

Q.2 Analyse possible causes of Mr Richards' added airway sounds and changed respiratory rate. Interpret the significance of these results and implications for his airway management.

On expectoration, Mr Richards' sputum is thick with brown discolouration. He has a weak cough with high risk of sputum retention.

Q.3 Review the range of methods used to mobilise and clear sputum from both lower and upper airways. Select the most suitable approach for Mr Richards.

Chapter 6

Sedation

Contents

Fundamental knowledge   59
Introduction   60
Drugs   60
Assessing sedation   62
Sedation scales   62
Sedation holds   64
Neuromuscular blockade   64
Implications for practice   65
Summary   66
Further reading   66
Clinical scenario   67

Fundamental knowledge

Psychological distress in the ICU (see Chapter 3)

Introduction

Critical illness, many interventions used in intensive care, and the intensive care environment itself can all cause distress and psychoses (see Chapter 3). Traditionally, sedation was usually used to facilitate invasive ventilation, with the arguable benefit that many sedative drugs induce amnesia. But sedation also deprives the individual of their autonomy, and to some extent their current awareness of being alive. Improved ventilator technology makes invasive ventilation more tolerable for conscious patients. Increasingly, sedative drugs have been viewed as 'chemical restraints' (Bray *et al.*, 2004), an intervention only justified when there is a specific indication, and within the limits of that indication.

Adverse effects vary between sedatives, but problems include:

- hypotension;
- reduced gut motility (malabsorption, constipation), especially with opioids;
- prevention of REM sleep;
- amnesia;
- delirium (Pandharipande *et al.*, 2004).

Although drugs are mentioned, this chapter focuses on nursing assessment and care, including for *neuromuscular blockade* (paralysing agents). As with any other drug, use outside manufacturers' licences makes individual users potentially legally liable for any harm caused (ICS, 2009a).

Drugs

Shehabi and Innes (2002) identify five groups of sedative agents:

- benzodiazepines
- opioids
- anaesthetics
- alpha 2 agonists
- antipsychotics.

Benzodiazepines (e.g. diazepam, lorazepam, midazolam)

Gamma-aminobutyric acid (GABA) is the main cerebral cortex inhibitory neurotransmitter, so GABA stimulation (by benzodiazepines) induces sedation, *anxiolysis* and hypnosis (Fullwood and Sargent, 2010).

Midazolam has largely superseded other benzodiazepines in ICU because it acts relatively rapidly and has the shortest *half-life*. Midazolam is largely hepatically metabolised and renally excreted, so failure of these organs may unpredictably increase half-life, especially with older people, who usually have reduced renal clearance. After some days, midazolam appears to accumulate in tissues, resulting in prolonged clearance time – some ICU patients take one week to wake (Shehabi and Innes, 2002). Concurrent use of opioids and midazolam substantially reduces dose requirements of both drugs (Shehabi and Innes, 2002).

The antagonist for benzodiazepines is flumazenil. Flumazenil's effect is far shorter than that of benzodiazepines (half-life under one hour) so, although useful to assess underlying consciousness, sedation is likely to return rapidly.

Opioids (e.g. morphine, fentanyl, remifentanil, alfentanil, sufentanil)

Opioids have sedative effects. Normally considered a 'side effect', for ICU management this combination of strong analgesia and sedation makes opioids useful. Preferred opioids vary between units. Morphine remains widely used, but the more expensive fentanils cause less accumulation and fewer side effects. Opioids are discussed in Chapter 7.

Anaesthetic agents (e.g. propofol, ketamine)

Propofol is the most widely used ICU sedative (Murdoch and Cohen, 2000). Its lipid emulsion easily crosses the blood–brain barrier, giving rapid sedation. This, together with its metabolites being inactive, makes its half-life short. Propofol reduces cerebral metabolism, so may be useful for treating epilepsy. It is relatively expensive, so some units restrict its use to when sedation is planned to one day. Long term it appears to be safe, but does not reduce the duration of mechanical ventilation compared with midazolam (Ho and Ng, 2008). Propofol is available in both 1 and 2 per cent concentrations, so labels should be checked carefully, especially if working on different units.

Propofol can cause:

- dose-related hypotension (Sessler and Varney, 2008);
- prolonged clotting (Fourcade *et al.*, 2004);
- hypertriglyceridaemia (Sessler and Varney, 2008);
- greenish urine, which, although probably clinically insignificant, may make relatives anxious.

It contains no preservative, but its lipid base may facilitate bacterial growth. Propofol has no analgesic effect, so concurrent analgesia should be given.

Ketamine is rarely used as it can cause nightmare-like hallucinations, but it can be useful in status asthmaticus as it bronchodilates (Cullis and Macnaughton, 2007).

Alpha 2 antagonists (e.g. clonidine)

Although not widely used, some centrally acting alpha 2 antagonists are sometimes used for sedation. Clonidine can be useful for withdrawal from prolonged sedation or alcohol/drug dependence (Cullis and Macnaughton, 2007). Clonidine is also sometimes used as an antihypertensive, which can be problematic if used for sedation in hypotensive patients.

Antipsychotics (e.g. haloperidol)

Many ICU patients experience delirium and acute psychoses (see Chapter 3). Antipsychotics are sometimes used to relieve these problems.

Assessing sedation

Over- and under-sedation are relative concepts, so open to subjective interpretation. Over-sedation delays weaning and recovery, compromises perfusion to, and so function of, all organs, and increases financial costs. Under-sedation arguably exposes patients to pain and stress. Achieving optimum sedation is a humanitarian necessity; professional autonomy and accountability make each nurse responsible for ensuring their patients are appropriately (i.e., not over- or under-) sedated. All ICU patients should be assessed for sedation level (Page, 2008) to facilitate titration of drugs to achieve optimal sedation.

Some ICUs have increasingly adopted no-sedation regimes (Strøm et al., 2010). Avoiding sedation avoids side effects, such as induced hypotension, which so often necessitates noradrenaline infusions. However, many ICUs using no-sedation also use physical restraints to prevent problems such as self-extubation. Few UK ICUs have adopted this strategy, although whether chemical restraint is ethically different from physical restraint is debatable.

How assessment is undertaken is much debated. Subjective assessments, such as gently brushing the tips of eyelashes, can usefully identify if someone is sedated deeply enough to tolerate traumatic interventions (e.g. intubation). Many scoring systems and methods have been developed to try to achieve objective assessment. Arbour et al. (2009) suggest that clinical scoring, rather than technologies, remains the 'gold standard' for assessing sedation. Many scales are used in practice, most being relatively simple lists, usually variants of the Ramsay scale. But using sedation scales does not reduce the time of mechanical ventilation (Williams et al., 2008), so risks being a 'paper exercise'. Some units use sedation protocols, although use of protocols alone does not guarantee improved patient outcomes (O'Connor et al., 2010).

Paralysis, whether from paralysing agents or pathology, prevents patients expressing awareness, invalidating almost all means of assessing sedation. So infusions of any paralysing agents should be stopped long enough before sedation assessment, to ensure they will not influence results.

Sedation scales

Many sedation scales have been developed. Lough (2008) suggests the four frequently used scores are:

- Ramsay;
- Riker Sedation-Agitation Scale (SAS);
- Motor Activity Assessment Scale (MAAS);
- Richmond Agitation and Sedation Scale (RASS).

Table 6.1 Ramsay scale

Awake levels:

1 patient anxious and agitated or restless or both
2 patient cooperative, orientated and tranquil
3 patient responds to command only

Asleep levels:

4 brisk response
5 sluggish response
6 no response

Source: Ramsay et al. (1974)

Ramsay

The Ramsay scale (Ramsay et al., 1974; see also Table 6.1), originally designed for drug research, is the oldest of scales discussed, remains the most widely used (Page, 2008), and is the basis for most scales, including University College Hospital (Singer and Webb, 1997), Brussels (Detriche et al., 1999), Riker (Riker et al., 2001) and the Richmond Agitation and Sedation Scale (RASS) (Ely et al., 2003). It offers a simple choice between six descriptions.

Bispectral index

Bispectral index (BIS) uses a forehead sensor for adapted EEG (electroencephalography) monitoring, deriving a numerical level of sedation between 1 and 100:

Awake patients	90–100
Conscious sedation (responds to noxious stimuli)	60–80
General anaesthesia	50–60
Deep hypnotic state	< 40
Very deep sedation	< 20
Absence of any brain activity	0

Although many ICU patients will be managed in the 60–80 range, < 60 is usually desirable if patients are paralysed. Similar EEG adaptations include evoked potentials, cerebral function monitors (CFMs) and cerebral function analysing monitors (CFAMs). Although Deogaonkar et al.'s study (2004) found BIS reasonably reliable, Avidan et al.'s (2008) large-scale study found patients remained aware during anaesthesia despite target-range BIS, while Arbour et al. (2009) found clinically significant differences between BIS and clinical scores, with risks of over- or under-sedation. Haenggi et al. (2009) concluded that BIS, event-related potentials and entropy cannot replace clinical sedation assessment with scoring systems, although Trouiller et al. (2009) suggest them as a useful adjunct to assessment.

Sedation holds

Stopping sedation daily, usually in the morning before ward rounds, enables thorough assessment of:

- neurological state;
- effectiveness of and need for sedation and analgesia;
- readiness to wean.

Sedation holds reduce physical and psychological complications associated with uninterrupted sedation (O'Connor *et al.*, 2009), enabling earlier discharge (Schweickert *et al.*, 2004). However, improved (patient-friendly) ventilator technology reduces the need for any sedation, so minimal or no sedation is increasingly becoming the norm. Sedation holds should be carefully planned to ensure adequate comfort for procedures such as X-rays, physiotherapy and line insertion, and be long enough for effects of sedatives previously given to fade. Times of sedation holds, and observed effects, should be recorded.

Sedations holds are usually excluded with:

- head injury;
- paralysis (from drugs or disease);
- patients in prone positions or on kinetic beds;
- patients awaiting procedures, such as CT scans or tracheostomy insertion.

Neuromuscular blockade

Improvements in ventilator technology have largely removed the need to prevent patients making respiratory effort. Neuromuscular blockade (chemical paralysis) is usually only used if there is a specific indication to prevent muscle work, such as hyperpyrexia (see Chapter 8).

Paralysing agents ('non-depolarising muscle relaxants') cannot cross the blood–brain barrier, so have no sedative or analgesic effects. Paralysed patients cannot alert staff if they are inadequately sedated, making it the most hazardous form of chemical restraint (Bray *et al.*, 2004). Some studies have found that up to two-fifths of patients remembered being paralysed (Arbour, 2000). Patients should not be paralysed and awake (ICS, 2007a), so complete sedation should be achieved before using paralysing agents.

Blocking release of acetylcholine (a neurotransmitter) at the neuromuscular junction causes skeletal (but not smooth) muscle relaxation. Paralysing agents may be classified as:

- depolarising
- non-depolarising.

Depolarising drugs act on motor end-plate, whereas non-depolarising drugs act on the post-synaptic end-plate. Whichever site is affected, acetylcholine transmission is blocked, causing muscle paralysis. Suxamethonium is a depolarising muscle relaxant; most other paralysing agents used in ICUs are non-depolarising.

Most paralysing agents are metabolised hepatically or excreted unchanged in urine, giving them a relatively long duration of effect. Atracurium and suxamethonium hydrolyse spontaneously in plasma, so are relatively short-acting. Atracurium is the most widely used paralysing agent in ICUs (Murdoch and Cohen, 2000), lasting 25–35 minutes (Pollard, 2005). Vecuronium, less frequently used, lasts 20–30 minutes (Pollard, 2005). Pancuronium causes less hypotension, so may be chosen where cardiovascular instability is especially problematic, but lasts 50–60 minutes (Pollard, 2005). Rocuronium lasts 3–40 minutes, with virtually no cardiovascular side effects or histamine release (Pollard, 2005), but is more expensive.

Paralysing agents should be stopped to assess sedation, but removing paralysis may cause undesirable physiological effects, so, like sedatives, paralysing agents should be stopped for no longer than is pharmacologically necessary.

Effectiveness of neuromuscular blockade should be assessed. The extrinsic eye muscle is the first muscle affected by paralysing agents, and the first to recover (Rang *et al.*, 2007), so brushing the eyelid indicates effectiveness. Extrinsic eye muscle paralysis may cause double vision and contribute to sensory imbalance. Paralysis is usually tested by absence of reflexes, such as peripheral electrical nerve stimulation. A relatively low (non-painful) voltage is usually sufficient to stimulate nerve reflexes. Users can benefit by trying out such tests on themselves, so they know what they are inflicting on their patients. The ulnar nerve is the most frequently used site (Arbour, 2000) and should cause thumb adduction. Arbour (2000) describes the 'train of four':

- 4 twitches = neuromuscular blockade occupies < 75 per cent of receptors;
- 3 twitches = 75 per cent blockade;
- 2 twitches = 75–80 per cent blockade;
- 1 twitch = 90 per cent blockade;
- 0 twitches = 100 per cent blockade.

BIS provides continuous monitoring of paralysis (Arbour, 2000), without inflicting potentially painful electric shocks.

Implications for practice

- Under- and over-sedation cause complications, so sufficient sedation should be provided to achieve comfort.
- Nurses should assess the efficacy of sedative and paralysing agents for their patients at least once every shift.
- There is no ideal sedation score; all staff should be familiar with whichever score is used on their unit.
- Daily sedation holds enable thorough reassessment, so should only be omitted by team decision.

- The sedation needs of each patient should be individually reviewed daily by the multidisciplinary team to meet each patient's need, evaluating:
  - humanitarian needs, to ensure patient comfort;
  - therapeutic benefits, to facilitate interventions;
  - side effects (e.g. hypotension), to ensure they are minimised.
- For brief procedures (e.g. intubation), the absence of blink reflexes confirms patients are adequately sedated.
- Paralysing agents should be stopped for sufficient time prior to assess sedation.
- Nerve stimulators are potentially painful/uncomfortable, so if used nurses should try tests on themselves (where safe to do so) so they are aware of what they are subjecting their patients to.

Summary

Sedation practices continue to change, with minimal sedation increasingly being replaced by no sedation. Sedation can relieve much psychological trauma caused by ICU admission, potentially providing physiological as well as humanitarian benefits. However, hypotension and other side effects can cause problems, while deep coma inhibits orientation and compliance with requests, removes patient autonomy and may contribute to PTSD.

Although chemical sedatives are prescribed by doctors, they are (normally) given by nurses; so the professional accountability of each nurse ensures that patients receive adequate (but not excessive) sedation.

The use of paralysing agents has declined; where used, there are usually specific therapeutic indications. Therefore, nurses should monitor and assess their effects.

Further reading

The ICS (2007a) issued brief but useful guidelines for sedation. Cullis and Macnaughton (2007) and Fullwood and Sargent (2010) are recent medical and nursing reviews. As with most drugs, the *British National Formulary* (*BNF*) and pharmacology texts provide useful information.

Clinical scenario

Peter Renton is a 30-year-old builder who was admitted to ICU ten days ago with crush injuries from an industrial accident. He has multiple lung contusions, is difficult to ventilate and his clinical observations and biochemical results suggest that he is developing acute kidney injury (AKI) and sepsis. In order to facilitate ventilation and other interventions, Mr Renton has been sedated with intravenous infusions of:

Midazolam 10 mg/hour for 10 days
Alfentanil 5 mg/hour for 10 days
Propofol 250 mg/hour for 7 days.

In addition, he received intravenous vecuronium at 10 mg/hour for 8 days, which was changed to bolus administration of pancuronium on day 8.

Q.1 Calculate the total amount of sedation given to Mr Renton in relation to the recommended dosage, drug metabolism and elimination (pharmacokinetics). Evaluate possible long-term complications and outline some nursing strategies that can minimise these.

Q.2 Review the appropriateness of sedation hold with Mr Renton. Plan how this is best managed, for example time of day, reduction in infusion rates, order in which to stop infusions, which infusions should continue, assessment of sedation level, goals of sedation.

Q.3 Consider the actions (pharmacodynamics) of vecuronium and pancuronium and provide the rationale for changing paralysing agents on Mr Renton's eighth day.

Chapter 7

Acute pain management

Contents

Fundamental knowledge   68
Introduction   69
Physiology   70
Psychology   70
Assessing pain   72
Managing pain   73
Opioids   73
Epidurals   74
Patient-controlled analgesia (PCA)   74
Non-opioids   76
Neuropathic pain   76
Anti-emetics   76
Implications for practice   76
Summary   77
Further reading   77
Clinical scenario   77

Fundamental knowledge

Anatomy and physiology of the nervous system, including sympathetic and parasympathetic, central and peripheral, motor and sensory

Spinal nerves – position of thoracic and lumbar nerves

Stress response (see Chapter 1)

Pain as a physical and psychological phenomenon

Local protocols/policies for epidural and PCA management

Pain is undesirable, a physical and psychological phenomenon that can cause physiological as well as psychological complications. Physiological problems caused by pain include:

- stress responses (see Chapter 1);
- reluctance to breathe deeply (if self-ventilating), contributing to atelectasis and respiratory failure;
- immunosuppression (Macintyre *et al.*, 2010).

Alleviating and relieving pain is fundamental to nursing care. Nurses therefore should understand:

- physiological and psychological processes of pain;
- how to assess pain;
- how to control pain.

Nurses should be familiar with indications, contraindications, usual doses, preparation, benefits and adverse effects of drugs they use. Much literature on pain management focuses on pharmacology, and specific information can be found in manufacturers' Summaries of Product Characteristics (SPCs) and pharmacopoeias (e.g. *British National Formulary* (*BNF*)), both of which should be available in all clinical areas. This chapter discusses some drugs, but focuses mainly on mechanisms and assessment of pain.

Causes of acute pain may be obvious (e.g. surgery), but patients may also suffer pre-existing chronic pain (e.g. arthritis). Chronic pain is usually less amenable to analgesia, and drugs that do work often create complications, such as immunosupression. Many interventions can cause pain, including:

- suctioning (the most commonly reported cause of pain in intubated patients);
- line insertion;
- drain removal;
- repositioning;
- physiotherapy.

Individual nursing assessment may identify ways to minimise discomfort, information that should be shared with colleagues (verbally, nursing records).

Many ICU patients are unable to perform even fundamental activities of living, so managing pain should include comfort measures, such as:

- smoothing creases in sheets;
- relieving prolonged pressure;
- turning pillows over;
- limb placement (e.g. with arthritis);
- reducing noise and light;
- touch, explanations, reassurance, empowerment.

Physiology

Pain signals, which may originate from physical or psychogenic stimuli, are transmitted to and received by the cerebral cortex, where they are perceived (interpreted) by higher centres in the brain. Pain is therefore necessarily individual to each sufferer, a complex interaction between physiology and psychology. Pain relief can therefore block either reception or perception of pain signals.

Pain is sensed by nociceptors, specialised nerve endings found throughout the body, especially in skin and superficial tissues. Two main types of nerves (A and C fibres) transmit pain signals. A fibres have myelin sheaths that conduct signals rapidly, whereas C fibres are unmyelinated and so conduct impulses slowly (Macintyre *et al.*, 2010). C fibres transmit dull, poorly localised, deep and prolonged pain signals, causing guarding movements and immobility. Sharp impulses from the fast A delta fibres are superseded by slower, dull and prolonged impulses from C fibres.

Melzack and Wall (1988) describe a 'gate' (in the substantia gelatinosa capping grey matter of the spinal cord dorsal horn), which may be:

- open
- closed
- blocked.

When open, impulses pass to higher centres (where they are perceived). A closed gate prevents impulses passing, leaving nothing to perceive. *Endogenous* chemicals control this gate (e.g. *serotonin* increases pain tolerance), so manipulating, supplementing or replacing these chemicals can control pain. The gate can also be blocked by other signals. A delta and C fibres share pathways, so A delta stimulation (e.g. skin pressure) can block the slower, dull, prolonged C fibre pain. Hence scratching itches, pressure bracelets and transcutaneous electrical nerve stimulation (TENS) can relieve pain.

Pain may be referred (e.g. phantom limb pain, cardiac pain in the left arm, appendix pain in the loin – see Figure 7.1), where embryonic nerve pathways were shared or where residual nerve pathways remain intact.

Psychology

Perception of signals received is influenced by various psychological factors, including:

- culture;
- anticipation – e.g. past experience, misinterpretation;
- emotional vulnerability – e.g. fear;
- distraction.

The word 'pain' derives from the Latin 'poena' (= punishment); perceiving pain as retribution may be partly a psychological coping mechanism, but also

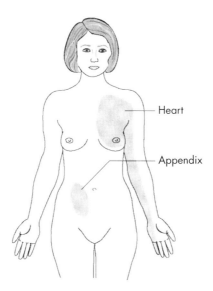

Heart

Appendix

Figure 7.1 Referred pain

encourages physiologically harmful, stoic attitudes of endurance. Culture also influences whether, when and how it is acceptable to admit to pain.

While recognising cultural influences, especially when pain is denied, stereotyping people is unhelpful and dehumanising. For example, older people may require less analgesia due to slower metabolism of analgesics and reduced pain sensation, but also grew up before the NHS existed, when stoicism was more widely expected. Pain is often underassessed and undertreated (Rakel and Herr, 2004; Ahlers *et al.*, 2010). Even if pain impulses were comparable, pain experiences are unique to each individual, necessitating individual assessment.

Anticipation is influenced by previous exposure to similar stimuli (e.g. endo-tracheal suction) and expectations. Readers may experience this for themselves when visiting dentists.

Critically ill patients are vulnerable. They feel, and are, disempowered. Such negative emotions exacerbate pain (Hawthorne and Redmond, 1998). Fear can create self-fulfilling prophecies (something hurts because we expect it to hurt), but uncertainty increases fear, so clear, honest explanations before actions, warning them how long they will have to endure it, help patients prepare for pain. Hayward's (1975) classic study found that information reduced pain, analgesia needs and recovery time.

Distraction may help people cope with pain by blocking the gate. Distraction and guided imagery can be useful nursing strategies, although impaired consciousness and verbal responses can limit their value in ICUs.

Assessing pain

Pain relief and providing comfort are fundamental to nursing. Ideally, the assessment of pain and effectiveness of pain management begins by asking patients, but communication may be limited by intubation, sedation, impaired psychomotor skills, and sometimes denial. Family/friends and nursing/medical notes may provide useful information, especially about chronic pain and individual coping mechanisms.

Pain experiences and analgesia needs frequently change significantly, necessitating regular reassessment. If patients are able to respond about their pain, they should be asked about:

- the site (including any radiation);
- the type (intensity, frequency, duration, radiation);
- whether anything triggers it;
- whether anything relieves it.

Nurses should observe whether pain is related to any activity, such as breathing (including artificial ventilation) or movement.

There is no ideal ICU pain assessment tool (Bird, 2003), but frequently used ones include:

- numerical scales (e.g. 0–3, 0–10, with higher numbers indicating worse pain);
- 'faces' (originally paediatric tools, but adapted for ICUs by McKinley et al. (2003));
- behavioural tools.

Changes in vital signs may be caused by acute pain, but can also have other causes. Non-verbal cues can be as reliable as verbal reports of pain (Feldt, 2000), so are especially useful if patients cannot talk. Sudden pain provokes a stress response (autonomic nervous system), with sudden:

- tachycardia (+ shallow breathing);
- hypertension;
- tachypnoea;
- vasoconstriction (clammy, pale peripheries);
- sweating.

Other non-verbal signs include:

- facial grimacing – clenched teeth, wrinkled forehead, biting lower lip, wide-open or tightly shut eyes;
- position – doubled up, 'frozen', writhing;
- pupil dilatation.

(Blenkharn et al., 2002; Murdoch and Larsen, 2004)

Impaired vision can make visual tools, such as faces, difficult to use (Bird, 2003).

The Behavioral Pain Scale (BPS) tool (Payen *et al.*, 2001) combines assessment of facial expression, upper limb movements and compliance with ventilation, so is useful for assessing pain in ventilated patients (Aïssaoui *et al.* 2005; Young *et al.*, 2006; Ahlers *et al.*, 2010). However, weakness/immobility and pathology may mask any or all of these signs, some of the criteria for assessing tolerance of ventilation are questionable, and it necessarily assumes patients are conscious enough to move limbs. The variant Behavioral Pain Scale – non-intubated (BPS-NI) is effective (Chanques *et al.*, 2009).

Managing pain

Opioids rightly remain the mainstay of acute pain management, but pain may be relieved through alternative or supplementary means. Pain is individual to each patient, so pain management should be individualised. Some generalisations can be made, provided practitioners remember to adapt generalisations to meet individual needs. Options will also be limited by what is available.

Where patients are conscious, discussing individual needs and preferences can provide nurses with valuable information, empower patients and reassure them. Where possible, open rather than closed questions should be used. Patient-controlled analgesia (PCA) is discussed below.

Opioids

Opioids are the mainstay of ICU analgesia.

Morphine remains the 'gold standard' opioid against which others are judged. It suppresses impulses from C fibres, but not A delta, so relieves dull, prolonged pain. Its relatively long effect makes bolus administration feasible, which also reduces problems from accumulation.

Diamorphine (heroin) is metabolised to morphine.

Fentanyl is twice as lipid-soluble as diamorphine (Hewitt and Jordan, 2004), so acts rapidly. Although more potent than morphine, it does not cause histamine release, so causes less hypotension. Fentanyl derivatives include alfentanil and remifentanil. Viscusi *et al.* (2007) found transdermal fentanyl to be as effective as intravenous morphine, although it does take about 24 hours to be fully effective. When patches are commenced, alternative analgesia should be provided for at least the first 24 hours.

Alfentanil's shorter duration (1–2 hours) makes continuous infusion safer; its metabolites are inactive, making it useful for patients with kidney injury, although liver failure prolongs its half-life.

Remifentanil is rapidly metabolised (by plasma), so has few, if any, complications from accumulation. It is, however, relatively expensive.

Low-dose *ketamine* can be useful for uncontrolled pain and, unlike most opioids, increases blood pressure (Chumbley, 2011).

Pethidine is rarely used because it is very short-acting, produces the toxic metabolite norpethidine, is highly addictive and provides no greater pain relief than morphine (Macintyre *et al.*, 2010).

Epidurals

Epidural opioids are usually more effective than intravenous ones (Marret *et al.*, 2007). Infusions usually combine opioids (fentanyl) with a local anaesthetic (bupivacaine). Local anaesthetics prevent nerve conduction of pain signals (Weetman and Allison, 2006), so produce an opioid-sparing effect.

The most common side effect of epidural analgesia is probably hypotension (Weetman and Allison, 2006), so when first mobilising patients it is usually advisable to use a hoist. Other common opioid-related side effects include pruritis (itching) from histamine release (Weetman and Allison, 2006). Unfortunately, a quarter of epidurals are misplaced, and more become dislodged (Ballantyne *et al.*, 2003), so are not always effective (McLeod *et al.*, 2001).

Each shift, nurses should check the epidural site – any infection is likely to be from skin-surface organisms, such as *Staphylococcus aureus* (Darouiche, 2006). Most Trusts have protocols and specific observation charts for managing epidurals. Most local protocols recommend hourly observation of:

- vital signs (HR, BP, RR, oxygen saturations)
- pain
- nausea
- sedation level
- level of sensory block.

Observation charts usually show 'dermatomes' – levels affected by each spinal nerve (see Figure 7.2). Where used, readers should be familiar with these.

Level of block is tested with cold spray or ice. A quarter of epidurals fail to provide effective analgesia, often due to catheter misplacement (Ballantyne *et al.*, 2003). Block should be sufficiently high to analgese, but not unnecessarily high or uneven. Blocks reaching T4 (nipple area) may paralyse respiratory muscles, so should be stopped immediately. Hypotension should *not* be managed by tilting the patient head-down, as this allows drugs to travel up the spine.

Removing epidural lines can cause infection and haematoma, so removal should be aseptic and only when clotting time is normal. The tip should be inspected to check it is intact; it is coloured (often blue) to make it distinctive. Heparin should usually be avoided before and after removal – times should be identified in local Trust policies.

Patient-controlled analgesia (PCA)

Giving patients control of administering their own opioids, within maximum preset lockout limits, usually achieves effective analgesia (McLeod *et al.*, 2001). PCAs usually contain morphine, although other opioids can be used; Michelet *et al.* (2007) found that adding small doses of ketamine with morphine reduced morphine consumption and improved respiratory function. However, about 12 per cent of people find them difficult to use (Mackintosh, 2007), so they are usually unsuitable if patients have:

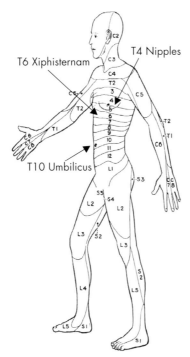

Figure 7.2 **Dermatomes**

- impaired psychomotor function;
- muscle weakness;
- visual deficits;
- confusion/forgetting how to control the machine.

Many Trusts produce specific observation charts for PCAs. These usually include:

- vital signs (HR, BP, RR, oxygen saturations)
- pain
- nausea
- sedation level.

As with epidurals, most Trusts recommend hourly observations.

PCA should be given through custom-made devices. These include a number of safety features, recording:

- set programs, including background rate and lockout time;
- amount delivered;
- unsuccessful attempts.

75

These should be recorded to enable continuing assessment. Unsuccessful attempts (demand within lockout time) indicate that analgesic needs are not being fully met, and so regimes should be reviewed.

Non-opioids

Non-opioids, such as paracetamol, inhibit the neurotransmitter prostaglandin E_2 (PGE$_2$). Some non-opioids (but not paracetamol) are anti-inflammatory, making them effective against musculoskeletal pain. Most have synergistic effects when combined with opioids (McCaffery and Pasero, 1999), achieving similar analgesia with smaller opioid doses, and so reducing adverse effects, such as constipation and itching. Non-steroidal anti-inflammatory drugs (NSAIDs) (e.g. ibuprofen) are mainly used for chronic musculoskeletal pain, but are sometimes used for post-operative pain. They can cause kidney injury.

Neuropathic pain

If pain appears resistant to other analgesics, the possibility of neuropathic pain (from damage to central or peripheral nerves) should be considered. Neuropathic pain is often difficult to control, but amitriptyline and gabapentin are often the best analgesics (Hayashida *et al.*, 2008; NICE, 2010b). Other drugs worth trying include tramadol (NICE, 2010b). Most neuropathic pain analgesics take days to become effective.

Anti-emetics

Opioids, given by any route, may induce nausea, both through delayed gastric emptying and by directly stimulating the vomiting centre in the brain. Nurses should observe for signs of nausea, assess likely causes and give appropriate prescribed anti-emetics. Most commonly used anti-emetics, such as ondansetron, cyclizine and prochlorperazine (stemetil), primarily affect the vomiting centre. Metoclopramide primarily increases gastric motility, so is useful where nausea is caused by gastric contents, but less useful when nausea is caused by vomiting centre stimulation (e.g. post-operative nausea and vomiting).

Implications for practice

- Promoting comfort and removing/minimising pain are fundamental to nursing.
- Pain is a complex phenomenon involving both physiological transmission of pain signals and cognitive interpretation.
- Pain is individual to each person, so requires individual nursing assessment.
- Currently there is no ideal pain assessment tool for ICUs, but verbal questions and visual observations can indicate comfort.
- Good pain management involves teamwork, so means of assessing and managing pain should be shared by the team. Where possible, this team

- should include the patient – discussing options and effectiveness, and offering PCA.
- Nociceptor signals (reception) are interpreted as pain in the cerebral cortex (perception); pain can be managed by removing either component.
- Opioids remain the mainstay of ICU analgesia, but supplementary ways to relieve pain and provide comfort should also be used.
- Simple analgesics, such as paracetamol, have opioid-sparing properties, and so reduce adverse effects of opioids.
- Analgesia should be given before tasks that are likely to cause pain.
- Nurses should evaluate effectiveness of pain relief to optimise its effect and minimise its complications.
- Nurses should observe for signs of nausea, assess likely causes and give appropriate prescribed anti-emetics.

Summary

Suffering is an almost inevitable part of critical illness, but this should not make pain acceptable. Pain is a complex phenomenon, involving both physiological transmission of pain signals and cognitive interpretation. Pain is culturally influenced and individual to each person, so should be assessed and managed individually. Promoting comfort and achieving effective pain management is fundamental to nursing, yet many patients continue to suffer unnecessary pain. Understanding physiological and psychosocial effects, together with the pharmacology of drugs used, enables nurses to plan effective pain relief. Acute pain often needs opioids, although non-opioid drugs can provide useful synergy with opioids, and non-pharmacological approaches should be considered. Evaluating and documenting effectiveness of pain relief help optimise its effects and minimise its complications.

Further reading

Classic books on pain management include Melzack and Wall (1988), McCaffery and Pasero (1999) and Hayward's (1975) classic study on post-operative pain. Wall and Melzack (1999) is a comprehensive reference text. Macintyre and Schug (2007) provide a useful handbook, while the Australian guidelines (Macintyre *et al.*, 2010) provide a comprehensive review. As with all drugs, the *BNF* provides useful summaries. Cade (2008) reviews assessment tools.

Clinical scenario

Rita Patel is a 38-year-old legal secretary, who was admitted to ICU for respiratory management following her second bariatric weight-loss surgical procedure. She has no immediate family in the area and has given her employer as next of kin. Miss Patel has a PCA of morphine sulphate

1 mg/ml; her pain is poorly controlled. She had previously had her pain controlled with pethidine and developed an urticaric rash. She dislikes the PCA and is requesting additional pethidine and medication to relieve itchiness.

Q.1 Identify the type, location and source of pain Miss Patel has been experiencing along with other influencing factors. Select the most appropriate pain assessment tools to use.

Q.2 Review the range of approaches used to administer analgesia in the ICU. Analyse the use of pethidine versus morphine in managing Miss Patel's acute pain and discuss alternative approaches and drugs that could be effective in managing her pain.

Q.3 Consider other non-pharmacological interventions that can be implemented to manage Miss Patel's pain effectively.

Chapter 8

Thermoregulation

Contents

Fundamental knowledge	79
Introduction	80
Pyrexia	80
Malignant hyperpyrexia	81
Measurement	81
Treatment	83
Hypothermia	83
Therapeutic hypothermia	84
Implications for practice	84
Summary	85
Further reading	85
Clinical scenario	85

Fundamental knowledge

Thermoregulation – hypothalamic control, shivering, sweating and heat loss through vasodilatation

Introduction

Human bodies can only function healthily within narrow temperature ranges. Body temperature, normally 36–37°C, is controlled by the thermoregulatory centre in the hypothalamus, responding to central and peripheral thermoreceptors. If cold, vasoconstriction and shivering responses conserve and produce heat; if hot, sweating and vasodilatation responses increase heat loss. Body temperature normally varies by up to 0.5°C during each day (Weller, 2001).

Body heat is produced:

- by metabolism
- in response to pyrogens.

Metabolism (chemical reactions) produces heat. Most post-operative pyrexias are caused by hypermetabolic tissue repair, not infection (O'Grady *et al.*, 1998; Perlino, 2001). Blood transfusion similarly usually causes low-grade pyrexia. With metabolic pyrexia people usually feel hot, as experienced during heavy exercise.

Infection causes pyrogens to be released; pyrogens (e.g. TNFα, *interleukin*-1) increase prostaglandin production, and prostaglandins increase the hypothalamus set-point (Bleeker-Rovers *et al.*, 2009), typically to higher temperatures than metabolism produces. As the hypothalamus attempts to increase heat production to match the higher set-point, people usually feel cold/shivery, so attempt to conserve warmth (e.g. extra bedding/clothing).

Infants are especially prone to rapid pyrexial fluctuations, due to hypothalamic immaturity, higher metabolic rates, and having more brown fat (which generates heat). Thermoregulatory impairment may cause febrile convulsions, so pyrexial children should be monitored frequently. The body surface area of children is proportionately larger than that of adults, making them also prone to more rapid heat loss.

Older people (most ICU patients) have lower body temperatures (Güneş and Zaybak, 2008), so early stages of pyrexia may be missed. Similarly, immunocompromise or immunosuppressive drugs may prevent pyrexia occurring with infection. So pyrexia may occur without infection, while infection may occur without pyrexia.

Pyrexia

The American Society of Critical Care Physicians (ACCP) defines clinically significant (i.e. probably from infection) temperatures as > 38.3°C (Isaac and Taylor, 2003), although hypermetabolism can cause severe hyperpyrexia.

Pyrexia can be protective, by:

- *inhibiting bacterial and viral growth* (Sessler, 2008) ('nature's antibiotic');
- *inhibiting pro-inflammatory cytokines* (Wong, 1998);
- *promoting tissue repair* through hypermetabolism.

But every degree centigrade also increases:

- oxygen consumption and
- metabolic waste – carbon dioxide, acids, water

by about 10 per cent. Nurses should therefore assess both the likely cause of pyrexia and its cost to the patient.

Hyperpyrexia (also called 'heatstroke' and 'severe hyperthermia') is a temperature above 40°C. At 41°C convulsions occur and autoregulation fails, death usually following at about 44°C, necessitating urgent ('first aid') neuroprotective cooling.

Malignant hyperpyrexia

Malignant hyperpyrexia, a genetic disorder of calcium channels in skeletal muscle (Brady *et al.*, 2009), may be triggered by drugs (e.g. anaesthetic agents such as suxamethonium, amphetamines) and stress (e.g. massive skeletal injury, strenuous exercise). Untreated malignant hyperpyrexia is fatal.

Precipitating causes should be removed. The only available drug to treat malignant hyperpyrexia is dantrolene sodium (1mg/kg) (Hopkins, 2008), which blocks calcium channels, relaxing skeletal muscle. Neuromuscular blockade (paralysis) may be used to prevent shivering (heat production).

Measurement

'Core temperature' is widely considered the 'gold standard'. The three core areas are those protected by thermoregulation to ensure survival – cranium, and thoracic and abdominal cavities (Stanhope, 2006). Core temperature therefore remains stable at 37°C ± 0.6°C (Washington and Matney, 2008). Ideally, temperature would be measured at the hypothalamus, which contains the thermoregulatory centre, but this is impractical. No core sites are completely non-invasive (Sessler, 2008), so the site chosen is necessarily a compromise between proximity to core and risks/benefits of invasiveness. Many sites, often called 'core', are merely approximations. Crawford *et al.* (2005) suggest that normal ranges for sites are:

- core: 36.8–37.9°C
- tympanic: 35.6–37.4°C
- forehead: 36.1–37.3°C
- axilla: 35.5–37.0°C
- rectal: 34.4–37.8°C
- oral: 36.0–37.6°C

although individual factors, critical illness and specific system function should also be considered.

Many thermometers and many sites are available, often provoking passionate views. Evidence can be found to both favour and disparage each type of thermometer and each measurement site. However, most clinically available thermometers are accurate (Sessler, 2008). Historically, temperature was usually measured orally, rectally or axillary, often with mercury-in-glass thermometers. Mercury-in-glass thermometers are now clinically almost obsolete (Sessler, 2008), as glass is hazardous and mercury neurotoxic, but many older studies compared other thermometers and sites with these, often unfavourably. Latman (2003) considers that no other currently available thermometers compare favourably with mercury-in-glass. The rectum was traditionally considered a core site, although given impaired bowel perfusion and function of many critically ill patients, this view is questionable. Rectal measurement, undignified and unreliable, is rarely justified in ICUs. Axillary measurement is theoretically unreliable for ICUs (Fulbrook, 1997; O'Grady *et al.*, 1998), but often used for disposable *chemical thermometers* (e.g. Tempadots™). Board (1995) found chemical thermometers accurate, but Creagh-Brown *et al.* (2005) found that over three-quarters of qualified nurses read them inaccurately. Their range is limited to 35.5–40.4°C (O'Toole, 1997), making them unsuitable for measuring hypothermia or hyperpyrexia. Chemical thermometers rely on visual interpretation, so can be subjective.

Pulmonary artery temperature, the closest measurable site to hypothalamic temperature, remains the 'gold standard' (O'Grady *et al.*, 1998). Catheters being highly invasive, temperature measurement alone does not justify their use. Debate persists about the accuracy of alternative sites and equipment.

Deep forehead (temporal artery) measurement may (Harioka *et al.*, 2000) or may not (Kistemaker *et al.*, 2006; Kimberger *et al.*, 2007) be reliable.

Tympanic measurement is widely used. The carotid artery supplies both the tympanic membrane and the nearby hypothalamus, so more accurately reflects core temperature than any other non-invasive device or site (El-Radhi and Patel, 2006; Stanhope, 2006; Kiekkas *et al.*, 2008). Like all thermometers, debate persists about whether they are (Giantin *et al.*, 2008) or are not (Lawson *et al.*, 2007) accurate. Common causes of under-readings are incomplete insertion. Dirty or damaged lenses also cause under-reading. Many tympanic thermometers offer optional adjustments of temperature to equivalents at other sites. Provided a tympanic (sometimes called 'ear') option is available, it is logical to set this, and ensure all thermometers are adjusted to the same setting, especially as 'offsets' for adjustment to other sites vary significantly between firms and models.

Probes on urinary catheters can measure *bladder* temperature. One-quarter of cardiac output flows through renal arteries, so if urine flow is good (60 ml/hour), bladder temperature indicates core temperature (Jung *et al.*, 2008). However, accuracy is affected by urine flow (Sessler, 2008), so if oliguria is present bladder thermometry is probably not suitable. Fallis (2005) found urine flow did not significantly affect bladder thermometry, but was measuring effects of furosemide.

Nasopharyngeal and *oesophageal* probes provide relatively non-invasive measurement, but are affected if air leaks past endotracheal cuffs. Either probe may cause distress and discomfort, so cannot be recommended.

Non-invasive skin probes, usually on patients' feet, measure *peripheral* temperature. Comparing differences between peripheral and central temperature indicates perfusion/warming – differences should be below 2°C if well perfused. Limb reperfusion should be monitored following vascular surgery to the leg.

Treatment

The appropriateness of treating pyrexia necessitates individual assessment and evidence-based practice. With pyrexias of infective origin, micro-organisms can often be destroyed more safely by antibiotics than by endogenous pyrexia.

Cooling may be:

- central (altering hypothalamic set-point);
- peripheral (increasing heat loss).

Peripheral cooling (reducing bedding, tepid sponging, fans) stimulates further hypothalamus-mediated heat production (shivering) and conservation (vasoconstriction). Shivering increases metabolism, increasing oxygen and energy consumption, while vasoconstriction traps heat produced in central vessels, creating hostile environments for major organs. Cooling also shifts the oxygen dissociation curve to the left, reducing oxygen delivery. Peripheral cooling is therefore fundamentally illogical (Marik, 2000). Paralysing and sedative drugs can reduce metabolism.

Antipyretic drugs (e.g. aspirin, paracetamol, NSAIDs) inhibit prostaglandin synthesis, so restoring normal hypothalamic regulation. Infective pyrexias usually respond to antipyretic drugs, while pyrexias from hypermetabolism or hypothalamic damage will not.

Sweat evaporation, vasodilatation and increased capillary permeability cause hypovolaemia and hypotension, necessitating additional fluid replacement. Electrolyte and acid/base imbalances should be monitored and treated.

If infection is suspected, appropriate cultures should be taken (e.g. blood) and empirical antibiotics prescribed. Suspected sources of infection (e.g. cannulae) should be removed if possible. Samples usually take days to culture, so recording samples sent on microbiology flow sheets helps ensure results are promptly acted upon.

Hypothermia

Traditionally, mild hypothermia was defined as 32–35°C, but temperatures below < 36°C are now widely regarded as being hypothermic; for example, this is the trigger used by the Modified Early Warning Score (MEWS) (Morgan *et al.*, 1997), a logical change within the context of approximations to core rather than oral measurement. Unless induced, significant hypothermia in ICUs is very rare; however, comparing central (or near-central) temperature with peripheral indicates perfusion, and can be especially valuable after vascular surgery.

Therapeutic hypothermia

Hypothermia reduces metabolism, so reducing oxygen demand and prolonging the time that cells can survive hypoxia. Each 1°C reduces metabolism by 6–7 per cent (Bernard and Buist, 2003). Hypothermia may also inhibit inflammatory cytokines (Peake *et al.*, 2008). Previously used for cardiac surgery, therapeutic hypothermia has been advocated for out-of-hospital cardiac arrests (Varon and Acosta, 2008) and cerebral protection during neurological injury/surgery (Jalan and Damink, 2001). Evidence however remains controversial, studies such as Harris *et al.* (2001) rejecting its use.

Problems from hypothermia (including therapeutic) include:

- reduced dissociation of oxygen from haemoglobin;
- peripheral shutdown, causing anaerobic metabolism;
- cardiac dysrhythmias (Bourdages *et al.*, 2010);
- impaired liver detoxification (Hussein, 2009);
- hyperglycaemia (Bernard and Buist, 2003).

Moderate to severe hypothermia (< 32°C) has 80 per cent mortality (Hinds and Watson, 2008).

Use should be limited to 32–34°C for 12–24 hours (Varon and Acosta, 2008), rewarming at 0.5–1°C/hour, or 1–2°C/day if intracranial hypertension exists (Varon and Acosta, 2008), although severe hypothermia may necessitate rewarming by 3°C per hour (Farley and McLafferty, 2008). The main side effect is shivering, which can be controlled with neuromuscular blockade (Varon and Acosta, 2008).

Implications for practice

- Pyrexia is a symptom, not a disease. Pyrexia should be managed in the context of individual patients (cost/benefit analysis).
- Current evidence for thermometers is limited and inconsistent, but tympanic and chemical thermometers are probably preferable options.
- Pyrexia may be metabolic or infective in origin.
- Clinically significant pyrexia (infection) is usually > 38.3°C.
- Pyrexia inhibits micro-organisms, but increases oxygen and energy consumption, while increasing metabolic waste.
- Infection should be treated with appropriate antibiotics.
- Peripheral cooling in infective pyrexia is usually illogical and counterproductive.
- Central cooling (antipyretic drugs) can restore normal hypothalamic thermoregulation.
- Evidence for therapeutic hypothermia is controversial and conflicting.

Summary

Pyrexia is a symptom, not a disease. Patients, not observation charts, should be treated. Low-grade pyrexia may be beneficial, so managing pyrexia should be individually assessed for each patient – cause, cost and benefit. Clinically significant pyrexia (> 38.3°C) usually indicates infection, and excessive cost, so should usually be reversed with paracetamol, while infection is treated with antibiotics. Unidentified infections should be traced through culture.

Further reading

Sessler has written many authoritative articles on thermometry and temperature, his (2008) providing a valuable recent (medical) review.

Clinical scenario

Fiona Clarke, a 35-year-old known asthmatic, was admitted to the ICU with severe dyspnoea and rash on upper body and arms. Mrs Clarke's core (central) body temperature is 38.2°C with shell (skin) temperature of 33°C. She has started to shiver.

Q.1 (a) List potential causes of Mrs Clarke's increased core temperature.
 (b) Identify the blood cells and mediators responsible.
 (c) Explain the shivering response and its effects on metabolism.
Q.2 Compare various approaches to temperature assessment in your own clinical area; include common sites used in temperature assessment as well as the equipment available. Which would be the most appropriate method to use to monitor Mrs Clarke's core temperature (consider accuracy, time resources, safety, comfort, minimal adverse effects)?
Q.3 Review effective nursing strategies for managing Mrs Clarke's temperature. Select the most suitable pharmacological interventions, laboratory investigations, physical cooling methods (their value, limitations, necessity) and comfort therapies.

85

Chapter 9

Nutrition and bowel care

Contents

Fundamental knowledge   86
Introduction   87
Nitrogen (protein)   87
Energy   87
Enteral nutrition   89
Parenteral nutrition   90
Refeeding syndrome   90
Bowel care   91
Diarrhoea   91
Constipation   93
Colostomies   94
Implications for practice   94
Summary   95
Further reading   95
Clinical scenario   95

Fundamental knowledge

Gut anatomy and physiology

Introduction

Nutrition is fundamental to health, yet Nightingale's (1859/1980) claim that thousands starve in hospitals continues to be relevant, a recent international study (Cahill *et al.*, 2010) finding that nutrition in intensive care is suboptimal. Starvation causes the body to use alternative energy sources – usually body protein (muscle), at daily rates of 1–2 per cent (Skipworth *et al.*, 2006) and increases risks of sepsis (Ros *et al.*, 2009). Critically ill patients lose 5–10 per cent of skeletal muscle mass each week (Griffiths, 2003), which will delay weaning and recovery. Early nutrition improves survival from critical illness (Doig *et al.*, 2009; Singer *et al.*, 2009). Feeding within 24–48 hours of disease/surgery significantly improves outcome (Artinian *et al.*, 2006).

Nitrogen (protein)

Metabolising (oxidising) 6.3 grams of protein produces 1 gram of nitrogen (Reid and Campbell, 2004). Serum nitrogen is transported mainly as ammonia (NH_3), which the liver converts to urea. So measuring urinary nitrogen indicates protein metabolism. Unless diet is especially protein-rich, excessive protein metabolism indicates malnourishment-induced muscle atrophy, which delays weaning. So:

- neutral nitrogen balance = dietary nitrogen matches urinary loss;
- negative nitrogen balance = excess urinary nitrogen *catabolised* for energy;
- positive nitrogen balance = protein building (*anabolism*).

McClave *et al.* (2009) suggest that protein is the most important macronutrient in critical illness, as it promotes wound healing, immunity and muscle-building.

Energy

Cells need energy to function. The energy used is adenosine triphosphate (ATP), produced by cell *mitochondria*. In health, glucose metabolism is the main source of ATP:

$$C_6H_{12}O_6 + 6O_2 \rightarrow 36 \text{ ATP} + \text{waste} (6 \text{ } CO_2 + 6 \text{ } H_2O).$$

Some energy is also derived from fats. Fat metabolism is more complex – Krebs' or the 'citric acid' cycle (see Figure 9.1). Each stage of *Krebs' cycle* releases ATP and two carbon atoms. Carbon combines with coenzyme A, forming acetyl-CoA, which enables further reactions. Fat metabolism produces much energy, but also much waste, each stage releasing acids (ketones, lactate), carbon dioxide and water. Carbon dioxide and water combine to form carbonic acid (H_2CO_3).

Hypoperfusion (shock) deprives cells of normal energy sources (oxygen and glucose) and waste removal. Anaerobic metabolism of alternative energy sources

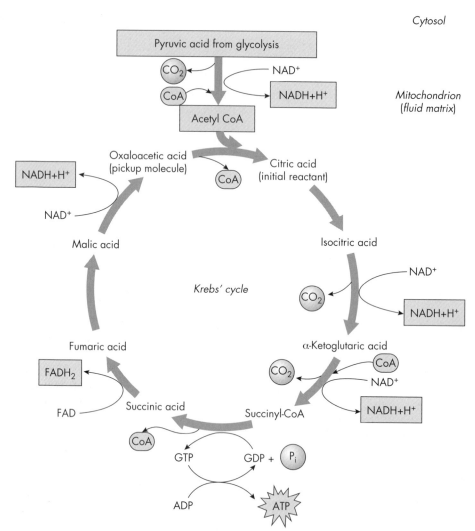

Figure 9.1 Krebs' (citric acid) cycle

(such as fat) increases waste, causing *hypercapnia* and *metabolic acidosis*, and creating increasingly hostile, acidic environments for cells.

Critical illness increases energy expenditure. Griffiths and Bongers (2005) suggest that total energy expenditure is 25 *kcal*/kg/day in severe sepsis and 30 in trauma, rising to 40 for sepsis and possibly 55 with some trauma cases by the second week. However, increased energy expenditure is often not matched by the body's ability to use energy sources from food. Assessing nutritional needs is a complex task, usually undertaken by dieticians.

Enteral nutrition

The gut contains many bacteria. Immunoglobulins (IgA, IgM) prevent bacterial translocation into blood, but hypoperfusion (shock) rapidly causes atrophy of gut villi, releases pro-inflammatory cytokines (Kudst, 2003), and enables bacterial translocation. Enteral nutrition increases blood flow to the gut, preserving normal function and reducing infections such as pneumonia (McClave et al., 2009).

Wide-bore gastric tubes (e.g. Ryles®) are easier to insert than fine-bore tubes, but cause more inflammation (Bowling, 2004). Placement can be confirmed by:

- insertion with ultrasound (e.g. Coretrak®);
- testing aspirate pH (NPSA, 2005);
- radiography.

Injecting air through tubes ('whoosh test') should not be used (NPSA, 2005), as transmitted sound can give falsely positive results. Nasal bridles reduce accidental tube removal (Gunn et al., 2009).

Nasojejunal tubes are seldom used, as there is little evidence to support benefits over gastric tubes (McClave et al., 2009). They should have alkaline aspirate, making it impractical to distinguish between jejunal and pleural aspirates. Position should therefore always be checked by radiography, before removing guidewires.

Gut surgery does not contraindicate enteral feeding (Hans-Geurts et al., 2007). Absence of bowel sounds should not be interpreted as paralytic ileus, as absent sounds may also be caused by absence of sufficient air in the gut to create sounds (McClave et al., 2009). Paralytic ileus seldom affects ileal motility, so if gastric feeding fails, jejunal tubes usually enable enteral nutrition. Jejunal tubes can regress into the stomach unless placed after the duodenojejunal flexure (Bowling, 2004).

Gastric residual volume (aspirate) is the most widely used method to evaluate feed tolerance (Gonzalez, 2008). The upper limit of aspirate that should be tolerated is often considered to be 200 ml, but ESPEN (European Society of Parenteral and Enteral Nutrition) advice adopts American guidelines:

- < 200 maintain feed;
- 200–500 maintain feed, but careful bedside evaluation;
- > 500 withhold feeds and reassess patient's tolerance.
          (Gonzalez, 2008; McClave et al., 2009; Montejo et al., 2009)

Fine-bore tubes can usually be aspirated, sometimes by injecting air to dislodge the tube from stomach folds (Metheny, 1993), although aspiration can cause collapse, blockage or rupture, so should not be routinely practised (Williams and Leslie, 2005). Gastric aspirate contains nutrients, digestive juices and electrolytes, but is also needed to stimulate peristalsis and ileal secretions, so volumes of up to 200 ml are usually returned. Williams and Leslie (2005) recommend reassessing but continuing feeding with aspirates of 200–500 ml.

For patients in ICUs, NICE (2006) recommends continuous feeding over 16–24 hours, with 24 hours recommended if insulin is infused. Most UK ICUs feed continuously. These recommendations are, however, ICU-specific and do not necessarily apply to patients in other areas.

Type and rate of feeds should be prescribed by dieticians, although most ICUs have protocols for commencing standard feeds at incremental rates. Feeds available include:

- standard – carbohydrate-rich;
- fibre – may reduce diarrhoea;
- 'respiratory' feeds – produce less carbon dioxide;
- 'renal' feeds – produce less (nitrogen) waste;
- pre-digested feeds – for malabsorption;
- immune-modulating/enhancing feeds – contain substrates that alter immune/inflammatory responses – e.g. glutamine.

The risk of aspiration can be reduced by prokinetics (e.g. metoclopramide, low-dose erthroymcin) (NICE, 2006; Nguyen et al., 2007) and nursing patients at 30–45° (McClave et al., 2009).

Parenteral nutrition

While enteral nutrition is preferable, supplementary or (total) parenteral nutrition (PN) may be necessary to prevent muscle atrophy. If normal nutrition is unlikely to be achieved within three days, parenteral nutrition should be commenced within 24–48 hours of admission (Singer et al., 2009), and if target enteral nutrition is not achieved within two days, it should be supplemented with parenteral (Singer et al., 2009).

PN can cause:

- gut atrophy, enabling translocation of gut bacteria;
- infection;
- hyperglycaemia;
- hypertriglycidaemia;
- impaired neutrophil function;
- lipid agglutination in capillaries (increased afterload);
- refeeding syndrome.

It is also costly. To minimise infection risks, PN should be given through a dedicated central line (Pratt et al., 2007; NCEPOD, 2010a), so when central lines are inserted, if PN is likely to be used, a line should be labelled for it, and not used for anything else.

Refeeding syndrome

During starvation, the body uses alternative energy sources ('auto-cannibalism'). Refeeding provides glucose, the normal energy source. This stimulates insulin production, which causes loss of important electrolytes and micronutrients into cells – especially phosphate (Fuentebella and Kerner, 2009), magnesium and calcium (Mehanna *et al.*, 2008). Complications can be reduced by introducing feeds slowly after prolonged starvation – half estimated requirement for 24–48 hours (NICE, 2006), with electrolyte and micronutrient supplements given where necessary. Prophylactic vitamin and phosphate supplements should be given (NCEPOD, 2010a).

Bowel care

In contrast to eating and oral care, bowel function is often a social taboo. Despite its importance for nursing care, it can often be given relatively low priority. ICU patients are prone to bowel dysfunction from:

- immobility;
- abnormal diet;
- abnormal peristalsis;
- fluid imbalances;
- effects of many drugs on the bowels (e.g. antibiotics, opioids, diuretics).

Commensal bacteria and yeasts in the colon assist digestion. Critical illness may facilitate their translocation across gut mucosa, causing endogenous infection. Translocation, and the controversial management of selective digestive decontamination, are discussed in Chapter 15.

Bowel care should include recording frequency, type and amount of faeces (Lewis and Heaton, 1997), and listening for bowel sounds (at least once each shift), although Baid (2009) questions the significance of bowel sounds. The Bristol Stool Form Chart (see Figure 9.2) provides objective descriptions.

Diarrhoea

Many ICU patients develop diarrhoea. Diarrhoea is simply more fluid entering the colon than can be reabsorbed, and may be caused by:

- *antibiotics* (destroy gut flora): 41 per cent of patients on antibiotics develop diarrhoea with enteral feeds, compared to 3 per cent without antibiotics (Guenter *et al.*, 1991);
- *excessive fluid* (colonic absorption is limited to about 4.5 litres each day);
- *reduced water reabsorption* from hypoalbuminaemia or hypoperfusion (both common in ICUs);
- *sorbitol* (used in some elixirs, such as paracetamol suspension): exerts higher *osmotic* gradients than plasma, drawing fluid into the bowel (Yassin and Wyncoll, 2005; McClave *et al.*, 2009).

Likely causes of diarrhoea should be identified and, where reasonably possible, treated. If treatment is not reasonably possible, nurses should attempt

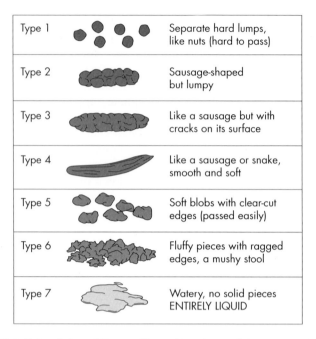

Type 1		Separate hard lumps, like nuts (hard to pass)
Type 2		Sausage-shaped but lumpy
Type 3		Like a sausage but with cracks on its surface
Type 4		Like a sausage or snake, smooth and soft
Type 5		Soft blobs with clear-cut edges (passed easily)
Type 6		Fluffy pieces with ragged edges, a mushy stool
Type 7		Watery, no solid pieces ENTIRELY LIQUID

Figure 9.2 Bristol Stool Form Chart (Lewis and Heaton, 1997)

to alleviate problems and risks. Enteral feeds seldom cause diarrhoea, so should not usually be stopped if diarrhoea occurs.

Diarrhoea can be a homeostatic way to remove pathological bowel bacteria, so reducing motility may cause/prolong infection. The most common pathogenic cause of healthcare-associated diarrhoea is *Clostridium difficile* (Weston, 2008). Pathogen removal should not be inhibited, but samples should be sent for culture, and appropriate antibiotics prescribed.

Diarrhoea not caused by pathogens may be managed by:

- reducing gut motility – e.g. codeine phosphate, loperamide;
- changing to fibre feeds;
- probiotics, such as *Saccharomyces boulardii* (McClave *et al.*, 2009).

Bowel contents are normally rich in electrolytes, including potassium and bicarbonate (Yassin and Wyncoll, 2005), so diarrhoea may cause *hypokalaemia* and *metabolic acidosis*. Metabolic imbalances should be treated.

Some ICU patients experience cramp pains when the gut recommences function or is overactive. This typically causes spasmodic pain (many patients will move their hands towards their abdomen) and irritability. Antispasmodic drugs, such as hyoscine nutybromide (Buscopan®) can provide symptom relief.

Diarrhoea is distressing and socially embarrassing for patients (and visitors), may excoriate skin, and can spread bacteria into wounds, lines or urinary catheters. Patients should therefore be reassured, washed and given clean linen. Faecal collection systems may reduce psychological distress and physiological risks such as infection (Echols *et al.*, 2004; Yassin and Wyncoll, 2005) and skin breakdown, but are relatively expensive.

Constipation

Constipation is variously defined; RCN (2008) criteria seem designed for chronic rather than acute problems, but include the popular definition of fewer than three defecations per week. Constipation may be due to:

- chronic problems with defecations;
- dehydration;
- immobility;
- drugs reducing gut motility (e.g. opioids).

However, gut failure from hypotension and hypoxaemia is probably the main cause (Gacouin *et al.*, 2010). As well as other problems, constipation can cause:

- discomfort
- agitation
- delayed weaning (Gacouin *et al.*, 2010).

Bowel management should include assessment of possible constipation through:

- identifying when bowels were last opened, and the type of stool passed;
- observing and palpating for abdominal distension;
- possibly, digital rectal examination ('PR');
- if hard stools are present in the rectum, giving stool softeners, enemas or (sometimes) performing manual evacuation of faeces.

RCN guidelines (2008) list contraindications and cautions for PR.
  Laxatives may be:

- bulk-forming, stimulating peristalsis (e.g. bran);
- direct peristaltic stimulants (e.g. senna);
- osmotic/softening (e.g. lactulose).

(Thorpe and Harrison, 2002)

Bulk-forming laxatives are usually impractical in ICUs and, increasing intra-abdominal pressure, reduce perfusion of abdominal organs. Osmotic laxatives should be avoided in hypovolaemic patients, or patients with poor gut perfusion. Stimulant laxatives, such as senna, are usually the best option. Normal gut transit time is often 12–24 hours, so senna is usually best given late at night. If laxatives fail, faecal softeners (e.g. glycerol suppositories) may be useful (Day, 2001).

Colostomies

Major bowel surgery often necessitates colostomy formation. Colostomy care is the same in ICUs as elsewhere, except that ICU patients can seldom care for their own colostomies. Colour and perfusion of stomas should be checked at least once every shift, and any concerns reported. Most Trusts employ stoma nurses, who should be actively involved.

Implications for practice

- Early and adequate nutrition hastens recovery and reduces endogenous infection.
- While multidisciplinary expertise is useful, nurses should both assess their patients' nutritional needs and coordinate care to ensure patients are adequately nourished.
- If the gut works, use it – enteral feeding is *usually* preferable.
- Nurses may need to initiate standard protocol feeding regimes, but dieticians should individually assess patients as soon as reasonably possible.
- Success in establishing feeds should be assessed through:
  - delivering the prescribed regime;
  - absence of high gastric aspirates or vomiting;
  - absence of diarrhoea;
  - absence of hyperglycaemia or other metabolic disturbances.

- Aspirates of up to 500 ml every four hours are often acceptable, although volumes of 100–200 ml are often an indication for prokinetics.
- If nasogastric feeding fails, other options include:
  - jejunal tubes;
  - percutaneous endoscopic gastrostomy/jejunostomy (PEG/PEJ) tubes.

- Diarrhoea is rarely caused by nasogastric feeding, so is not an indication to stop feeds.
- Bowel function should be assessed on admission, and reviewed each shift. Frequency, type and amount of stool should be recorded.
- The Bristol Stool Form assessment provides a useful way to quantify bowel evacuations.
- Senna is usually the best laxative for ICU use, and is usually best given at night.
- Overactive bowels can be slowed with drugs such as codeine phosphate or loperamide.
- Bowel spasm distress may be relieved by antispasmodics.
- Faecal collection systems are expensive, but can reduce distress to patients from frequent faecal incontinence and the subsequent washes and changes, and reduce infection risks for others.
- Stoma nurse specialists should be involved in the care of all patients with newly formed stomas.

Summary

Malnutrition causes much ill-health, delays recovery and increases mortality. Early and appropriate nutrition is fundamental to care. Protecting the gut may prevent sepsis. Nurses should therefore assess nutritional needs. Feeding should be enteral whenever possible.

Many ICU patients are unable to identify a need to defecate, or report constipation, yet are prone to bowel dysfunction. Nurses should therefore monitor bowel function. Diarrhoea frequently occurs in ICU patients, usually being caused by disease or treatments.

Further reading

Most ICU texts include substantial chapters on nutrition, and articles on nutrition frequently appear in medical and nursing journals. Major guidelines and reports include McClave *et al.* (2009), Singer *et al.* (2009) and NCEPOD (2010a). Williams and Leslie (2004, 2005) provide useful nursing reviews of enteral feeding. Thomas and Bishop (2007) is the key (dieticians') text. Websites such as that of the British Association of Parenteral and Enteral Nutrition (BAPEN) contain current and often useful material. The RCN (2008) provides guidelines on bowel care.

Clinical scenario

Richard Lewis is 71 years old, weighs approximately 70 kg, and has an arm span of 1.88 metres. He was admitted to the ICU 15 days ago following emergency surgery for a perforated appendix. He is a smoker and has a tracheostomy to facilitate weaning from mechanical ventilation. His glycaemic control maintains his blood sugar at 4.7 mmol/litre with intravenous insulin infusion of 0.5 iu/hour.

Mr Lewis is fed via a nasojejunal (NJ) tube in his right nostril. He receives 75ml/hour of enteral nutrition combining two pre-digested feeds of 750 ml Peptamen® (1 kcal/ml) with 1 litre Nutrison Protein Plus® (1.25 kcal/ml). He has diarrhoea > 800 ml/day, which is infected with *Clostridium difficile* and being treated with oral vancomycin.

Q.1 Calculate Mr Lewis's body mass index (BMI). Assess his nutritional status and requirements in the ICU. Identify other information needed to complete assessment.

Q.2 Analyse Mr Lewis's feeding regime, including total daily calories, the potential benefits and risks of the feeding approach and type of enteral feed.

Q.3 Consider strategies to manage Mr Lewis's diarrhoea and prevent cross-infection. Review the range of faecal containment systems available in your clinical area and other resources used to manage patients' diarrhoea. Evaluate effectiveness of these strategies.

Chapter 10

Mouthcare

Contents

Fundamental knowledge	96
Introduction	97
Anatomy	97
Plaque	98
Infection	98
Assessment	99
Replacing saliva	100
Teeth	100
Lips	101
Pressure sores	101
Dentures	101
Implications for practice	101
Summary	102
Further reading	102
Clinical scenario	102

Fundamental knowledge

Oral anatomy
Composition of dental plaque

Introduction

Hygiene is a fundamental activity of living. Poor oral care in ICUs contributes to ventilator-associated pneumonia (VAP) (Mori *et al.*, 2006), so most recent studies, such as Cason *et al.* (2007), Ross and Crumpler (2007) and Chao *et al.* (2009), focus on how improved care can reduce VAP. Other evidence is sparse and weak (Berry *et al.*, 2007). However, there has been less interest in wider aspects of oral care in ICUs, such as reducing long-term dental decay (O'Reilly, 2003).

Oral hygiene provides psychological comfort (O'Reilly, 2003). The mouth is used for communication – lip-reading is possible despite intubation, while, following extubation, oral discomfort may make speech difficult. The mouth is also associated with intimate emotions (smiling, kissing). Patients with, or thinking they have, dirty mouths or halitosis may feel (psychologically) isolated.

Providing oral hygiene merely replaces activities ICU patients would perform for themselves, if able. Mouthcare should therefore:

- maintain hygiene;
- keep the oral cavity moist;
- promote comfort;
- protect from infection;
- prevent trauma;
- prevent dental decay.

Anatomy

Saliva is release from glands (see Figure 10.1). Secretion increases with:

- oral pressoceptor stimulation (from anything in the mouth, including endotracheal tubes);
- oral chemoreceptor stimulation (especially acids);
- thoughts of food;
- smelling food (in environment, on clothing);
- lower gut irritation.

However, ICU patients may develop dry mouths (xerostomia) from:

- absence of oral intake;
- reduced saliva from drugs (e.g. morphine, diuretics) and sympathetic nervous system stimulation;
- drying (convection) from mouths wedged open by oral endotracheal tubes.

Therefore, saliva secretion may be excessive or diminished. Saliva contains many chemicals, including immune defences, so excesses or deficits can cause colonisation/infection and ulceration. Normally slightly acidic (pH 6.75–7.0 (Marieb and Hoehn, 2007)), Treloar (1995) found mean salivary pH of 5.3 in ICU patients, which is more likely to cause tooth decay.

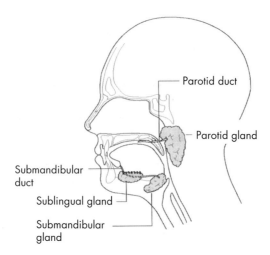

Figure 10.1 Oral (buccal) cavity

Saliva may be serous (containing ptyalin, which digests starches) or mucous (containing mucin, a lubricant). Sympathetic vasoconstriction and dehydration reduce salivary gland perfusion, making saliva viscous and mucin-rich – dry mouths are familiar from 'fight or flight' responses. Endogenous sympathetic stimulation from stress may be compounded by *exogenous* catecholamines (adrenaline/noradrenaline). Saliva production also decreases with age – most ICU patients are old.

Plaque

Plaque (sugar, bacteria and other debris) metabolises to acids, especially lactic acid. Plaque can contain 10^8–10^{11} bacteria per gram (Murray *et al.*, 2009). Accumulated plaque calcifies into calculus or tartar, disrupting seals between gingivae and teeth. Gingivitis (sore, red and bleeding gums) occurs within ten days of plaque formation (Kite and Pearson, 1995).

Plaque is not water soluble, so mouthwash solutions are not a substitute for brushing. Oral neglect enables bacteria to multiply around teeth and dissolve bone (periodontitis/periodontal disease). Periodontitis is the main cause of adult tooth loss, so neglect in ICU can have rapid and enduring effects.

Infection

Micro-organisms grow readily in ICU patients' mouths because:

- mouths are warm, moist and static;
- saliva accumulates at the back of throats, especially if gag/swallowing reflexes are impaired;

- blood and plaque provide protein for bacterial growth (O'Reilly, 2003);
- normal flora are often destroyed by antibiotics;
- immunosuppression facilitates growth.

Infection is usually bacterial, but candidiasis, the most common fungal infection, can be recognised by white spots (Clarke, 1993). Herpes simplex, the major oral virus (susceptible to aciclovir cream), creates sores and cysts around the mouth and lips. Most oral fungi, including candidiasis, are susceptible to nystatin.

Excessive or purulent secretions should be removed with suction. Yankauer catheters are often best for the front of the cavity, but deep oral suction is often easier with a soft catheter. Removal of tenacious secretions may necessitate lubricating the mouth with clean water from a 5 ml syringe, usually best directed at the side of the mouth. Frequency of moistening or removing secretions should be assessed individually for each patient.

Micro-organisms may bypass low-pressure endotracheal cuffs. Scannapieco *et al.* (1992) found respiratory pathogens in 64 per cent of ICU patients, compared with 16 per cent of dental clinic patients. Endotracheal tube tapes are often heavily contaminated with bacteria (Hayes and Jones, 1995). Oral trauma, such as from suction, enables pathogens to enter the bloodstream. So ICU nurses should regularly reassess oral health and hygiene.

Assessment

Oral assessment should include each aspect of the cavity:

- lips
- gums
- teeth
- tongue
- hard palette
- soft tissue
- salivary production
- evidence of any infection
- evidence of any cuts/purpura/blood.

These should be assessed against risk factors from:

- overall condition
- underlying pathology
- treatments (including effects of drugs).

Viewing the oral cavity requires a good light (e.g. pentorch).

Most assessment tools are lists (e.g. Jenkins, 1989; Heals, 1993; Treloar, 1995; Jiggins and Talbot, 1999; Rattenbury *et al.*, 1999; Xavier, 2000). While lists can provide a useful structure, assessment should be individualised to each patient, and there is little evidence of either sustained effectiveness from (Kelly *et al.*, 2010) or validity of (Berry *et al.*, 2007) any tool. Many are relatively lengthy, and risk becoming one more time-consuming 'tick-box exercise' that fails to be translated into nursing care.

Replacing saliva

Many mouthcare solutions and other aids have been marketed, but few remove or prevent plaque. There are artificial saliva solutions, but these are seldom used in ICUs. *Sterile water* can provide moisture, but has no cleansing properties, so is an adjunct rather than a replacement for other care. Some mouthwashes are antibacterial: *chlorhexadine* prevents bacterial and fungal growth, and so reduces VAP (Chan *et al.*, 2007a; Gastmeier and Geffers, 2007).

Foam sticks are useful for moistening the mouth between cleaning (O'Reilly, 2003), but do not remove debris from surfaces or between teeth, so plaque accumulation progresses (Grap *et al.*, 2003). Frequency of moistening mouths should be individualised to patients.

Excess fluid, whether patients' own saliva or instilled water/mouthwashes, should be removed, which usually necessitates suction.

Teeth

Teeth should be brushed at least twice daily to reduce caries (de Oliveira *et al.*, 2010). However, toothbrushing does not reduce VAP (Munro *et al.*, 2009). Between brushing, additional comfort cleaning/refreshing will usually be needed. Toothbrushes (with or without toothpaste) remain the best way to clean patients' teeth (Rello *et al.*, 2007; Kelly *et al.*, 2010), loosening debris trapped between teeth and removing plaque. Technique should reflect brushing one's own teeth: brush away from gums to remove, rather than impact, plaque in gingival crevices. Manipulating toothbrushes in others' mouths, especially when they are orally intubated, can be difficult, so small-headed ('paediatric') toothbrushes are often most effective for brushing others' teeth (Jones, 2004). Angling toothbrushes at 45° to gingival margins, using very small vibratory movements, collects and removes plaque (Dougherty and Lister, 2004). With limited mouth opening (trismus), interspace toothbrushes may be better for removing plaque. Toothbrushes can clean heavily coated tongues, and gums and tongue of endentitious patients (O'Reilly, 2003).

Fluoride toothpaste is preferable (Rattenbury *et al.*, 1999), although patients may find the taste of their usual brand comforting. Most toothpastes dry the mouth (Jones, 2004), so should be rinsed out thoroughly – sterile water from a 5 ml syringe, and continuous suction, are usually the best way to achieve this. Yankauer catheters can stimulate a cough/gag reflex, so should be used sparingly; soft catheters are usually more effective for mouthcare.

Vigorous brushing may cause bleeding, especially if patients have coagulopathies (e.g. DIC); oral care should therefore be planned holistically. If nystatin is prescribed, this should be administered following mouthcare.

Lips

Lips are highly vascular, with sensitive nerve endings. Mucosa being exposed, they can dry quickly. Lips are even more closely associated with communication (e.g. lip-reading) and intimacy (e.g. kissing) than the mouth. Lipcare can therefore prevent drying/cracking, while providing psychological comfort. Lip balm, in the form of white petroleum jelly or yellow soft paraffin, is often used to keep lips moist (Bowsher *et al.*, 1999). Contrary to circulating myths, petroleum jelly neither explodes nor burns (Winslow and Jacobson, 1998).

Pressure sores

Any body surface area may develop pressure sores (see Chapter 12). Treloar's (1995) small study found multiple lip, tongue and mucosal lesions, as well as very dry mouths, in ICU patients. Endotracheal tubes and tapes place pressure on various tissues, including the mouth. Gingival surfaces are more susceptible to sores than teeth (Liwu, 1990), and tube tapes can lacerate lips. Pressure from tapes can be reduced by placing them away from lip corners, supporting pressure points with gauze or sponge pads, and moving tapes and tubes (Clarke, 1993). Teeth can usually be cleaned most effectively when changing endotracheal tapes.

Dentures

About half of older people do not have their own teeth (Watson, 2001). Intubation and impaired consciousness normally necessitate removal of any dentures, but property should be checked on admission so that dentures are not lost. Nursing records should include whether patients normally wear partial or complete dentures, and relevant care.

Dentures may easily be damaged or warp, especially if left dry or if cleaned in hot water (Clarke, 1993). Dentures should usually be left to soak overnight in cold water (Xavier, 2000; Clay, 2002; O'Reilly, 2003). Toothpaste should not be used on dentures, as it can damage their surfaces (Clarke, 1993). Patients, or their families, may be able to supply their normal cleaning agents, which, if available, should be used (Xavier, 2000).

Implications for practice

■ Mouthcare should be individually assessed, rather than following routine/rituals.
■ Toothbrushes (with or without toothpaste) are the best means for providing mouthcare.
■ Teeth should (usually) be brushed with toothpaste twice daily, with additional comfort cleaning between, according to individual assessment.
■ Fluoride toothpaste helps prevent decay.
■ Rinse toothpaste out thoroughly, using sterile water and continuous suction.
■ Mouthwashes or moist swabs moisten the mouth but do not remove plaque.

■ If antibacterial washes or gels are needed, consult pharmacists.
■ If patients wear dentures, maintain their normal care if possible, and record where they are stored.
■ White petroleum jelly or yellow soft paraffin protects lips from cracking.

Summary

Mouthcare is too easily forgotten in the physiological crises of critical illness, but problems developing from patients' time in the ICU can cause long-term or permanent oral/dental disease. The current paucity of material on mouthcare in ICUs makes evidence-based practice difficult.

Further reading

Kelly *et al.* (2010) review oral care, albeit from stroke care perspectives. Chan *et al.* (2007a) provide a meta-analysis, although as with much recent literature they focus on preventing VAP.

Clinical scenario

Michael Dodd is a 22-year-old gentleman who has a past medical history of poorly controlled asthma. He presents with left lower lobe pneumonia. This is his third admission to the ICU for respiratory support. He weighs 90 kg, is receiving enteral nutrition at 75 ml/hour and has been mechanically ventilated for seven days. Mr Dodd's oral endotracheal tube length is 23 cm at the lips, positioned on the right side of his mouth and balancing on his teeth. He has visible dental decay at gum margins with white spots on his tongue and hard palate.

Mr Dodd's intravenous drug therapy includes sedative infusions of propofol and midazolam, antibiotic infusions of vancomycin and rifampicin and hydrocortisone. He has a temperature of 38.5°C, Hb 10.4 g/dl, WBC 9.3×10^9/litre^3, CRP 207 mg/litre.

Q.1 List the equipment needed to inspect and assess Mr Dodd's oral status to include gums, tongue, salivary glands, teeth, palate, lips and jaw.
Q.2 Identify Mr Dodd's risk factors for developing oral complications. Use a published oral assessment tool to calculate and interpret his oral assessment score.
Q.3 Develop a plan for Mr Dodd's mouthcare, including frequency of interventions, method of brushing teeth and tongue, lip lubrication and use of any topical lotions or creams.

Chapter 11

Eyecare

Contents

Fundamental knowledge   103
Introduction   104
Ocular damage   104
Assessment   105
Interventions   106
Implications for practice   107
Summary   107
Further reading   108
Clinical scenario   108

Fundamental knowledge

Anatomy – cornea, lens, tear production, blink reflex

Introduction

Patients are seldom admitted to ICU for ocular pathologies, but one-third to two-thirds of critically ill patients suffer eye surface disease (Dawson, 2005), especially dryness, redness, and discharge (Oh *et al.*, 2009). Exposed eye surfaces are at increased risk of infection (*keratitis*) – at least one-fifth of ICU patients develop exposure *keratopathy* (Rosenberg and Eisen, 2008). Abrasion can occur from bedding, endotracheal tube tapes and other equipment, while positive pressure ventilation increases intraocular pressure, so causing potential 'ventilator eye'. This chapter does not discuss specialist ocular pathophysiologies, but reasons for and types of eyecare needed by most ICU patients.

In health, the eyelid protects the eye surface. Tear production and frequent blinking maintains health and moistens eye surfaces. While many ICU patients can maintain their own ocular health, some may develop complications. Problems can occur from:

- increased intraoccular pressure or periorbital oedema (especially prone positioning);
- impaired blink reflex, such as from paralysis (disease or chemical);
- decreased tear production;
- patient being unable to move their head;
- eye infection.

If patients are unable to maintain their own ocular health, nurses should meet this need for them.

Nurses may feel squeamish about touching eyes, but eyecare maintains physiological and psychological health. Ocular abnormalities often make patients and relatives anxious. For most people, vision is the most used sense, eye contact helping communication. So visual deficits contribute significantly to sensory imbalance. ICU nurses should therefore evaluate:

- visual appearance;
- eyecare performed;
- how care is described.

Eyecare in ICU varies greatly, with limited supporting evidence (Dawson, 2005). Substantive research being needed, suggestions here necessarily remain tentative.

Ocular damage

The cornea, the eye's outer surface, has no direct blood supply, otherwise sight would be impaired. It is therefore vulnerable to drying, trauma and lacerations (e.g. from pillows, endotracheal tapes, dust and particles). Blink reflexes and tear production, which normally protect and irrigate corneal surfaces, may be absent/weak. Drugs (e.g. atropine, antihistamines, paralysing agents) also inhibit tear production. If blink reflexes are absent, eyelids should be closed or corneas protected with a cover (Imanaka *et al.*, 1997).

Bacteria can cause *blepharitis* – inflammation of eyelash follicles and sebaceous glands, resulting in redness, swelling and crusts of dried mucus collecting on the lids. Crusts may cause corneal trauma on eyelid closure with blinking. If ocular infection is suspected, it should be reported and recorded; swabs may need to be taken and topical antibiotics prescribed.

Incomplete eyelid closure or loss of blink reflexes cause corneal drying (exposure keratopathy), and can cause infection (keratitis) or corneal ulceration (Suresh *et al.*, 2000; Dawson, 2005). The cornea is richly supplied with sensory nerves (Patil and Dowd, 2000), making lacerations very painful. Corneal damage exposes deeper layers to infection, while avascularity delays healing, often leaving opaque scar tissue. Ocular trauma may remain unrecognised until patients regain consciousness, finding their vision permanently impaired.

Normal intraocular pressure is 12–20 mmHg (average 15 mmHg). Drainage of aqueous humour, and so intraocular hypertension, subconjunctival haemorrhage and other damage, may be caused by positive intrathoracic pressure (positive pressure ventilation), tight ETT tapes, oedema, poor head alignment or prone positioning. Hypercapnia increases intraocular pressure (Patil and Dowd, 2000), a potential complication of permissive hypercapnia. ICU patients are therefore at high risk of intraocular hypertension. More than half the patients in Suresh *et al.*'s (2000) small study (n=34) developed 'ventilator eye'. Head elevation (e.g. 30° if supine) assists venous drainage.

Contact lenses are removed preoperatively, but with emergency admissions may still be in place. Contact lenses or glasses, if removed, should be stored safely, and recorded in nursing notes in case of loss.

Assessment

Structured eye assessment tools are not generally used in ICUs, and with the proliferation of paper assessment tools might prove counterproductive if introduced. However, nurses should assess the condition of their patients' eyes through:

- existing documentation;
- visual observation of patients;
- knowledge of normal ocular anatomy;
- verbal questions (to patients or family).

Cues to consider include:

- contact lenses/glasses;
- abnormalities (e.g. eyelids, lashes, exophthalmos); whether abnormalities are unilateral/bilateral;
- periorbital oedema;
- patient positioning, venous drainage;

- muscle weakness ('droopy eye');
- eye closure – whether lids cover cornea completely;
- if eyes look infected/inflamed;
- if eyes look sore ('redeye' – often a sign of acute bacterial conjunctivitis);
- tear production (excessive/impaired) – moist/dry eyes;
- blink reflex (absent, impaired, slow);
- eye pain (flinching during eyecare/interventions);
- visual impairment (double, cloudy, difficulty focusing);
- how the patient feels (e.g. are eyelids heavy?).

Closed questions are often easier for intubated patients to answer.
Unless patients have specific ocular disease, eyecare should:

- maintain ocular health;
- replace lost functions;
- ensure comfort;
- protect from trauma/infection.

To perform eyecare:

- tilt the head backwards (Russell, 2008) – this helps nurses see what they are doing and keeps solutions in the eye;
- use a good light (Russell, 2008), but avoid shining light directly into patients' eyes.

Frequency of eyecare should be individualised to needs.
While assessing and caring for patients' eyes, nurses can also make neurological assessment of:

- pupil size and reaction;
- accommodation for near and long vision: place a finger near the patient's nose; when moved away, pupils should diverge.

Ocular damage may invalidate any or all of these tests.

Interventions

Dry eyes should be lubricated, although optimal solution or frequency remains unclear (Dawson, 2005). *Artificial tears* seem a logical replacement if tear production is inadequate. *Chloramphenicol* eye-drops are often used to treat acute bacterial conjunctivitis (Høvdin, 2008). Eye-drops should be dropped into the outer side of the lower fornix (see Figure 11.1), which is less sensitive than the cornea (Russell, 2008). Over-vigorous use of eye-drops on corneas resembles water torture. To minimise infection risk, solutions should be stored in a clean area. If reusable, they should be labelled with date and time of opening. Local hospital policies will identify how long solutions can be used after opening.

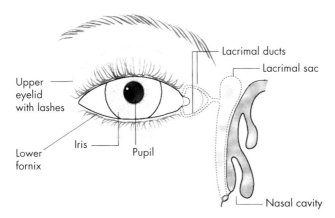

Figure 11.1 External structure of the eye

If eyelid *closure* is incomplete, and patients cannot blink, corneal surfaces should be kept moist and covered. Cleaning should be performed with sterile water, eye surfaces being very susceptible to infection. Saline can irritate and sting, so it is generally best to use sterile water or commercial eye-drops. Excess moisture should be removed delicately, but no method is ideal – cotton wool and gauze can both scratch delicate corneal surfaces, while sticks on cotton buds can cause trauma. Many people are especially squeamish about eyes, so relatives may become especially anxious when eyes are covered.

Implications for practice

- Many ICU patients suffer 'ventilator eye'.
- Care for each patient should be individually assessed.
- If patients are unable to maintain their own ocular health, eyecare should keep eyes clean, moist and covered.
- Nursing semi-recumbent helps venous drainage.
- Prone positioning can damage eyes; elevating the bedhead by as little as 10° and careful head alignment can reduce complications.
- Eyecare solutions are potential media for infection, so should be changed regularly (check unit/hospital policy; if not specified, change at least one each shift).
- Exposed corneas are vulnerable to trauma, so keep pillow edges, endotracheal tape and other equipment away from eyes.

Summary

Although patients are seldom admitted for ocular conditions, diseases and treatments can expose ICU patients to ocular damage. Yet eyecare in ICU is often given low priority, and there is little reliable and substantiated literature to guide interventions. Preventative eyecare should be commenced on admission

(Oh *et al.*, 2009). Care inevitably relies heavily on custom, practice, rituals and anecdotal support. As part of their fundamental patient care, nurses should support/provide what their patients need. Nurses should therefore assess their patients' ocular health and risks, planning individualised care accordingly.

Further reading

Eyecare in ICU is much under-researched, and little other specialist literature exists. Ocular literature rarely discusses care of critically ill patients, although the Joanna Briggs Institute (2002) has synthesised what little knowledge is available. Patil and Dowd (2000) and Suresh *et al.* (2000) are among the few relatively recent medical articles. Oh *et al.* (2009) is one of the few recent studies, although the large number of chemically paralysed patients in their study limits its applicability to the UK. *The Royal Marsden NHS Trust Manual of Clinical Nursing Procedures* (Dougherty and Lister, 2008) offers sound advice for nursing care.

Clinical scenario

Jonathan Hopkins is 48 years old and works as a computer programmer. Mr Hopkins wears non-gas-permeable contact lenses and has a severe astigmatism in one eye. He recently required treatment for recurrent conjunctivitis. He was admitted with community-acquired pneumonia. In the first 24 hours he received respiratory support via facial mask CPAP of 10 cmH$_2$O with FiO$_2$ of 0.5.

Q.1 Identify factors that can cause ocular damage or complications with Mr Hopkins' vision.

Q.2 Mr Hopkins developed bacterial keratitis and corneal ulceration associated with exposed cornea from an over-tightened head harness securing his CPAP face mask. Consider how this affected his recovery in relation to his perceptions, vision, communication interactions and pain. Reflect on the legal, ethical and professional responsibilities towards Mr Hopkins. (Has substandard practice or negligence occurred? If yes, who might be responsible?)

Q.3 Review eyecare in your own clinical area. Are the ocular assessment and associated interventions:

- systematic (in both approach and documentation);
- based on a local or published guideline;
- knowledge and/or evidence-based;
- effective at identifying risk patients, and before complications occur?

Chapter 12

Skincare

Contents

Fundamental knowledge	109
Introduction	110
Pressure sores	110
Assessment	111
Prevention	112
Necrotising fasciitis	112
Implications for practice	113
Summary	113
Further reading	114
Clinical scenario	114

Fundamental knowledge

Structure and anatomy of skin
Functions of skin
Pressure sore (decubitus ulcer) formation
Stages of wound healing

Introduction

Incidence of pressure sores in ICUs varies widely, with half of ICU patients having sores in some studies (Elliott *et al.*, 2008); most studies suggest up to one-fifth of ICU patients develop pressure sores (Pender and Frazier, 2005; de Laat *et al.*, 2006). Pressure sores increase:

- morbidity (human costs);
- mortality;
- financial costs (prolonged stay, additional treatments, litigation).

(Dowsett and White, 2010)

Pressure sores increase morbidity, and possibly mortality, so maintaining skin integrity is fundamental to care, although potentially difficult to achieve with high-risk hypotensive and immobile patients, especially if turning risks compromising vital organ function. Epidermal cells take one month to migrate from basal layers to skin surfaces (Casey, 2002), so healing is slow, exposing deeper tissues to potential infection.

ICU patients are at high risk for developing pressure sores because of:

- prolonged peripheral hypoperfusion
- oedema
- anaerobic metabolism
- immunocompromise
- malnutrition.

This chapter revises pressure sore development, identifies some assessment systems available, and describes some ways of preventing pressure sores. Wound dressings are not discussed, as rapid changes in practice and availability make inclusion in this book impractical. Necrotising fasciitis, a dermatological condition often proving fatal, is also discussed. Much literature originates, or is sponsored/promoted by, people and commercial companies with vested interests, so should be treated cautiously.

Pressure sores

When external pressure exceeds capillary pressure, perfusion fails, leading to necrosis. Capillary occlusion pressure, the amount of pressure required to occlude capillaries, is often cited at 30–32 mmHg. This originates from Landis's 1930 study, which measured 21–48 mmHg in normotensive volunteers (mean 32 mmHg) (Lowthian, 1997). ICU patients are not volunteers, and seldom normotensive. So 20–25 mmHg is generally a safer upper limit for any unrelieved pressure on any tissue. Visible signs of pressure sores may appear on skin surfaces, but pressure in solid tissue near bony prominences can be 3–5 times that exerted on skin (Houwing *et al.*, 2000).

Pressure sores can be caused by intrinsic factors (Waterlow, 1995):

- age
- malnutrition
- dehydration
- incontinence
- medical condition
- medication

and extrinsic ones:

- unrelieved pressure
- shearing
- friction.

Extrinsic factors are usually more easily modified.

Excessive moisture or dryness hastens skin breakdown. Urine is acidic, so leaks around urinary catheters excoriate skin. Perspiration makes skin excessively moist, and contains urea. Faeces also contain acids. Diarrhoea, inability to alert nurses to the need for bedpans, and gathering sufficient staff to turn patients can result in anal areas being exposed to evacuated faeces, causing excoriation. Barrier creams can reduce risks of breakdown, so are useful adjuncts to, but not substitutes for, nursing care. Prompt hygiene and 'comfort' washes reduce risks, and lubricating dry skin (e.g. with aqueous cream) can prevent breakdown.

Traditionally, pressure sores are associated with skin over bony prominences – elbows, heels, sacrum. These are risk areas for ICU patients, but other possible sites for sores include:

- head (especially the back);
- ears;
- lips/mouth (around ETTs);
- beneath invasive equipment (e.g. hubs of arterial lines);
- skinfolds (e.g. breasts, groin, abdomen);
- chest and face if prone positioned.

Hair may hide sores on backs of heads, until blood is found on pillows. Nurses should therefore proactively assess all risk areas.

Assessment

Pressure areas should be regularly assessed (at least once each shift), and assessment tools can provide useful cues, but become counterproductive if they are viewed as just another paper exercise. Many assessment tools have been developed. The Braden Scale (Bergstrom *et al.*, 1987) is the most widely used assessment in the USA (Ayello and Braden, 2002). Pender and Frazier (2005) found it unreliable for ICUs, while Suriadi *et al.* (2006) found it had high sensitivity (identified patients at risk), but low specificity (many false positives). The most widely used tool in the UK is Waterlow (1985, updated 2005). Most UK nurses are familiar with it, and it reliably predicts risks of pressure sore development in ICUs (Sayar *et al.*, 2009), although most ICU patients fall in the 'high-risk' score.

Prevention

Pressure ulcers have traditionally been viewed as a sign of poor care, and many Trusts now require clinical incident forms to be completed if pressure ulcers develop. The DH (2009a) has set a target of eliminating avoidable pressure sores. Pressure on skin can be decreased either by changing position or increasing surface area over which pressure is spread. Two-hourly pressure area care owes more to ritual than logic, and is probably seldom practised in any clinical area; average time between turns in UK ICUs is 4.85 hours (Goldhill *et al.*, 2008), frequency not being related to staffing numbers (Badacsony *et al.*, 2007).

Many aids have been marketed, although most ICUs mainly use either *low air loss mattresses* (e.g. Nimbus®) or *tilting/kinetic beds* – see Chapter 27. Choice of mattress or other aids may be restricted by:

- weight limits for equipment (including hoists);
- pathology – e.g. head or spinal injury patients require a firm mattress to maintain spinal alignment;
- cost, if equipment needs to be hired.

Many other pressure-relieving aids, such as Prevalon™ boots, are also marketed; advice on what is available locally, and what is best for each patient, can be provided by tissue viability nurses.

Most hospitals employ tissue viability nurses to disseminate information and provide an immediate resource for staff, but it is also valuable to identify a link specialist among ICU staff to:

- provide information for all unit staff;
- apply information to special needs and problems of ICU patients;
- audit skincare;
- link to wider resources (e.g. tissue viability nurse).

Necrotising fasciitis

Necrotising fasciitis is rare, although incidence is increasing (Angoules *et al.*, 2007). Infection usually follows minor skin damage (Hasham *et al.*, 2005), beginning as cellulitis. Infection spreads rapidly (3–5 cm each hour) through connective tissue, especially extremities or the perineum (Jallali, 2003), progressing to systemic inflammatory response syndrome (SIRS) and multi-organ dysfunction syndrome (MODS). Depending on how quickly and effectively it is treated, about one-quarter of patients will die (Hasham *et al.*, 2005).

Necrotising fasciitis should be treated with urgent surgical debridement (Hasham *et al.*, 2005) and intravenous antibiotics (Copson, 2003), while organ dysfunction necessitates system support. Hyperbaric oxygen can improve oxygen delivery to tissues (Jallali, 2003) but is not available in most hospitals. Extensive infection may leave residual deformity (Hinds and Watson, 2008), and amputation may be necessary (Jallali, 2003).

Tissue necrosis produces gases (hydrogen, methane, hydrogen sulphide, nitrogen) and putrid discharge. Some infections (e.g. streptococcal) have no odour, but many smell of rotting flesh, which, together with the grey colour, is distressing for patients, visitors and staff. Air-fresheners may help mask odours, although chemicals should not enter exposed wounds. Gross (oedematous) swelling of flesh may make patients almost unrecognisable, so visitors should be warned to expect distressing appearances.

Implications for practice

- ICU patients are 'high risk' for pressure sore development.
- Sores develop if external pressure exceeds capillary occlusion pressure; 20–25 mmHg is usually a safe upper limit for sustained pressure. ICU patients can therefore develop sores in many places, including the backs of heads.
- Pressure areas should be checked at least once every shift.
- No ideal assessment tool exists for ICUs, but whatever is used should be familiar to all staff.
- Pressure area aids should allow tissue perfusion, so pressures should be below capillary occlusion pressure (20–25 mmHg) for part of each cycle.
- Hospital tissue viability nurses, and unit link nurses for tissue viability, can be a valuable resource.
- Necrotising fasciitis is a rare, but potentially devastating, infection that progresses rapidly and should be treated aggressively.

Summary

Skin has many functions; the cost of skin breakdown can be measured in mortality, humanitarian terms (morbidity), increased length of stay in the ICU, increased financial costs and litigation.

Various scoring systems have been designed to assess skin integrity, but none is ideal for ICUs, and the best system is only as good as the staff using it. Anthony *et al.* (2008) found conflicting evidence for efficacy of scores, and that nurses' clinical judgement was closer to expert opinion than scoring systems, and suggested that nurses may be wasting time conducting risk assessment scoring. Pressure sores continue to occur in ICUs. The culture of guilt surrounding pressure sores is unhelpful to everyone; despite good nursing, sores will occur, so nurses should assess and minimise risk factors to reduce the incidence.

Further reading

General nursing journals frequently carry articles on skincare, the *Journal of Wound Care* specialising in the topic. Most anatomy texts include detailed chapters on skin. Goldhill *et al.* (2008) and the parallel article, Badacsony *et al.* (2007), provide recent evidence of skincare issues in ICUs. Anthony *et al.* (2008) studied the usefulness of scoring systems, with provocative conclusions.

Website

Braden Scale: www.bradenscale.com/braden.pdf

Clinical scenario

Norman Robinson is a 60-year-old gentleman who tripped on an uneven paving stone and sustained a superficial abrasion to the lateral aspect of his left knee. Within 24 hours, his leg was increasingly painful and oedematous, and he was unable to extend his knee or bear weight. Two days after this fall, Mr Robinson was diagnosed with necrotising fasciitis and had aggressive surgical debridement. This involved 'degloving' his left leg and the application of skin grafts taken from his right leg. He was admitted to the ICU following surgery for mechanical ventilation and organ support. Mr Robinson is increasingly oedematous with extensive (offensive-smelling) wound exudate from both legs and constant diarrhoea. He weighs 93 kg and is 1.68 m tall.

Other results include pyrexia of 38.5°C, tachycardia 115 bpm, MAP 73 mmHg, CVP 20 mmHg and urine output greater than 60 ml/hour over the last four hours. Blood investigation revealed creatinine 218 μmol/litre, urea 18.4 mmol/litre, albumin 17 g/litre, platelets 61×10^{-9}/litre, Hb 8.5 g/dl, WBC 14×10^{-9}/litre. Microbiological examination of tissue from his left leg shows large presence of *Staphylococcus aureus* and beta haemolytic group A *Streptococci*. Appropriate antibiotics have been prescribed.

Q.1 Identify Mr Robinson's risk factors for developing further skin breakdown.

Q.2 Consider the range of pressure-relieving equipment in your clinical area, select appropriate mattress type, aids and other interventions to optimise skin integrity.

Q.3 Review wound assessment and documentation for Mr Robinson. How should his exudative wounds and skin grafts be managed to minimise other complications and promote wound healing?

Chapter 13

Children in adult ICUs

Contents

Fundamental knowledge	115
Introduction	116
A: Airway	116
B: Breathing	117
C: Circulation	117
D: Disability (neurological)	118
E: Exposure	118
Drugs	119
Transfer	119
Legal aspects	120
Meningitis	120
Implications for practice	121
Summary	121
Support groups	122
Further reading	122
Clinical scenario	122

Fundamental knowledge

Local policies about consent and child protection
Location and contents of paediatric equipment and
resources in the workplace

Introduction

Paediatric intensive care units (PICUs), provided in the UK by regional centres, improve survival (Ramnarayan *et al.*, 2010). However, when children initially become critically ill they are often in their local hospital. Children are usually only admitted to ICUs if additional care to that available on paediatric wards is needed, and until retrieval teams from PICUs arrive to transport patients to specialist centres (DH, 1997; Hallworth and McIntyre, 2003). The occasional emergency paediatric admission creates two main problems for staff in general (adult) ICUs:

- when children are admitted, their condition is usually at its most critical/ unstable;
- admission is so infrequent, most staff in general ICUs have little or no experience of paediatric nursing.

This chapter therefore focuses on initial management and stabilisation of critically ill children, using the ABCDE format likely to be used when stabilising children for transfer. However, pandemic influenza planning in 2009 anticipated significant numbers of children being cared for on general ICUs (see Chapter 16). In a position statement, the NMC (2009) acknowledged that nurses might have to care for people in unfamiliar settings or areas of practice, requiring that nurses act 'responsibly and reasonably'. This chapter will not discuss neonates, who would be admitted to special care baby units (SCBUs). Meningitis, which can also occur in adult patients, is discussed.

Children, especially young children, are still developing. Physical growth necessitates higher metabolic rates, increasing oxygen and nutritional demands, while increasing physiological waste. Many vital signs, such as heart rate, are therefore higher than in adults, with different 'normal' ranges for different ages. But the crisis that has necessitated ICU admission is also likely to make many vital signs abnormal. Unless familiar with paediatric ranges, nurses need to assess which signs are significant, and often need to rely on trends.

A: Airway

Proportionally increased oxygen demand, carbon dioxide production and smaller airways make children prone to respiratory problems. Infants normally breathe though their noses (Duncan, 2009), so any nasal obstruction necessarily obstructs the airway. Children's tongues are relatively larger than their oropharynx, making airway obstruction more likely (Patel and Meakin, 2000). Relatively minor inflammatory responses, or mucous, can obstruct airways, so intubation is likely to be an early priority. Paediatric endotracheal tubes, and suction equipment, are necessarily smaller than adult versions, making tubes more prone to obstruction by mucous, and removal more difficult due to smaller and more flimsy catheters. Marsh (2000) suggests normal endotracheal tube sizes for children over one year are:

$$\text{internal diameter (mm)} = \frac{\text{age} + 4}{4}$$

or approximately the diameter of the child's finger. Tibballs (2003) recommends 6FG suction catheters for neonates, 8FG for infants and small children, and 10FG for older children. Being especially prone to hypoxia, children should always be preoxygenated before suction.

Children under 8 years of age have significantly narrower airways than adults. Traditionally uncuffed tubes have been used for younger children (Patel and Meakin, 2000), although Weiss *et al.* (2009) and Resuscitation Council UK (2010) recommend using cuffed tubes for all children. Cuffed tubes are likely to be a half size smaller, and increase cricoid oedema and subglottic stenosis. Initially, oral tubes are usual, but once stabilised, tubes are usually changed to nasal (Duncan, 2009), which are more comfortable and less likely to be displaced. Nasal tubes can however cause nasal sores, so skin should be inspected regularly.

B: Breathing

Children have little physiological reserve, small respiratory systems and high metabolic rates, making them very susceptible to hypoxia. Oxygen should therefore be given quickly to any hypoxic child. Davies and Hassell (2001) suggest that normal respiratory rates are:

- ▪ < 1 year   30–40 breaths/minute;
- ▪ 2–5 years   20–30 breaths/minute;
- ▪ 5–12 years 15–20 breaths/minute;
- ▪ > 12 years 12–16 breaths/minute.

These rates will usually be mimicked on ventilator settings. Otherwise, paediatric ventilation is similar to that used with adults, only with proportionally smaller volumes. Saturation and arterial blood gas values are similar to those of adults.

C: Circulation

Unless born with congenital abnormalities, children usually have healthy cardiovascular systems, so blood pressure monitoring is often less valuable than with adults, but should reflect a healthy adult range. Cardiovascular changes usually indicate respiratory dysfunction (Davies and Hassell, 2001), such as hypoxia. Normal cardiovascular vital signs are shown in Table 13.1.

Children in shock are more likely to survive if given aggressive fluid resuscitation (Morgan and O'Neill, 1998; Thomas and Carcillo, 1998). If not already established, vascular access will therefore be a priority. Children's immature nervous systems are less sensitive to inotropes (Wilkinson, 1997), so proportionally larger doses may be needed. Paediatric resuscitation algorithms differ slightly from adult ones, so should be displayed prominently in bed areas where children and nursed. Fluid balance assessment should include any nappies, dressings or other losses.

Table 13.1 Normal cardiovascular vital signs in children (Cockett, 2010)

Age	Heart rate (bpm)	Systolic BP	Diastolic BP	Mean arterial pressure
Newborn (3 kg)	100–180	70–70	25–24	40–60
Infant	100–160	85–105	55–65	50–90
Toddler	80–110	95–105	55–65	50–100
Preschool	70–110	95–110	55–65	50–100
School age	65–110	95–110	55–70	60–90
Adolescent	60–90	110–130	65–80	65–95

High metabolic rates make children especially susceptible to hypoglycaemia, and critically ill children may not have eaten for some time. Blood glucose should therefore be assessed, especially if fitting occurs (Davies and Hassell, 2001).

D: Disability (neurological)

Immature vital centres, and other brain functions, make children prone to exaggerated responses, such as fitting (Stokes *et al.*, 2004). Among other causes, fitting may be due to hypoxia or hyperthermia, so stabilising vital signs reduces such complications, Neck muscles of young children are weak, and their head is disproportionately large, so children are prone to spinal cord injury. Children are especially susceptible to meningitis (see page 120).

Midazolam and morphine are the most frequently used sedatives and analgesics in paediatric ICUs (Jenkins *et al.*, 2007). Traditionally, propofol has often been avoided, because of concerns about 'propofol syndrome' (metabolic acidosis, lipidaemia, cardiac failure, dysrhythmias, death), although propofol syndrome rarely occurs (Jenkins *et al.*, 2007).

Parents usually help provide children with comfort and reassurance, but the admission is usually emotionally traumatic for parents (Teare and Smith, 2004). Parents often experience guilt and anger, however illogical both may be. Even more than relatives of adult patients, they need information and emotional support. Parents with other children experience additional stress (Clarke, 2000) and conflicting loyalties.

E: Exposure

Up to the age of six, febrile convulsions are common, usually caused by infection (Bethel, 2008). Very young children are prone to extremes of temperature because they have:

■ an immature hypothalamus;
■ larger body surface area in proportion to body mass;
■ brown fat (which insulates more effectively than white fat).

They can therefore rapidly develop pyrexia or hypothermia. Limited immunity exposes them to greater risk of infection. Temperature should therefore be monitored regularly, and problems treated promptly.

Like all patients, children should be thoroughly examined ('exposed') for any other signs of injury; in children this may include non-accidental injury.

For transfer, children should be 'mummy wrapped' in insulating blankets, with woollen hats and gloves. As well as retaining heat, this also protects vascular access and makes them easier to handle during transfer.

Drugs

Unlike most adult doses, paediatric drugs dosages are usually prescribed according to patients' weight or body surface area. Weight will usually have been recorded on admission. If children have not been weighed recently, parents may know or have some health records. If no other source is available, weight can be estimated in children over one year of age by adding four to their age, and doubling the sum:

weight (kg) = (age + 4) × 2.

Until one year of age, 10 kg is usually a fair estimate of likely weight. Most units keep paediatric formularies and quick reference guides with paediatric equipment.

Morphine remains the 'gold standard' opioid for children, although other standard opioids are also used. Ketamine, not an opioid, causes less cardio-vascular instability, and with children seldom causes the nightmare-like hallucinations it can with adults (Dallmeyer, 2000).

Chloral hydrate is often used for sedation (Jenkins *et al.*, 2007). This is given nasogastrically, has no analgesic effect, and is not licensed for use with children aged under 2 years. It can cause nausea, but is less likely to if diluted with water (Dallmeyer, 2000). Triclofos, a chloral hydrate derivative, causes less nausea and vomiting. Propofol is not licensed for paediatric use, and is contraindicated for children under 17 years of age receiving intensive care (*BNF*, 2009).

Drugs are sometimes given intraosseously, but nurses should only use this route if competent to do so.

Transfer

Specialised PICU care is desirable (Cogo *et al.*, 2010), so early transfer will normally be planned. Most likely adverse events during transfer are:

- loss of monitoring (batteries);
- loss of intravenous access;
- accidental extubation;
- blocked endotracheal tube;
- exhaustion of oxygen (ml of oxygen required = minute volume × time of transfer in minutes);

- incomplete kit;
- ventilator malfunction;
- pump battery failure.

Equipment should be carefully checked before transfer, as apart from communication problems, most problems 'on the road' are related to equipment (Fortune and Playfor, 2009).

Legal aspects

Children have different status in law from that of adults. Some laws specify ages at which people can act independently of their parents, although ages differ for different laws. In the wake of the Gillick case and the Children Act 1989, concepts of legal 'minors' have changed from age-related to competence-related (Dimond, 2008). Nurses should clarify what rights children and others do, and do not, have. If in any doubt, advice should be sought from their Trust's legal department.

Each year 2–3 per cent of children in the UK are abused, one in each thousand of these resulting in serious injury (Russell and McAuley, 2009). Vague history, or bruising that is not adequately accounted for, may indicate non-accidental injury. Head injury, especially subdural haemorrhages in infants, is the most common reason for abused children to need intensive care (Russell and McAuley, 2009). Suspected abuse should be reported, but is emotionally, legally and politically contentious, so should be referred to senior staff. Written records and verbal reports should remain factual.

Meningitis

Infection can cause inflammation of the meninges, or subarachnoid space. Viral meningitis is more common and less serious than bacterial meningitis. Bacteria usually responsible for childhood meningitis are:

- *Streptococcus pneumoniae*
- *Neisseria meningitides*
- *Haemophilus influenza* type b (*Hib*).

Incidence peaks under one year of age, before immunity matures, with a lesser peak during adolescence (Maclennan, 2001). Meningitis can progress rapidly, death following within hours of mild non-specific febrile symptoms. Neck stiffness is often the earliest specific symptom. One in seven survivors suffers permanent disability, especially hearing loss (Peate, 2004). Prompt and appropriate treatment is therefore vital.

Meningitis is usually diagnosed by lumbar puncture – infected cerebrospinal fluid (CSF) contains protein and leucocytes. Lumbar puncture is contraindicated with raised intracranial pressure, as it may cause *tentorial herniation* ('coning'). Treatment is mainly intravenous antibiotics, with aggressive system support.

Meningitis usually causes photophobia, so children should be nursed in a dark room.

Meningitis is a notifiable disease, so all contacts should be traced. Antibiotics are usually given to everyone who had prolonged contact with bacterial meningitis during the previous week.

Implications for practice

- Children are rarely admitted to adult ICUs, but when they are, they are usually in crisis, awaiting transfer to regional PICUs. An ABCDE approach is useful to stabilise the child for transfer.
- Respiratory failure is the most common cause for admission.
- Primary cardiovascular disease is rare; cardiovascular failure is usually secondary to hypoxia.
- Most units have a room or trolley with readily accessible paediatric equipment, including:

  - paediatric drug formularies;
  - paediatric resuscitation guidelines;
  - regional PICU protocols.

- Staff should familiarise themselves with local paediatric equipment.
- Paediatric drug doses are almost always far smaller, usually varying with size/age. Before giving any drugs, nurses should carefully check prescriptions and amounts, seeking further advice if concerned about anything.
- Parents usually suffer guilt and anxiety, so need information and support, and should be actively included in the child's care.
- Waiting rooms should cater for siblings – toys, small chairs and information booklets.
- If unsure of children's legal status, or concerned about non-accidental injury, seek advice from senior staff.
- Meningitis usually begins with non-specific fever-like symptoms, but bacterial meningitis can be rapidly fatal. Neck stiffness is usually the earliest specific symptom.
- Meningitis is a notifiable disease; anyone having prolonged contact with bacterial meningitis during the previous week should be given prophylactic antibiotics.

Summary

Paediatric admissions to adult ICUs are rare, but when they occur they are usually brief, with the aim of stabilising for transfer. This is challenging and stressful for staff with little or no familiarity with paediatric nursing. Principles of nursing critically ill children are largely similar to those for nursing adults, with proportionally smaller volumes and sizes. Adult ICU nurses are however usually unfamiliar with these sizes, so should carefully check all prescriptions and calculations, seeking advice if they have any concerns.

Parents and siblings usually experience extreme psychological crises, needing information and support. Family should be prepared, and involved in care as much as possible.

Support groups

Childline: 0800 1111
Meningitis Research Foundation: 0808 800 3344
National Meningitis Trust, Fern House, Bath Road, Stroud, Gloucestershire GL5 3TJ: 01453 768000
NSPCC Child Protection Helpline: 0808 800 5000
Families Anonymous: 0845 1200 660
Doddington and Rollo Community Association, Charlotte Despard Avenue, Battersea, London SW11 5HD: 0845 1200 660; office@famanon.org.uk

Further reading

Before and around the time of *A Bridge to the Future*, there were a number of paediatric critical care books written in whole or part for staff in general ICUs. Recently, most books and articles have focused on paediatric critical care. One of the more useful books for general ICU nurses is Cockett and Day (2010). Although written for A&Es, Bethel (2008) has some useful chapters applicable to ICUs. Murphy *et al.* (2009) provide useful case studies.

Clinical scenario

Annabel White is a healthy 16-year-old who ingested an unknown amount of alcohol at a local nightclub. On admission to the adult ICU, Miss White is conscious but disorientated with a self-ventilating respiratory rate of 39 breaths/minute, tachycardia (164 beats/minute) with hypotension (80/40 mmHg). Blood investigations reveal metabolic acidosis and hypoglycaemia. Miss White's parents are aware of her admission but not yet present.

Q.1 Review local hospital policies on paediatric admissions to ICUs. What documentation is needed and who should be informed about Miss White's admission?

Q.2 Miss White is non-compliant with interventions, for example oxygen therapy, positioning and assessment. Consider issues regarding her autonomy, legal age of competence and consent. Can she refuse treatment? Who should advocate for Miss White and give consent on her behalf?

Q.3 Consider the impact of the ICU environment on Miss White and the impact of her presence on other ICU patients and staff. Outline nursing strategies that may be used to promote compliance and stabilise her condition.

Chapter 14

Older patients in ICUs

Contents

Introduction	124
Ageing	124
Physiological effects	125
Outcomes	126
Ageism	127
Implications for practice	128
Summary	128
Further reading	128
Clinical scenario	129

Introduction

Most patients in hospital (Young and Sturdy, 2007) and ICUs (Pisani, 2009) are over 65. As UK society ages, numbers of older people in ICUs are increasing (Ridley, 2005). Healthcare should be provided according to clinical need, regardless of age (DH, 2001; International Council of Nurses, 2006). Yet limited material appears about older people in specialist literature, making them a potentially neglected majority. Comparing quantity and quality against paediatric critical care literature illustrates the relative neglect.

Age is not a disease, and diseases suffered by older people are not unique to their cohorts. Physiological ageing, multiple pathology and polypharmacy often complicate their physical needs, while negative attitudes by society, hospitals and staff may limit access to services or mar their psychological care (DH, 2001). Admission of old people to ICUs raises ethical questions:

- Should there be age limits for ICU admission?
- With limited resources, should resources be allocated between different groups?
- Should age be a factor in resource allocation?
- Is there a need for specialist input from Health Care of Older People (HCOOP) teams?
- If only one bed was available but two patients needed ICU admission, how would readers react to that bed being given to the older patient?

Most old people are healthy, but healthy people are not admitted to ICUs. This chapter outlines effects that physiological ageing can have on major body systems, before focusing on wider social and attitudinal issues.

Ageing

Ageing can be:

- *chronological* (number of years lived);
- *sociological* (role in society, e.g. retirement);
- *physiological* (physical function).

(de Beauvoir, 1970)

Chronological ageing, often over 65, is statistically simple and clear, so is adopted by much medical literature, especially quantitative research, and (with qualification) by the DH (2001), but it is usually medically arbitrary, failing to recognise each person's uniqueness and individuality. So nurses should approach each person as an individual, rather than chronological stereotype.

Ageing almost inevitably brings decline in most physiological functions, although rates of decline vary between systems and individuals. *Reserve function* – the difference between actual level of function and minimum function needed for homeostasis – provides a barrier against disease. Progressive decline in reserve function increases the likelihood of chronic and multiple disease in later years, such as diabetes mellitus.

Underlying chronic conditions, including chronic pain such as arthritis, are more common among older people. Arthritis may be visually apparent, but individual assessment may identify other needs, enabling nurses to avoid inflicting accidental pain.

Physiological effects

Hypertension, reduced stroke volume and cardiac output, and other chronic *cardiovascular* changes are partly age-related (Vanhoutte, 2002; Richardson *et al.*, 2004), but mainly from acquired damage, especially from smoking (Fogarty and Lingford-Hughes, 2004). Older people may suffer various cardio-vascular diseases, including:

- dysrhythmias, especially atrial fibrillation (see Chapter 22);
- coronary artery disease;
- heart valve disease;
- atherosclerosis;
- peripheral vascular disease.

However caused, poor perfusion affects all other body systems.

Nearly all aspects of *respiratory* function significantly decline with age (Mick and Ackerman, 2004; Richardson *et al.*, 2004), making acute respiratory failure more likely (Behrendt, 2000).

Central nervous system degeneration progresses throughout life, although cerebral atrophy makes older people more able to compensate for increased cerebral volumes, making them more likely to survive intracranial hypertension. Neurophysiological changes are complex, but older people are at greater risk from the three Ds:

- dementia
- delirium
- depression.

Anxiety disorders are common in older people (Wetherell *et al.*, 2005). Up to half of hospitalised people over 70 develop delirium (Danter, 2003), so confusion should always be treated as acute and reversible until proven otherwise. Reality orientation can be useful, but may provoke aggression; alternative approaches, such as validation therapy (Feil, 1993), seek to empower rather than control people. But most approaches rely on verbal responses, limiting their value for intubated, sedated patients. Communication can be problematic with all ICU patients, but acute limitation may be compounded by dysphasia, hearing loss, impaired vision or impaired memory. Communication needs should therefore be individually assessed – relatives may be a valuable source for information or achieving communication.

Renal problems typically associated with ageing (e.g. incontinence, prostatic obstruction) are alleviated by catheterisation. Age-related decline in renal function (Richardson *et al.*, 2004) may cause abnormal biochemistry, such as elevated serum creatinine, but like most other critically ill patients, acute kidney injury (AKI) is usually caused by hypovolaemia. Drug clearance is reduced (Richardson *et al.*, 2004), making older people potentially more sensitive to the effects of many drugs.

With advancing age, *skin* becomes thinner, fragile and poorly perfused, making it prone to sheering pressure sores, with wounds taking longer to heal (Richardson *et al.*, 2004). Most pressure sores occur in older people, hence the weighting for age on Waterlow and other assessment scales. Pressure area aids can reduce incidence of pressure sores, but optimising endogenous factors (nutrition, perfusion) reduces risks. Reduced capillary perfusion impairs cutaneous drug absorption (e.g. glyceryl trinitrate (GTN)/fentanyl patches) and removal of metabolic waste.

Gastrointestinal function declines with age (Eliopoulos, 2001), but the gut's large functional reserve normally sustains adequate function (Firth and Prather, 2002), although gastric emptying may be slower (Richardson *et al.*, 2004).

Liver dysfunction is mainly pathological rather than chronological (Eliopoulos, 2001). Reduced ability to metabolise drugs may necessitate reduced doses and more careful monitoring of plasma drug levels.

Older people are more frequently *malnourished* than younger people (Devlin, 2000) due to factors such as poverty, poor mobility, maldentition, reduced gut motility, digestive problems, lack of facilities or chronic bowel dysfunction. These may delay recovery, weaning and rehabilitation.

As *muscles and bone atrophy*, they are replaced by fat. Fat repels water, so older people are more prone to dehydration. As calcium metabolism declines, less is absorbed, while stored (skeletal) calcium is leached, reducing bone density, so making bones more brittle and liable to fracture. Muscle weakness contributes to delayed weaning from ventilation and prolongs rehabilitation.

Outcomes

Most studies about older ICU patients measure mortality, increasingly to hospital discharge or later. For example, Ford *et al.*'s (2007) study of post-operative octogenarians found one-fifth died in ICU and one-third died in hospital, but mortality was higher if vasoactive drugs were needed. These outcomes are broadly similar to those of other groups of patients (see Chapter 50). Underlying physiological function does affect outcome (Boumendil *et al.*, 2004), so physiological rather than chronological age-related criteria for ICU admission may be justified. Morbidity is less often studied, although critically ill older people are more likely to develop PTSD (Wallen *et al.*, 2008) and dementia (Ehlenbach *et al.*, 2010), which raises the challenge of whether, and if so how, morbidity can be reduced.

Chronological age alone should not determine ICU admission (NCEPOD, 2010b). While few units now have overt age-related admission criteria,

NCEPOD (2010b) found low admission rates among older people, which suggests covert (subjective) criteria may remain, making healthcare for critically ill older adults a lottery.

NCEPOD (2010b) suggests older people arguably have specialist needs, which benefit from input by teams specialising in HCOOP, although evidence is drawn from other specialities. Their findings suggest older people receive good care in ICUs, even though anecdotal evidence suggests that HCOOP teams generally have little input into ICU care.

Ageism

'Ageism', the 'notion that people cease to be people … by virtue of having lived a specific number of years' (Comfort, 1977: 35), may be overt (e.g. refusing services to people over a certain age) or covert (e.g. attitudes).

Overt chronological age criteria for critical care admission are now rare (DH, 2001) and unacceptable (Preston *et al.*, 2008). Hubbard *et al.* (2003) suggest people are not denied access to critical care because of age, and the World Health Organization (WHO, 2007), responding to fears of a global influenza pandemic, acknowledged the 'fair innings' arguments for prioritising services towards younger people, instructing that age-based rationing should only be adopted after widespread public consultation. However, predictive scoring (e.g. APACHE (Knaus *et al.*, 1985)) can create covert ageism – APACHE II scores chronological age to account for physiological ageing, as well as scoring pathophysiologies. APACHE scores of older people are therefore disproportionately increased, and do not reflect length of stay or severity of disease (Laskou *et al.*, 2008).

Older people may have sensory or expressive communication difficulties. While staff should optimise communication, they should beware of insidious prejudice, stereotyping or other negative attitudes, such as speaking loudly to all old people, rather than assessing whether they have any deficit, and if so how to compensate for it.

Many older people grew up before the National Health Service existed, so remember a very different society (and social values); doctors (and nurses) were presumed to always know best. Their beliefs and values may therefore differ significantly from those of nurses caring for them; different generational values may cause misunderstandings. Nurses should empower choices, which with older people may take more encouragement.

Bereavement, social mobility and physical immobility may leave older people isolated and deprived of social support (families, friends). Friends/family may treat the older person as a burden. Psychological isolation can become self-fulfilling, encouraging older people to adopt child-like dependent behaviour and/or appear confused. Stereotypes may be widespread, and insidious in their effect, but nursing care should be individualised to each person (Meyer and Sturdy, 2004). Deeny (2005: 325) suggests 'care of critically ill older people … may cause us to modify physical environments, reflect on professional attitudes, revise education and training and be more collaborative with older people advocacy groups and experts from outside critical care'.

Implications for practice

- Older patients already form about half of UK ICU admissions; numbers will probably increase, so ICU nurses should actively consider needs and quality of care.
- Function of all body systems declines with age, but most older people are healthy. When acute ill-health necessitates ICU admission, care should anticipate recovery.
- Reduced function, and possible multipathology, necessitates individualised, holistic care.
- Confusion should be treated as acute and reversible, until proven otherwise.
- Sensory or expressive communication limitations may be acute or chronic, so should be individually assessed, and individualised strategies planned to overcome limitations.
- In-service and post-registration education should include significant focus on nursing older people in ICUs.
- Ageism, insidious throughout society, can easily, and insidiously, influence care; reflecting on and evaluating nursing care (individually and in groups) helps identify areas for development.

Summary

Definitions of 'old' are arbitrary. Chronological ageing is widely used, but arguably a poor indicator of healthcare needs. Many ICU patients are 'old', and appear to have similar mortality rates to those of younger patients. Morbidity and needs are less often studied, making older people a potentially neglected majority. The paucity of literature on older patients in ICUs makes this one of the most neglected aspects of ICU nursing.

Pathologies experienced by older people are largely those suffered by younger patients. Multiple pathologies, system dysfunction and slower metabolism make physiological needs of older patients complex. ICU admission can also threaten psychological and social health. Nurses can humanise potentially threatening and ageist ICU environments to meet the needs of older patients.

Further reading

De Beauvoir (1970) provides highly readable, challenging sociological perspectives. Medical studies of age-related outcomes frequently appear, but otherwise literature on older people in ICUs is infrequent. Material from specialist journals, such as *Age and Ageing* and *Nursing Older People*, can often be applied to ICUs. Redfern and Ross (2006) remains the classic text on nursing older people, with much material that is transferable to ICUs.

Clinical scenario

Albert Rose is an active and independent 89-year-old who was admitted to the ICU following emergency laparotomy for a perforated bowel. He has an ileostomy and two abdominal drains with a total of 2 litres blood loss in the first four hours. He is mechanically ventilated with an Hb of 8.2 g/dl and Hct (haematocrit) of 29 per cent.

Q.1 Review the main age-related physiological changes and expected normal values for an 89-year-old in the ICU. What are the implications of these changes in managing Mr Rose's treatments?

Q.2 Analyse the significance of Mr Rose's Hb value on his recovery. Examine the benefits and adverse effects of blood transfusion with older ICU patients. Should Mr Rose be transfused?

Q.3 Consider possible outcomes for Mr Rose following discharge from hospital. Formulate a strategy to promote his physical and mental recovery.

Chapter 15

Infection control

Contents

Fundamental knowledge	130
Introduction	131
Sources	131
Organisms	131
Bacteria	132
Fungi	134
Ventilator-associated pneumonia (VAP)	134
Laboratory screening	134
Controlling infection	135
Implications for practice	137
Summary	137
Further reading	137
Clinical scenario	138

Fundamental knowledge

Standard precautions
Asepsis
Immunity (see Chapter 25)
Common healthcare-associated infections
Local infection control guidelines

Introduction

Infection and its prevention have been the focus of much media and political attention in recent years. Infection often causes hospital admission, and can cause morbidity and mortality. Mutation of organisms into multi-resistant strains has escalated in the last decade (Larson *et al.*, 2010). Critically ill patients are immunocompromised, so more susceptible to infection. Many studies, reviews and policies have recently been published, such as *Saving Lives* (DH, 2007a). Some changes in practices should reduce incidence, but solutions often remain elusive.

One-quarter of all hospital infections occur in ICUs (Allen, 2005), while more than a quarter of patients admitted to ICUs have infections, nearly half of which are healthcare-associated (Dhillon and Clark, 2009). Critical illness causes immunocompromise, making patients in ICUs more susceptible to infections, and up to ten times more likely to develop healthcare-associated infection (HAI) than general ward patients (Lim and Webb, 2005). This chapter presents a summary of the problems infection causes for ICU patients, brief descriptions of the main problem organisms, and strategies that can help reduce incidence of infection. Necessarily, this chapter only highlights key aspects; staff should be familiar with local policies and protocols.

Sources

Infection can be:

- endogenous
- exogenous.

Endogenous infection, from organisms already harboured by patients, in ICUs usually occurs through the *respiratory tract* (e.g. ventilator-associated pneumonia, VAP), but can also occur through the *skin*, especially through central venous lines (Pratt *et al.*, 2007), or the *gut* (Hall and Horsley, 2007).

Exogenous infection is usually through *contact* (staff, procedures, equipment), but can also be *airborne*.

Exogenous cross-infection causes up to one-third of healthcare-associated infections, at least half of which are preventable (Harbath *et al.*, 2003).

Organisms

Bacteria remain the most common cause of infections, so form the focus of organisms discussed in this chapter. However, significant viral and fungal infections in ICUs are increasingly common, so some of these organisms are also included. Viruses are not discussed here, but are in other chapters (see the index for specific organisms). Other types of organisms, such as prions (the cause of Creutzfeldt-Jakob disease), are seldom significant in ICUs, so are not discussed in this book.

Bacteria that are commensals (harmless) to healthy people may become pathogens to vulnerable ICU patients. 'Infection' only occurs when people develop pathological responses to micro-organisms. Destroying commensals with antibiotics enables opportunist infection from organisms colonising (but not necessarily infecting) healthier people. Critically ill patients are immuno-compromised, so most infections are *opportunist* – from organisms that rarely infect healthy people.

Bacteria may be gram 'positive' or 'negative' (Pitt, 2007). Although derived from laboratory staining, this crude distinction remains useful; gram positive generally reside on skin, in air or the environment, whereas gram negative are generally from the bowels, soil or water (Pitt, 2007). Gram positive organisms include:

- *Staphylococci*
- *Clostridium*
- *Enterococci*
- *Streptococci.*

Gram negative organisms include:

- *Acinetobacter*
- *Enterobacter*
- *Escherichia coli*
- *Helicobacter pylori*
- *Klebsiellae*
- *Proteus*
- *Pseudomonas*
- *Serratia.*

Gram negative organisms have thinner cell walls, so produce endotoxins for protection. Endotoxin stimulates inflammatory responses.

Gram negative organisms tend to colonise moist areas, whereas gram positives are usually transmitted by direct contact or are airborne spread (Barrett, 1999). Infection control has therefore changed from concern about moist reservoirs to airborne and direct contact risks.

Bacteria

Most strains of *Staphylococci aureus* remain meticillin-sensitive (*MSSa*), but meticillin-resistant *Staphylococcus aureus* (*MRSa*) has becomes problematic. Between one-third and half the population are colonised with *S. aureus* (Lim and Webb, 2005), making a large reservoir for potential infection. Although *MRSa* may be acquired in ICUs, it is more likely to be present before admission (Howie and Ridley, 2008), so patients should be routinely screened on admission to the ICU (DH, 2007a). Spread should be contained by:

■ identifying infection (routine screening of all admissions);
■ collaboration with Local Infection Control departments;
■ informing wards before discharge.

Also, there should be a thorough ('deep clean') of bed areas after discharge – domestic services usually provide this service. Whether patients with *MRSa* should be isolated remains controversial (Cepeda *et al.*, 2005; Garvey and Belligan, 2009); current guidelines suggest isolation should be considered, depending on facilities and risk (Coia *et al.*, 2006).

Pseudomonas is the second commonest cause of VAP (Kerr and Snelling, 2009). It especially colonises moist environments, such as washbasins (Cholley *et al.*, 2008). Skin colonisation is brief, but highly pathogenic (Pittet and Boyce, 2001), and colonisation of respiratory and urinary tracts frequently occurs (Bertrand *et al.*, 2001).

Enterococci are normal gut flora, but the third most common cause of HAI (Gould, 2008), especially urinary tract infections (Heintz *et al.*, 2010). *Enterococci* are hardy organisms, surviving more than one week in the environment (Zirakzadeh and Patel, 2006). Vancomycin-resistant *Enterococci* (*VRE*) usually inhabit the gut although may be detected elsewhere, and are resistant to most antibiotics. Although pathogenicity is relatively low, it can transfer resistance to *MRSa*, and co-infection is fairly common (Zirakzadeh and Patel, 2006), so it poses a major threat to already critically ill patients. *VRE* infections are usually managed by barrier nursing. Rectal/stoma swabs may be taken for screening.

Clostridium difficile infections frequently make headline news. Typically transmitted from faeces, only about 3 per cent of adults carry *C. difficile* in their gut, but colonisation rates increase significantly in the over-65s (Hall and Horsley, 2007). First identified in 1935, the organism remained relatively unproblematic until 2001, when the 027 strain mutated (Pépin *et al.*, 2005; Kelly and LaMont, 2008).

C. difficile is resistant to most broad spectrum antibiotics, most infections occurring when other gut flora are destroyed by antibiotics (Shannon-Lowe *et al.*, 2010). Proton pump inhibitors (PPIs) also seem to favour growth (Cunningham and Dial, 2008). Infection is usually treated with oral vancomycin or metronidazole (Shannon-Lowe *et al.*, 2010).

Infection typically causes explosive diarrhoea, spreading spores into the environment. *C. difficile* spores are virtually impossible to eliminate (Wren, 2009). Alcohol handrubs are ineffective (Wren, 2009). Chlorine-based cleaners should be used to decontaminate infected environments (Hall and Horsley, 2007), and probiotics such as *S. boukardii* may be useful (Kelly and LaMont, 2008).

Acinetobacter is normally found in water and soil. Multi-resistant strains of *A. baumannii* (*Acb*) (Munoz-Price and Weinstein, 2008) have caused most hospital *Acinetobacter* infections (Pitt, 2007). *Acinetobacter* readily colonises surfaces and the skin of staff (Preller and Wilson, 2009); infection is more likely to be found in ICU with prolonged ventilation (Pitt, 2007).

Fungi

Fungal infection and mortality among critically ill patients is rising (Soni and Wagstaff, 2005). The most common fungal infection in ICUs is from *Candida*. In France it is the third most common cause of *nosocomial* bloodstream infections (Bougnoux *et al.*, 2007). Although *Candida albicans* remains the most prominent species, widespread use of fluconazole has favoured increased infection rates from other species, including *C. glabrata*, *C. parapsilosis* and *C. tropicalis* (Hajjeh *et al.*, 2004). ICU patients are especially susceptible to oral and skinfold fungal colonisation/infection, so these areas should be inspected carefully, and maintaining hygiene contributes to reducing infection.

Ventilator-associated pneumonia (VAP)

One-quarter of ICU patients develop VAP (Blot *et al.*, 2011), typically from multi-resistant organisms (Giantso *et al.*, 2005), and usually within five days of ICU admission (Blot *et al.*, 2011). VAP significantly increases mortality (Stolz *et al.*, 2009). Treating VAP is problematic, but Dodek *et al.*'s (2004) systematic review recommended:

- orotracheal intubation;
- changing ventilator circuits only for each new patient;
- closed endotracheal suction systems, changed for each new patient and as clinically indicated;
- heat/moisture exchangers (HMEs), unless specifically contraindicated;
- weekly changes of HMEs;
- semi-recumbent positioning (30–45°) unless contraindicated.

Other means suggested to reduce VAP are:

- chest physiotherapy (Ntoumenopoulos *et al.*, 2002);
- kinetic therapy (Kennedy, 2004);
- draining subglottic secretions (Lorente *et al.*, 2007; Pneumatikos *et al.*, 2009; Lacherade *et al.*, 2010);
- early tracheostomy (Möller *et al.*, 2005).

However, evidence for interventions reducing ICU stay, hospital stay or mortality is often weak, conflicting or non-existent.

Laboratory screening

Nurses collect most specimens sent for microscopy, culture and sensitivity (MC+S). Records of when specimens were sent should be kept – a pathology flow sheet is useful. Each shift, nurses should review what has been sent, request any outstanding results, and alert medical staff to any concerns.

Blood cultures, usually taken by medical staff, are useful for identifying septicaemia. Preliminary reports may be available after 24 hours, as some organisms can be visually identified after this time. Confirmed, detailed reports are normally available after completing the culture at 48 hours, by which time sensitivity will usually also be identified. Debate persists about indications for blood cultures, many units taking cultures if patients' temperatures exceed an identified limit – often 38–38.4°C. Such figures reflect greater likelihood of infective rather than metabolic pyrexia (see Chapter 8), but are not always reliable. Blood cultures are an investigation of suspected infection in any sick patient (ICS, 2007b).

Controlling infection

Antibiotics generally remain the best way of treating existing infections, although prevention is better than cure. Unfortunately, compliance with infection control measures remains suboptimal (Gammon *et al.*, 2008). Appropriate antibiotics should be prescribed by medical staff, usually with advice from microbiology. Duration of treatment with antibiotics should be identified and clearly recorded, usually on drug charts. Nurses should inform medical staff if prescriptions are due for review. Some antibiotics have narrow therapeutic ranges (e.g. gentomycin, vancomycin), necessitating blood tests to check serum levels; staff should check local protocols, and clarify the appropriate time before and/or after antibiotic dose.

Invasive cannulae cause one-third of HAIs, with central lines remaining the single main cause of nosocomial septicaemia (Pratt *et al.*, 2007). Vascular access and other invasive devices are necessary with sicker patients, but unneeded devices should be removed. Peripheral cannulae should be routinely replaced every 48–72 hours (Pratt *et al.*, 2007). Central lines should not be routinely changed (Pratt *et al.*, 2007) and dressings should remain in place for seven days provided they are clean and intact (Pratt *et al.*, 2007). Infection risks increase when dressings or lines are changed, so administration sets for continuous infusions should be used for 72 hours unless there is a specific contraindication (Pratt *et al.*, 2007). Insertion dates of all invasive equipment should be clearly recorded.

Moving *equipment* between patients can also spread infection. Where dedicated equipment is not practical (e.g. portable X-ray, 12-lead ECG), it should be cleaned after use.

Airborne bacteria may be transmitted through:

- dust
- skin scales
- droplets.

Airborne infection is significantly reduced by use of in-line suction catheters (see Chapter 5). Other ways to reduce airborne infection on ICUs include:

- planning higher-risk procedures at times of least disturbance;
- careful disposal of linen (e.g. bringing linen skips/bags to bedsides, carefully rolling linen inwards to trap skin scales);
- air-flow systems.

Hand hygiene remains the simplest, easiest, cheapest and most important way to reduce transient colonisation (Pratt *et al.*, 2007), and should be performed before each patient-care episode (Pratt *et al.*, 2007). Alcohol rubs are the 'gold standard' for hand hygiene (WHO, 2005), being better antimicrobials than soap, and more convenient (Girou, 2003), although some organisms, such as *C. difficile*, may survive alcohol rubs. Sufficient amounts should be dispensed (this varies between products), spread fully over hands, and allowed to dry. Local Infection Control departments can advise on amounts and times for products used.

Hand hygiene often misses the parts most likely to touch patients – thumbs, fingertips and backs of hands (Ayliffe *et al.*, 2001). The RCN (2005) described good technique. Hands should be dried thoroughly after washing as moisture, including wet alcohol, facilitates bacterial growth. Patients and relatives have been encouraged to challenge staff about hand hygiene (NPSA, 2004a); staff have a professional duty to challenge anyone about to touch patients without performing adequate hand hygiene. Anyone (staff or family) visiting any patient on an ICU should clean their hands before entering the unit. Alcohol rubs should be placed by each entrance to the unit, with prominent signs informing people to prevent infection by cleaning their hands.

Personal protective equipment (PPE – aprons, gloves) reduces colonisation/infection from patients to staff. Aprons also reduce transmission of bacteria from clothing, so should be worn by anyone having patient contact. Colour-coded aprons for each bedspace encourage staff to change aprons when moving between patients. Gloves significantly reduce cross-infection (Pratt *et al.*, 2007; Garvey and Belligan, 2009), so should be worn whenever manipulating invasive devices.

Documentation helps identify when actions are required. Useful documentation includes charts for:

- equipment changes
- specimens sent and results.

Inadequate staffing (quantity and quality) increases cross-infection (Allen, 2005; Coia *et al.*, 2006; Hugonnet *et al.*, 2007; Knoll *et al.*, 2010).

Pneumonia in ICU patients usually originates from nasal, oropharyngeal or gastric flora (Torres *et al.*, 2009). *Selective oral/digestive decontamination* (SOD/SDD) can prevent pathogen colonisation, and so VAP (Gastmeier and Geffers, 2007), but whether mortality is (de Smet *et al.*, 2009; Torres *et al.*, 2009) or is not (Chan *et al.*, 2007a) increased continues to be debated. SOD/SDD may increase bacterial resistance (Oostdijk *et al.*, 2010), and it is not commonly practised in the UK due to fears of encouraging *C. difficile* (Chandler and Hunter, 2009).

Implications for practice

- Hand hygiene should be carried out before and after each aspect of care, and before approaching and after leaving each bed area.
- Alcohol handrubs should be available at each bed area, and be used before and after any patient contact. Staff should know how much to use, and how long it takes to dry. Some infections, such as *C. difficile*, are resistant to alcohol, necessitating handwashing.
- All taps should have elbow-operated levers at elbow height; taps should not be turned on by hand.
- Towel dispensers should provide individual paper towels that will not drape in moist sink units.
- Nursing/medical documentation should include easily accessible flow sheets of specimens sent, and results. Each entry should be dated and signed.
- Equipment (e.g. HMEs) should be changed according to manufacturers' instructions; catheter mounts should be changed at the same time as humidifiers.
- Invasive techniques and disconnection of intravenous lines should, when possible, avoid times of dust disturbance (e.g. floor cleaning, damp dusting).
- Strict asepsis must be observed when breaking/bypassing normal non-specific immune defences, such as when handling intravenous circuits, treating open wounds, or undertaking procedures involving the trachea, stomach or jejunum.
- Hospital infection control nurses and other specialists should be actively involved in multidisciplinary teamwork.
- Colour coding bed areas (aprons, equipment) discourages inappropriate movement between bedspaces.

Summary

Infection is not always preventable, but it incurs high costs in human life, morbidity and budgets. Antibiotics and other medical treatments can reduce morbidity and mortality, but preventing infection is humanly (and financially) preferable.

Hand hygiene remains the most important way to prevent infection. Hygiene is helped by adequate and appropriate facilities, including accessible alcohol handrubs, aprons and unit guidelines/protocols. All multidisciplinary team members should be actively involved in making decisions, nurses having an especially valuable role in coordinating and controlling each patient's environment.

Further reading

Pratt *et al.* (2007) is the national guideline for infection control, while Coia *et al.* (2006) provide national guidelines for controlling *MRSa*. Ridley's (2009) Intensive Care Society book gathers key issues for medical practice, while Weston (2008) provides nursing perspectives. Articles frequently appear in many specialist and general journals, while the Department of Health website provides current national guidance. Staff should be familiar with local policies.

Clinical scenario

Nadeen Persad is a 32-year-old with chronic kidney disease who was successfully resuscitated following cardiopulmonary arrest. She requires admission to the ICU for closer monitoring. An ICU doctor and nurse (who is four months' pregnant) go with appropriate transfer equipment to retrieve the patient while an ICU bed is prepared for the admission. On arrival at the ward, the ICU doctor and nurse are informed that Mrs Persad has active pulmonary *Tuberculosis* and *Acinetobacter* in her diarrhoea.

Q.1 Consider the common transmission modes and pathogenicity of *Tuberculosis* and *Acinetobacter*. Specify the infection control precautions to be followed in order to minimise potential cross-transmission of the micro-organisms to other patients and staff when transferring and admitting Mrs Persad to the ICU.

Q.2 In addition to the prepared bed area, the ICU has two protective isolation rooms available – airflow in one room is under positive pressure and the other room is under negative pressure. Provide a rationale for which area or room Mrs Persad should be admitted into.

Q.3 Management of Mrs Persad's infections focused on three main areas:

- containment (e.g. screening of staff, visitors);
- prevention of cross-transmission (both exogenous and endogenous – to other patients; to other sites within Mrs Persad; minimising vectors etc.);
- eradication (specific antibiotics, administration routes etc.).

Design a nursing care plan for her while on the ICU, incorporating published infection control guidelines, local clinical guidelines and a holistic nursing approach. Integrate professional, psychosocial, psychological and physical aspects into this plan.

Chapter 16

Pandemic planning

Contents

Fundamental knowledge   139
Introduction   140
Twentieth-century pandemics   140
Influenza   141
Rationing   142
Treating victims   143
Prevention   144
Implications for practice   144
Summary   145
Further reading   145
Clinical questions   145

Fundamental knowledge

Community-acquired infections and their transmission
Pathology of pneumonia
Source isolation precautions

Introduction

Throughout history there have been epidemics, some of which have caused high mortality. These epidemics have almost invariably been caused by viruses, usually influenza, which have mutated, often from other species, to become highly contagious and pathogenic. Over half the known human pathogens have originated in other species (Stein, 2009). Recent epidemics have prompted historical analysis, which suggests semi-predictable patterns to epidemics. It is therefore anticipated that an epidemic is likely to occur soon. During the last decade there have been two anticipated epidemics ('bird flu' and the 2009 'swine flu') for which extensive preparations were made. Arguably, preparations exceeded the effects of the diseases, at least in the UK, creating dangers of complacency towards future outbreaks. This chapter reviews the historical evidence, explores what has been learned from recent preparations and outbreaks, and suggests likely implications for future practice.

Twentieth-century pandemics

Since the sixteenth century there has been an average of three pandemics each century, at intervals of 10–50 years (WHO, 2007). Records and evidence from the twentieth century are considerably larger than those from previous centuries. The worst pandemic of the twentieth century was the 1918 'Spanish flu' (H1N1), which began in 1918. Although populations were vulnerable due to generally poorer health, debilitation in the aftermath of the First World War, and lack of knowledge about the virus, the virus seems to have been an especially lethal strain – emerging from birds into humans and swine simultaneously (Zimmer and Burke, 2009). More than a quarter of the world's population were infected, killing 50–100 million people (Stein, 2009). Infections persisted for years, with often devastating long-term effects, such as the encephalitis lethargica of 1917–1923 described by Sacks (1990). Survival was highest among socially isolated populations (Stein, 2009). Partly due to the extent, and partly because survivors, evidence and records were available once microbiological research could seek answers, this outbreak has become the one against which all modern pandemics are measured (Saidi and Brett, 2009).

Further influenza pandemics occurred in 1957 (H2N2; 'Asian flu') and 1968 (H3N3 'Hong Kong flu'), each killing about one million people. Like the 1918 outbreak, mortality was highest among young adults (15–34 age groups) (Saidi and Brett, 2009). Both outbreaks brought a second wave, the one from the 1968 virus occurring 16 months after the first UK cases (DH, 2009b). Noticeably, pandemics are about a generation apart, suggesting that exposure during previous epidemics conferred some immunity on older populations. Intervals between most pandemics are 10–40 years (Saidi and Brett, 2009). As the last pandemic was in 1968, this makes another pandemic already overdue.

The 2003 outbreak (H5N1; 'bird flu' or severe acute respiratory syndrome – SARS) originated in Hong Kong, spreading rapidly to 30 countries (notably Toronto in Canada), infecting 8,241 and killing 784 people (Fowler *et al.*, 2003) – an approximate mortality of 1 in 10. The virus diversified, developing several distinct sublineages (Pareek and Stephenson, 2007), which delayed production and distribution of specific vaccines and treatments (WHO, 2008). While mortality was low, morbidity was significant – survivors (at one year) experienced reduced respiratory function and poorer quality of life (Hui *et al.*, 2005). Avian viruses do not replicate efficiently in humans, but swine viruses do (Stein, 2009), which made the 2009 'swine flu' (H1N1; originally called SOIV = swine origin influenza virus) more likely to infect large numbers than the 2003 outbreak. A pandemic was declared on 11 July, and strain was placed on paediatric ICUs, but elsewhere disruption was limited. H1N1 caused 138 deaths in England (Donaldson *et al.*, 2010), infection being highest among teenagers (Kelly *et al.*, 2009).

Influenza

Influenza A develops new strains every 2–3 years (Saidi and Brett, 2009). Most infections cause mild respiratory disease, although each year people do die from influenza, usually among the more vulnerable groups, especially older people. Influenza vaccinations for vulnerable groups, and healthcare workers, are now standard practice. Vaccinations are not however without risks, and many healthcare staff appear reluctant to receive vaccination, considering that personal risks outweigh benefits. For example, there have been (unsubstantiated) claims that H1N1 vaccines cause Guillain-Barré syndrome (Nachamkin *et al.*, 2008).

Incubation times for influenza are brief – H5N1 incubation occurs in seven days or less (Writing Committee of the Second World Health Organization Consultation on Clinical Aspects of Human Infection with Avian Influenza A (H5N1) Virus, 2008), so widespread transmission can occur before those spreading it become symptomatic.

Some immunity develops following exposure, but whether it is lasting is questionable. Pandemics have appeared approximately one generation apart, infection being highest in children (Miller *et al.*, 2010) and younger adults, presumably as they lack immunity from exposure during previous pandemics (Chowell *et al.*, 2009; Miller *et al.*, 2010). Unlike seasonal influenza, pandemic influenza disproportionately affects children; more than one-third of patients admitted to UK hospitals in the 2009 H1N1 outbreak were children (Walunj *et al.*, 2010), while median age of those dying in Mexico was 18 years (Saidi and Brett, 2009). Unlike most ICU patients, victims are therefore:

- young
- suffering single or dual organ failure (lungs, often complicated by cardio-vascular).

Kidney injury often occurred, more than one-fifth of patients needing renal replacement therapy (Brauser, 2010). With the 2009 outbreak, most deaths occurred in people with pre-existing chronic disease (Fajardo-Dolci *et al.*, 2010), although AKI increased both length of stay and mortality (Brauser, 2010). The 2003 outbreaks caused infections and deaths among healthcare workers, in many cases probably from occupational exposure (Manocha *et al.*, 2003; Lapinsky and Granton, 2004). However, the 2008 epidemic caused no secondary infections among healthcare workers in Mexico (Perez-Padilla *et al.*, 2009).

The World Health Organization (WHO, 2008) classification of pandemic stages is:

- phase 1–5: predominantly animal infections; few human infections;
- phase 4: sustained human-to-human transmission;
- phases 5–6: pandemic – widespread human infection;
- post peak: possible recurrent events;
- post pandemic: disease activity at seasonal level.

This enables responses to be graded against the threat.

Rationing

Recent outbreaks have caused severe respiratory failure and ARDS, mainly in young adults and children (Perez-Padilla *et al.*, 2009). Pandemic influenza is likely to cause overwhelming need for invasive ventilation, exceeding availability of ICU and PICU beds. The principle of 'saving most lives' (WHO, 2008) is likely to guide local, national and international practice. Contingency planning for recent threatened pandemics included:

- creating beds for invasive ventilation in areas such as operating theatres;
- using staff from other wards/departments, who have transferable skills.

Although contingency planning should enable some increase in resources, it is unlikely to prove sufficient (Saidi and Brett, 2009; Sprung *et al.*, 2010), making rationing of resources inevitable. Non-emergency operations and other treatments are likely to be suspended. If demand continues to exceed supply, triaging admissions to exclude the following is almost inevitable (Bailey *et al.*, 2008):

- those who are too well;
- those who are too sick to benefit; or
- those with co-morbidities likely to limit short-term survival.

This will however raise ethical questions of who should be denied resources (WHO, 2008). For example: are treatments more likely to be denied to older people on grounds of chronological age? – what the WHO (2008) refers to as the 'fair innings' argument. Planning for pandemics that may prove less problematic than anticipated inevitably diverts resources from other areas of healthcare, denying resources to existing patients to prepare for potential future demands (WHO, 2007). National, professional and local guidance is likely to be issued, but this inevitably deals with generalisations, and cannot always solve specific dilemmas faced by nurses 'by the bedside'.

While contingency planning is laudable, creating 'temporary ICUs' will almost inevitably mean less than ideal environments. Staff drafted from elsewhere are likely to feel stressed/frustrated. New ways of working may be necessary; for example, an experienced ICU nurse may have to oversee a relatively large number of patients, prescribing care for staff with transferable skills, but not experienced or confident in ICU nursing, to carry out. Similarly, medical staff and professions allied to medicine may be drafted in to face similar stressors. Coupled with the risks of occupational exposure to a potentially fatal and highly virulent virus, staff may be sick or opt not to work. Rankin's (2006) survey of the 2003 Toronto outbreak found that:

- two of the 44 victims were nurses exposed through their work;
- at least 79 nurses missed 15 days or more due to sickness;
- nurses worked long hours (sometimes 14–15 hours a day) to cover hospitals;
- nurses became 'social lepers';
- the worst aspect for nurses was fear of the unknown.

In Taiwan in 2003 nearly three-quarters of the nursing workforce felt their job put them at risk, although only a minority wanted to leave their jobs (Shiao *et al.*, 2007); UK cultural differences might draw different responses – Saidi and Brett (2009) estimate that up to half of staff may be absent.

Problems will be compounded by a reduction in normal sources of supply. Elsewhere, both inside and beyond hospitals, workforces will be depleted. What this will affect most is unpredictable, but shortages of drugs, oxygen, equipment, linen or transport could occur, necessitating further local rationing. Social isolation improves survival from epidemics (Stein, 2009), so curfews and restrictions on mobility may be imposed. A pandemic is therefore likely to prove difficult, for many reasons, but adequate contingency planning can reduce some of the stresses and burdens.

Some experience of implementing disaster planning has been gained through major terrorist attacks, such as 9/11 (2001, New York) and 7/7 (2007, London), but these attacks were of limited duration, affecting finite numbers of victims. When pandemics surface, initial and secondary waves are expected, but duration and effects are largely speculative.

Treating victims

Austerity necessitates prioritisation, so adopting an ABCD approach to assessment, treatment and care is helpful.

Airway: Respiratory failure usually necessitates intubation and invasive ventilation. While such airway management is familiar to ICU nurses, many victims are likely to be young children. As numbers of children exceed PICU resources, adult ICUs are likely to care for significant numbers. Nurses and other staff in adult ICUs usually have very limited experience of caring for children (see Chapter 13).

Breathing: Conventional artificial ventilation (pressure control or pressure support) is likely to be needed. NIV is unlikely to be effective, and places others at risk from aerosol spread. Aerolised viruses place staff and visitors at risk, so closed circuits should be maintained as far as possible, with filters, masks and eye-shields used to minimise risks. For the 2009 outbreak, FFP2 masks were recommended for normal procedures, and FFP3 for aerosol-producing procedures. Unless patients have chronic airway problems, peak inflation pressures should be low (< 20), and aggressive weaning and transfer to lower-dependency areas should be possible after a very few days.

Cardiovascular: Shock commonly complicates severe respiratory failure from influenza, and myocarditis may occur. Steroids should be avoided, as they may cause shedding of virus particles. Experience from the 2009 outbreak suggests that little fluid is needed.

Disability: Severe disease usually necessitates sedation, and occasionally paralysis. Drugs used are unlikely to differ from standard practice, remembering that nasogastric clonidine is often used for sedating children, and that paediatric doses of nearly all drugs are smaller than adult ones, and usually weight-related. Glucose supplements and early enteral feeding are likely to be beneficial.

Prevention

The virulence of epidemic influenza will necessitate precautions to minimise risks to staff and family. Although specific precautions are likely to be given for each threatened epidemic, other patients, staff and visitors should be protected by source isolation, including:

- isolation rooms, preferably with negative pressure;
- if patients are not intubated, the wearing of high-efficiency masks by staff and visitors, such as the N-95 respirator, to prevent air-droplet and airborne acquisition (File and Tsang, 2005);
- contact precautions, including long-sleeved fluid-repellent, waterproof double gown, gloves, hat and overshoes;
- non-reusable goggles or face shields.

Implications for practice

- Historical evidence suggests that pandemic influenza is likely to occur soon.
- Pandemic influenza is likely to affect much of the population.
- Disease is likely to cause life-threatening respiratory failure in large numbers of young adults and children.
- Shortage of beds, staff, equipment and other supplies will necessitate rationing and triage that may make many staff ethically uncomfortable.
- Social strains outside hospitals are likely to impact on health services.
- Pandemic planning aims to minimise avoidable mortality and morbidity.
- Risk of transmission to staff is high, so Infection Control and Occupational Health departments should be involved to provide advice and monitoring.

Summary

All Trusts have disaster plans, but on the rare occasions these have been needed they have generally been used for brief occurrences, such as the September 2001 Twin Towers attack in New York or the July 2007 bombing in London. Tragic as these events were, casualties were limited to a very brief time-span. Pandemics persist, without certainty of their geographical or chronological limitations.

Mild outbreaks of influenza are an annual occurrence. The influenza virus frequently mutates, making prediction of strains, and therefore vaccination, problematic. In the twentieth century, pandemics generally occurred once per generation, the last pandemic occurring in 1968. A pandemic within the next few years therefore seems likely. In 2003 and 2009 outbreaks occurred that failed to become the threatened pandemic. These, and historical analysis, have provided some experience of likely problems and solutions, but have also encouraged some public scepticism and complacency. A pandemic is likely to overwhelm healthcare resources, necessitating rationing, triage and ethically uncomfortable choices. Planning aims to limit the impact of the looming disaster.

Further reading

Zimmer and Burke (2009) provide a historical review, but guidelines are likely to change with each threatened pandemic, so the most appropriate reading will be currently available evidence. Readers should check websites such as:

- Department of Health;
- World Health Organization;
- professional organisations such as the Nursing and Midwifery Council (NMC) and General Medical Council (GMC);
- bodies such as the Royal College of Nursing (RCN) and British Medical Association (BMA);
- local Trust intranet.

Sprung *et al.* (2010) provide ICU-specific guidelines for epidemic or mass disasters.

Clinical questions

Q.1 Find out about and read the current contingency plans for your Trust and ICU.

Q.2 Identify what resources, including equipment, are available in your unit to cope with pandemic influenza.

Q.3 List at least six significant effects that activation of these plans would be likely to have on your own current daily work.

Part III

Monitoring

Chapter 17

Respiratory monitoring

Contents

Fundamental knowledge   149
Introduction   150
Visual monitoring   150
Tactile monitoring   151
Auscultation   151
Waveform analysis   153
Indexed measurements   157
Pulse oximetry   157
End-tidal carbon dioxide   158
Implications for practice   159
Summary   159
Further reading   159
Acknowledgement   159
Clinical scenario   160

Fundamental knowledge

Haemoglobin carriage of oxygen (see Chapter 18)
Respiratory anatomy
Normal mechanics of breathing – muscles, negative pressure
Cough reflex and physiology

Introduction

There are many ways to assess and monitor breathing. As with all patients, respiratory rate and depth remain important, but artificial ventilation necessitates additional monitoring. This chapter includes:

- auscultation
- ventilator observations (including waveform analysis).

Assessments primarily used by other professions, such as chest X-rays and bronchoscopy, are not discussed. As with all observations, trends should be assessed, and interpreted holistically, in the context of individual patients.

Visual monitoring

Respiratory history is usually gained from individual handover and inter-disciplinary notes – medical, nursing, physiotherapy. Additional valuable fundamental information can be gained visually:

- Skin colour and texture (and any clamminess) indicates perfusion – especially lips and tongue.
- Finger clubbing and abnormal chest shape indicate chronic problems.
- For self-ventilating patients, accessory muscle use indicates respiratory distress.
- Shallow breathing may reflect reduced demand, but with tachypnoea indicates other problems – possibilities include pain or limited airflow.
- Unequal chest wall movement – causes should be investigated, but could include pneumothorax.

Other signs of respiratory problems include:

- inability to complete sentences without pausing for breath;
- sudden confusion – more often caused by hypoxia than non-respiratory factors;
- cyanosis – a late sign, appearing only with desaturation < 85–90 per cent, and not appearing with severe anaemia (< 3–5 grams/decilitre (g/dl) (Darovic, 2002a; Lumb, 2005)).

Sputum should be observed for:

- volume
- colour (see Table 17.1)
- consistency (e.g. frothy, tenacious, watery)
- purulence
- haemoptysis.

Type and amounts of sputum, and frequency of suctioning, should be recorded.

Table 17.1 **Sputum colour – possible causes**

Colour	Possible cause
Black	Tar (cigarette smoking)
	Old blood
	Coal (in ex-miners)
	Smoke inhalation (rescued from fire)
	Saliva staining (e.g. iron therapy)
Pink	Fresh blood (frothy pink sputum often indicates pulmonary oedema)
Cream, green	Infection
Yellow	Infection
	Allergy (e.g. asthma)

Tactile monitoring

Movement of sputum in larger airways can create vibration on the chest wall, which may be felt by placing a flat hand palm-down across the sternum ('tactile crepitations'). Although not as reliable as auscultation, this can quickly identify a need for suction, but if no vibration is felt, lung fields should be auscultated.

Auscultation

Breath sounds are created by air turbulence, and are useful to assess:

- intubation (bilateral air entry)
- bronchial patency/bronchospasm
- secretions
- effect of suction (before and after).

Breath sounds should be assessed at the start of each shift. Stethoscopes are usually best placed over:

- right and left main bronchi, then
- mid lobe (usually just to the side of the nipple), then
- bases of lungs (front, side or back)

comparing sounds from both lungs (see Figure 17.1). All sounds are created in bronchioles, but transmitted, and dulled, through lower airways. Chest (and abdominal) sounds can be deceptive, so should not be absolutely relied upon.

Sounds may be normal, abnormal, diminished or absent. Abnormal sounds may be heard on inspiration, expiration, or on both phases, so having identified abnormal sounds, nurses should listen to further breaths to identify on which phases sounds occur. Names of sounds vary between texts (Wilkins *et al.*, 2004), but normal sounds are often called:

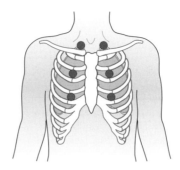

Figure 17.1 Auscultation sites for breath sounds (anterior chest wall)

- *bronchial*: high pitch, loud, air blowing through a tube (the trachea);
- *bronchovesicular*: medium pitch, heard at lung apices;
- *vesicular*: low pitch and volume, like rustling wind, heard in most parts of lungs.

Abnormal sounds include:

- *stridor*: monophonic inspiratory wheezes from severe laryngeal or tracheal obstruction;
- *wheeze (rhonchi)*: obstruction of lower airways; inspiratory wheezes indicate constant obstruction (e.g. COPD), whereas expiratory wheezes indicate bronchospasm;
- *crackle (rales, crepitations)*: on inspiration only, this indicates atelectasis, but if present on both inspiration and expiration is likely to be sputum;
- *pleural rub*: grating sound caused by friction between inflamed pleural surfaces from pleural disease (e.g. pneumonia, pleurisy).

Absent sounds may indicate absent airflow due to:

- obstruction (sputum plug)
- pneumothorax
- atelectasis
- emphysema

or lack of transmission to the chest wall (e.g. obesity, small tidal volume, pleural effusion, pneumothorax).

Artefactual sounds include:

- heartbeat
- gut movement
- clothing
- friction of stethoscope against equipment (e.g. cotsides)

- chest hair (crackles)
- airflow in special beds.

Interpreting breath sounds is a skill. Listening to healthy lungs (your own) is an essential baseline. Readers unfamiliar with listening to abnormal breath sounds should ask a respiratory physiotherapist or other expert to auscultate with them. Recordings of breath sounds (see 'Further reading') are also valuable.

Waveform analysis

Each breath has three active phases:

- inspiration
- inspiratory hold (or 'plateau')
- expiration.

See Figure 17.2. A fourth phase is passive:

- expiratory hold.

Inspiration affects, and is affected by, bronchial muscle stretch; so patients with COPD cannot fully dilate bronchi during short inspiratory time. Most gas exchange occurs during plateau (peak inflation pressure). Expiration is passive recoil; short expiration time of muscle spasm (asthma) causes gas trapping (and distress).

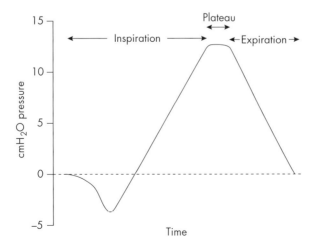

Figure 17.2 Breath waveform

Most ventilators can display three waveforms:

- pressure
- flow
- volume

all plotted against time. From these, two loops are usually available:

- pressure:volume
- flow:volume.

Waveform indicates effectiveness of modes and settings (Branson, 2005).

Pressure graphs (see Figure 17.3) indicate compliance. The slope should be linear. Increased slope near the end of inspiration indicates reduced compliance (hyperinflation). If the slope reduces during inspiration, compliance is increasing, indicating lung recruitment (Macnaughton, 2006). High pressure can cause barotrauma (see Chapter 4), so settings usually aim to maximise volume while minimising pressure. Ventilators include pressure limits and alarms, but pressure graphs provide detailed visual information about pressure.

Flow graphs (see Figure 17.4) are useful for assessing triggered (patient-initiated) breaths. Triggering is shown below the baseline, and should be followed by rising inspiratory flow (above the baseline). Triggers without inspiratory flow indicate wasted work of breathing, so sensitivity should be reduced. Expiratory flow normally returns below the baseline; if it fails to return to the baseline, gas-trapping (auto-PEEP; bronchospasm) is occurring.

Reducing settings (respiratory rate, tidal volume, pressure support) reduces flow. Flow may also be improved (smaller waveform) by bronchodilators.

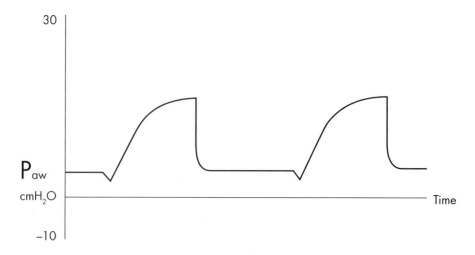

■ *Figure 17.3* **Pressure waveform**

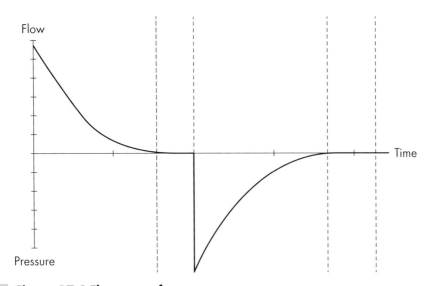

Figure 17.4 Flow waveform

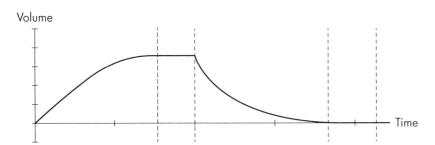

Figure 17.5 Volume waveform

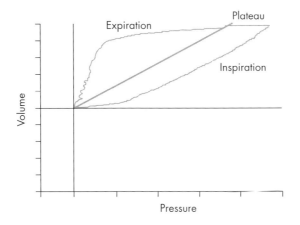

Figure 17.6 Pressure:volume loop

Volume graphs (see Figure 17.5) are possibly the least useful waveform, as tidal and minute volumes are measured elsewhere on ventilators, but loss of volume indicates air leaks.

Pressure:volume loops (see Figure 17.6) indicate compliance, and are probably the most valuable visualisation of ventilation. At the start of inspiration, alveolar (and so lung) compliance is poor, causing significant increase in pressure with little increase in volume. After a critical point, alveoli inflate easily, causing volume to rise significantly, with little further increase in pressure. A reversed picture on expiration gives normal pressure:volume loops a rhomboid shape. Mandatory breaths are anticlockwise, spontaneous clockwise (Pipbeam, 2006). Although pressure and volume measured are throughout the lung fields, it may be helpful to think of the loop display as a single alveolus. Abnormal shapes include the following:

- Jagged ('sawtooth') lines, which indicate fluid; if on inflation, these are probably secretions, but if seen on inspiration and expiration they may be caused by either secretions or water in the circuit.
- 'Beaking' (extending far to the right at the end of inspiration) indicates over-distension, usually resolved by reducing pressures (e.g. PEEP, pressure support, tidal volume).
- Wide loops indicate excessive ventilation, usually resolved by reducing tidal/minute volume.
- Flattened (increased tilting to the right) indicate worsening compliance (Pipbeam, 2006), while increasing tilts to the left indicate improving compliance.
- Incomplete leaks indicate either air leaks or gas trapping – the flow waveform should be checked to confirm there is a problem.

Changing settings to adjust the shape (width) of the loop can maximise volume while minimising pressure. In pressure-driven modes, this loop may not show abnormalities as ventilation will be reduced to maintain pre-set pressures.

Flow:volume loops (see Figure 17.7) indicate air-trapping (auto-PEEP) and air leaks (Pipbeam, 2006):

- bronchoconstriction/dilatation (changes in flow);
- loss of volume if expiratory wave fails to return to the start of inspiration on the horizontal axis (= leak);
- loss of flow if expiratory wave fails to return to the start of inspiration on the vertical axis (= gas trapping);
- jagged lines indicate fluid in circuits (secretions, water).

Manufacturers' booklets often provide usefully illustrated guides to what is available, and readers not familiar with observing waveforms should set up a ventilator circuit with a test lung, viewing various modes, and manipulating the test lung to mimic coughs, a triggered breath and resistance.

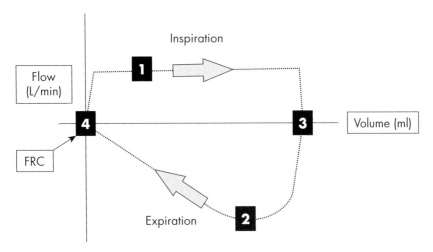

Figure 17.7 Flow:volume loop

Attempts to rationalise weaning have encouraged quantification of respiratory function, usually indexed to patient size. Two examples are oxygen index (OI):

$$= \frac{FiO_2 \times MAP \times 100}{PaO_2}$$

and rapid shallow breathing index (RSBI):

$$= \frac{\text{respiratory rate } (f)}{\text{tidal volume } (V_t) \text{ in litres}}.$$

Advocates claim that an oxygen index above 26 or RSBI below 100 indicates likely successful weaning, but reliability of either measurement remains unclear; Monaco *et al.* (2010) suggest RSBI is not clinically useful to predict weaning. Trachsel *et al.*'s (2005) paediatric study found that oxygen index predicted outcome.

Pulse oximetry

Pulse oximetry is non-invasive and continuous, so is a useful means to monitor oxygenation. However, oximetry measures saturation of haemoglobin – the oxygen stored in the haemoglobin 'bank'. Because oxygen dissociation from haemoglobin is complex, the relationship between SO_2 and partial pressure of oxygen in arterial blood (PaO_2) varies – see the oxygen dissociation curve in Chapter 18.

Limitations of oximetry include:

■ *Poor perfusion*: pulse oximetry calculates saturation by measuring light absorption through a finger or other tissue. Only two per cent of total light absorption is by blood, so poor blood flow causes unreliable signals ('noisy signal'). Most oximeters in ICUs show capillary pulse waveforms (*plethysmograph* or 'pleth'), which should reflect arterial pulses. Poor waveforms indicate insufficient signal (blood supply), probably making readings spurious. Repositioning probes, or warming peripheries, may improve accuracy.

■ *Anaemia*: oximetry measures percentage saturation of haemoglobin, not quantity of haemoglobin, or oxygen, available. Saturation should always be interpreted in relation to haemoglobin levels.

■ *Dark colours*: either on the skin or in blood (e.g. bilirubinaemia) absorb more red light, causing under-readings of 3–5 per cent (Wahr and Tremper, 1996). Trends remain constant, but patients' saturation may be slightly higher than oximeters indicate (blood gas analyser saturation is more accurate). Whether this is clinically significant is debatable. Nail varnish is frequently identified as a concern, but does not significantly affect readings (Rodden *et al.*, 2007; Hinkelbein and Genzwuerker, 2008).

■ *Burns*: heat from the light bulb in the probe can cause burns, especially in patients with poor peripheral perfusion. Probe sites should be changed at least four hourly (MDA, 2001), or more frequently if indicated by manufacturers' recommendations or patients' circulatory status and/or skin integrity.

■ *Oxygen dissociation*: pulse oximetry measures the saturation of haemoglobin by oxygen, not the partial pressure in plasma (measured by ABGs), which will determine oxygen delivery to cells (see Chapter 18).

End-tidal carbon dioxide

End-tidal carbon dioxide ($etCO_2$; capnography) enables continuous non-invasive breath-by-breath monitoring of expired concentrations, end-tidal approximating to residual alveoli levels. End-tidal carbon dioxide usually differs < 1 kPa from arterial blood gas measurement (Hinkelbein *et al.*, 2008), but as normocapnia ranges for arterial blood are 4.6–6.1 kPa, an extra kilopascal is significant. Differences are increased with dead space, and displayed figures are usually higher than blood gas tensions. Some monitors are unable to display $etCO_2$ in kilopascals (kPa), displaying instead either as a percentage (%) or millimetres of mercury (mmHg). Units of measurement will be displayed on the monitor and should be checked.

Harvey and Thomas (2010) suggest capnography should be standard monitoring for ventilated patients in ICUs. When carbon dioxide causes particular concern (e.g. inverse ratio ventilation, permissive hypercapnia, head injury, high-frequency ventilation and other alternative modes), it may show useful trends.

Implications for practice

- Information should be interpreted holistically – in the context of other relevant observations, underlying disease, and treatments.
- Respiratory monitoring should meet clinical needs while minimising risks, where appropriate non-invasive or minimally invasive modes should be selected.
- ICU nurses should undertake and document visual, tactile and auscultatory respiratory assessment on all patients.
- Ventilator waveform display indicates airway response to ventilation, enabling optimal adjustment of settings; pressure:volume loops indicate compliance, so are usually the most useful single waveform.
- Pulse oximetry provides a continuous guide of oxygenation, but is limited by the amount of haemoglobin to carry oxygen and factors that affect oxyhaemoglobin dissociation.
- Capnography provides a useful trend of carbon dioxide removal, although it is significantly less accurate that arterial measurement.

Summary

Respiratory monitoring is fundamental to intensive care. Much can be assessed non-invasively, by listening and looking. Ventilators provide much information, especially if waveforms are displayed. Readers should take early opportunities to become familiar with available means of respiratory monitoring on their units. Whatever means is used, observations can only be as reliable as those making and interpreting the observations. ICU nurses should therefore understand the physiology and mechanics of lung function and pathophysiology. Respiratory monitoring is fundamental to care underlying many of the pathologies discussed in the third section of this book.

Further reading

Most texts describe widely used methods of monitoring. Classic texts include Lumb's (2005) respiratory physiology. For staff wishing to develop skills of X-ray interpretation, Corne and Pointon (2010) is a useful resource. Wilkins *et al.*'s (2004) guide to lung sounds is augmented by a useful CD of the sounds.

Acknowledgement

The section on waveform analysis is based largely on a workshop by Jane Roe and Rosie Maundrill presented at the BACCN 2008 National Conference.

Clinical scenario

Kathleen Fogarty is a 58-year-old lady who was admitted to the ICU for mechanical ventilation to support deteriorating respiratory function. The cause of her recent deterioration is unknown, but possible diagnoses include bronchospasm, basal pneumonia or aspiration of upper airway secretions.

Mrs Fogarty has a visible and widespread drug-related erythematous rash, worse at extremities, and extensive oral ulcerations. Her sputum is thick, mucopurulent, yellow-green and copious. On auscultation, she has expiratory phase and late expiratory wheeze, vesicular breath sounds diminished in apices, and crackles in right base. Her $etCO_2$ is 6.5 kPa and SpO_2 is 94 per cent.

Q.1 Identify and interpret Mrs Fogarty's abnormal lung sounds; explain their relevance to other results and her recent deterioration.

Q.2 Review additional investigations or monitoring required to fully assess Mrs Fogarty's respiratory function.

Q.3 Evaluate the nurse's role with respiratory monitoring in your own clinical area. Consider the range of monitoring approaches available and the nurse's role in interpreting and acting on results, troubleshooting, training and supervising.

Chapter 18

Gas carriage

Contents

Fundamental knowledge   161
Introduction   162
Pressure of gases   162
Oxygen carriage   163
Haemoglobin   163
Oxygen dissociation   164
Cell respiration   164
Oxygen debt   166
Oxygen toxicity   166
Carbon dioxide carriage   166
Heliox   167
Haemoglobinopathies   168
Implications for practice   169
Summary   169
Support groups   169
Further reading   169
Clinical scenario   169

Fundamental knowledge

Pulmonary anatomy and physiology (including vasculature)
Normal respiration (including chemical and neurological
   control and mechanics of external respiration)
Dead space
Haemoglobin – anatomy and physiology (erythropoietin,
   erythropoiesis, oxygen binding)

Introduction

Textbooks such as this necessarily focus on one aspect at a time (reductionism). But body systems function as parts of the whole body, not in isolation. Cardiovascular and respiratory functions are particularly closely interdependent: delivering oxygen and nutrients to tissues, while removing carbon dioxide and other waste. Respiration should achieve adequate tissue oxygenation, so gas movement across lung membranes forms *external respiration*, while gas movement between tissue cells and capillaries forms *internal respiration*.

This chapter explores internal respiration, identifying various factors that affect tissue perfusion and oxygenation. The structure of haemoglobin, and its effect on oxygen carriage and the oxygen saturation curve are identified. Carbon dioxide carriage and some haemoglobinopathies (carbon monoxide poisoning, sickle cell, thalassaemia) are also discussed. Aspects of arterial blood gas results are identified, but most are discussed more fully in the next chapter.

Pressure of gases

Transfer of gases across capillary membranes is determined by pressure gradients, so differences between partial pressure of intracellular and capillary oxygen levels determines tissue oxygenation. Partial pressure of arterial oxygen (PaO_2) therefore indicates oxygen available for diffusion to cells.

Air is approximately 21 per cent oxygen and 79 per cent nitrogen, with negligible amounts of other gases – only 0.04 per cent is carbon dioxide. Representing the whole of inspired air as 1, the fraction of oxygen in inspired air (FiO_2) is 0.21. The common practice of recording FiO_2 as 21 for patients not receiving supplementary oxygen is technically incorrect (an FiO_2 of 21 is 2100 per cent oxygen).

Barometric, and so alveolar, pressure (at sea level) is 101.3 kPa. Total atmospheric pressure includes water vapour. Pressure of water vapour is variable in air, but fully saturated air at 37°C (both normally achieved during inspiration) has 6.3 of its 101.3 kPa pressure from water vapour, leaving 95 kPa for all gases. If normal air were to reach alveoli, the partial pressure of oxygen is 21 per cent of 95 kPa (see Table 18.1).

Table 18.1 Partial pressures of gases at sea level

	Concentration in air (%)	Pressure in air (kPa)	Pressure in alveoli* (kPa)
Water vapour		variable**	6.3
Oxygen	21	21.27 in dry air	13.3
Carbon dioxide	0.03	0.03 in dry air	5.3
Nitrogen	79	80 in dry air	76.4

Notes:
* provided 37°C, hence constant water vapour.
** depends on temperature.

However, air reaching alveoli is initially diluted by 'dead space' air – air remaining in the airways from the last breath out. 'Dead space' air is relatively carbon dioxide rich and oxygen poor. This further dilutes the partial pressure of oxygen. Gases transfer across semipermeable membranes (alveoli) by pressure gradients, so as long as oxygen tensions (the partial pressure) are higher in alveoli than pulmonary capillaries, oxygen diffuses into blood. Similarly, higher carbon dioxide tensions in pulmonary capillaries than in alveoli enable transfer into alveoli.

Physiological adult dead space is about 150 ml, with additional pathological dead space when alveoli are not perfused. Artificial ventilation dead space begins at the inspiratory limb ('Y' connector) of ventilator tubing. Small breaths or large dead space therefore lower alveolar partial pressure of oxygen.

Oxygen carriage

Oxygen is carried by blood in two ways:

- plasma (3 per cent)
- haemoglobin (97 per cent).

Oxygen is not a very soluble gas, so at normal (sea-level) atmospheric pressure 3 ml of oxygen dissolve in each litre of blood, insufficient to maintain life. Haemoglobin solves this problem, by having a high affinity for oxygen, and so readily transporting the vast majority of oxygen in our blood. However, it is the small amount of dissolved oxygen that exerts the partial pressure in blood (e.g. PO_2), and can diffuse into cells. Maintaining partial pressure of oxygen therefore in part depends on adequate dissociation of oxygen from haemoglobin.

Tissue oxygen supply is therefore affected by:

- haemoglobin level
- oxygen saturation of haemoglobin
- oxygen dissociation
- perfusion pressure.

Perfusion pressure is discussed in other chapters.

Haemoglobin

Erythrocytes are mainly haemoglobin. With average diameters of 7 nanometers (μm), erythrocytes are slightly smaller than capillaries (8–10 micrometers). The poor solubility of oxygen is thus overcome by placing haemoglobin, and oxygen, close to capillary walls.

Physiological normal levels for haemoglobin (Hb) are 13–18 g/dl (male) and 11.5–16.5g/dl (female). But while dilution reduces oxygen-carrying capacity, haemoglobin also determines viscosity of blood. Less viscous blood flows more easily through small vessels (capillaries), so optimum oxygen delivery to cells is a paradoxical balance between:

■ high haemoglobin (more viscous blood) – carries more oxygen;
■ low haemoglobin (less viscous blood) – flows more easily through capillaries.

Survival from critical illness is highest when haemoglobin is 7–9 g/dl (Hebert *et al.*, 1999), although specific groups, such as older people, may benefit from higher levels (Boralessa *et al.*, 2003), possibly 8–10 g/dl.

Oxygen dissociation

While haemoglobin transports oxygen efficiently, its high affinity for oxygen limits dissociation: only 20–25 per cent of available oxygen normally unloads, making normal venous saturations (SvO_2) 70–75 per cent. The SaO_2–SvO_2 difference therefore indicates tissue uptake (consumption) of oxygen, with low SvO_2 indicating tissue hypoxia (Wagstaff, 2009). Large differences indicate high demand, with the possibility that demand is not being met, so consider increasing:

■ supply (FiO_2)
■ carriage (Hb).

Small differences indicate low uptake, which may be from:

■ low demand
■ low delivery (e.g. poor perfusion, oedema).

Oxygen dissociates readily if haemoglobin is fully or highly saturated, but lower saturations reduce dissociation. This variable relationship between SaO_2 and PaO_2 is shown in the S-shaped oxyhaemoglobin dissociation curve (see Figure 18.1).

Factors that can change ('shift') oxyhaemoglobin dissociation include:

■ temperature
■ pH
■ 2,3 DPG (diphosphoglycerate) levels (see pages 207 and 333)
■ haemoglobinopathies.

Shifts to the left reduce, while shifts to the right increase, dissociation (see Table 18.2). If dissociation is reduced, saturation (SaO_2) may remain high, despite low partial pressures (PaO_2).

Cell respiration

The purpose of respiratory function is to supply tissue cells with sufficient oxygen to enable aerobic metabolism in mitochondria. Measuring mitochondrial respiration is not practical, so cruder parameters (e.g. arterial gas tensions) are measured instead. However, measured parameters only partly indicate delivery of oxygen to cells, and removal of carbon dioxide.

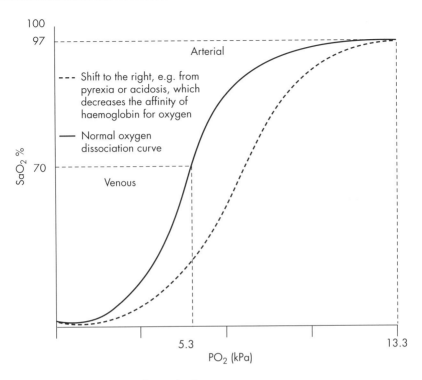

■ *Figure 18.1* **Oxygen dissociation curve**

Table 18.2 **Some factors affecting oxygen dissociation**

Curve shifts to right (increased oxygen dissociation from haemoglobin) with:
■   increased temperature
■   acidosis (pH) – the *Böhr effect*
■   increased CO_2
■   increased 2,3 DPG (diphosphoglycerate)

Curve shifts to left (decreased oxygen dissociation from haemoglobin) with:
■   reduced temperature
■   alkalosis
■   (some) haemoglobinopathies (e.g. HbF)
■   carbon monoxide
■   decreased CO_2
■   decreased 2,3 DPG

Partial pressures of oxygen progressively fall with further stages of internal respiration: normal capillary pressure of 6.8 kPa gives tissue pressure of 2.7 kPa, and mitochondrial pressure of 0.13–1.3 kPa. Conversely, intracellular carbon dioxide tensions are higher. These pressure gradients create *internal respiration*.

Oxygen debt

In hypoxic conditions, oxygen and glycogen are withdrawn from haemoglobin and myoglobin (muscles), creating a 'debt' that is normally repaid once high oxygen demand ceases. So, after completing strenuous exercise we continue to breathe deeply. Anaerobic metabolism for intracellular ATP production produces lactic acid.

Prolonged critical illness can cause cumulative oxygen debt which, with recovery, flushes toxic acids and cytokines into the circulation, causing potential reperfusion injury (see Chapter 24).

Oxygen toxicity

Hyperoxia releases free oxygen *radicals* (Rousseau *et al.*, 2005), so prolonged exposure to high concentrations of oxygen can damage lung tissue. High-concentration oxygen also 'washes out' nitrogen from lungs – nitrogen, being an inert gas, and the majority (79 per cent) of air, distends alveoli. Increasing oxygen concentration reduces nitrogen, potentially causing atelectasis. PEEP helps prevent atelectasis from nitrogen washout. Although precise concentrations and times are disputed, prolonged use of high-concentration can cause oxygen toxicity, and therefore lung damage. Hinds and Watson (2008) suggest oxygen toxicity occurs with FiO_2 above 0.6 for more than 24 hours. However, severe critical illness may necessitate risking oxygen toxicity to preserve cell (and so the patient's) life.

Carbon dioxide carriage

Air contains virtually no carbon dioxide (0.04 per cent). Metabolism produces 200 ml of carbon dioxide every minute. Carbon dioxide diffuses by concentration gradients from cells into capillary blood, and from pulmonary capillaries into alveoli. Normal concentrations of blood carbon dioxide are 48 ml/dl (arterial) to 52 ml/dl (venous). Carbon dioxide is normally the most important 'drive' for the respiratory centre in the brainstem. Carbon dioxide is also vasoactive, stimulating vasoconstriction.

Carbon dioxide carriage is relatively simple compared with oxygen carriage. It is carried in blood in three ways:

- plasma (10 per cent)
- haemoglobin (20 per cent)
- bicarbonate (70 per cent).

Plasma: Carbon dioxide is approximately 20 times more soluble than oxygen, so is readily carried in solution by plasma.

Haemoglobin: Carbon dioxide is carried as carbaminoglobin. Carbon dioxide binds to globin, not haem, so (unlike carbon monoxide) does not displace oxygen.

Bicarbonate: Most carbon dioxide carriage is in plasma bicarbonate.

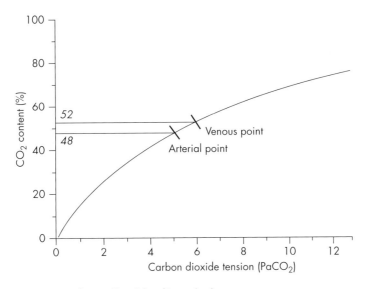

Figure 18.2 Carbon dioxide dissociation curve

Many blood gas analysers measure the total carbon dioxide carried (tCO_2). Diffusion of carbon dioxide occurs through simple tension gradients, making the carbon dioxide dissociation curve virtually linear (see Figure 18.2). Like the oxygen dissociation curve, carbon dioxide dissociation can move to the right or left. Rightward shifts (lowering carbon dioxide content per unit of pCO_2) occur with raised oxygen concentrations in blood – the '*Haldane effect*'.

Hypercapnia improves cardiac output and peripheral tissue perfusion (Akça *et al.*, 2002), typically causing a flushing appearance to facial skin.

Heliox

Like air, Heliox contains 21 per cent oxygen, but replaces air's nitrogen with helium. Helium has a low density (three times less than air and eight times less than oxygen) so, being less affected by airway resistance, reduces work of breathing (Harris and Barnes, 2008). With airway obstruction, where work of breathing is excessive, Heliox may enable adequate oxygenation. It should be given through a non-rebreathing mask so it is not diluted with room air (Kass, 2003). Benefits should occur within minutes, buying time to resolve the underlying problem (Calzia and Stahl, 2004). Its value beyond one hour is limited (Ho *et al.*, 2003). Use and availability are often limited by its relative expense, although costs of alternatives, and need for urgent intervention, may make it cost-effective. It has been advocated for use with COPD (Tassaux *et al.*, 2005; Eves and Ford, 2007). Few ventilators (invasive or non-invasive) are designed to work with Heliox (Calzia and Stahl, 2004), and it may affect ventilator monitoring. As Heliox must be at least 70 per cent helium to be effective, maximum oxygen concentration is 30 per cent (Strandvik *et al.*, 2006).

Heliox is inert, colourless, odourless and tasteless. It disperses quickly, so should not significantly affect anyone nearby. It does however affect patients' vocal cords, so they should be warned about a temporary high-pitched, squeaky voice.

Haemoglobinopathies

Critical illness may be complicated by haemoglobinopathies, such as those described below.

Sickle cell (HbS) is a genetically inherited chromosomal abnormality, causing the abnormal haemoglobin to 'sickle' (change to an elliptical shape) in hypoxic conditions. Sickling occludes small capillaries, causing intense ischaemic pain, necrosis and tissue infarction. Crises may be fatal. Traditionally associated with the 'malaria belt' (sickling provides some protection against the malarial parasite), people with sickle cell disease now live worldwide. Sickle cell disease means both haemoglobin chromosomes are affected (HbS, HbS). Sickle cell trait affects one chromosome (HbS, HbA). Although sickle cell disease is more serious than trait, both should be regarded as at risk during critical illness.

Crisis management should provide:

- analgesia
- oxygen
- fluids
- blood (exchange) transfusion to reduce HbS.

Thalassaemia ('Cooley's anaemia') is a hereditary genetic mutation, traditionally found in people of Mediterranean or south-east Asian ancestry. Lack of haemoglobin necessitates transfusion. But as blood transfusion causes iron overload, chelation (e.g. deferasirox) is also needed (Porter, 2009).

Carbon monoxide (FCOHb) levels in blood are normally negligible (< 1 per cent), although levels in smokers are higher (Blumenthal, 2001). Half-life of carbon monoxide is 4–5 hours in air, but only 40 minutes if breathing 100 per cent oxygen (BTS, 2008), so pure oxygen should be given to patients with carbon monoxide poisoning.

Methaemoglobin (MetHb) is caused by the iron in haemoglobin changing from a ferrous to ferric state, reducing oxygen carriage. A few drugs can cause methaemoglobin, including *nitric oxide* (NO), a gas occasionally used to dilate pulmonary capillaries and so improve oxygenation.

Foetal haemoglobin (HbF) has a higher affinity for oxygen than normal adult haemoglobin (HbA), so reducing tissue oxygenation. Conversion to adult haemoglobin normally begins in utero, and is normally completed by 1–2 years of age (Farrell and Sittlington, 2009), but foetal haemoglobin can (abnormally) persist throughout life.

Implications for practice

- Oxygen is vital for life, so adequate oxygen delivery to cells, as well as adequate oxygen carriage by haemoglobin, should be achieved.
- Oxygen dissociation from haemoglobin is affected by various factors (see Table 18.2), including pH and temperature.
- PaO_2 measures plasma oxygen, whereas SaO_2 measures oxyhaemoglobin. Variable relationships between these two can be seen from arterial blood gas analysis.
- Prolonged high-concentration oxygen (> 60 per cent for > 24 hours) can cause toxic lung damage, so should be avoided if possible. Where it cannot be avoided, PEEP should be used to compensate for nitrogen washout.
- Heliox may provide adequate oxygenation despite airway obstruction, so can usefully create time for other interventions.
- Sickle cell disease can cause life-threatening crises, usually prevented by adequate oxygenation and hydration.
- Sickle cell crisis usually needs opioid analgesia.

Summary

Oxygen is primarily carried by haemoglobin (SO_2), but partial pressure in plasma (PO_2) creates the pressure gradient for transfer to tissues. Complex, changeable, relationships between SO_2 and PO_2 are shown by the oxygen dissociation curve, which may be 'shifted' to the right or left by various factors. Haemoglobinopathies affect oxygen carriage.

Support groups

The Sickle Cell Society, 54 Station Road, London NW10 4UA: 020 8961 7795
UK Thalassaemia Society, 19 The Broadway, London N14 6PH: 0800 731 1109

Further reading

Most physiology texts contain useful chapters on gas carriage. Hebert *et al.*'s (1997) classic study remains the basis for guiding most blood transfusions. The British Thoracic Society (BTS, 2008) acute oxygen therapy guidelines are useful, even though specifically excluding applicability to ICUs. Rees *et al.* (2010) review sickle cell disease.

Clinical scenario

Nina Walker is 36 years old and was admitted to the ICU with a head injury and fractured spine at C5 from falling downstairs. The first blood gas taken was from a central vein, while Miss Walker was self-ventilating via a face mask with FiO_2 0.6, in flat supine position wearing a hard collar. The second blood gas is arterial, taken 12 hours post-intubation and mechanical ventilation using spontaneous mode and FiO_2 0.25. Miss Walker's respiratory rate is 16 bpm, her Hb is 9.8 g/dl and core temperature at 12 hours is lower at 35.7°C.

Blood gas and electrolyte values are:

	On admission to ICU Central venous blood FiO_2 0.6 Temperature 35.9°C	12 hours later Arterial blood FiO_2 0.25 Temperature 35.7°C
pH	7.27	7.51
PaO_2 (kPa)	3.30	13.36
$PaCO_2$ (kPa)	6.84	3.80
HCO_3^- (mmol/litre)	21.1	25.3
BE (mmol/litre)	−2.5	+0.3
Lactate (mmol/litre)	3.3	1.9
SO_2 (%) (SvO_2/SaO_2)	48.5	97.9

Q.1 Using the oxygen dissociation curve (Figure 18.1) verify Miss Walker's percentage O_2 saturation of haemoglobin for both blood gas results (plot the position of her PO_2 incorporating her Hb, temperature and other arterial blood gas values). Repeat this using the carbon dioxide dissociation curve (Figure 18.2) to calculate CO_2 content percentage.

Q.2 Explain any shifts in the oxygen dissociation curve and haemoglobin's affinity for O_2 at Miss Walker's cellular (tissue) and alveolar membrane for both venous and arterial blood gases. How does the level of carbon dioxide in blood affect oxygen transport?

Q.3 Review alternative assessment approaches that can be used by nurses to monitor effectiveness of oxygen transport to Miss Walker's tissues (consider and specify types of visual observation, laboratory investigations, blood oximetry values such as O_2Hb, COHb, HHb, MetHb, RHb).

Chapter 19

Arterial blood gas analysis and acid/base balance

Contents

Fundamental knowledge	171
Introduction	172
Acid/base definitions	172
pH measurement	172
Respiratory balance	173
Metabolic balance	174
Renal control	175
Chemical buffers	175
Acidosis	176
Tonometry	176
Taking samples	176
Interpreting samples	177
Compensation	181
Five steps	182
Implications for practice	182
Summary	182
Further reading	183
Clinical scenarios	183

Fundamental knowledge

Cell metabolism (oxygen consumption, ATP
   production, carbon dioxide production)

Introduction

Arterial blood gas analysis provides valuable information about acid/base balance, and respiratory and metabolic function. Analysers provide additional useful information about various metabolites and electrolytes. Therefore arterial blood gas sampling and analysis is a core skill for ICU staff. Analysers and 'normal ranges' vary between units, so using sample printouts from your unit may be helpful. The UK measures gases in kilopascals (kPa) – the Système Internationale (SI) unit. The USA uses mmHg: 1 kPa is 7.4 mmHg.

Acid/base definitions

Acids can release hydrogen ions; bases (alkali) can accept (buffer) hydrogen ions. Strong acids (e.g. hydrochloric) release many free hydrogen ions, whereas weak acids (e.g. carbonic) release few. Acid/base balance is the power of hydrogen ions (pH) measured in moles per litre ('power' in the mathematical sense, for the negative logarithm). The power of hydrogen ions can be controlled (balanced) either through *buffering* or exchange. Hydrogen (H^+), a positively charged ion (cation), can be buffered by a negatively charged ion (anion), such as bicarbonate (HCO_3^-).

pH measurement

Chemically, the pH scale ranges from 0–14, making pH 7 chemically neutral. Arterial blood is normally slightly alkaline (pH 7.35–7.45). Blood pH < 7.35 is acidotic, while pH > 7.45 is alkalotic. If arterial acid/base balance is ideal (pH 7.4), each litre of blood contains 0.000 04 *millimole* (or 40 nanamoles, nmol) of hydrogen. Keeping the vast range of hydrogen ions substances can release or accept within a scale of 0–14 is achieved using a negative logarithm. Unfortunately, few people think logarithmically.

A logarithm expresses numbers as a (mathematical) power:

$$10^1 = 10$$
$$10^2 = 10 \times 10 = 100$$
$$10^3 = 100 \times 10 = 1000$$
$$10^4 = 1000 \times 10 = 10,000$$

Each addition to the power (log) causes a tenfold increase in the actual number. Bacteria and blood cells, being very numerous, are usually measured using the log of 10. Negative logarithms similarly represent very small divisions by subtraction from the log:

$$10^0 = 1$$
$$10^{-1} = 0.1$$
$$10^{-2} = 0.01$$

Changing pH by one represents a tenfold (logarithmic) change in hydrogen ion concentration (acidity), while changing pH by 0.3 doubles or halves concentrations:

> pH 7.7 = 20 nmol/litre H^+
> pH 7.4 = 40 nmol/litre H^+
> pH 7.1 = 80 nmol/litre H^+
> pH 6.8 =160 nmol/litre H^+

Cell metabolism produces acids, so hydrogen moves from intracellular to extracellular fluid through concentration gradients, intracellular (where hydrogen is produced) concentrations being highest (normally 7.0 (Atherton, 2003)). Interstitial and venous pH is normally 7.35 (Marieb and Hoehn, 2007).

Blood pH outside 7.0–7.8 is usually fatal (Marieb and Hoehn, 2007), although Selby and James (1995) report rare survival from pH 6.4. Arterial pH below 7.0 usually leads to coma and death, while levels above 7.8 overstimulate the nervous system, causing convulsions and respiratory arrest.

Acid/base balance is controlled through these functions:

- respiratory
- metabolic (renal function, chemical buffers).

Respiratory balance

Carbon dioxide dissolves in water to form carbonic acid:

$$CO_3 + H_2O \leftrightarrow H_2CO_3$$

a weak (pH 6.4), unstable acid. In lungs, carbonic acid, being unstable, dissociates back into water and carbon dioxide, so normal blood levels are normally maintained by adapting ventilation (rate and depth of breathing). Carbonic acid is the main acid in blood, levels depending on carbon dioxide concentrations (PCO_2). Carbon dioxide is therefore considered a *potential* acid (lacking hydrogen ions, it is not really an acid), so:

- *respiratory acidosis* is failure to remove sufficient carbon dioxide (i.e. high $PaCO_2$);
- *respiratory alkalosis* is excessive removal of carbon dioxide (i.e. low $PaCO_2$).

(See Figure 19.1.)

Hypercapnia stimulates respiratory centres to increase ventilation (rate and depth), removing more carbon dioxide. So although respiration cannot remove hydrogen ions, it can inhibit carbonic acid formation, restoring homeostasis. Respiratory acidosis is caused by *hypo*ventilation. Respiratory alkalosis is caused by *hyper*ventilation. Chonghaile *et al.* (2008) found hypercapnic acidosis

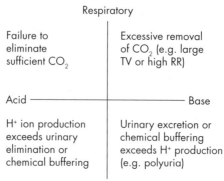

Respiratory

| Failure to eliminate sufficient CO_2 | Excessive removal of CO_2 (e.g. large TV or high RR) |

Acid ————————————— Base

| H^+ ion production exceeds urinary elimination or chemical buffering | Urinary excretion or chemical buffering exceeds H^+ production (e.g. polyuria) |

Metabolic

Figure 19.1 Origin of acid/base imbalance

reduced lung injury from *E. coli* (*Escherichia coli*) pneumonia, although whether this has clinical significance is unclear.

In health, respiratory response to acidosis is rapid, exerting up to double the effect of combined chemical buffers (Marieb and Hoehn, 2007). Doubling or halving alveolar ventilation can alter pH 0.2, returning life-threatening pH of 7.0 to 7.2 or 7.3 in 3–12 minutes (Guyton and Hall, 2005).

Metabolic balance

Metabolic balance is more complex. Acids are:

- ingested (e.g. wine, most crystalloid IVIs)
- produced (metabolism)
- removed through the kidneys and
- buffered by chemicals.

Bases (e.g. bicarbonate) are:

- produced
- reabsorbed (renally)
- ingested/infused (e.g. antacids).

Metabolic acidosis may be from:

- tissue acids (especially lactic or ketoacids) or
- hyperchloraemia.

Ketoacids are from alternative metabolism (starvation, insulin-lack). Lactate (see page 181), the main cause of metabolic acidosis in ICUs, indicates anaerobic metabolism, usually from perfusion failure. *Hyperchloraemia* increases dissociation of hydrogen ions from body water, so causing metabolic acidosis. Hyperchloraemic acidosis is caused by excessive saline infusion (Ochola and Venkatesh, 2009), although whether hyperchloraemia causes significant problems is questionable (Handy and Soni, 2008).

Hydrogen (H⁺) ions, an essential component of any acid, are removed by the kidney or buffered by bases. Acidosis therefore occurs if:

- hydrogen production exceeds removal (excessive production; kidney injury);
- buffer production is insufficient (especially, liver failure).

Metabolic alkalosis is caused by excessive removal/buffering of hydrogen (H⁺) ions or excessive production/absorption of bases due to:

- polyuria;
- hypokalaemia (causing excess H⁺ in urine);
- gastric acid loss (e.g. excessive nasogastric drainage, vomiting);
- excessive buffers (e.g. colonic reabsorption from constipation).

Renal control

Other than insignificant transdermal loss, hydrogen ions are only removed from the body in urine, being actively exchanged into glomerular filtrate when other cations (mainly sodium) are reabsorbed. The extent of active hydrogen ion excretion into urine is seen on urinalysis: normal blood (from which urine is formed) pH is 7.4, while normal urinary pH is 5.0.

Kidneys usually excrete 30–70 mmol of hydrogen ions daily, but after a week or more can remove 300 mmol daily. Kidney injury therefore causes metabolic acidosis.

Chemical buffers

Chemical buffers respond rapidly, within seconds, balancing hydrogen ions by binding acids to bases. They do not eliminate acids from the body.

Bicarbonate is the main chemical buffer of extracellular fluid, responsible for half of all chemical buffering. Hydrogen ions are essential to produce bicarbonate (HCO_3^-). Bicarbonate can combine with hydrogen to produce carbonic acid:

$$HCO_3^- + H \leftrightarrow H_2CO_3$$

Phosphate (PO_4^{3-}) is the least important buffer in blood, but the main urinary, interstitial and intracellular buffer.

Plasma proteins. Albumin is the main plasma protein, although histidine (in haemoglobin) is also a significant buffer. Hypoalbuminaemia, common in critical illness, therefore reduces metabolic buffering.

Chemical buffers are produced in many places, but especially in the liver, therefore hepatic failure causes metabolic acidosis.

Acidosis

Acidosis (blood pH < 7.35) may be:

- respiratory = failure to excrete sufficient carbon dioxide (= high pCO_2);
- metabolic = failure to excrete/buffer sufficient H^+ ions (= base excess below –2; low HCO_3^-).

Acidosis:

- increases respiratory drive;
- shifts the oxygen dissociation curve to the right, increasing oxyhaemoglobin dissociation ('Böhr effect'); treating acidosis rather than underlying causes therefore deprives hypoxic tissues of available oxygen (Winser, 2001);
- reduces blood carriage of carbon dioxide (Cavaliere *et al.*, 2002);
- is negatively inotropic, and reduces effectiveness of infused inotropes;
- impairs enzyme activity (Shangraw, 2000).

Acidosis is a symptom, not a disease. Many critically ill patients tolerate arterial pH significantly below 7.2 (Forsythe and Schmidt, 2000), as seen with permissive hypercapnia (see Chapter 27). Treatment should focus on underlying pathologies. Oxygen delivery to peripheries should be optimised, without increasing cell metabolism.

Bicarbonate infusions to reverse acidosis can cause many problems, including the following:

- They exacerbate intracellular acidosis (sodium bicarbonate is an extracellular ion, but also forms carbon dioxide, which can transfer into cells) (Cooper and Cramp, 2006).
- Alkalosis reduces oxygen dissociation from haemoglobin (shifts the oxygen dissociation curve to left).

Bicarbonate infusions should only be used in immediately life-threatening situations, such as pH < 7.1 or cardiopulmonary resuscitation exceeding 20–25 minutes (Winser, 2001).

Tonometry

Hypoxic tissues metabolise anaerobically, which produces many hydrogen ions. The gut being highly vascular, gastric (intramucosal) pH (pHi) may indicate acidaemia, although so far tonometry has proved more useful for research than practice (Beale *et al.*, 2004). For accuracy, feed should be aspirated before measurement (Marshall and West, 2003), which limits its clinical usefulness.

Taking samples

Blood gas samples should not be taken within 20–30 minutes of any changes to ventilation, or any interventions that affect respiratory function (Hennessey and Japp, 2007). Arterial lines provide easy access for obtaining samples for blood gas analysis. Transcutaneous gas analysis is non-invasive, but more useful for neonates than adults. Intra-arterial electrodes enable continuous gas tension monitoring, PiO_2 correlating well with arterial samples (PaO_2) (Abraham *et al.*, 1996). However, equipment is costly, and intra-arterial monitoring has not (yet) established itself in ICU practice. Continuous gas analysis is currently impractical and too costly for widespread clinical use (Ault and Stock, 2004), but future technological improvements may make this, or transcutaneous gases, practical alternatives.

Potential sampling errors that may affect results include:

- *Dilution* from saline flush, if insufficient fluid is withdrawn from the 'dead space' of arterial lines; blood should be clearly free of saline, but sampling ports are usually close to the cannula, making 0.5–1 ml usually sufficient discard.
- Excessive *negative pressure* may damage cells (haemolysis), causing potassium release; if pressure is needed, it should be gentle, steady and minimal.
- *Air* in samples causes falsely low readings, so should be expelled (Szaflarski, 1996). Samples should be covered immediately to prevent atmospheric gas exchange.
- *Delay in analysing* causes inaccuracies, as blood cells in samples continue to metabolise: potassium and carbon dioxide levels increase, pH and oxygen fall. As ICUs usually have analysers on the unit, this rarely causes significant problems, but usually justifies interrupting routine calibrations.
- *Erythrocyte sedimentation* may cause either concentrated plasma or concentrated cells to enter the analyser, affecting many results, especially haemoglobin; samples should be mixed continuously, rotating with a thumb roll, not vigorous shaking (which causes haemolysis).

When taking samples, these pitfalls should be avoided, but they should also be considered when interpreting results, especially if the sample has been obtained by someone else.

Interpreting samples

Like all skills, interpreting results improves with practice, and benefits from using a systematic approach. There are four main sections to blood gas results, each with a very few key measurements:

- pH
- respiratory ($PaCO_2$, PaO_2, SaO_2)
- metabolic (HCO_3^-, SBC)
- 'add-ons' (electrolytes, metabolites).

Not all results are always printed together, and there will be other (usually less valuable) results, some of which are included below.

This chapter describes key measurements, some analysers offering additional results. Standard abbreviations used for some other measurements are listed in Table 19.1. Electrolytes and metabolites, measured by most analysers, are listed in Table 19.2 and discussed in Chapter 21. Having a printout from a patient you have recently cared for will be useful while reading through this section.

Temperature

Debate persists between temperature correction ('pH-stat') and analysing all samples at 37°C ('alpha-stat'). Temperature affects dissociation of gases, so PaO_2, $PaCO_2$, pH, base excess, and HCO_3^- results differ with different temperatures – seen by reanalysing samples at different temperatures. However, even if staff have confidence in the measured temperature, temperature differs in different parts of the body. Analysing all samples at the machine default of 37°C is easier and safer (Bisson and Younker, 2006), so most ICUs no longer temperature-correct gases (Smith and Taylor, 2005). But consistency of all staff is more important than abstract debate.

pH

Normal: 7.35–7.45.

Table 19.1 Some abbreviations commonly found on blood gas samples

Abbreviation	Meaning
F	fractional concentration in dry gas
I	ideal
P	pressure, or partial pressure
Q	volume of blood
A	alveolar
a	arterial
c	capillary
v	venous

Table 19.2 Normal levels of electrolytes and metabolites often measured by blood gas analysers

Electrolyte/metabolite	Normal range
Sodium (Na^+)	135–145 mmol/litre
Potassium (K^+)	3.5–4.5 mmol/litre
Calcium (Ca^{++}, also written $Ca2^+$)*	1.1–1.3 mmol/litre
Chloride	95–105 mmol/litre
Glucose	4.1–6.1 mmol/litre
Lactate	< 2 mmol/litre

Note: * Blood gas analysers measure ionised calcium, not total calcium; biochemistry laboratories measure total calcium. See Chapter 21 – 'Blood results'.

pH measures overall acidity or alkalinity of blood; it does not differentiate between respiratory and metabolic components. (NB: Ph = *pharmacopoeia* or *phenyl*.)

PaCO$_2$

Normal: 4.6–6.1 kPa (BTS, 2008).

Carbon dioxide dissolves in water, forming carbonic acid (see page 173). High carbon dioxide tension (high PaCO$_2$) therefore indicates respiratory acidosis, while low carbon dioxide tension indicates respiratory alkalosis.

tCO$_2$ (or ctCO$_2$)

Normal: 21.6–22.5 mmol/litre (48–50 vols%).

Although most carbon dioxide is carried in bicarbonate, nearly one-third is carried either in solution (as carbonic acid) or by haemoglobin. TCO$_2$ measures the total carbon dioxide in plasma. This measurement is generally of limited use.

PaO$_2$

Normal: 12.0–14.6 kPa (BTS, 2008).

PaO$_2$ measures partial pressure of oxygen in plasma. This is a very small (normally about 3 per cent) of oxygen in blood, but as gas exchange relies on pressure gradients, partial pressure of oxygen determines tissue oxygenation.

Saturation

Normal: 97 per cent.

Arterial saturation indicates percentage saturation of haemoglobin by oxygen, and is the same as SpO$_2$ measured by pulse oximeters (see Chapter 17). Blood gas analysers use many colours to calculate saturation, while pulse oximeters use only two, so analysers are more accurate, especially if carbon monoxide is present. Venous saturation is discussed in Chapter 18.

A-a gradient

Normal: 2–3.3 kPa (depending on age).

Alveolar-arterial (A-a) gradient indicates whether 'shunting' is occurring. Measurement is only reliable if FiO$_2$ is entered into the analyser. Many analysers do not display A-a gradient; significant shunting is probably occurring if high concentrations of inspired oxygen are needed.

HCO₃

Normal: 22–28 mmol/litre.

Bicarbonate is the main buffer in blood, so low bicarbonate indicates metabolic acidosis, while high levels indicate metabolic alkalosis. While most bicarbonate is produced by the metabolic system, some is also produced from carbon dioxide:

$$CO_2 + H_2O \leftrightarrow H_2CO_3 \leftrightarrow HCO_3^- + H$$

(carbon dioxide + water form carbonic acid, which can dissociate to bicarbonate and a hydrogen radical).

Normally negligible, the respiratory component becomes increasingly significant with increasingly abnormal $PaCO_2$. Actual bicarbonate (ABC, the amount measured) therefore includes both metabolic and respiratory production. Microchip calculation enables removal of the respiratory component by adjusting the measurement to standard conditions (temperature 37°C and $PaCO_2$ 5.3 kPa), giving a *standardised bicarbonate* (SBC, HCO_3^-std). So although a derived measurement, SBC gives more reliable indication of metabolic function than HCO_3^-.

Base excess (BE)

Normal: ±2.

Base excess measures metabolic acid/base balance, indicating moles of acid or base needed to restore one litre of blood to pH 7.4. Unlike pH, base excess is a linear scale, so easier to understand. Neutral is zero, positive base excess is too much base (alkaline; metabolic alkalosis), while negative base excess is insufficient base (metabolic acidosis).

Base excess is calculated from bicarbonate levels, so although base excess is viewed as a metabolic figure, carbon dioxide affects bicarbonate. Standardised base excess (SBE, BE-std) more accurately indicates metabolic balance.

Anion gap

Normal: 10–18.

This measures the difference (gap) between measured cations and measured anions:

$$(Na^{+K}) - (Cl^- + HCO_3^-).$$

In health, cations and anions are balanced, but there are more anions than cations not measured by analysers, hence the gap. The anion gap is largely an archaic way of assessing acid/base balance, and is not included on many analysers. Increased gaps may be caused by:

- metabolic acidosis from metabolic acid production (hyperchloraemia causes a normal gap) (Durward, 2002);
- dehydration (Williams, 1998);
- increased minor anions (e.g. lactate, ketones, renal acid) (Williams, 1998);
- drugs given in organic salts (e.g. penicillin) (Williams, 1998);
- decreased minor cations (magnesium, calcium – rare) (Williams, 1998).

Reduced gaps may be caused by:

- hypoalbuminaemia (Williams, 1998);
- severe haemodilution (Williams, 1998);
- increased anion gap metabolic acidosis = excess acid (through ingestion, the body's own production, or an inability to excrete) (Cooper, N., 2004).

Normal anion gap metabolic acidosis indicates loss of base (Cooper, N., 2004).

Lactate

Normal: < 2 mmol/litre.

Metabolism normally produces about 0.8 mmol/kg/hour of lactate (Cooper, 2003), but anaerobic metabolism significantly increases production. Lactate is converted into lactic acid (pH 3.4), causing/increasing metabolic acidosis. Raised lactate indicates perfusion failure, with significant mortality once lactate reaches 4 (Trzeciak *et al.*, 2007; Callaway *et al.*, 2009). Whether sepsis predicts mortality in most pathologies (Vandromme *et al.*, 2010) or only sepsis (Ansen *et al.*, 2009) is disputed.

Compensation

Homeostasis aims to keep blood pH 7.4. Overall pH of blood is the balance of both respiratory and metabolic function (see Figure 19.1 on page 174). If able, the body compensates for a problem with one by an equal and opposite reaction with the other.

When analysing samples, identify:

- if pH is normal (7.35–7.45);
- respiratory acid/base balance (pCO_2);
- metabolic acid/base balance (bicarbonate, base excess).

If pH is normal, but respiratory and metabolic balances are abnormal and opposite, compensation is succeeding. If pH is abnormal, compensation is incomplete (if metabolic and respiratory balances are opposite) or absent (if metabolic and respiratory balances are not opposite).

Critical illness often causes acidosis – respiratory (respiratory failure) or metabolic (e.g. kidney or liver failure). Alkaloses are usually compensatory. Respiratory compensation occurs quickly (within minutes), but metabolic compensation takes hours or days to be fully effective (and to fully stop). So metabolic compensation only occurs in response to prolonged respiratory complications. Metabolic 'overshoot' may be seen in ICUs where artificial ventilation resolves the primary respiratory acidosis, but metabolism continues compensation for a problem no longer present.

Five steps

From the four sections identified at the start of this section, core blood gas analysis can be achieved in five steps:

1   pH – is it normal? If not, is acidosis or alkalosis present?
2   Respiratory ($PaCO_2$ = ventilation + respiratory acid/base balance; PaO_2 + SaO_2 = oxygenation).
3   Metabolic acid/base balance (HCO_3^-, SBC).
4   Is compensation occurring? If so, which way? Is it fully or partly successful? (Short cut: acidosis is usually the problem; alkalosis is usually compensation.)
5   'Add-ons' (electrolytes, metabolites).

Implications for practice

- Acidosis is usually caused by disease, alkalosis usually by compensation.
- Survival is only possible within a very narrow range of blood pH.
- Analyse ABGs systemically, using the five-step approach.
- Standardised bicarbonate and base excess levels should be used rather than HCO_3^- and BE figure.
- Gases should not be temperature-corrected unless there is an exceptional reason.

Summary

Blood gas analysis remains one of the most valuable means of monitoring respiratory and metabolic function. ICU nurses both take and interpret arterial blood gas samples, so need to know potential sources of error (sampling, transporting), standard unit practices (e.g. whether or not to enter patients' temperature) and how to interpret results, in a logical sequence, in the context of their patient. 'Normal' figures may vary slightly, but principles remain applicable. Electrolytes and metabolites, not discussed here, are included in Chapter 21.

Further reading

Chapters on acid/base balance are included in many physiology, ICU and clinical chemistry/biochemistry texts. Hennessey and Japp (2007) and Foxall (2008) provide useful handbooks, with many scenarios for practice. Articles periodically appear in journals, Coggan (2008) being a useful recent example. Introductory articles periodically appear in nursing and medical journals, such as Baylis and Till (2009). Lian (2010) is also useful, but being from the USA uses mmHg.

Clinical scenarios

Patient 1: 36-year-old female who is unconscious from taking an aspirin overdose.

Patient 2: 45-year-old male, a known alcoholic with a history of vomiting, had developed difficulty breathing.

Patient 3: 62-year-old male with a history of congestive cardiac failure with 15 per cent *ejection fraction*, had developed pneumonia and bilateral pleural effusions.

Patient 4: 75-year-old female, had a dynamic hip replacement, and developed a chest infection, reduced respiratory function and possible pulmonary embolism.

Arterial blood gas analyses on admission of these four patients to the ICU:

	Patient 1	*Patient 2*	*Patient 3*	*Patient 4*
FiO_2	0.6	0.35	0.28	0.4
pH	7.25	7.55	7.48	7.29
PaO_2 (kPa)	9.32	11.9	12.6	7.49
$PaCO_2$ (kPa)	8.10	4.6	3.05	11.05
HCO_3^- (mmol/litre)	21.2	34.4	20.1	33.7
BE (mmol/litre)	1.9	6	−6.3	12.4
Lactate (mmol/litre)	1.5	0.7	0.8	0.5

Q.1 Identify the acid/base status of the four blood gases (acidosis, alkalosis, respiratory, metabolic, compensated or uncompensated).

Q.2 Analyse the likely causes of the acid/base disturbances. Consider their effect on other organs/systems and how the ICU nurse can assess, anticipate and minimise any potentially adverse effects.

Q.3 Review potential sources and direction of analytical errors (e.g. air bubbles in blood sample can falsely decrease PO_2) that can occur with these blood gas analysis results.

Chapter 20

Haemodynamic monitoring

Contents

Fundamental knowledge	184
Introduction	185
Skin assessment	185
Arterial blood pressure	185
Non-invasive blood pressure measurement	186
Intra-arterial measurement	186
Central venous pressure	188
Dangers	190
Removal	191
PICCs	191
Cardiac output studies (flow monitoring)	191
Ultrasound	195
Other technologies/NIRS	195
Implications for practice	196
Summary	196
Further reading	196
Clinical scenario	196

Fundamental knowledge

Experience of using invasive monitoring (including 'zeroing')
Cardiac physiology: atria, ventricles, valves
Cardiac cycle: systole, diastole
Relationship between cardiac electrical activity (ECG) and output (pulse, blood pressure)
How breathing affects venous return
V/Q mismatch
Oxygen dissociation (see Chapter 18)

Introduction

The purpose of the cardiovascular system is perfusion, supplying cells with oxygen and glucose needed for normal anaerobic metabolism (energy) and removing metabolic waste (carbon dioxide, metabolic acids, water). Without perfusion, cells die. Haemodynamic monitoring therefore aims to indicate perfusion.

More invasive (e.g. cardiac output monitoring) modes generally provide more information, but create more problems/risks. Options chosen therefore depend on balancing benefits against burdens. Monitoring equipment is diagnostic, not therapeutic, so once risks outweigh benefits, or maximum time limits are reached, it should be removed.

'Normal' figures are cited here as a guide, but many assume 'average' 70 kg patients, and individuals can have wide healthy variations, so trends are more important than isolated measurements.

Skin assessment

Pale, discoloured, cyanosed or clammy skin indicates poor perfusion (whether from hypovolaemia, vascular disease or excessive vasoconstriction). Although non-invasive and easily visible, skin discolouration may be acute or chronic, and has limited value in critical illness. Peripheral warmth and pulses indicate perfusion, and are especially important to assess after vascular surgery. Excessively warm and flushed peripheries indicate excessive vasodilatation (e.g. sepsis).

Capillary refill measures peripheral perfusion. Capillary refill is assessed by pressing on a finger pad or nailbed for 5 seconds. On releasing pressure, initial blanching should vanish within 2 seconds (Jevon, 2007). Delayed capillary refill indicates peripheral perfusion failure, from hypotension, hypovolaemia or excessive peripheral vascular resistance, but should not be used to imply perfusion of main organs (Pamba and Maitland, 2004).

Arterial blood pressure

This is the pressure exerted on arterial walls. Pressure is determined by flow and resistance. Flow is affected by driving force (cardiac output, or left ventricular ejection) and viscosity. Resistance (afterload) is both vascular (constriction, atherosclerosis) and interstitial (e.g. oedema). Capillary blood flow ('*microcirculation*') is reduced if blood viscosity increases (see Chapter 21).

Systolic pressure indicates perfusion, although mean arterial pressure (MAP) is a better measure of this. Systolic pressure increases with distance from the heart, so pedal arterial lines usually measure higher systolic pressures than radial ones.

Diastolic pressure is the pressure exerted on the arterial wall during the resting phase of the cardiac cycle. Abnormally low diastolic pressure (< 80 mmHg) indicates either hypovolaemia or vasodilatation. Once CVP is optimised with fluids, vasopressors (e.g. noradrenaline) may be needed.

185

Of the three pressures, MAP is least affected by differences between arteries or artefact, such as damp traces (Darovic, 2002b; Safar *et al.*, 2003), so with poor arterial traces, MAP usually remains reliable. 'Normal' MAP is about 90–105 mmHg. The sepsis care bundle suggests a minimum acceptable MAP is 65 mmHg, although hypertensive patients may need higher pressures to perfuse organs.

Pulse pressure, the pressure created by each pulse (systolic minus diastolic), indicates vessel response to pulse. Stereotypical normal pulse pressure is:

120 – 80 = 40 mmHg.

High (wide) pulse pressures usually indicate vascular disease, such as atherosclerosis (Haider *et al.*, 2003), while low (narrow) pulse pressures usually indicate arterial hypovolaemia, which may be caused by:

- systemic hypovolaemia;
- poor cardiac output;
- excessive vasodilatation (e.g. SIRS).

Other haemodynamic monitoring (e.g. CVP) may indicate likely causes.

Non-invasive blood pressure measurement

Cuff pressure monitoring provides adequate information for most hospitalised patients, but greater frequency and accuracy is usually needed in the ICU. A common error is to use cuffs that are the wrong size for patients. Smaller cuffs over-read, while larger cuffs under-read. Non-invasive blood pressure is 'dampened' by tissues between arteries and skin surfaces. Intra-arterial measurement should be more accurate, often being 5–20 mmHg above non-invasive pressure measurements.

Intra-arterial measurement

Direct (invasive) arterial pressure monitoring provides:

- continuous measurement;
- visual display;
- access to arterial blood for sampling.

Pulse waveform (see Figure 20.1) indicates cardiac function:

- The area beneath the wave indicates pulse volume.
- The upstroke indicates myocardial contractility; normally it should be almost vertical; shallower upstrokes indicate poor flow; changes in shape can indicate response to inotropes (Easby and Dalrymple, 2009).
- Downstrokes are normally almost vertical, like the upstroke; more gentle downslopes occur with vasoconstriction (Easby and Dalrymple, 2009).

- The *dicrotic notch* (closure of the aortic valve) normally occurs about one-quarter to one-third of the way down the downstroke; its position indicates peripheral vascular resistance (high dicrotic notch = vasoconstriction, low = vasodilatation (Easby and Dalrymple, 2009)); poorly defined or absent dicrotic notches indicate aortic valve incompetence.
- Extensive systemic vasodilatation and low systemic vascular resistance (e.g. SIRS) can cause an *anacrotic notch* on upstrokes, with widening of the dicrotic notch.

Breathing can cause 'arterial swing', but significant arterial swing usually indicates hypovolaemia, where inspiration causes significantly reduced stroke volumes. Rises in late inspiration can also be caused by cardiac overload.

Disconnection, or significant oozing around arterial cannulae, can cause rapid blood loss, so security of connections should be checked, sites covered by transparent bio-occlusive dressings, and (if possible) placed where easily observed. Waveform display should be continuously monitored, with alarms normally set to give early warning of problems such as hypertension, hypotension and disconnection. Although rare, arterial lines can occlude arteries, so care should include checking colour, warmth and capillary refill of extremities beyond cannulae.

Errors can be caused by:

- *transducer level* – (should be at heart level; small changes in height cause large errors in measurement);
- *occlusion* – patency should be maintained with continuous infusion (normally at 300 mmHg) with 'normal' saline (Kannan, 2008; Mitchell *et al.*, 2009);

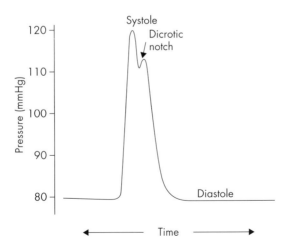

Figure 20.1 Arterial trace

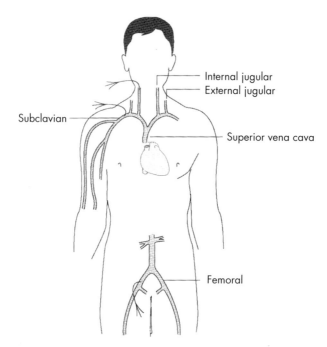

Figure 20.2 Main central venous cannulation sites

■ *drugs* – no drug should be given through arterial lines (bolus concentrations can be toxic), so lines and all connections/taps should be clearly labelled and identified (NPSA, 2008a).

Central venous pressure

Central lines, or central venous catheters (CVCs), are widely used in ICUs, for both monitoring and access (see Figure 20.2). Transducers should be 'zeroed' at midaxilla level – open the port from the monitor to air, and press calibration ('zero'). Ideally, pressure should be measured:

■ From the distal (tip) lumen, with no other infusions running simultaneously through that lumen. When distal lumens are unavailable, differences from other lumens are usually insignificant.
■ With the patient supine – because most ICU patients are usually nursed semi-recumbent, CVP is frequently measured in other positions. Transducer level can vary significantly between staff (Figg and Nemergut, 2009). More upright positions reduce pressure. Measurements taken when patients are on their sides are unreliable.
■ With the transducer placed midaxilla (phlebostatic axis: intersection of lines from midsternal fourth intercostal space and midaxilla).

Central venous pressure (CVP) directly measures pressure in the vena cava (usually, superior), so is determined by:

- blood volume returning to the heart ('filling pressure' or 'preload');
- function of the right atrium and ventricle;
- intrathoracic pressure.

Normal CVP for self-ventilating patients is 0 to +8 mmHg (mean +4 mmHg). Normal range increases with positive intrathoracic pressure (by 3–5 cmH$_2$O) and with PEEP/CPAP.

Low CVP usually indicates fluid loss (e.g. haemorrhage, excessive *diuresis*, gross *extravasation*), although Marik *et al.* (2008) deny that CVP indicates circulating blood volume. Various factors can cause high CVP:

- hypervolaemia (e.g. excessive fluid infusion, kidney injury);
- cardiac failure (e.g. right ventricular failure, pulmonary embolism, mitral valve failure/regurgitation, tamponade);
- increased intrathoracic pressure (e.g. positive pressure ventilation, PEEP/CPAP);
- lumen occlusion/obstruction (e.g. cannula against vein wall; thrombus);
- high blood viscosity (rare, but possible following massive blood transfusion);
- artefact (e.g. fluids infusing through transduced lumen).

If causes of high pressure are not obvious, nurses should seek advice. Very high pressures (> 18 mmHg) may indicate pulmonary oedema.

Central venous pressure being far lower than arterial, waveforms are more difficult to analyse, but should show three phases: 'a' (with 'x' descent), 'c' and 'v' (with 'y' descent) (see Figure 20.3):

a: initiated by right atrial contraction, so is absent with atrial fibrillation, and peaked with diseases such as right ventricular failure and pulmonary hypertension (Wagih and Arthurs, 2008);

x: atrial pressure falls with atrial relaxation (systolic contraction), so will be absent with tricuspid regurgitation (Wagih and Arthurs, 2008);

c: initiated by right ventricular contraction and tricuspid valve closure, so should follow the QRS wave on ECGs;

v: initiated with right atrial filling (so corresponds with T waves on ECGs); peaked with tricuspid valve disease;

y: pressure falls with tricuspid valve opening (ventricular filling).

Breathing causes 'respiratory swing':

- rising with positive pressure ventilator breaths (increased intrathoracic pressure);
- falling with self-ventilating breaths (negative pressure).

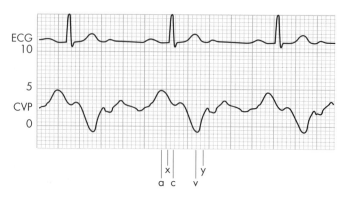

■ *Figure 20.3 CVP waveform*

Where transducer monitoring is not available, manometers can measure CVP. Mercury being neurotoxic, manometers use isotonic fluids (e.g. 5% glucose). Readings are therefore in centimetres of water (cmH_2O) rather than millimetres of mercury (mmHg):

$1 \ cmH_2O = 0.74 \ mmHg$
$1.36 \ cmH_2O = 1 \ mmHg.$

Differences, negligible with low pressures, accumulate with higher ones.

Dangers

Inserting central lines can puncture any surrounding tissue (lung puncture = pneumothorax, arteries, myocardium). Insertion may also accidentally be retrograde (e.g. passing up, rather than down, the internal jugular vein). Nurses assisting during insertion should observe patients and monitors (ECG, airway pressures), reporting any concerns. Once inserted, lines should be stitched and position checked by X-ray before use.

Once inserted, problems include:

■ infection
■ dysrhythmias
■ air emboli.

Infection is usually from skin commensals (Safdar and Maki, 2004). Curtis (2009) suggests about 1 in 20 become infected, while the DH (2007b) suggests that CVCs are responsible for more than two-fifths of sepsis, although evidence for such statements is often very old. Rates are higher with femoral lines (Waldmann and Barnes, 2004). Heparin-coated lines reduce thrombosis and infection (Long and Coulthard, 2006), but chlorhexidine and silver sulfadiazine impregnation does not reduce infection (Camargo *et al.*, 2009). Provided they are intact and not soiled, dressings should only be changed every seven days (Smith, M., 2007).

Dysrhythmias can be precipitated by many causes, including mechanical irritation from catheters introduced into the heart. ECG should be continuously monitored, and any unexplained dysrhythmias reported and recorded.

Air emboli of 50–100 ml are fatal (Polderman and Girbes, 2002). The small bubbles often seen in intravenous lines are not harmful, but (self-ventilating) negative intrathoracic pressure of 4 cmH$_2$O could draw 90 ml of air in one second through an 18-gauge needle (Polderman and Girbes, 2002). Central lines should, whenever possible, be easily visible and checked regularly, especially with self-ventilating patients. Nurses should regularly check all connections are secure.

Removal

Central lines should be removed with patients positioned head-down (RCN, 2003b), so any accidental air emboli do not rise to cerebral circulation. Self-ventilating patients should breathe out and hold their breath (out) during removal, so intrathoracic pressure equals atmospheric pressure.

PICCs

Peripherally inserted central cannulae (PICCs) are used more in wards and the community than in ICUs. They pose a far lower infection risk than other central lines, but:

- provide limited access (most a single lumen, some are double);
- debatably, may not provide reliable CVP;
- are often misplaced (Tan *et al.*, 2009);
- are prone to block (Tan *et al.*, 2009).

Cardiac output studies (flow monitoring)

CVP measures cardiac preload, but *flow monitoring* provides more information about heart, and vascular, function. Direct and derived measurements, with commonly used abbreviations, are described below, with normal ranges summarised in Table 20.1. Not all measurements are available with all systems. Most measurements are derived, relying on information such as:

- haemoglobin
- central venous pressure.

Indexing output to body surface area (m^2 – by entering height and weight) makes figures comparable between patients of different weight, so is generally used. Like other derived measurements, incorrect data fed into machines causes incorrect results. All systems are less reliable with irregular rhythms (e.g. atrial fibrillation).

Table 20.1 Normal flow monitoring parameters (not all parameters are available on all machines)

CI	2.5–4.2 litres/minute/m²
CO	4–8 litres/minute
CVP (self-ventilating)	0 to +8 mmHg (right atrial level)
DO$_2$	900–1100 litres/minute
DO$_2$I	520–720 ml/minute/m²
EVLW	5–7 ml/kg (3500–4000 ml for 70 kg)
LCWI	3.4–4.2 kg/m/m²
LVSWI	50–60 gm/m/m²
PAP	10–20 mmHg
PPV	< 10 per cent
PVR	< 250 dynes/second/cm⁵
PVRI	255–285 dynes/second/cm⁵/cm²
RCW	0.54–0.66 km/m/m²
RVSWI	7.9–9.7 gm/m/m²
SVV	< 10 per cent
SV	about 70 ml at rest (range 60–120 ml)
SVI	35–70 ml/beat/m²
SvO$_2$	75 per cent
SVR	800–1200 dynes/second/cm⁵
SVRI	2000–24000 dynes/second/cm⁵/m²
VO$_2$	200–290 litres/minute
VO$_2$I	100–180 ml/minute/m²

Pulmonary artery catheters (PACs; also called pulmonary artery flotation catheters – PAFCs – and 'Swan Ganz') have largely been replaced by less invasive alternatives (Wiener and Welch, 2007). Any readers encountering one should only use it if they are competent to do so; many older ICU texts describe PAFCs. Some measurements below are only available with PAFCs.

Less invasive options include:

- *PICCO* – peripherally inserted continuous cardiac output;
- *LidCO®* – lithium-derived cardiac output;
- *FloTrac®*;
- transoesophageal *Doppler*.

All four analyse pulse waveform (contour) to derive measurements. Comparability and reliability of all technologies has been much studied and disputed, but most measurements are reliable (Lamia *et al.*, 2008). However, irregular rhythms, such as atrial fibrillation, and some drugs, such as paralysing agents, can make measurements unreliable.

Non-invasive means include:

- thoracic electrical bioimpedance;
- partial carbon dioxide rebreathing;
- radial pulse applanation tonometry.

Thoracic electrical bioimpedance (TEB) uses ECG-like electrodes, measuring differences in thoracic resistance (bioimpedance) to high-frequency, very low-magnitude electrical currents. Aortic flow supplies less than 1 per cent of thoracic bioimpedance, so high signal-to-noise ratio may cause significant inaccuracies. Whole-body electrical bioimpedance is accurate (Cotter *et al.*, 2004), but TEB less so (Chaney and Derdak, 2002), and the latter has not been widely adopted in UK ICUs.

Partial carbon dioxide rebreathing causes patients to periodically rebreathe (carbon dioxide-rich) gas. Capnography then measures differences between breathing and non-rebreathing carbon dioxide tensions. As acid/base buffering keeps venous carbon dioxide tensions essentially constant, differences in arterial carbon dioxide reflect cardiac output. Both animal and human studies show good correlation with thermodilution measurements. Readings are available at 3-minute cycles. However capnography relies on constant respiratory rate to tidal volume ratio, so use of partial carbon dioxide rebreathing to measure cardiac output is confined to ventilated patients (without triggering). It should not be used if rebreathing carbon dioxide may cause problems.

Radial pulse applanation tonometry is not suitable for critically ill patients, as it does not reflect responses to fluid bolus or changes of inotropes (Compton *et al.*, 2008).

Cardiac output (CO)
Normal: 4–8 litres/minute

Cardiac index (CI)
Normal: 2.5–4.2 litres/minute/m^2

Cardiac output is the volume of blood ejected over one minute. Cardiac index may be increased by compensation for critical illness and/or inotropes. Low cardiac index indicates myocardial dysfunction.

Stroke volume (SV)
Normal: About 70 ml at rest (range 60–120 ml)

Stroke volume index (SVI)
Normal: 35–70 ml/beat/m^2

Stroke volume is the volume of blood ejected with each contraction of the heart, so HR × SV = CO. Stroke volume relies on adequate preload and muscle contractility; if stroke volume is poor, preload (CVP) should be optimised with fluids before using inotropes.

Systemic vascular resistance (SVR)
Systemic vascular resistance index (SVRI)
Normal: SVR 800–1200 dynes/second/cm^5
       SVRI: 2000–24000 dynes/second/cm^5/m^2

Systemic vascular resistance ('afterload') is the resistance met by cardiac output from blood vessels. Blood pressure is the sum of HR × SV × SVR. Excessive vasodilatation (distributive shock, such as SIRS) reduces SVR. SVR monitoring is therefore useful for inotrope/vasopressor therapy.

Left cardiac work (LCW)
Left cardiac work index (LCWI)
Normal LCWI: 3.4–4.2 kgm/m^2

Left ventricular stroke work (LVSW)
Left ventricular stroke work index (LVSWI)
Normal LVSWI: 50–60 gmm/m^2

Managing severe left ventricular failure is a delicate balance between maintaining adequate cardiac output and myocardial oxygenation. Insufficient work deprives the brain of oxygen; excessive work deprives the myocardium of oxygen.

Right cardiac work (RCW)
Right cardiac work index (RCWI)
Right ventricular stroke work (RVSW)
Right ventricular stroke work index (RVSWI)
Normal: RCW 0.54–0.66 km/m/m^2
        RVSWI: 7.9–9.7 gm/m/m^2

Measuring right ventricular function assists management with right heart failure.

Pulmonary artery pressure (PAP)
Normal: $\dfrac{8\text{–}15}{15\text{–}25}$ mmHg

Pulmonary vascular resistance (PVR)
Pulmonary vascular resistance index (PVRI)
Normal: PVR < 250 dynes/second/cm^5
        PVRI 255–285 dynes/second/cm^5/cm^2

Pulmonary hypertension may be caused by ARDS, pulmonary oedema, pulmonary embolism and other pathologies. Pulmonary hypotension with high central venous pressure indicates right-sided heart disease, such as tricuspid valve stenosis/regurgitation or right ventricular infarction (usually inferior myocardial infarction) or septal defects (rare in adults).

Delivery of oxygen (DO$_2$)
Delivery of oxygen index (DO$_2$I)
Normal: DO$_2$ 900–1100 litres/minute
        DO$_2$I 520–720 ml/minute/m^2

This indicates whether oxygen reached its target – the tissues.

Consumption of oxygen (VO_2)
Consumption of oxygen index (VO_2I)
Normal: VO_2 200–290 litres/minute
        VO_2I 100–180 ml/minute/m^2

Oxygen is needed by all cells, so delivery has little value unless tissues extract it.

Stroke volume variation (SVV)
Normal: < 10 per cent

Stroke volume varies with changes in intrathoracic pressure (breathing). In health, provided heart rhythm is regular, variations are small, but hypovolaemia increases variations. SVV > 10 per cent indicates need for fluids, provided the chest is not open (Wyffels *et al.*, 2010).

Hypotension with SVV < 10 per cent is usually an indication for inotropic support. SVV is unreliable with irregular rhythms, especially atrial fibrillation, as changes in ventricular filling time significantly alter stroke volumes.

Pulse pressure variation (PPV) is similar to SVV, and similarly is normally < 10 per cent.

Extravascular lung water (EVLW)
Normal: 5–7 ml/kg (3500–4000 ml for 70 kg)

Aggressive fluid management may cause pulmonary oedema, progressing to ARDS. Calculating EVLW therefore enables optimisation of fluid management (Sakka *et al.*, 2002) and inotrope therapy (Salukhe and Wyncoll, 2002).

Ultrasound

Ultrasound enables visualisation and measurement of the heart and blood flow through central vessels, so is valuable for medical diagnosis. Among the most frequent measurement from cardiac ultrasound is *ejection fraction*. The average healthy adult left ventricle can hold about 130 ml of blood, but only ejects 70–90 ml. The volume ejected can therefore be expressed as a fraction, or more often percentage, of total ventricular volume. A normal healthy ejection fraction is 0.6–0.75, or 60–70 per cent. Smaller ejection fractions usually indicate extensive left ventricular damage, usually from myocardial infarction.

Other technologies/NIRS

Technological developments continue to offer new means and alternatives for monitoring. For example, Nanas *et al.* (2009) recommend near infrared spectroscopy (NIRS) for assessing microcirculation (tissue oxygen deficits).

Implications for practice

■ Skin colour, warmth and capillary refill time indicate peripheral perfusion.
■ Diastolic blood pressure and pulse pressure indicate systemic vascular resistance.
■ Mean arterial pressure (MAP) indicates perfusion pressure.
■ Intra-arterial blood pressure monitoring is usually more accurate than non-invasive measurement, provided arterial traces do not look dampened.
■ Low CVP indicates hypovolaemia; high CVP may be from fluid overload, cardiac failure, positive intrathoracic pressure, user error or catheter obstruction.
■ Indexed measurements are adjusted to body surface area (m^2), so are usually used.
■ SvO_2 (compared with SaO_2) indicates oxygen uptake.
■ SVR is useful for assessing effects of vasopressors.
■ SVV and EVLW enable optimisation of fluid therapy.

Summary

Haemodynamic monitoring necessarily forms a major aspect of intensive care nursing. Means described here can provide much information to guide therapy. All modes, especially invasive ones, have complications, so should only be used if benefits outweigh problems. Nurses should actively assess and, where possible, initiate appropriate monitoring. Equipment should only be used by staff competent to do so, and within manufacturers' guidelines and time limits.

Further reading

NPSA (2008a) highlight problems and recommend good practices with arterial lines.

Manufacturer's booklets and websites can be useful resources for cardiac output (flow monitoring) analysers. Many medical articles explore specific aspects, while Easby and Dalrymple (2009) review broader aspects.

Clinical scenario

Ellen Harrison, 62 years old, is admitted to the ICU with a chest infection and possible sepsis. She is sedated, mechanically ventilated with intravenous infusions of noradrenaline at 0.4 µg/kg/minute and milrinone at 248 ng/kg/minute. Mrs Harrison is 1.75 m tall and weighs 75 kg (body surface area of 1.90 m^2). A pulmonary artery catheter is floated to provide additional information and tract responses to drug infusions.

Her haemodynamic profile reveals:

BP	140/50 mmHg (MAP 80 mmHg)	
HR	112 bpm	
Rhythm	Sinus tachycardia with self-terminating runs of unifocal ventricular ectopics	
CVP	16 mmHg	
CO	5.6 litres/minute	CI 2.9 litres/minute/m^2
SV	61 ml	SVI 32 ml/beat/m^2
SVR	744 dynes/second/cm^5	SVRI 1416 dynes/second/cm^5/m^2
PVR	157 dynes/second/cm^5	PVRI 300 dynes/second/cm^5/m^2
LVSWI	23 gm/m/m^2	
RVSWI	4 gm/m/m^2	
PAP	38/20 mmHg (mean PAP = 27 mmHg)	
PCWP	14 mmHg	
SvO$_2$	81 per cent	

Q.1 (a) Identify nursing interventions that can assist in preventing complications associated with PA catheters.

   (b) Why is a chest X-ray performed after the insertion of a PA catheter?

   (c) Note symptoms that may indicate pulmonary infarction.

Q.2 Compare Mrs Harrison's haemodynamic values to normal parameters. Reflect on the likely cause and implications of abnormal results, for example on Mrs Harrison's perfusion and oxygen delivery; will she be warm, cool, dilated, constricted?

Q.3 Consider the clinical implications of Mrs Harrison's haemodynamic values and how they may guide changes in her vasoactive drug infusions rates. Devise a plan of care to include rationales for choice of prescribed drugs and/or fluid therapies and haemodynamic goals.

Chapter 21

Blood results

Contents

Introduction   199
Haematology   199
Biochemistry   204
Implications for practice   210
Summary   211
Further reading   211
Clinical scenario   211

Introduction

Blood is a transport mechanism, so contents reflect body activity. Recognising abnormal values and knowing what to do about them enables early and appropriate interventions. This chapter outlines main haematology and biochemistry results. Liver function tests are outlined in Chapter 41 and cardiac markers (e.g. troponin) are included in Chapter 29.

Although results are discussed individually below, low levels may be caused by:

- dilution;
- loss;
- failure of supply or production;

while high levels may be from:

- dehydration (haemoconcentration);
- excessive intake/production;
- failure to metabolise or remove (e.g. hepatic or renal dysfunction).

Dilution (from large-volume intravenous infusion) and haemoconcentration (from excessive drainage or fluid shifts) are not identified specifically below, but should always be considered as possible causes of abnormal results.

Erroneous results may be caused by sampling errors:

- venepuncturing limbs where IVIs are running;
- insufficient blood;
- incorrect bottles;
- incorrect inversion times for bottles (resulting in insufficient mixing of additives);
- incorrect labelling;

so results appearing inconsistent with patients' clinical state should be checked.

Many treatments of abnormalities are identified, but other treatments are possible. Treatments identified are those normally used on ICUs, so are not necessarily appropriate in other settings.

Haematology

Blood has three types of cells:

- erythrocytes (red blood cells – RBCs);
- leucocytes (white cells);
- platelets;

Table 21.1 Erythrocyte results

RBC	males	$4.5–6.5 \times 10^{-12}/\text{litre}$
	females	$3.9–5.6 \times 10^{-12}/\text{litre}$
Hb	males	13–18 gr/dl
	females	11.5–16.5 g/dl
PCV/Hct	males	40–52%
	females	36–48%
MCV (mean cell volume)		$80–95 \ \mu m^{-3}$
MCD (mean cylindrical diameter)		$6.7–7.7 \ \mu m$
MCHC (mean corpuscular haemoglobin concentration)		32–35 g/dl
MCH (mean corpuscular haemoglobin)		28–32/g

so, a full blood count includes:

- haemoglobin (oxygen carriage);
- white cell count (WCC – immunity), with specific types of white cells also measured;
- platelets and other clotting measurements.

Albumin, total (plasma) protein and clotting are also discussed. All blood cells are produced by bone marrow, so diseases or treatments causing bone marrow suppression affect counts of all cells. Tests that can be performed on erythrocytes are summarised in Table 21.1.

Haemoglobin (Hb)

Normal: 13–18 g/dl (men) 11.5–16.5 (women).

Polycythaemia (raised levels), usually an adaptive response to chronic hypoxia, can be caused by living at high altitudes, but in the UK is usually caused by chronic lung, or sometimes cardiac, disease.

Critical illness usually causes low levels from:

- blood loss
- dilution
- reduced *erythropoiesis*
- premature haemolysis from disease (e.g. sepsis) and filtration

and sometimes anaemia or other causes, including iatrogenic.

Haemoglobin transports most oxygen in arterial blood, so low haemoglobin reduces oxygen-carrying capacity. Oxygen delivery to cells is a paradox between oxygen carriage (erythrocytes) with oxygen delivery (plasma). Blood is plasma and cells; plasma is mainly (90–95 per cent) water, and most blood cells (99 per cent) are erythrocytes. Higher haemoglobin concentrations therefore make blood thicker, while lower levels make it more dilute. Dilute blood flows more easily through capillaries, from which tissue cells receive oxygen. So dilute blood carries less oxygen, but delivers it more effectively. Moderate anaemia improves survival from critical illness, survival being highest with Hb 7–9 g/dl (Hebert *et al.*, 1999), although in older people anaemia increases mortality and morbidity (Eisenstaedt *et al.*, 2006). Many intensivists aim for levels of 8–10 in most older patients.

Because most blood cells are erythrocytes, packed cell volume (PCV), or haematocrit (Hct), also indicates erythrocytes, as a percentage of total volume.

Treatment: Low Hb (< 7 g/dl) can be treated by blood transfusion.

White cell count (WCC)

Normal: $5–10 \times 10^3$/microlitre.

Although often called white blood cells, most white cells live outside the bloodstream. For example, only 2–3 per cent of neutrophils (by far the largest type of white cell) are in the bloodstream (Storey and Jordan, 2008). White cells use the bloodstream to move about; inflammation attracts white cells back into blood so they can move to infected areas. Hence new infections cause rapid rises in WCC.

However, increases may be caused by non-infective triggering of the immune system, while immunodeficiency can cause a lack of response to infection. Severe/prolonged infection may deplete reserves, hence low counts (<4) may indicate severe sepsis. Infection cannot therefore be excluded if counts are normal or low.

Low counts (leucopaenia) can be treated with granulocyte colony-stimulating factor (G-CSF), but this takes some days to work so, although useful for oncology, it has little value in critical illness.

There are two main groups of leucocytes:

- granulocytes
- agranulocytes

identified by whether or not cell membranes contain granules. Granulocytes tackle acute infections, whereas agranulocytes provide longer-term defences. Both main groups have further sub-types of cells. Normal counts are identified in Table 21.2.

Treatment: Usually, underlying causes are treated (e.g. infection with anti-biotics). Low neutrophil count may be an indication for protective isolation (reverse barrier nursing).

Table 21.2 Normal white cell counts

White cell type	x 10^9/litre	per mm^3	%
neutrophils (polymorphs)	2.5–7.5	2500–7500	50–70
basophils	< 0.2	< 200	≤ 3
eosinophils	0.04–0.44	40–400	≤ 5
lymphocytes	1.5–4.0	1500–4000	≤ 12–50
monocytes	0.2–0.8	200–800	3–15

Note: UK uses x 10^9/litre.

Granulocytes

There are three types of granulocytes:

- neutrophils (polymorphoneuclear, so 'polymorphs')
- basophils
- eosinophils

identified by laboratory staining.

Most leucocytes (50–70 per cent) are neutrophils. Neutrophils are the first and main defence against infection, destroying bacteria by phagocytosis, resulting in pus. With infection, neutrophil count rises before other types of leucocytes.

Basophils and eosinophils are not usually significant in critical illness, but both may indicate allergic reactions (Storey and Jordan, 2008).

Agranulocytes

There are two types of agranulocytes:

- lymphocytes – T and B cells
- monocytes.

Agranulocytes are an important part of immunity, lymphocytes recognising and tackling antigens, and monocytes migrating into tissues. But they have limited value for critical illness, while excessive/inappropriate lymphocyte reactions can cause *anaphylaxis*.

Platelets (thrombocytes)

Normal: 150–400 × 10^9/litre.

Platelets circulate for about ten days. Normally kept inactive by endovascular chemicals (e.g. prostacyclin), they are activated by platelet-activating factor (PAF; released by the endothelium of damaged blood vessels) to assist clotting.

Platelet counts are often low in critical illness, from:

- loss from bleeding;
- impaired production;
- anti-platelet drugs (e.g. aspirin, clopidogrel).

However, impaired blood flow and immobility exposes ICU patients to high risk of deep vein thrombosis (DVT), and pulmonary embolism (PE). ICU patients should therefore be prescribed prophylactic anticoagulants, titrated against clotting studies, and given thromboembolism deterrent stockings (TEDS™) unless there are specific contraindications to either (Cayley, 2007).

Treatment: Platelets can be transfused if indicated.

Albumin and total protein (TP)

Normal: Albumin 35–50 g/litre.
Total protein (TP): 60–80 g/litre.

Plasma proteins create most of the colloid osmotic pressure that retains normal plasma volume within the bloodstream. Proteins also:

- bind drugs and chemicals (see calcium, page 208);
- transport substances (e.g. bilirubin);
- are antioxidants;

so plasma protein, especially albumin, deficiency causes excessive extravasation, hypovolaemia, oedema and many other complications. Although there are many plasma proteins, more than half total protein concentration is albumin, and albumin exerts three-quarters of plasma protein colloid osmotic pressure.

Hypoalbuminaemia and low levels of other plasma proteins are multifactorial, caused by:

- *catabolism* provoking protein metabolism;
- malnutrition (see Chapter 9);
- liver hypofunction (see Chapter 41).

Normal albumin half-life is 18–20 days (Maloney *et al.*, 2002), so although protein levels can be viewed as a marker of illness/recovery, changes take many days to occur. Low albumin correlates with muscle weakness (Schalk *et al.*, 2005) and increases mortality (Palma *et al.*, 2007).

Treatment: Exogenous albumin has only transient effects. Early nutrition (see Chapter 9) provides proteins needed in critical illness for tissue repair (McClave *et al.*, 2009).

Clotting

Normal: APTT 25–35 seconds.
PT 10–12 seconds.
INR 0.9–1.1.

In addition to platelet count, clotting is usually measured by:

- activated partial thromboplastin time (APTT or PTT), which measures the intrinsic clotting pathway;
- activated prothrombin time (APT or PT), which measures the extrinsic clotting pathway;
- international normalised ratio (INR), which indicates overall clotting time (intrinsic + extrinsic pathways).

Treatment: With anticoagulant therapy target INR should normally be about 2.5 (Baglin *et al.*, 2006).

D-dimers

Normal: < 250 ng/ml (μg/litre), sometimes reported as 'negative'.

D-dimers are fibrin degradation products, released by fibrinolysis (clot break-down). Raised levels therefore indicate either significant clot to breakdown (DVT or PE) or reduced (renal) clearance. Negative D-dimers can exclude DVT or PE (Task Force, 2008a), but positive levels cannot confirm diagnosis (Rathbun *et al.*, 2004), so this test is not often used.

Treatment: Treat the disease – e.g. with intravenous heparin.

Biochemistry

The main urea and electrolyte (U+E) results used in ICUs, and the ones discussed here, are:

- C-reactive protein (CRP)
- sodium (Na^+)
- chloride (Cl^-)
- potassium (K^+)
- glucose ($C^6H^{12}O^6$)
- phosphate (PO_4^{3-})
- magnesium (Mg^{++} or Mg^{2+})
- calcium (Ca^{++} or Ca^{2+})
- creatinine
- urea.

C-reactive protein (CRP)

Normal: 0–10 mg/ml.

CRP is an acute phase protein, serum levels rising within 4–6 hours after an inflammatory trigger (McWilliam and Riordan, 2010). Causes of inflammation are inferred from individual patient contexts; in ICU, CRP usually indicates sepsis (Póvoa, 2002; Warren *et al.*, 2002). Failure to reduce within 48 hours of antibiotics probably indicates treatment failure (McWilliam and Riordan, 2010).

Treatment: Treat the disease – e.g. SIRS with system support.

Sodium (Na⁺)

Normal: 135–145 mmol/litre.

Sodium is the main intravascular cation. In critical illness, abnormal levels usually indicate hydration status:

- acute *hypernatraemia* = (usually) dehydration (Fisher and Macnaughton, 2006; Reynolds *et al.*, 2006);
- hyponatraemia = haemodilution (Reynolds *et al.*, 2006), such as fluid overload (e.g. renal failure) or shifts from cells (where sodium concentration is normally 14 mmol/litre).

Abnormal levels are neurotoxic, levels below 120 causing encephalopathy, and levels above 160 causing fitting. Hypernatraemia (> 150) strongly predicts mortality (O'Donoghue *et al.*, 2009).

Treatment: Hyponatrameia is treated by giving sodium, usually as 0.9% sodium chloride ('normal saline'), relying on the kidney to remove excess water while conserving salt. Hypernatraemia usually indicates dehydration, rehydration being achieved with water, usually as 5% glucose.

Chloride (Cl⁻)

Normal: 95–105 mmol/litre.

As 0.9% sodium chloride is hyperchloraemic (154 mmol/litre chloride), excessive saline infusions can cause hyperchloraemic acidaemia. Hyperchloraemia can also impair mental function and cause abdominal discomfort, headaches, nausea and vomiting.

Treatment: Hyperchloraemia is usually from excessive saline infusions, which should be discontinued. Hypochloraemia is rare, and rarely problematic.

Potassium (K⁺)

Normal: 3.5–4.5 mmol/litre.

Most (98 per cent) body potassium is inside cells (Greenlee *et al.*, 2009). Serum potassium is used for cardiac conduction; *hypokalaemia* impairs conduction, so can provoke bradycardia and escape dysrhythmias, while *hyperkalaemia* can cause tachydysrhythmias. With patients at risk of cardiac dysfunction (most ICU patients), it is safer to maintain levels at 4–5 mmol/litre, slightly higher than normal physiological levels. Laboratory results may be > 1 mmol/litre higher than ABGs, as clots form in sample bottles, releasing potassium into serum (Parry *et al.*, 2010).

Most (90 per cent) potassium loss is renal, so serum potassium levels usually reflect urine output: polyuria causes hypokalaemia, while oliguria causes hyperkalaemia. Haemofiltration causes rapid potassium loss, unless physiological levels are added to *dialysate*/replacement. Intracellular fluid contains about 150 mmol/litre, so extensive cell damage (such as major trauma) or large fluid shifts can cause hyperkalaemia. Haemolysis causes potassium leak from damaged blood cells, so haemolysed samples give high levels. Due to haemolysis, laboratory samples give higher levels than blood gas analysers (Parry *et al.*, 2010).

Treatment: Life-threatening hyperkalaemia (> 6 mmol/litre) should be urgently treated with intravenous glucose and insulin infusion, which transfers potassium into cells (Nyirenda *et al.*, 2009). Concurrent intravenous calcium (gluconate or chloride) stabilises cardiac conduction (Nyirenda *et al.*, 2009). Less severe hyperkalaemia (5–6 mmol/litre) may be treated with calcium resonium, given orally or rectally. If hyperkalaemia is caused by fluid shifts from severe dehydration, patients should be aggressively rehydrated. Salbutamol also transports potassium into cells (Kemper *et al.*, 1996), but supporting evidence is largely paediatric, and the side effect of tachycardia probably makes this unwise in adults.

Hypokalaemia is treated with potassium supplements. Strong potassium concentrations (such as 40 mmol in 100 ml) are often infused in ICUs, but must be given through a central line, as peripheral infusion is very painful and likely to cause severe thrombophlebitis. Strong potassium concentrations should only be used in critical care areas (NPSA, 2002) where continuous ECG monitoring, potassium analysers and high staffing levels are available.

Glucose (C₆H₁₂O₆)

Normal: 4–8 mmol/litre (but target may be higher – e.g. < 10 mmol/litre).

Glucose is the main source of intracellular energy (see Chapter 24), needing insulin to transport it into cells. Insulin deficiency or resistance therefore causes hyperglycaemia. In critically ill patients, stress responses and various drugs (e.g. corticosteroids, adrenaline) reduce insulin production and increase insulin resistance.

Glycaemic control has raised much controversy and conflicting evidence over the last decade. Insulin may (Dandona *et al.*, 2007) or may not (Brundage *et al.*, 2008) be anti-inflammatory, and may reduce organ damage (Langley and Adams, 2007) and ventilator days (Scalea *et al.*, 2007), but may increase pro-inflammatory cytokines (Brundage *et al.*, 2008). Following van den Berghe *et al.*'s (2001) influential studies, tight glycaemic control (aim: 4.6–6.1) was widely adopted, but while some studies found tight glycaemic control reduced mortality (Egi *et al.*, 2006; Scalea *et al.*, 2007; Ascione *et al.*, 2008), evidence is accumulating that it either has no effect on mortality (Ligtenberg *et al.*, 2006) or even increases it (Preise *et al.*, 2009; NICE-SUGAR Study Investigators, 2009). Tight glycaemic control has caused more hypoglycaemia (Wiener *et al.*, 2008; Bilotta *et al.*, 2009), which may be fatal or may contribute to depression (Dowdy *et al.*, 2008). Dellinger *et al.* (2008) recommend all patients receiving IV insulin should receive a glucose *calorie* source. Increasingly, glucose targets in ICU have risen from van den Berghe *et al.*'s (2001) 4.4–6.1 to Preise *et al.*'s (2009) 7.8–10.0, although 7.8 is arguably too high for a lower limit.

Arterial blood glucose is 0.8–1.67 mmol/litre higher than capillary/venous (Barrett *et al.*, 2010). Whether this is clinically significant is debatable, especially if glycaemic control is managed solely by arterial blood gases. Kessler (2009) recommends avoiding capillary (fingertip) measurement in critically ill patients, as results can be:

- falsely high with low haematocrit, high bilirubin, severe lipidaemia;
- falsely low with high haematocrit, hypoxia;
- also false with vasopressors, oedema, shock.

Treatment: Hypoglycaemia is treated by giving glucose. Hyperglycaemia in ICUs is managed with sliding-scale insulin infusions.

Phosphate (PO_4^{3-})

Normal: 0.8–1.45 mmol/litre.

Most (80 per cent) phosphate is in bones (Gaasbeek and Meinders, 2005). Serum phosphate:

- produces ATP (cell energy);
- produces 2,3 DPG (assists oxygen dissociation from haemoglobin);
- buffers acids (phosphate is the main intracellular buffer, although only a minor buffer in serum);
- reduces free fatty acids.

Hyperphosphataemia, rare in ICUs except when patients have chronic kidney disease, stimulates parathyroid hormone production, so may cause calcium imbalance, and so dysrhythmias, but is otherwise rarely problematic.

Polyuria and haemofiltration contribute to the hypophosphataemia seen in many critically ill patients. Hypophosphataemia causes:

■ muscle weakness, including respiratory muscles (which may delay weaning) (Fisher and Macnaughton, 2006);
■ intracellular acidosis;
■ intracellular hypoxia.

Treatment: Hypophosphataemia is usually treated by phosphate infusion (often 50 mmol over 24 hours), ideally infused through a central line. Oral supplements are also available.

Magnesium (Mg⁺⁺ or Mg²⁺)

Normal: 0.7–1.0 mmol/litre.

Serum magnesium ('nature's tranquilliser') is a calcium antagonist, stabilising cell membranes and reducing conduction – vasodilates, delays atrioventricular cardiac conduction.

Hypomagnesaemia, usually from malnutrition or excessive diuresis, occurs in many ICU patients (Dubé and Granry, 2003), and may cause tachydys-rhythmias (Dubé and Granry, 2003), muscle weakness (Astle, 2005) and other problems. Hypermagnesiumaemia (> 3mmol/litre) is very rare, and rarely a problem in ICUs, but may cause cardiac and/or respiratory arrest.

Treatment: In critical care, magnesium is usually infused intravenously; this can cause bradycardia and hypotension. Oral magnesium supplements are also available.

Calcium (Ca⁺⁺ or Ca²⁺)

Normal: total calcium 2.25–2.75 mmol/litre (laboratory results).
         ionised levels 1.0–1.5 mmol/litre (ABG results).

Like magnesium, only 1 per cent of body calcium is in blood, but serum calcium facilitates:

■ cardiac conduction
■ muscle cell contraction
■ cell function
■ clotting.

About half serum calcium is normally protein-bound, and half free (*ionised*, or unbound). Only free (unbound) calcium is active. ICU patients almost invariably have low plasma protein (albumin) levels, which reduces protein-binding sites. Laboratories may 'correct' calcium levels to reflect the amount of physiologically active (ionised) calcium.

Table 21.3 Main biochemistry results

	Normal	(Normal) source	Loss	Main significance	Likely treatments if low	Likely treatments if high
CRP	< 10 mg/litre	liver (acute phase protein)		inflammatory marker	not significant*	treat cause, not symptom
sodium	135–145 mmol/litre	diet	gut; urine loss regulated by aldosterone	sodium is the main extracellular cation	give sodium (e.g. 0.9% sodium chloride IVI)	sign of dehydration – give water
chloride	95–105 mmol/litre	diet	with salt	combines with sodium to form salt	not significant*	stop saline infusions
potassium	3.5–4.5 mmol/litre	diet (also cells – trauma, fluid shifts)	90% urine, 10% stools; lost with haemofiltration if not added to dialysate	cardiac conduction	potassium supplements glucose IVI	50 iu actrapid + 50 ml 50%
glucose	4.6–6.1 mmol/litre	diet	glycolysis	cell energy: $C_6H_{12}O_6 + 6\,O_2 \rightarrow$ 36 molecules of ATP	glucose supplements	insulin
phosphate	0.80–1.45 mmol/litre	diet	urine/haemofiltration	cell energy (adenosine triphosphate has 3 phosphate moledules) and 2,3 DPG	phosphate supplements	not significant, very rare*
magnesium	0.75–1.0 mmol/litres	diet (especially greens)	urine/haemofiltration; gut loss (e.g. vomiting, loose stools/stoma)	energy; calcium antagonist – vasodilates bronchodilates, cardiac conduction	magnesium supplements	not significant; very rare*
calcium (total)	2.2–2.6 mmol/litre	diet	urine	cardiac conduction, clotting, cell repair	calcium supplements	rare*; can be treated with calcium antagonists (e.g. magnesium) or calcium channel blockers
calcium (ionised)	1.0–1.5 mmol/litre					
urea	3–9 mmol/litre	protein metabolism	urine	marker of renal function	not significant*	treat disease (AKI), not symptom
creatinine	60–120 micromol/litre	muscle metabolism – 50–100 micromol/day	urine	marker of renal function	not significant*	treat disease (AKI), not symptom

Note: * with acutely ill (ICU) patients; in other specialities significance and treatments may differ.

Treatment: Hypocalcaemia is treated with calcium supplements. Hypercalcaemia is rare, and rarely significant in ICUs.

Creatinine

Normal: female 50–90 micromol/litre.
         male 70–120 micromol/litre.

Creatinine, a waste product of muscle metabolism (hence gender differences), is normally cleared in urine. With kidney injury, levels usually rise steadily 50–100 micromol/day (Skinner and Watson, 1997). Glomerular filtration rate (GFR) is often estimated from creatinine levels. Normal GFR is > 90 ml/minute/ 1.73m^2; although an estimate, GFR may give earlier indications of impending failure than reported creatinine levels.

Treatment: Low levels of creatinine are not significant. Raised creatinine (and urea, or low GFR) indicates kidney injury, so renal replacement therapy may be needed.

Urea

Normal: 3–9 mmol/litre.

Urea is a waste product of (any) protein metabolism, normally cleared in urine. High urea and creatinine usually indicate kidney injury, but if uraemia disproportionately exceeds creatinine (ratio is usually approximately 1:20) excessive protein metabolism is more likely, especially from digestion of blood following gastrointestinal bleeds. Uraemic patients are often disorientated/ delirious; whether this is caused by urea or other neurotoxins is debated.

Treatment: As for creatinine.

Implications for practice

- Low results are caused by: dilution, loss or failure of supply/to produce.
- High levels are caused by: dehydration (haemoconcentration), excessive intake/production, or failure to clear.
- Optimum Hb for most critically ill patients is 7–9 g/dl.
- Key electrolytes in critical illness are usually potassium (aim 4–5 mmol/litre if cardiac history/problems), phosphate (aim > 0.8 mmol/litre) and magnesium (aim > 0.7 mmol/litre).
- Benefits of tight glycaemic control (aim 4.4–6.1 mmol/litre) are disputed, as it has caused deaths from hypoglycaemia; a safer upper target is probably < 10 mmol/litre.

Summary

Blood is the transport system of the body, so abnormal results indicate problems, but may also cause further complications. Nurses usually download results before medical staff, so understanding main results and how abnormalities should be managed enables earlier treatment.

Further reading

Higgins (2007) provides an accessible book about laboratory investigations. While most medical/nursing articles explore specific aspects, occasionally overview articles appear in medical and sometimes nursing journals.

Clinical scenario

Henry Duff is a 68-year-old known diabetic. He was admitted two days ago with bleeding gastric ulcers and has frequent episodes of melaena. He is self-ventilating on 28 per cent oxygen via nasal cannulae, with a respiratory rate of 18–28 breaths/minute. He has an intravenous infusion of Omeprazole (80 mg over 10 hours) in progress. Mr Duff appears to be hallucinating, reports visual disturbances, is confused and at times agitated, and has the following blood results.

Haematology		Biochemistry		Arterial blood gas	
Hb	9.2 g/dl	CRP	102 mg/litre	pH	7.48
WBC	18.7×10^{-9}/litre	Na^+	162 mmol/litre	$PaCO_2$	4.33 kPa
Neutrophils	15.2×10^{-9}/litre	K^+	4.7 mmol/litre	PaO_2	9.55 kPa
Lymphocytes	2.5×10^{-9}/litre	Cl–	130 mmol/litre	HCO_3^-	25.7 mmol/litre
Platelets	234×10^{-9}/litre	HCO_3^-	25 mmol/litre	Base excess	1.1 mmol/litre
MCV	90 μm^3	Glucose	10.5 mmol/litre	Lactate	1.5 mmol/litre
		PO_4^{-3}	0.74 mmol/litre		
INR	1.2	Mg^{2+}	0.72 mmol/litre		
APTT ratio	1.58	Ca^{2+}	2.38 mmol/litre		
		Urea	18.6 mmol/litre		
		Creatinine	136 μmol/litre		
		Bilirubin	36 mmol/litre		
		ALT	38 iu/litre		
		Alk Phos	129 iu/litre		
		Albumin	16 g/litre		
		Gamma GT	132 iu/litre		

Q.1 Interpret Mr Duff's blood results and note the clinical significance of abnormal values. Consider which of the abnormal blood results may be caused by Mr Duff's pathophysiology, and which may be caused by sampling errors.

Q.2 Explain the potential causes of Mr Duff's hypernatraemia. Identify interventions and therapies that should be implemented to resolve abnormality.

Q.3 Review other blood tests that could aid the assessment process for Mr Duff's condition, and provide a rationale for these suggestions.

Chapter 22

ECGs and dysrhythmias

Contents

Fundamental knowledge 213
Introduction 214
Basic principles of
 electrocardiography (ECG) 215
Action potential 218
Lead changes 218
ST abnormalities 218
QT abnormalities 219
U waves 219
General treatments 219
Ectopics 220
Atrial dysrhythmias 222
Atrioventricular blocks 226
Bundle branch block 228
Ventricular dysrhythmias 228
Asystole 231
Pulseless electrical activity 231
Implications for practice 232
Summary 232
Further reading 232
Clinical questions 233

Fundamental knowledge

Myocardial physiology – automaticity, conductivity,
 rhythmicity
Normal limb electrode placement

213

Normal cardiac conduction (SA node, AV node,
    Bundle of His, Purkinje fibres)
Physiology of normal sinus rhythm
Current Resuscitation Council guidelines
Experience of using continuous ECG monitoring
    and taking 12 lead ECGs

Introduction

Some dysrhythmias are immediately life-threatening; others may compromise cardiac function by reducing stroke volume, and increasing tachycardia and myocardial hypoxia. Dysrhythmias are usually symptoms of underlying problems, and may be acute or chronic. Chronic dysrhythmias (atrial fibrillation being especially common) should be controlled, but can rarely be reversed. Most acute dysrhythmias should actively be reversed if possible, necessitating close haemodynamic monitoring and support. This chapter focuses on acute rather than chronic problems.

Although ICU nurses seldom see the range of dysrhythmias encountered in coronary care units, ECG monitoring is standard, so nurses should be able to:

- identify dysrhythmias;
- identify likely causes from patients' histories;
- know usual management and treatment for commonly occurring dys-rhythmias.

As with almost all problems, early intervention reduces complication and improves survival and outcome, so ICU nurses should develop expertise in this fundamental aspect of critical care monitoring.

Some commonly used drugs are mentioned, but practices vary, so users should consult Summary of Product Characteristics (SPC) or pharmacopoeias for detailed information on drugs.

Normal conduction begins in the sino-atrial node, passing through atrial muscle to the atrioventricular node, then passing from the atrioventricular node through the ventricular conduction pathway and into ventricular *myocytes*. There are therefore three key stages in normal cardiac conduction and the ECG:

- atrial (P wave);
- atrioventricular node (PR interval);
- ventricular (QRS complex, ST segment, T wave).

The etymologically more accurate 'dysrhythmia', rather than the more popular 'arrhythmia', is used here as, except for asystole, rhythms are problematic rather than absent.

Basic principles of electrocardiography (ECG)

An ECG is a time/voltage graph of myocardial electrical activity, representing three-dimensional events in two. This section summarises basic principles for revision. Any parts unfamiliar to readers should be revised further before proceeding (e.g. from Hampton, 2008a).

- On ECG graph paper, each small square is 1 mm × 1 mm, and each large square is 5 mm × 5 mm.
- Horizontal axes represents time.
- ECGs are normally recorded at 25 mm/second, making each large square = 0.2 seconds, each small square = 0.04 seconds.
- Vertical axes represent voltage; a calibration square (normally 10 mm = 1 mV = 2 large squares) usually appears at the beginning or end of ECG printouts, and often on bedside monitors.
- A normal sinus rhythm complex (see Figure 22.1) is labelled PQRST.
- P = atrial *depolarisation* (activity).
- QRS = ventricular depolarisation.
- T = ventricular *repolarisation* (end of activity).
- sinoatrial (SA) and atrioventricular (AV) nodes have both sympathetic and parasympathetic nerve fibres, so are affected by brainstem control and vagal stimulation; hence suction can cause bradycardia/ectopics/blocks.

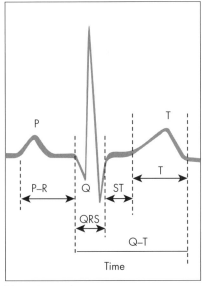

Normal wave form

Figure 22.1 Normal sinus rhythm

■ Limb electrodes are normally colour-coded (red, yellow, green, black) and most units now use five-electrode monitors:

- red = right arm
- yellow = left arm
- green = left leg/hip
- black = right leg/hip
- white = 4th intercostal space to right of sternum (modified chest lead 1: MCL-1).

■ Electrical 'views' remain unchanged anywhere along limbs, or on a line between the limb joint and heart, so electrodes may be placed anywhere along the view line:

- lead I = right arm to left arm (bipolar)
- lead II = right arm to left leg (bipolar)
- lead III = left arm to left leg (bipolar)
- aVR = right arm (unipolar)
- aVL = left arm (unipolar)
- aVF = foot (left leg; unipolar).

■ Limb lead II follows the normal 'vector' (or 'axis') of cardiac conduction, so is usually the default lead for single-lead monitors and rhythm strips on 12-lead ECGs.

■ Chest (precordial) leads examine electrical activity from right atrium, through right ventricle, septum, left ventricle, to left atrium (see Figure 22.2):

- C (or V) 1 (red): 4th intercostal space, to right of (patient's) sternum
- C2 (yellow): 4th intercostal space, left of sternum
- C3 (green): between C2 and C4
- C4 (brown): 5th intercostal space, midclavicular line
- C5 (black): between C4 and C6
- C6 (purple): 5th intercostal space, midaxilla.

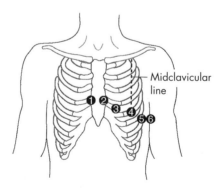

■ *Figure 22.2 Chest lead placement*

■ Normal times: P wave = 0.08 seconds (2 small squares)
PR interval* = 0.12–0.2 seconds (3–5 small squares)
QRS = maximum 0.12 seconds (3 small squares)
T wave = 0.16 seconds (4 small squares)
QT interval = < ½ preceding R-R interval, maximum 0.4 seconds (2 large squares).

* Measure PR intervals from beginning of the P wave to start of QRS.

■ Sinus rhythm = technically, any rhythm originating from the sinoatrial node, although in practice the term is often used to describe regular rhythms of 60–100 beats per minute (bpm) originating from the SA node.

Table 22.1 provides a framework for ECG interpretation.

Table 22.1 Framework for ECG interpretation

Recording the ECG:
Are electrodes correctly placed (red = right arm, yellow = left arm, green/black = left leg)?
Is there a clear baseline (isoelectric line)?

Regularity:
Is the rate regular?
If not, is rate:
■ regularly irregular (is there a pattern)?
■ irregularly irregular (no pattern)?

P wave:
Does the P wave appear before the QRS?
Is there one P wave before every QRS?
Is the shape normal?
Are P waves missing?

PR interval:
Is the PR interval 3–5 small squares?

QRS complex:
Is the QRS width within 3 small squares?
Is the QRS positive or negative?
Is the axis normal?
Does the QRS look normal?

ST segment:
Does the isoelectric line return between the S and the T?
If not, is it:
■ elevated (> 1 mm above isoelectric line)?
■ depressed (< 0.5 mm below isoelectric line)?

T wave:
Does the T wave look normal?
Is the QT interval < ½ preceding R-R interval, and maximum 0.4 seconds?

Tachycardia (> 100 bpm):
Narrow complex (usually with P waves) = atrial (supraventricular).
Broad complex (without P wave) = usually ventricular.

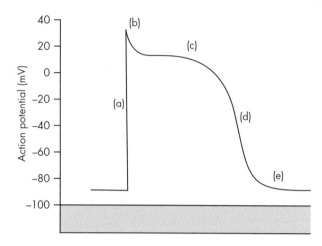

(a) Rapid depolarisation: influx via fast sodium channel (phase 0).
(b) Fast calcium channel open (phase 1).
(c) Plateau: slow calcium channel open (phase 2).
(d) Rapid depolarisation: potassium channel open (phase 3).
(e) Resting phase (phase 4).

Figure 22.3 Action potential

Action potential

At rest, the electrical charge (polarity) of myocyte membranes is about –90 millivolts (mV). Active movement of cations (positively charged ions) across the cell membrane changes this charge, making the cell electrically excitable (depolarisation). When normal cation concentrations are restored, the charge is stabilised and electrical activity ends (repolarisation). Action potential is created by overlapping but sequential prominence of 'channels' in myocyte membranes – sodium, calcium, potassium; the calcium channel creates both the peak and main duration of depolarisation, while activity ends with potassium influx. Hence, deranged serum calcium or potassium often causes ectopics and dysrhythmias. Figure 22.3 shows an action potential graph.

Lead changes

Each lead views cardiac conduction differently, so sites of infarctions may be diagnosed through lead changes (see Table 22.2).

Usual lead placement does not view posterior myocardium clearly, but posterior infarction is best seen in C1 and C2.

ST abnormalities

From the S wave, ECG complexes should return almost vertically to the isoelectric line. Any ST elevation or depression should be noted and, if new, reported. Many monitors detect ST abnormalities.

Table 22.2 Likely lead changes with myocardial infarction

Part of heart	Coronary artery	Leads affected
Anterior	LAD or Cx	V2–V4
Anterolateral	LAD	V4–V6, I, aVL
Lateral	LAD or Cx	I, II, aVL, V6
Inferior	RCA or Cx	II, III, aVF
Inferolateral	RCA or Cx	II, III, aVF, aVL, V4–V6
Inferoseptal	Cx	II, III, aVF, V1–V3
Posterior	Cx or RCA	V1, V2

ST elevation (2 mm in chest leads, 1 mm in limb leads) in two or more consecutive leads usually indicates acute myocardial infarction. Classification of *acute coronary syndromes* into:

■ ST elevation (STE-ACS); also called ST elevation myocardial infarction (STEMI);
■ non-ST elevation (NSTE-ACS); also called non-ST elevation myocardial infarction (NSTEMI); and
■ unstable angina (UA)

is discussed in Chapter 29.

ST depression usually indicates ischaemia.

QT abnormalities

The QT interval represents ventricular depolarisation. Prolongation therefore represents prolonged ventricular excitability, which may progress to ventricular dysrhythmias, such as *torsades de pointes* (see page 230) (Mudawi *et al.*, 2009). 'Prolonged QT syndrome' is often genetic, but can be triggered by electrolyte abnormalities (potassium, calcium, magnesium) and drugs (e.g. tricyclic antidepressants) (Adam and Osborne, 2009). QT intervals are often 'corrected' to what they would be if heart rate were 60 bpm: corrected QT = QTc.

U waves

U waves are seldom present, and if present seldom seen, and if seen are seldom significant. They appear like a second, smaller T wave, and are not usually pathological, but may indicate electrolyte abnormality, especially *hyperkalaemia* or *hypercalcaemia* (Meek and Morris, 2008a).

General treatments

Underlying causes (e.g. electrolytes – especially potassium and calcium) of dysrhythmias should be resolved, but otherwise asymptomatic dysrhythmias seldom require treatment. Haemodynamic compromise (hypotension) necessitates action.

Myocardial hypoxia is often present, so oxygen is usually a first-line treatment.

Most *drugs* ('chemical cardioversion') used either suppress myocardial automaticity or change AV node conduction (some increasing, others decreasing). New dysrhythmias may be caused by drugs, so drug charts should be reviewed – pharmacists are a useful source for advice about side effects. If possible, problem drugs should be discontinued – e.g. salbutamol may cause tachycardia; metochlopramide may cause bradycardia. Bradycardic dysrhythmias may need positive *chronotropes* (e.g. atropine). Tachycardic dysrhythmias are often caused by overexcitability. Amiodarone is often the first-line drug, as it reduces ventricular and supraventricular tachycardias. Ventricular conduction may be blocked with:

- beta-blockers (esmolol, sotalol, propanolol), which inhibit beta receptors (see Chapter 34);
- calcium channel blockers (e.g. diltiazem).

Poor cardiac output may necessitate positive inotropes, such as dobutamine (see Chapter 34).

If drugs fail, electrical cardioversion may restore stable rhythms. 'Overpacing', using faster pacing rates, may also restore stable rhythms, but is not generally used in most ICUs. Pacing can be used for bradycardias, but such problems (and so treatment) are rare in ICUs.

Problems likely to persist should be referred to cardiologists, as later ablation (destruction of abnormal pacemakers or conduction pathways) or other treatments may be needed.

Ectopics

Two key questions should be answered about ectopics:

- Where do they originate?
- What is their timing?

There are three possible answers to the first question:

- atrial
- junctional/nodal
- ventricular

and, provided underlying rhythms are regular, two possible answers to the second:

- *premature* (before expected impulses) or
- *escape* (expected complexes are absent, so ectopic impulses 'escape' into gaps).

With irregularly irregular rhythms (e.g. atrial fibrillation), timing of ectopics cannot be identified.

Premature complexes indicate overexcitability. Escape ectopics indicate failed conduction. Likely causes of overexcitability or failed conduction include:

- damaged conduction pathways (infarction, oedema, hypoxia);
- drugs/stimulants;
- electrolyte imbalance (especially potassium; also calcium, magnesium);
- acidosis.

Treatment: Occasional ectopics seldom need treating, but underlying causes should (if possible) be resolved. Potassium imbalance is the most likely single cause, so serum potassium is usually maintained at 4–5 mmol/litre. Calcium and magnesium imbalances can also cause ectopics.

Frequent premature ectopics should be treated before they progress to dysrhythmias. Generally amiodarone is the drug of choice in ICUs, although calcium channel blockers, beta-blockers and other drugs (e.g. digoxin) may be used. Escape ectopics provide a pulse that would otherwise be missed, so are 'a friend in need' and should never be treated, although causes of the failed normal conduction should be resolved. Drugs used vary with focus and cause.

Atrial ectopics

Atrial ectopics (see Figure 22.4) have:

- abnormal P waves
- possibly different PR intervals
- normal QRS, ST and T.

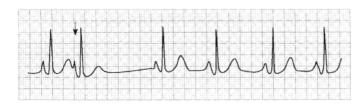

Figure 22.4 Premature atrial ectopic

Junctional/nodal ectopics have:

- no P wave (or occasionally inverted P waves, which may be before or after the QRS);
- normal QRS, ST and T.

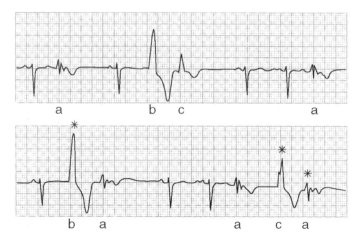

Figure 22.5 Multifocal ventricular ectopics

Ventricular ectopics (see Figure 22.5) have:

- no P wave;
- (usually) broad QRS (3 small squares).

Complexes from a single focus ('unifocal') look alike; ectopics with different shapes originate from different foci ('multifocal'). A sequence of three or more ectopics is sometimes called a *salvo*.

Atrial dysrhythmias

Sinus arryhthmia

Sinus arrhythmia (see Figure 22.6) occurs in a few young, usually athletic, people. Inspiration significantly increases venous return (Meek and Morris, 2008b), and so heart rate. Large tidal volumes from ventilators could mimic reversed sinus arrhythmia, but large tidal volumes are seldom used. Sinus arrhythmia is rarely seen in ICU, rarely problematic, and should not be treated.

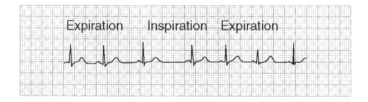

Figure 22.6 Sinus arrhythmia

Sinus bradycardia

Although any sinus rate below 60 bpm is technically sinus bradycardia, significant problems usually only develop with rates below 50.

Treatment: Sinus bradycardia is only treated if symptomatic or problematic – rare in ICU. Obvious causes should be removed, so oxygen should be optimised. Rate may be increased with atropine or other drugs, but if problems persist pacing may be needed.

Sinus tachycardia

Tachycardia is any sinus rate > 100 bpm. Although normal in young children, tachycardia is abnormal with adults, but many critically ill patients have compensatory mild tachycardias. Most positive inotropes are also positive chronotropes (= increase heart rate). Faster tachycardias (> 160 bpm) reduce stroke volume, so causing hypotension (Hinds and Watson, 2008), and are often not sinus. In practice, the term 'supraventricular tachycardia' is usually used for rates above 140–160 bpm.

Supraventricular tachycardia (SVT)

SVT (see Figure 22.7) is any tachycardia originating above the ventricles, although it usually implies rates exceeding 140–160 bpm. More specific terms, such as 'atrial tachycardia' (i.e. originating in the atrium, but not sinus), are sometimes used.

Treatment: In ICUs, SVT is usually treated with amiodarone. Other drugs, such as beta-blockers, may sometimes be tried.

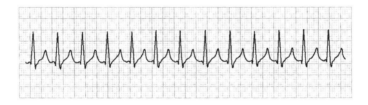

Figure 22.7 Supraventricular tachycardia

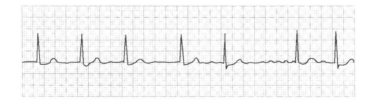

Figure 22.8 Atrial fibrillation

Atrial fibrillation (AF)

Atrial fibrillation (see Figure 22.8) is classified as:

- first diagnosed (regardless of duration or symptoms);
- *paroxysmal*: spontaneous termination, usually within 48 hours, can persist for seven days;
- persistent: not self-terminating;
- long-standing: more than one year;
- permanent ('accepted'): no cardioversion attempted.

(Task Force, 2010a)

New-onset AF may be provoked by disease or surgery – 4 per cent of all in-hospital patients develop AF (Walsh *et al.*, 2007). If not self-resolving, AF should be reversed if possible. Permanent/established ('chronic') AF should be controlled.

AF causes chaotic atrial activity, seen by either a chaotically wavy or almost flat line between ventricular electrical activity. QRS complexes, ST segments and T waves are normal (unless there are other cardiac problems), but timing (space) between ventricular contractions (QRS complexes) is erratic – irregularly irregular.

Treatment: New-onset AF is usually treated by amiodarone (Zimetbaum, 2007; Musco *et al.*, 2008). Other drugs, or cardioversion, are occasionally used. Controlling permanent AF necessitates both:

- rate control (aim < 100 bpm)
- anticoagulation (aim INR 2.5).

Traditionally, rate control was most often achieved with digoxin (a cardiac *glycoside*). Musco *et al.* (2008) recommend beta-blockers for rate control. Dronedarone has recently been approved by NICE.

Atrial flutter

Atrial flutter (see Figure 22.9) causes rapid waves with distinctive sawtooth shapes ('F' waves), typically 300 bpm. This rate exceeds possible AV nodes conduction, so a regular block occurs, usually of an even ration (e.g. 2:1, 4:1, 6:1 or 8:1); 4:1 AV block with atrial rates of 300 creates ventricular responses of 75 bpm. But blocks can change suddenly, creating gross tachycardia (2:1 block = ventricular rate 150/minute) or bradycardia.

Treatment: Generally, electrical cardioversion is usually preferred, but chemical cardioversion (e.g. amiodarone) may restore sinus rhythm. Where pacing wires are already inserted, such as following cardiac surgery, 'over-pacing' may be preferred.

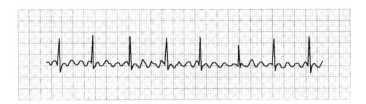

Figure 22.9 Atrial flutter

Wolff-Parkinson-White syndrome (WPW)

Wolff-Parkinson-White syndrome (see Figure 22.10) is caused by a rare congenital abnormality. An abnormal extra atrioventricular conduction pathway, the Bundle of Kent, can cause impulses to re-enter atria, causing a 'circus movement' and sudden, gross, life-threatening tachycardia. Circus movement broadens bases of QRS complexes ('delta' waves).

Treatment: Chemical (e.g. amiodarone) or electrical cardioversion are usually used to stabilise crises. Later, ablation of the Bundle of Kent will usually be needed.

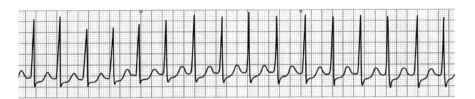

Figure 22.10 Wolff-Parkinson-White syndrome

Junctional (or 'nodal') rhythm

Juntional (or 'nodal') rhythm (see Figure 22.11) describes impulses originating in the AV node or atrioventricular junction. Rate is often (but not always) slower than sinus/atrial rhythms. P waves are not usually seen, but if present are inverted, and may appear after QRSs. Irritation (oedema, mechanical – e.g. central lines in the right atrium) may cause junctional ectopics. Oedema from cardiac surgery often causes transient junctional rhythms (hence epicardial pacing wires).

Treatment: Junctional rates are often sufficient to support life, but should be closely monitored. If bradycardia becomes symptomatic, treat as sinus bradycardia above (atropine, pacing).

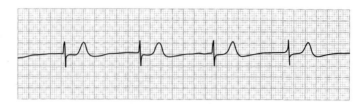

Figure 22.11 Junctional (or 'nodal') rhythm

Atrioventricular blocks

Any conduction pathway may be blocked by:

- infarction
- oedema
- ischaemia.

If oedema or ischaemia resolve, blocks usually disappear. Infarction usually causes permanent block. Blocks may occur at the atrioventricular node (first, second or third degree) or in one of the bundle branches.

First-degree (AV node) block

First-degree (AV node) block (see Figure 22.12), delayed atrioventricular node conduction, prolongs PR intervals beyond 0.2 seconds (five small squares). Despite delay, every impulse is conducted, so a QRS complex follows each P wave. Acute blocks may be caused by disease or drugs. Chronic first-degree block is usually from age-related sclerosis of the atrioventricular node, and rarely problematic.

Treatment: Acute block should be monitored, but only treated if bradycardia causes problems. Chronotropes (e.g. atropine) or pacing can resolve symptomatic bradycardia.

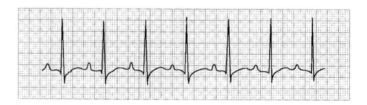

Figure 22.12 First-degree block

Second-degree block

Second-degree block, or incomplete heart block, occurs when at regular intervals there is an unconducted P wave. There are two types of second degree block:

- type 1 (also called 'Mobitz type 1' or 'Wenkebach'): progressive lengthening of PR intervals until an atrial impulse is unconducted (see Figure 22.13);
- type 2 (also called 'Mobitz type 2' or sometimes just 'Mobitz'): constant PR intervals, with regular unconducted P waves (e.g. 2:1; see Figure 22.14).

Type 2 is less common, but more serious, than type 1, as it is more likely to progress into third-degree block or asystole (Jevon, 2009).

Treatment: If new and/or symptomatic, optimise oxygen and remove causes (e.g. any drugs blocking conduction). Chemical cardioversion may help, but pacing is often needed.

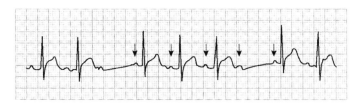

■ *Figure 22.13* Second-degree block (type 1)

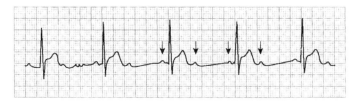

■ *Figure 22.14* Second-degree block (type 2)

Third-degree block

Third-degree block, or complete heart block (see Figure 22.15), causes complete atrioventricular dissociation. Any atrial activity (e.g. P waves) is unrelated to QRS complexes; some P waves may be 'lost' in QRS or T waves. However, patients with third-degree block more often have atrial fibrillation. Ventricular pacemakers usually cause broad, regular, but slow QRS complexes – often 30 bpm). Cardiac output and blood pressure are usually compromised.

Treatment: Unless transient, pacing is almost invariably needed. Until pacing is commenced, optimise oxygen.

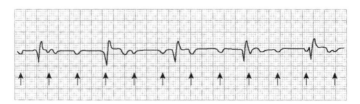

Figure 22.15 Third-degree block

Bundle branch block

Bundle branch block (see Figure 22.16) occurs when conduction through one of branches from the Bundle of His, or one or more of the left hemibranches, is blocked. This creates two QRS complexes – a normal one from the intact branch, and a broadened ventricular-shaped complex from impulses spreading across the septum. This RSR, or biphasic QRS, wave creates the characteristic M or W shapes on ECGs.

Left bundle branch block causes a W in early, and an M in late chest leads; right bundle branch block reverses this picture The mnemonics WiLLiaM and MaRRoW may be useful:

- WiLLiaM: W in C1 and M in C6 = LBBB;
- MaRRoW: M in C1 and (often) W in C6 = RBBB.

New left bundle block (i.e. not on previous ECGs), together with chest pain, indicates myocardial infarction and is classified as ST-ACS (ST wave elevated myocardial infarction – see Chapter 29), necessitating urgent pPCI. New right bundle branch block often necessitates management of heart failure, but may be treated with PCI.

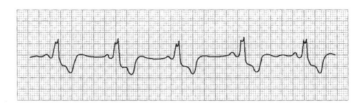

Figure 22.16 Bundle branch block

Ventricular dysrhythmias

Ventricular impulses originate in ventricular muscle, so usually travel from muscle fibre to muscle fibre rather than through conduction pathways, making progress relatively slow, giving them typically broad QRS complexes. Impulses originating in or near conduction pathways may have narrow complexes. Rates typically commence slowly (about 30 bpm), but myocardial hypoxia rapidly accelerates rate, often to gross tachycardia.

Bigeminy and trigeminy

Bigeminy and trigeminy (see Figure 22.17) are sinister extensions of ventricular ectopics, occurring regularly. Bigeminy is one ventricular ectopic every other complex; trigeminy is one ventricular ectopic every third complex. Ectopics are usually unifocal, usually from hypoxia or digoxin toxicity.

Treatment: Trigeminy is not usually treated. Provided underlying causes are resolved, bigeminy can be treated with rhythm stabilisers.

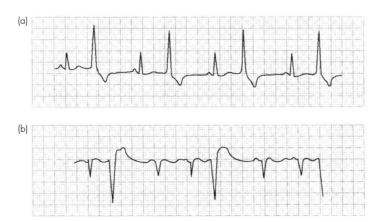

Figure 22.17 Bigeminy and trigeminy

Ventricular tachycardia

Ventricular tachycardia (see Figure 22.18) is a regular rhythm, with rapid unifocal impulses (typically 200–250 bpm). Asymptomatic VT rarely persists, either reverting or progressing after a few minutes.

Treatment: Ventricular tachycardia with a pulse may respond to drugs (e.g. amiodarone), but pulseless VT is a shockable rhythm, necessitating immediate resuscitation.

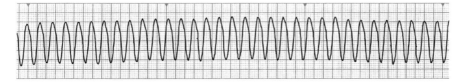

Figure 22.18 Ventricular tachycardia

Torsades de pointes

Torsades de pointes (see Figure 22.19), a rare type of multifocal ventricular tachycardia, causes ECG traces to 'twist' around isoelectric baselines, creating an irregular broad-complex tachycardia. If prolonged or untreated it leads to ventricular fibrillation. It may be caused by drugs (e.g. amiodarone, vancomycin, soltolol), severe electrolyte imbalance (especially hypokalaemia, hypomagnesaemia), subarachnoid haemorrhage, myocardial infarction, angina, bradycardia, sinoatrial block or congenital abnormality.

Treatment: Electrolyte imbalances or underlying causes should be treated, and drugs that prolong QT intervals should be stopped. Drugs include magnesium (Kaye and O'Sullivan, 2002). If drugs fail, temporary atrial or ventricular pacing or cardiopulmonary resuscitation may be necessary.

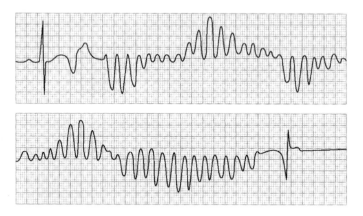

Figure 22.19 Torsades de pointes

Ventricular fibrillation (VF)

Ventricular fibrillation (see Figure 22.20) is almost invariably fatal in 2–3 minutes. VF may be coarse or fine; fine VF may appear like asystole, so increasing gain on ECGs shows whether 'f' waves are present.

Treatment: Ventricular fibrillation is a shockable rhythm, necessitating immediate resuscitation.

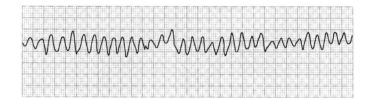

Figure 22.20 Ventricular fibrillation

Asystole

Asystole (= ventricular standstill), literally absence of systole, appears as an uninterrupted isoelectric line, although progression from dysrhythmias to asystole may persist for considerable time ('dying' heart), with occasional atrial or ventricular complexes. Chest wall movement from breathing (including mechanical ventilation) typically causes slow undulations to the isoelectric line.

Absence of any cardiac function is an arrest situation. Before initiating arrest calls, staff should take ten seconds to assess patients (pulse, ECG): absence of complexes on ECGs may be caused by:

- disconnection/failed electrodes (e.g. dry gel) – typically causes a perfectly horizontal isoelectric line;
- fine VF – increasing height ('gain') of ECG may reveal fibrillation.

Treatment: Asystole is not a shockable rhythm. Cardiac compressions and drugs (following the Resuscitation Council algorithm) are essential to maintain effective circulation. Drugs include:

- adrenaline (1 mg)
- atropine (3 mg).

If P waves are present, external or transvenous pacing may be used. Resuscitation is seldom successful.

Pulseless electrical activity (PEA)

Pulseless electrical activity results in whatever electrical activity is seen not being translated into pulses and arterial blood pressure traces. ECG traces are usually abnormal, often showing tachycardia and with low-amplitude complexes. PEA is typically caused by one of the '4Hs and 4Ts', listed below, to 'consider' on the 2010 Resuscitation Council algorithm:

- hypoxia
- hypovolaemia
- hyper-/hypokalaemia
- hypothermia
- tension pneumothorax
- tamponade
- toxic/therapeutic disturbances (drug overdose)
- thrombi (PE, MI).

Causes are usually obvious from patients' histories.

Treatment: PEA is not a shockable rhythm. Cardiac compressions and drugs should be given. Underlying causes should be reversed.

Summary

Critical illness exposes ICU patients to various symptomatic dysrhythmias, so ICU patients are usually continuously monitored; ICU nurses should therefore be able to recognise common dysrhythmias and initiate appropriate action. Many drugs are used in cardiology, but most acute problematic dysrhythmias respond to amiodarone. ICU staff should already be familiar with basic electrocardiography, so this chapter has discussed dysrhythmias most likely to be seen in ICUs, together with standard treatments. Staff should be familiar with current Resuscitation Council guidelines.

Further reading

Current Resuscitation Council guidelines should be familiar and available, and can be downloaded from the UK Resuscitation Council website. The European Society of Cardiology produces guidelines for many common dysrhythmias, which can be downloaded from their website. There are many books, articles and internet resources for ECG interpretation. Hampton (2008a) provides a useful overview, with supplementary detail in Hampton (2008b) and examples for practice in Hampton (2008c). Houghton and Gray (2008) is also useful.

Clinical questions

Q.1 Describe how you would perform a 12-lead ECG on an ICU patient who is awake. Include how you would explain procedure, position the patient and apply electrodes to ensure an accurate and optimal ECG tracing.

Q.2 For continuous bedside ECG monitoring in the ICU, which lead (e.g. I, II, III, aVF, aVR, C1) is usually chosen for waveform analysis? Justify your choice in relation to cardiac physiology and note the expected waveform.

Q.3 Reflect on situations where external carotid massage has been performed for tachycardia. Appraise desired effects, limitations, safety issues and nurse accountability. What other strategies can be used to reduce life-threatening tachycardia in emergency situations?

Chapter 23

Neurological monitoring

Contents

Fundamental knowledge   234
Introduction   235
Intracranial pressure   235
Cerebral blood flow   237
Cerebral oedema   238
Glasgow Coma Scale   238
Pupil size and response   239
Limb assessment   240
Jugular venous bulb saturation (S_jO^2)   241
ICP measurement   241
Other technologies   242
Implications for practice   242
Summary   243
Further reading   243
Clinical scenario   243

Fundamental knowledge

Brainstem function
Cerebral blood supply – carotid arteries, Circle of Willis
Cerebral autoregulation
Sedation (see Chapter 6)

Introduction

Many ICU patients have acutely altered neurological function, whether from chemical sedation, disease of other organs/systems, or specific neurological disease/damage. Patients unconscious on admission may have suffered hypoxic brain damage, which can only be fully assessed on waking. Some ICUs specialise in neurosurgery or neuromedicine, but most units receive patients with head injuries and cranial pathologies. Many conditions, such as meningitis or hepatic failure, can increase intracranial pressure, causing both acute confusion and physiological complications. Nurses should therefore assess and monitor neurological function.

The nervous system can be differentiated between central and peripheral. The central nervous system is the brain and spinal cord. Peripheral nerves link the spinal cord to all other organs and tissues. Either, or both, parts of the nervous system may be dysfunctional, and therefore assessment should measure whichever part of the nervous system is a cause for concern.

The simplest way to assess neurological function is whether someone is responding appropriately and in their normal manner. Unfortunately, diseases and treatments prevent normal responses in many ICU patients, but with conscious patients their actions and communication (non-verbal as well as verbal) should be assessed. Acute neurological changes may be caused by abnormal biochemistry, especially glucose; so biochemistry should be assessed. Other non-invasive assessments can indicate:

- consciousness (Glasgow Coma Scale (GCS));
- cranial nerve function (pupil responses, gag, cough, facial movements);
- spinal nerve function (limb movement).

Invasive neurological monitoring is largely limited to neurological centres, although is sometimes used elsewhere. However neurological function is assessed, it should be understood by staff and beneficial to patients. Assessments recorded and reported should remain factual, and any limiting factors noted with the report. For example, intubated patients cannot make a verbal response, and pupil size or muscle strength may be evaluated differently by different observers. Where assessors are uncertain about their evaluation, they should seek a second opinion.

Intracranial pressure

Most of the total adult intracranial volume (average 1.7 litres) is brain tissue, the remaining 300 ml normally being equally divided between blood and cerebrospinal fluid (CSF) (Hickey, 2003b). Because the skull is rigid and filled to capacity with essentially non-compressible contents (the *Monro-Kellie hypothesis*), increasing one component necessarily compresses others. Small and transient increases of intracranial contents may be compensated for by displacing blood and CSF into the spinal column, so coughing, straining or sneezing do not usually cause problems; this is known as *compliance*. But sustained pressure, once compliance is exhausted, inevitably causes intracranial hypertension (see Figures 23.1 and 23.2). Any pressure on vital centres may affect vital signs, so neurological assessment should be evaluated in the context of vital signs, especially pulse and blood pressure.

Normal adult intracranial pressure (ICP) is 0–15 mmHg. Increased intra-cranial contents, such as cerebral oedema or bleeding, increase intracranial pressure, causing neurological dysfunction. Sustained intracranial pressures of 20–30 mmHg may cause injury. Cerebral autoregulation fails when ICP exceeds 40 mmHg (Hickey, 2003b). Sustained intracranial pressure over 60 mmHg causes irreversible ischaemic brain damage and is usually fatal (Bahouth and Yarbrough, 2005). Progressive cell damage (see Chapter 24) causes a vicious circle of intracranial hypertension and tissue injury (see Figure 23.3).

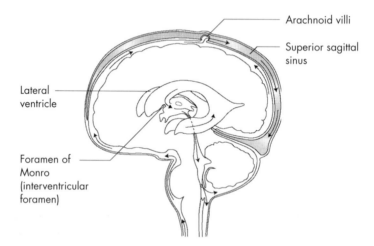

Figure 23.1 Cross-section of the cranium

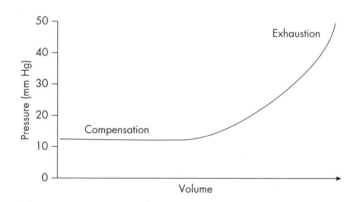

Figure 23.2 Pressure:volume curve

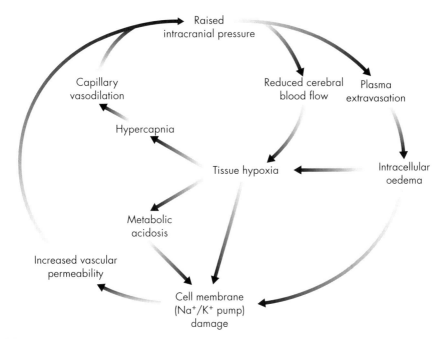

Figure 23.3 Intracranial hypertension and tissue injury:
a vicious circle

Cerebral blood flow

The brain normally receives about 15 per cent of cardiac output. The single main factor affecting cerebral perfusion is mean arterial pressure. Brain cells have high metabolic rates, yet unlike most cells have no ATP (energy) stores. Therefore, without constant supplies of oxygen and glucose, ischaemic damage rapidly occurs. In health, autoregulation maintains relatively constant cerebral blood flow, if necessary depriving other tissues to supply the brain. But cerebral damage can cause autoregulation to fail, resulting in excessively high or low cerebral perfusion pressure (CPP). CPP is also limited by the inability of the skull to expand, and so CPP is the difference between mean arterial pressure (MAP) and intracranial pressure:

CPP = MAP–ICP.

Many monitors can calculate CPP from ICP. The arterial transducer should be at aortic root level, not head level. It can also be estimated by non-invasive transcranial Doppler (Edouard *et al.*, 2005).

CPP should be high enough to fully perfuse the brain, without increasing intracranial pressure – generally 65–70 mmHg (Werner and Engelhard, 2000), although with traumatic brain injury (TBI) target CPP is 60 mmHg (Robertson,

2001). Initial symptoms of insufficient or excessive CPP may include acute confusion and fitting, but sustained high or low CPP are likely to cause strokes.

Cerebral oxygenation is also influenced by oxygen carriage (e.g. hypoxia, anaemia). So management of intracranial hypertension should consider total trends and factors affecting cerebral demand and supply, rather than focusing on single measurements or parameters. Hypoxia ($PaO_2 < 7$ kPa) causes metabolic acidosis, which increases cerebral blood flow (Ross and Eynon, 2005).

Hypocapnia ($PaCO_2 < 4$) may cause cerebral vasoconstriction, and so ischaemia, while hypercapnia increases intracranial pressure. Ventilation should therefore aim for $PaCO_2$ 4.5–5.0 kPa (Hunningher and Smith, 2006).

Cerebral oedema

Intracranial hypertension is usually caused by cerebral oedema (May, 2009), which can be:

- interstitial
- intracellular
- (usually) vasogenic.

Interstitial and intracellular oedema formation is discussed in Chapter 33.

Vasogenic hypertension is caused when blood–brain barrier failure causes excessive blood flow into capillaries, which forces plasma proteins across capillary walls. Proteins in tissue spaces draw further fluid into already oedematous tissue.

Glasgow Coma Scale

Normal: 14–15.

The Glasgow Coma Scale (GCS) is an established means of assessing level of consciousness by evaluating eye, verbal and motor responses. It does not measure peripheral nerve function or effectiveness of chemical sedatives, and in the ICU eye responses may be impaired by disease or drugs. Although it does not measure pupil reaction or cardiovascular function, these are both affected by brainstem function, so are important adjuncts to GCS assessment.

Each response (eye, verbal, motor) scores a minimum of one point, so the minimum GCS score is 3 and the maximum 15. Scores below 14 indicate impaired consciousness:

13 = mild impairment
9–12 = moderate impairment
3–8 = severe impairment (coma).

Scores of 8 or below indicate high risk of airway obstruction from impaired consciousness, so intubation is usually indicated (Riley, 2009). Assessment should include distinguishing purposeful from reflex responses – e.g. eyes opening spontaneously may be a reflex.

Although overall scores add three components together, scores for each component should also be recorded, eye responses being less reliable for predicting outcome than verbal and motor responses (Teoh *et al.*, 2000).

Response to painful stimuli may already have been observed, such as localising irritation from oxygen masks or endotracheal tubes/suction. Inflicting pain conflicts with fundamental values of nursing, so should only be used when therapeutic benefits outweigh humanitarian considerations. Pain may also cause physiological harm, such as increasing intracranial pressure and stress responses. As peripheral stimuli may elicit spinal reflex responses of guarding or withdrawal, central stimuli should be used to assess consciousness (Cree, 2003). Central stimuli include:

- suborbital pressure (running a finger along the bony ridge at the top of the eye);
- trapezium squeeze (pinching the trapezius muscle, between head and shoulders);
- sternal rub (grinding the sternum with the knuckles);
- mandibular pressure – pushing upwards and inwards on the angle of the patient's jaw for a maximum 30 seconds (Waterhouse, 2005).

Peripheral stimuli, such as nail-bed pressure, can elicit central responses (Lower, 2003), such as grimacing, or peripheral reflexes (see page 240).

Different stimuli may be appropriate for different patients and situations. Painful stimuli should not be inflicted if patients respond to clear commands (Dougherty and Lister, 2008). The trapezium squeeze should not be used if patients have a neck injury, although the opposite shoulder to one-sided injury should be considered. Suborbital pressure should be avoided with skull fractures. Sternal rub should not be used repeatedly, as bruising and skin damage can be caused, and with cervical spine injury may be below the lesion and so fail to elicit a response. Mandibular pressure is more difficult, and may dislocate the jaw, so is usually the least useful stimulus. If response from one stimulus is unclear, other stimuli should be attempted.

Neurological crises may occur rapidly, secondary damage occurring before intermittent measurement (e.g. GCS) detects deterioration. Frequency of GCS monitoring varies greatly. In ICUs, GCS is generally assessed each shift, or more frequently if there are neurological concerns.

Pupil size and response

Normal: PERTL; normal size varies with light level.

Normally, pupils constrict in light and dilate in darkness. Pupil response is best assessed in a darkened area (if possible) to dilate the pupils. Both eyes should be assessed for:

■ pupil size (in millimetres);
■ whether both pupils are equal (PE).

Eyelids may need to be gently raised. A bright light (e.g. pentorch) should then be moved from the corner to the centre of the eye, assessing:

■ how briskly pupils react to light (RTL).

One-fifth of people have unequal pupils (Patil and Dowd, 2000), so minor inequalities are normal (Waterhouse, 2005). Dilated, fixed or (significantly) unequal pupils are usually a late sign of intracranial hypertension (Waterhouse, 2005). Pupil reaction is controlled by the occulomotor nerve (cranial nerve III) and is normally brisk, so sluggish responses indicate either brainstem damage or cranial nerve III dysfunction. Drugs affecting pupils include atropine eye-drops (dilate) and opioids (pinpoint constriction).

Limb assessment

Normal: equal + strong.

Limb movement requires both peripheral nerve and muscle function. Peripheral motor nerves may respond to either:

■ painful peripheral stimuli, transmitted through sensory nerves and causing spinal reflexes; or
■ central nervous stimuli (response to commands).

Both legs and both arms should be tested together, by:

■ asking patients to lift their limbs;
■ holding feet/hands and asking patients to push you away;
■ asking patients to grip your hands;
■ if unable to move limbs, testing ability to localise sensation – initially light sensations such as touch, but if these elicit no response, painful peripheral stimuli may be needed (e.g. fingernail pressure).

Assessment should evaluate:

■ strength (strong, medium, weak);
■ coordination;
■ any unilateral weakness.

Many people are slightly stronger on their dominant side, and for GCS assessment the stronger motor response should be scored, but significant weakness on one side may indicate a stroke or other problem, so should be noted and reported. Ability to raise legs when lying supine in bed also indicates significant muscle strength, and probable ability to breathe without ventilator support.

If not overridden by central nervous control, peripheral stimuli should cause guarding/defensive spinal reflexes, such as *flexion* (withdrawal). Central nervous system damage may cause abnormal peripheral responses, such as *extension* (pushing towards the stimulus) or *decorticate posture* (limbs flexed rigidly outwards).

Jugular venous bulb saturation (SjO₂)

Normal: 60–65 per cent.

Jugular vein catheterisation (using retrograde insertion of a CVP-like catheter with oximeter) enables oxygen saturation and content measurement; on X-ray the tip should rest at the border of the first cervical spine. Probes can also be introduced through ICP microtransducer burrholes (Kiening *et al.*, 1996). Like mixed venous saturation, jugular bulb saturation indicates global cerebral oxygen delivery.

Low levels are often artefactual, but may indicate cerebral hypoperfusion. High, and rising, SjO_2 often indicates increased cerebral blood flow, and very high levels (> 85 per cent) usually indicate imminent death.

Although SjO_2 can monitor total (global) cerebral oxygenation, it cannot identify where ischaemia or bleeds are occurring (Clay, 2000). SjO_2 is rarely measured outside specialist neurological ICUs.

ICP measurement

Normal: 0–15 mmHg.

Intraventricular catheters, usually fibre-optic, can be connected to most ICU monitors to display a waveform (see Figure 23.4).

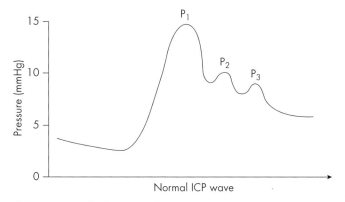

■ *Figure 23.4* **Normal ICP waveform**

Mean intracranial pressure is usually recorded. Arterial pulses affect intracranial pressure, creating waves that should have three peaks (Hickey, 2003b):

- P1: *percussion wave*: sharply peaked, with fairly constant amplitude, produced by arterial pressure transmitted from choroids plexus to ventricles.
- P2: *tidal wave*: shape and amplitude are more variable, but like an arterial waveform it ends on the dicrotic notch. P2 indicates cerebral compliance (Ross and Eynon, 2005).
- P3: *dicrotic wave*: from aortic valve closure.

Like other pressure-monitoring waves, dampened shape indicates unreliable measurement. Probes are normally reliable, but once inserted cannot be recalibrated. Suspected inaccuracy (doubtful waveforms) can be tested by lowering the patient's head, which should increase pressure, and so waveform amplitude.

Other technologies

Intracranial monitoring is necessarily invasive, and penetrating the skull for monitoring largely limits its use to specialist neurological centres. Almost inevitably, technological developments will bring some less- or non-invasive device that is sufficiently accurate for wider use. Geeraerts *et al.* (2008) found non-invasive ocular sonography correlated with invasive ICP.

Implications for practice

- Abnormal blood glucose levels are a common cause of acute behavioural changes.
- Nearly all units receive patients with head injuries, so need some means to assess and monitor neurological status.
- Because the skull is rigid, any increase in contents (bleeding, oedema) increases intracranial pressure, impairing cerebral perfusion.
- Where specialised neurological monitoring is unavailable, intracranial pressure can be assessed using:
  - Glasgow Coma Scale (with pupil responses);
  - spinal reflexes;
  - blood tests (glucose, electrolytes, gases);
  - mean arterial pressure.
- ICP should be 0–15 mmHg, but transient rises are insignificant.
- CPP should be sufficient to perfuse the brain, without increased intracranial pressure – 60 mmHg is usually aimed for.
- Continuous display is valuable for evaluating effects of all aspects of care.

Summary

Intracranial hypertension can occur in many ICU patients; monitoring neurological status (outside neurological ICUs) often relies on the Glasgow Coma Scale (GCS), which assesses level of consciousness rather than cerebral perfusion. More invasive methods of assessment inevitably incur greater risks, but may provide more useful information to guide treatment. As with monitoring any aspect of patient care, benefits and burdens of each approach should be individualised to patients, and justified by the extent to which they can safely be used and usefully guide treatments and care given. Management of patients with intracranial hypertension is discussed in Chapter 36.

Further reading

The *Marsden Manual* (Dougherty and Lister, 2008: chapter 26) provides useful, authoritative guidelines on GCS assessment. Hickey (2003a) remains the key text for neurological nursing. May (2009) reviews intracranial hypertension. Specialist journals include the *Journal of Neuroscience Nursing*, *Annals of Neurology* and *Journal of Neurology, Neurosurgery and Psychology*.

Clinical scenario

Michael Roberts is a 54-year-old who was admitted to the ICU unconscious. He sustained a head injury from a fall downstairs at home and was found by his partner. Mr Roberts is a known insulin-dependent diabetic who drinks approximately eight units of alcohol a day and has epilepsy. On examination Mr Roberts had a large scalp haematoma over the right parietal region, another over his right eye and bruising to his right elbow.

Mr Roberts' initial results are:

Glasgow Coma Scale (GCS) 6 (E1, V1, M4)
All limbs flexing spontaneously without any stimuli
Both pupils' response to light is sluggish, equal size at 4 mm
Respiration rate 26 bpm, audible gurgling breath sounds
SpO2 100 per cent on 15 litres of oxygen
BP 232/120 mmHg
HR 100 bpm
Capillary refill < 2 seconds with warm peripheries

Mr Roberts was intubated and sent for a head CT scan, which revealed a large right subdural haematoma with midline shift (9 mm) to the left side of his brain, widespread subarachnoid haemorrhage, fracture to right parietal skull and several focal intracerebral contusions. He underwent emergency craniotomy for evacuation of the subdural haematoma and insertion of an ICP bolt. He was invasively ventilated, and sedated with propofol and fentanyl infusions.

Mr Roberts' post-operative results are:

GCS 4 (E1, V1, M2)
Right pupil not assessed as eye closed from local swelling; left pupil sized at 2 mm and sluggish response to light
ICP 35 mmHg
BP 132/65 mmHg
HR 68 bpm
Capillary refill < 2 seconds
Central temperature 34.4°C
Blood sugar 14 mmol/litre

Q.1 Explain why the GCS is used in Mr Roberts' initial and post-operative neurological assessment and what his score represents. Consider how accuracy can be ensured, the frequency of assessment and the most appropriate type of stimuli for Mr Roberts.

Q.2 Calculate Mr Roberts' cerebral perfusion pressure (CPP = MAP–ICP) and explore its physiological implications (i.e. for cerebral perfusion and autoregulation, and effect on other body systems, especially those controlled by the autonomic nervous system). What is the likely cause and significance of his temperature and blood sugar results?

Q.3 Review complications and risks associated with ICP monitoring; consider how these may be managed with Mr Roberts.

Part IV

Micropathologies

Chapter 24

Cellular pathology

Contents

Fundamental knowledge   247
Introduction   248
Cell membranes   248
Mitochondria   249
Cell death   249
Inflammatory responses   249
Acute phase proteins   251
Radicals   251
Implications for practice   252
Summary   252
Further reading   252
Clinical scenario   253

Fundamental knowledge

Oxygen delivery to cells
Glycolysis

Introduction

Focus on visible macrophysiology (systems and organs) has increasingly been replaced by recognition that disease processes originate primarily at micro-physiological levels – organ/system failure follows widespread cell failure. Cell function relies on chemical reactions, which require both oxygen and energy. Absence of oxygen and energy sources (mainly blood glucose) therefore quickly leads to cell damage and failure. Inflammation is cell tissue's homeostatic response to protect itself, but exaggerated and inappropriate inflammatory responses cause life-threatening disease, such as systemic inflammatory response syndrome (SIRS – see Chapter 32). Restoring oxygen and energy supplies to failing cells may enable cell survival, reversing critical illness.

There are hundreds of chemicals that, in health, the body produces to help maintain homeostasis but that, in ill-health, can contribute to or cause critical illness. A few of the most significant chemicals are identified in this chapter, which therefore outlines pathological mechanisms underlying most critical illnesses. Readers may find sections in this chapter more useful as reference points for later use. This chapter begins with brief revision of cell physiology. If unfamiliar, this should be supplemented from anatomy texts.

Cell membranes

Cell membranes are a single layer of phospholipid, interspersed with proteins and cholesterol. This phospholipid creates an oil-like film that is both flexible and self-sealing, and that separates internal structures of cells from their external environment. Although some passive movement of fluid and solutes does occur across cell membranes, most movement is actively regulated by various 'pumps', 'channels' or 'gates' in cell membranes. Probably the best known is the sodium-potassium pump, but many others exist, including calcium channels mentioned in Chapter 22. Calcium channel blockers manipulate this channel in cardiac

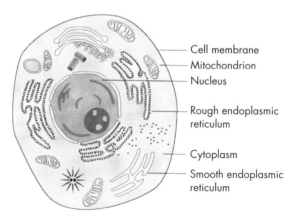

Cell membrane
Mitochondrion
Nucleus
Rough endoplasmic reticulum
Cytoplasm
Smooth endoplasmic reticulum

Figure 24.1 Cell structure

and vascular cells. Active movement through these pumps and channels maintains normal, healthy intracellular environments. Cell failure affects all parts of cells, including membranes.

Mitochondria

Mitochondria produce adenosine triphosphate (ATP), the type of energy that cells use. ATP is normally mainly produced from metabolism of glucose and oxygen (Krebs' cycle):

$$C_6H_{12}O_6 + 6O_2 \rightarrow 36 \text{ ATP molecules} + \text{waste}$$

While normal aerobic metabolism produces 36 ATP molecules from each gram of glucose, anaerobic metabolism (typically caused by perfusion failure – shock) produces only two ATP molecules (Nathan and Singer, 1999), together with two mmol of lactic acid (Nunn, 1996) – hence the significance of lactate measurements with shock/sepsis. Poor perfusion also fails to remove metabolic waste (acids and carbon dioxide), creating a toxic environment for failing cells. Oxygen radicals (see page 251) accelerate cell and organ failure. Cells with high metabolic rates (including cardiac and brain cells) are especially vulnerable to hypoxic damage (Clay *et al.*, 2001).

Cell death

Cells may die either through *apoptosis* (cell shrinkage; programmed cell death) or *necrosis* (cell swelling). Apoptosis is normal cell death; necrosis is pathological.

In health, damaged or redundant cells initiate apoptosis, a non-inflammatory process that causes changes within cells, causing them to shrink (Mach *et al.*, 2009). This ensures safe containment of intracellular contents, which if they escaped into surrounding tissues would be potentially toxic.

Necrosis is an inflammatory process. Lack of ATP (cell energy) causes pumps in cell membranes to fail (Kam and Ferch, 2000). This causes an influx of sodium, followed by water, while preventing escape of intracellular water, so causing intracellular oedema and further membrane damage. Cell membrane failure also increases calcium influx, which accumulates in the energy-producing mitochondria, so damaging organelles (Hunter and Chien, 1999). If not reversed, increasingly toxic intracellular environments progress to necrosis, and provoke inflammatory responses – release of pro-inflammatory chemical mediators such as tumour necrosis factor alpha (TNFα) and interleukins. Cell necrosis causes many pathologies seen in ICUs, so underlies discussion in many subsequent chapters.

Inflammatory responses

This homeostatic mechanism forms part of non-specific immunity. Damaged tissue releases pro-inflammatory cytokines (especially TNFα and interleukin 1), which provoke endothelium release of vasoactive chemicals, including histamine (a vasodilator) and leucotrienes (which increase capillary permeability). Increased blood flow and leakier capillaries enable leucocytes and other defences to migrate into infected tissue, and destroy invading bacteria. When confined to an area of local damage, this homeostatic response promotes healing; but when extensive inflammatory responses occur, extensive vasodilatation and massive capillary leak cause life-threatening SIRS.

Inflammatory responses release many chemical vasoactive mediators, which:

- vasodilate
- increase capillary leak
- activate other defences, such as mast cells.

There are many chemical mediators. Appropriate responses to threats, such as infection, help restore health. Imbalanced responses can either be insufficient, in which case diseases can cause harm or death, or excessive, in which case the response becomes pathological. Critical illness usually provokes excessive inflammatory responses; key mediators are discussed below.

Cytokines ('cell killers') are mainly mediators of the immune system, mostly released by leucocytes. TNFα (also called cachectin) is usually the first cytokine to be released, and initiates the cytokine cascade. TNFα stimulates growth of new surface receptors (adhesion molecules) on vascular endothelial cells, enabling leucocyte adhesion, accumulation and phagocytosis (Abbas *et al.*, 1994). TNFα:

- depresses cardiac function (negatively inotropic);
- initiates immune responses (including pyrexia);
- promotes clotting;

thus causing hypotension, pyrexia and thrombi.

Interleukins are a diverse group of chemicals, with varying effect, many pathogenic. They have been implicated in various autoimmune disorders (Raeburn *et al.*, 2002). Interleukins 1, 6 and 8 are major mediators of critical illnesses.

Nitric oxide is the main endogenous vasodilator released by vascular endothelium. It is released in response to tissue hypoxia, so once sufficient blood flow delivers oxygen, the mechanism triggering its release is removed. Excessive nitric oxide release, such as occurs during sepsis, causes inappropriate vasodilatation, and so hypotension. With tissue ischaemia, such as angina, nitric oxide release can be increased by nitrates, such as glyceryl trinitrate and isosorbide mono-/dinitrate.

Leukotrienes are mediators also released by leucocytes. Excessive leukotriene release in sepsis causes capillary leak – extravasation of blood water resulting in tissue oedema and hypovolaemia.

Acute phase proteins

Infection initiates early release of proteins, including fibrinogen, alpha-1 protinase inhibitor, C-reactive protein (CRP – see Chapter 21) and serum amyloid-associated protein to assist phagocytosis.

Radicals

Any biochemical reaction can release *free radicals* (e.g. micro-organism lysis by neutrophils, Krebs' cycle). Free radicals are molecules with one or more unpaired electron in their outer orbit; this makes them inherently unstable, reacting readily with other molecules to pair the free electron. Reaction of two radicals eliminates both, but reactions between radicals and non-radicals produce a further radical. Reactivity is indiscriminate, so although their lifespan lasts only microseconds, chain reactions may be thousands of events long, causing the autocatalysis underlying most critical illnesses.

Pierce *et al.* (2004) suggest that two free radicals are especially significant:

- nitrogen oxygen species (NOS)
- reactive oxygen species (ROS).

ROS, also called oxygen free radicals or oxygen radicals, are formed during reduction of oxygen to water, and have been implicated in hundreds of diseases (Pierce *et al.*, 2004). Oxygen radical reactions form toxic chemicals such as superoxide, hydrogen peroxide (H_2O_2) and hydroxyl (Mak and Newton, 2001) – hydrogen peroxide damages cell membranes and DNA (deoxyribonucleic acid) (Pierce *et al.*, 2004).

Oxygen metabolism occurs intracellularly, inevitably releasing some radicals. The few radicals normally produced are destroyed by antioxidants, such as vitamin E, vitamin C and albumin. Massive production of oxygen free radicals overwhelms endogenous antioxidant defences. Despite many studies, antioxidant therapy has few benefits; Haji-Michael (2000) argues that only selenium and glutamine have proven benefits. Neutrophil activation increases oxygen free radical production.

Hypoxic vascular epithelium releases endogenous nitric oxide, a vasodilator. Increasing blood flow delivers more oxygen to the hypoxic tissue. Nitric oxide release is stimulated by nitrates, such as glyceryl trinitrate and isosorbide dinitrate. Excessive nitric oxide production causes massive vasodilatation, one factor causing SIRS.

Reperfusion injury is caused when oxygen radicals and other toxic chemicals are flushed from any ischaemic tissue via the re-established circulation into the myocardium (Burke and Virmani, 2007). These chemical mediators can cause myocardial stunning, resulting in transient ventricular tachycardia, other dysrhythmias and ectopics. Although reperfusion injury can occur following any ischaemia, and is relevant to many pathologies discussed in the remainder of this book, it becomes especially significant following myocardial infarction,

251

accounting for up to half of final infarct size (Yellon and Hausenloy, 2007). Drugs to reverse these mediators are being researched, such as BAY 58–2667 (Krieg *et al.*, 2009).

Implications for practice

■ Most critical pathologies originate at microcellular rather than macrosystem level; knowing about these processes enables nurses to understand pathologies and treatments covered in most other chapters (e.g. pressure sores, oxygen toxicity, fluid and electrolyte balance).

■ Cells need energy and oxygen. Microcirculatory resuscitation requires:

● oxygen delivery to cells (tissue perfusion);
● nutrition;
● ventilation.

■ High FiO_2 (above 0.5–0.6) is potentially toxic, so should not be used for more than a few hours.

■ Reperfusion injury can cause secondary damage, so recovery requires close observation of effects (e.g. dysrhythmias) and prompt intervention.

Summary

Cell function is complex, and knowledge of cell function and potential medical interventions is rapidly increasing. Knowing about cell dysfunction is a useful basis for understanding pathophysiologies described in the remainder of this section. The microscopic nature of cell function and dysfunction makes these less easy to understand than function and dysfunction of major organs. This chapter has therefore given an overview of cellular pathology and some of the more significant mediators.

Most critical illnesses originate and progress at cellular level; macroscopic symptoms are accumulations of microscopic problems. Treatments should therefore focus on underlying mechanisms of disease rather than more easily observed effects. Understanding these microscopic mechanisms enables nurses to monitor and assess effects of treatments.

Abnormal figures (e.g. disordered arterial blood gases) may be tolerated to assist cell recovery (e.g. permissive hypercapnia – see Chapter 27). It is probable that future drug development will increasingly target micropathophysiology.

Further reading

Current attempts to target problems from cell dysfunction prompt frequent articles in medical and scientific journals, although complexities of this aspect of science limit the value of most articles for most nurses. Fewer articles have appeared in nursing journals, but Mach *et al.* (2007) review apoptosis. Normal cell physiology can be revised from recent and appropriate anatomy texts, such as Marieb and Hoehn (2007).

Clinical scenario

David Mitchell, 33 years old with a history of poorly controlled asthma, is admitted to the ICU following a respiratory arrest. On endotracheal suction his sputum is thick and mucopurulent, and arterial blood gases indicate severe respiratory acidosis.

His blood results include abnormalities in white blood cells and are:

WBC	27.3×10^{-9}/litre
Platelets	277×10^{-9}/litre
Neutrophils	23.4×10^{-9}/litre
Eosinophils	1.6×10^{-9}/litre
Basinophils	0.8×10^{-9}/litre
Monocytes	0.7×10^{-9}/litre
Lymphocytes	0.7×10^{-9}/litre
Hb	7.6 g/dl
CRP	372 mg/litre

Arterial blood gases are:

pH	7.26
$PaCO_2$	8.08 kPa
PaO_2	8.78 kPa
HCO_3^-	24.2 mmol/litre
Base excess	0.1 mmol/litre
Lactate	2.3 mmol/litre

Q.1 Draw and label a diagram of the typical eucaryotic cell. Include structures (and make brief notes on their functions) such as nucleus, cytoplasm, cytoskeleton, microtubules, endoplasmic reticulum, Golgi complex, ribosomes, mitochondria, lysosomes, cell surface (or surface membrane) with its various structures and components (e.g. desmosomes, tight junctions, gap junctions, antibody response and hormone binding sites).

Q.2 Analyse Mr Mitchell's WBC differential results; do they indicate inflammatory response or infection (e.g. consider functions of each cell type; which cells increase in response to bacteria or have digestive function, and which respond to allergens)?

Q.3 Mr Mitchell develops systemic hypotension and acute lung injury. Review the cellular processes that caused this from his respiratory condition (e.g. effect of hypoxia and hypercapnoea on cellular function, mitochondrial ATP production, cell membrane potential, mediators triggered, function and systemic effects of these mediators, causes of capillary permeability, role of basophils, implications of associated histamine release).

Chapter 21 identifies normal reference ranges.

Chapter 25

Immunity and immunodeficiency

Contents

Fundamental knowledge	254
Introduction	255
Immunity	255
Immunodeficiency	256
HIV and ARC	256
Problems	257
Ethical and health issues	258
Implications for practice	258
Summary	258
Support groups	259
Further reading	259
Clinical scenario	259

Fundamental knowledge

Physiology of normal immunity

Introduction

The immune system enables us to resist many potential pathogens, but most critically ill patients are immunocompromised. This chapter describes normal immunity, illustrating dysfunction through human immunosuppressive virus (HIV) and AIDS-related complex (ARC).

Immunity

Immunity may be:

- non-specific (innate)
- specific (adaptive).

Non-specific immunity is any defence mechanism not targeting specific micro-organisms. Much human non-specific immunity is present at birth. Specific immunity is necessarily acquired through exposure to various organisms or antibody vaccination.

Non-specific immunity includes:

- stickiness of mucous membrane and cilia (trapping airway particles smaller than two micrometres);
- body 'flushes' (tears, saliva), many including antibacterial lysozyme;
- sebrum (from sebaceous glands) preventing bacterial colonisation of skin;
- acidity/alkalinity of gastrointestinal tract;
- pyrexia (see Chapter 8);
- inflammatory response – increases and activates phagocytes and *complements*;
- interferon – inhibits viral replication and enhances action of killer cells;
- lactoferrin – binds iron (needed by microbes for growth);
- the steroid hormone cortisol (hydrocortisone) released from the adrenal glands and the glucocorticoid hormone cortisone released from the liver.

Non-specific chemical defences inhibit bacteria and viruses, but can cause or complicate disease, for example:

- inflammatory responses complicate most critical illnesses;
- stress ulceration is more likely with critical illness;
- graft versus host disease (GvHD – see Chapter 43) threatens viability of transplanted tissue (foreign protein), necessitating immunosuppression.

Logically, immunosupression would help recovery, but in sepsis, and probably most critical illnesses, steroids do not help recovery (Annane *et al.*, 2009).

Specific immunity involves recognition of specific antigens by antibodies (lymphocytes, part of the agranulocyte group of white cells – see Chapter 21). T-lymphocytes respond to (non-specific) protein by producing various cytokines;

B-lymphocytes are antigen-specific. Excessive or inappropriate responses can cause:

- allergy
- anaphylaxis or
- autoimmunity, if the body's own tissue is identified as the antigen.

Immunodeficiency

Failure of the immune system is usually either secondary to autoimmune pathologies (e.g. HIV, leukaemia, hepatic failure) or drug-induced (e.g. steroids, ciclosporin/tacrilimus, chemotherapy). The immune system can also be overwhelmed by infection or complex surgery/invasive treatment, exposing patients to opportunistic infections (e.g. *MRSa*), which may colonise, but not infect, healthier people (e.g. staff). Older people (most ICU patients) have decreased immunity due to age-related reduced T-cell function (Schwacha and Chaudry, 2000).

HIV and ARC

Since initial reports of HIV in 1981, some people have been colonised by the virus while remaining disease-free. HIV+ therefore means the virus is present, regardless of whether infection exists. Once the virus causes pathological responses, the person has acquired immune deficiency syndrome (AIDS), more often called AIDS-related complex (ARC).

In the 1980s, survival of ventilated HIV+ patients was poor, so ICU admission was often denied. However, partly due to highly active antiretroviral therapy (HAART), mortality has fallen from 70 to 39 per cent (Vizcaychipi *et al.*, 2007), survival to hospital discharge continuing to improve (Powell *et al.*, 2009), and outcome being comparable to other medical admissions to ICUs (Dickson *et al.*, 2007).

In the West, infection among 'high-risk' groups has declined, although needle sharing still causes about one-tenth of all UK HIV+ infections (Bennett and Baker, 2001). Worldwide, transmission is mostly heterosexual (Simon, 2006), and incidence among heterosexual non-drug users in the UK is increasing. UK incidence varies greatly, but tends to be highest in large inner-city areas.

HIV is usually divided between type 1 (HIV-1) and type 2 (HIV-2). HIV-1, prevalent in the West, is further divided into subtypes M (main), N and O (Simon, 2006). Initially, the virus replicates rapidly: 10^9–10^{10} daily, but after serocoversion, viral titre drops dramatically (Leigh Brown, 1999). HIV-1 assays can identify antibodies within 20 minutes (Simon, 2006), but seroconversion takes some weeks to occur.

HIV primarily attacks CD4 (T helper) lymphocytes, causing progressive problems with immunodeficiency. Once inside host cells, HIV transmits genetic information as a single *ribonucleic acid* (RNA) strand. Using the enzyme reverse transcriptase, it then replicates RNA into a DNA copy (hence 'retrovirus'). This clumsy arrangement is complicated by inaccuracies of enzyme replication, causing on average one mutation each replication cycle (Wainberg, 1999).

Problems

Autoimmune dysfunction exposes patients to opportunistic infections and other problems:

- respiratory failure;
- cardiovascular failure;
- gastrointestinal dysfunction;
- central nervous system damage;
- psychological stressors.

Respiratory failure remains the main cause of ICU admission (Wittenberg *et al.*, 2010), usually caused by bacterial pneumonia (Barbier *et al.*, 2009). The virus *Pneumocystis jirovici*, previously called *Pneumocystis carinii* pneumonia (*PJP*; sometimes still abbreviated as *PCP*) remains the single main microorganism causing respiratory failure (Miller *et al.*, 2006), although incidence is declining (Wittenberg *et al.*, 2010). *P. jirovici* forms cysts in alveoli and interstitial lung tissue, which often progress to ARDS. Tuberculosis (TB) infection increasingly complicates ARC (Huang *et al.*, 2006), a problem aggravated by development of resistant strains (Gandhi *et al.*, 2010). With HIV+ patients living longer, more are developing respiratory failure from asthma and emphysema (Huang *et al.*, 2006). Unsurprisingly, lower tidal volumes improve outcomes (Davis *et al.*, 2008).

Cardiovascular failure is often from sepsis, but prolonged anti-retroviral therapy can cause dyslipidaemias, insulin resistance and diabetes (Huang *et al.*, 2006).

Gastrointestinal dysfunction includes malnourishment and increased motility – diarrhoea, vomiting and nausea. Early nutrition, often with vitamin supplements, significantly improves outcome. Anti-emetics and antidiarrhoeal drugs can restore comfort and dignity. Mouthcare provides comfort and helps prevent opportunist infection.

Central nervous system damage and encephalitis are usually seen at postmortem. Many patients suffer both cognitive and behavioural changes, such as memory loss, apathy, poor concentration, and (very) early dementia. HAART has not reduced incidence of neurological disease (Wittenberg *et al.*, 2010). Cognitive changes can be especially distressing for families and friends.

Psychological stressors include the stigma surrounding HIV/ARC and anxieties about dying. Psychological distress needs human care and interaction, spending time with people, and allowing them to express their needs. Isolation may reinforce stigmatisation or provide valuable privacy for patients and their families or friends.

Ethical and health issues

HIV and ARC have raised more ethical dilemmas and issues than any other disease in recent years. Often, HIV status is undiagnosed on admission to the ICU (Huang *et al.*, 2006; Dickson *et al.*, 2007). Non-consensual touch is (legally) assault, so undertaking tests on patients unable to give informed consent, or receive the counselling that would usually be given before HIV testing, risks charges of assault. Although this applies to any tests, most tests in the ICU are justifiable as being in patients' best interests. Treatment for HIV is relatively long term, and knowing HIV status would often not alter the care given, so tests should usually wait until patients are fully conscious and can make informed decisions.

Relatives may discover diagnosis of HIV/ARC from death certificates, having been unaware, and perhaps disapproving, of the deceased's lifestyle. Duty of confidentiality to patients is absolute (apart from specific legal requirements), extending beyond the death of patients. Dilemmas raised through clinical practice can usefully be discussed among unit teams, contributing to professional growth of all involved. Goffman (1963) and Sontag (1989) raise provocative insights. Support agencies are identified below.

Implications for practice

■ Many ICU pathologies and treatments impair immunity, so high standards of infection control are needed to protect patients from opportunistic infections.

■ Respiratory failure is the main reason for patients with ARC being admitted to ICUs; outcome is comparable to most other patient groups, so HIV/ARC should not prejudice admission.

■ Informed consent should be gained before testing for HIV.

■ People with HIV/ARC may experience prejudice and stigma. Nurses have a duty of care to all their patients, and should promote positive attitudes among other staff.

■ ARC often causes various gastrointestinal symptoms. Nurses should assess nutritional needs and bowel function, feeding early, and providing appropriate care and support.

■ HIV+ patients and their families may need additional psychological support; many Trusts employ specialist HIV nurses.

Summary

Most patients in ICUs are immunocompromised. Treatments and interventions increase infection risks, but proactive infection control can reduce risks from nosocomial infection.

HIV and ARC have created medical and ethical challenges for healthcare. The unique role of nurses in the ICU team enables them to challenge and resolve stigmas and negative attitudes to meet the psychological and physiological needs of their patients.

Support groups

National AIDS helpline: 0800 012 322
Terrence Higgins Trust: 0845 1221 200
Body Positive: 0800 566 6599

Further reading

Ethical dilemmas raise issues from wider contexts; Goffman's (1963) classic work on stigma (written before HIV was identified) and Sontag's (1989) outstanding investigative journalism offer valuable sociological insights, raising many ethical issues. Extreme reactions to the stigma of a fictional killer virus are effectively illustrated in the film *Outbreak* (Warner Brothers, 1995). Many experiential accounts exist, such as Gunn's (1992) poetry chronicling the deaths of friends from ARC. Useful ICU-specific material includes Huang *et al.* (2006), Dickson *et al.* (2007), Powell *et al.* (2009) and Wittenberg *et al.* (2010).

Clinical scenario

Vanessa Warring, a 27-year-old single mother of two small children, was admitted to intensive care for ventilatory support following rapidly deteriorating respiratory function from right lung pneumonia. Miss Warring refused consent for an HIV test pre-intubation. Microbiology results confirmed presence of *Pneumocystis* pneumonia (*PCP*). Her CD4 count on admission was < 20 cells/mm³. Over the next ten days, Miss Warring continued to deteriorate despite therapy, she became colonised with several opportunistic organisms and it was obvious that she was dying. Her children were being cared for by a social worker.

Q.1 Explain the differences in immune response between HIV-positive and HIV-negative people on exposure to *Pneumocystis jiroveci*. (Why is an HIV-positive person more likely to develop *PCP*?) List other opportunistic organisms, and their source, that are likely to infect Miss Warring.

Q.2 Analyse the interventions available to support Miss Warring's system; include the value and limitations of these interventions (e.g. protective isolation, drug therapies of antibiotics, antiviral, antifungal, nutrition, psychological support, therapeutic relationships).

Q.3 Consider the ethical and legal issues associated with this situation. Should Miss Warring's children be tested for HIV? Who should make this decision and how would this be justified?

Chapter 26

Disseminated intravascular coagulation (DIC)

Contents

Fundamental knowledge   260
Introduction   261
Pathophysiology   261
Progression   262
Signs   262
Treatment   262
Related pathologies   263
Nursing care   264
Deep vein thromboses (DVTs)   264
Implications for practice   265
Summary   265
Further reading   265
Clinical scenario   265

Fundamental knowledge

Normal clotting – intrinsic, extrinsic and common
    coagulation pathways

Introduction

Disseminated intravascular coagulation (DIC) is secondary to other pathologies, causing uncontrolled systemic activation of coagulation, just as SIRS is uncontrolled systemic activation of inflammatory homeostatic responses. Half of deaths from polytrauma are from major haemorrhage, and between a quarter and half of patients with sepsis develop DIC (Zeeleder *et al.*, 2005). Pathophysiology and treatments are described, together with three related syndromes:

- haemolytic uraemic syndrome (HUS);
- thrombotic thrombocytopaenia purpura (TTP);
- heparin-induced thrombocytopaenia and thrombosis syndrome (HITTS).

Most hospitalised patients are at risk of venous thromboembolism (VTE) (Cohen *et al.*, 2008). Venous stasis from immobility, and procoagulant pathologies, place ICU patients at very high risk of deep vein thrombosis (DVT), the single main cause of pulmonary emboli. VTE prophylaxis, which is usually 'routine' for all ICU patients, is also discussed.

Pathophysiology

As with SIRS, pro-inflammatory cytokines are released by a trigger (Ho *et al.*, 2005; Zeeleder *et al.*, 2005), causing inappropriate systemic clotting, coagulation and fibrinolysis. Although gram negative bacteria cause most cases of DIC, other possible triggers include:

- viruses (especially varicella, hepatitis, cytomegalovirus (CMV));
- trauma;
- vascular disorders (aortic aneurysm);
- severe burns;
- obstetric complications (amniotic fluid embolus, abruptio placentae);
- hepatic failure (low-grade DIC);
- cancer;
- reaction to toxins/drugs;
- immunological disorders (severe allergic reactions, haemolytic transfusion reaction, transplant rejection).

(Hambley, 1995; Levi and ten Cate, 1999)

There is no single diagnostic test for DIC (Ho *et al.*, 2005; Levi *et al.*, 2009); the best laboratory tests are D-dimers and fibrin degradation product (FDP) (Yu *et al.*, 2000), although with major haemorrhage, confirming suspected diagnosis is usually less important than prevention, especially as management of DIC and major haemorrhage are broadly similar. *Thromboelastography* (TEG) shows quality, not quantity, of platelets.

Progression

DIC causes four main complications:

- haemorrhage
- hypotension
- microvascular obstruction and necrosis
- haemolysis.

Procoagulant material from cell injury enters the systemic circulation, activating widespread inappropriate clotting. Proteolysis stimulates further coagulation and fibrinolysis, causing intravascular formation of fibrin (Levi and ten Cate, 1999). Excessive fibrin deposits consume clotting factors (hence 'consumptive coagulopathy') and cause inappropriate clotting. Fibrin meshes:

- obstruct blood flow (especially to arterioles, capillaries and venules), causing capillary ischaemia, metabolic acidosis and tissue necrosis;
- haemolyse erythrocytes that manage to penetrate fibrin meshes;
- trap platelets (hence low platelet counts).

Consumption of clotting factors leaves insufficient for haemostasis, so patients bleed readily (typically from invasive cannulae and trauma, such as from endotracheal suction). DIC progresses rapidly, often occurring within a few hours of the trigger.

Signs

Early symptoms of DIC are typically non-specific, such as:

- *breathing* – mild hypoxia, dyspnoea;
- *circulation* – petechial bleeding (especially trunk), mucocutaneous bleeding (especially gut), purpura, minor renal dysfunction;
- *disability* – mild cerebral dysfunction (e.g. confusion);
- *exposure* – skin rashes, mottled, cool.

As DIC progresses, symptoms become more severe. DIC prolongs *clotting times*, with high levels of fibrin degradation products, such as D-dimers, and reduced levels of antithrombin and many clotting factors, especially fibrinogen, platelets and antithrombin. Patients bleed from multiple sites, including arterial and venous cannulae.

Treatment

DIC is always secondary to an underlying problem, so resolving underlying causes (if possible) usually stops DIC (Levi *et al.*, 2009).

Clotting factors should be replaced with the following:

- platelets should be transfused if patients are actively bleeding, but not prophylactically for low platelet counts (Levi *et al.*, 2009);

- fresh frozen plasma;
- cryoprecipitate (Green, 2003);
- fibrinogen;
- recombinant factor VII;
- vitamin K/tranexamic acid.

Heparin may be useful (Levi *et al.*, 2009) to dissolve microthrombi and so release clotting factors, but has no proven efficacy (Ho *et al.*, 2005). Giving antithrombin is not effective for DIC caused by sepsis (Ho *et al.*, 2005; Afshari *et al.*, 2007).

Severe acidosis may be actively reversed. System failure often necessitates support (e.g. ventilation, inotropes, haemofiltration). Various other symptoms may also require treatment (e.g. antibiotics and cytoprotective drugs to prevent gastric bleeding). The pro-inflammatory state often also causes vasodilatation and so hypotension. Aggressive fluid resuscitation is often necessary, but will further dilute already scarce clotting factors.

Related pathologies

Haemolytic uraemic syndrome (HUS) is a rare disorder in adults, although relatively common in children, similar to DIC, causing:

- haemolytic anaemia
- thrombocytopaenia
- acute kidney injury (AKI) (usually from microthrombi).

It is often caused by *E. coli* infection (Amirlak and Amirlak, 2006). Pathology and causes of HUS are unclear, but are often associated with bacterial or viral infections. Mortality can reach 12 per cent (Inward, 2008); urgent plasma exchange is essential (Short *et al.*, 2001).

Thrombotic thrombocytopaenia purpura (TTP), also rare, resembles HUS (Short *et al.*, 2001), extending to systemic and central nervous system involvement. Symptoms typically include purpura, neurological deficits, multifocal neuropsychiatric disturbances and kidney injury. TTP is usually treated by plasmapheresis and supportive therapies (Novitzky *et al.*, 2008). Platelets may exacerbate TTP, so should not be transfused unless there is life-threatening haemorrhage (British Society for Standards in Haematology, Blood Transfusion Task Force, 2003).

Heparin-induced thrombocytopaenia and thrombosis syndrome (HITTS; HIT) is caused by heparin therapy, especially unfractioned rather than low molecular weight heparin (Warkentin, 2003). Like DIC, HITTS can become fulminant, causing major organ infarction (e.g. myocardial, cerebral). Platelets may cause acute arterial thrombosis, so should not be given (British Society for Standards in Haematology, Blood Transfusion Task Force, 2003). Unfraction heparin is now rarely used, making HITTS a relatively rare phenomenon in ICUs.

Nursing care

Bleeding can occur anywhere, internally or externally. Nurses should therefore:

- observe skin for bruising, petechial or purpuric haemorrhages;
- observe any invasive sites for oozing/bleeding (e.g. intravenous cannulae, drains, wounds);
- observe and test any body fluids for blood (nasogastric aspirate, vomit, stools, urine).

Daily urinalysis may also reveal protein. Any abnormal findings should be reported.

Although DIC is a medical problem, and treatments will be medically prescribed, nursing care can significantly reduce complications from trauma, sepsis and bleeding. Many nursing interventions may provoke haemorrhage:

- endotracheal suction
- turning
- cuff blood pressure measurement
- enemas
- rectal/vaginal examinations
- plasters/tape
- shaving
- mouthcare.

Some interventions may be necessary, although alternative approaches should be considered. For example, as wet shaves are likely to cause bleeding, electric shavers may be safer. Similarly, foam sticks are less traumatic than toothbrushes. Lubrication of skin and lips (e.g. with yellow soft paraffin) helps prevent cracking. Invasive cannulae and procedures should be minimised to reduce risks of haemorrhage.

Small bleeds, which may be physiologically insignificant, can cause great distress and sometimes fainting. Visitors should be warned about the possible sight of blood, escorted to the bedside, and observed until staff are satisfied about their safety. If patients sense their relatives are distressed, they may themselves become distressed, aggravating their disease.

Deep vein thromboses (DVTs)

Risk of thromboembolism is significantly increased with immobility and infection (NICE, 2007a). DVTs delay hospital discharge (Parnaby, 2004) and can be fatal – pulmonary emboli are almost invariably from DVTs (BTS, 2003).

Development of DVTs is significantly reduced with subcutaneous low molecular weight heparin and anti-thrombotic stockings ('TEDS™') (NICE, 2007a). Unless there are specific contraindications, such as excessively prolonged clotting, all patients in ICUs should have:

- daily subcutaneous low molecular weight heparin;
- daily clotting screens (target INR 2.5 (Baglin *et al.*, 2006));
- knee-length anti-thrombotic stockings;
- twice daily removal and remeasuring of stockings.

DIC is not a contraindication to VTE prophylaxis in critically ill, non-bleeding patients (Ho *et al.*, 2005; Levi *et al.*, 2009).

Implications for practice

- DIC is a rare, but often fatal, complication of critical illness.
- If patients have prolonged/deranged clotting, nurses should be especially vigilant to minimise any interventions that may cause trauma/bleeding.
- Unless specifically contraindicated, all ICU patients should receive DVT prophylaxis (anticoagulants, TEDS™).
- TEDS™ should be removed twice daily, and remeasured before being replaced.

Summary

DIC is a rare complication caused by a variety of pathological processes. Early treatments with anticoagulants have been largely superseded by more conservative (temporary) approaches of replacing clotting factors and treating symptoms to buy time while underlying pathologies are treated. Nursing care should focus on avoiding complications of trauma, while minimising anxiety to both patients and relatives.

Patients in ICUs are at especially high risk of developing DVTs due to often prolonged immobility and pro-coagulant diseases and syndromes. DVT prophylaxis is, and should be, routine for all ICU patients, unless there are specific contraindications. Prophylaxis generally includes daily subcutaneous injection of low molecular weight heparin, knee-length anti-thrombotic stockings, and daily clotting screens.

Further reading

Levi *et al.* (2009) provide authoritative guidelines for DIC. NICE (2007a) guidelines for DVT prophylaxis should be followed.

Clinical scenario

Gary Williams is 56-year-old Afro-Caribbean man admitted with a coagulopathy of unknown cause. Initial investigations revealed deranged clotting, 15–20 ml/hour of cloudy urine with casts, fever (37.7°C), tachypnoea (44 breaths/minute) and tachycardia (124 beats/minute), with hypotension (84/58 mmHg) and severe metabolic acidosis. He has bloodshot eyes and rectal bleeding.

Mr Williams' blood investigation values include:		Laboratory reference range:
INR	1.5	0.9–1.1
APTT ratio	3.78	0.85–1.15
Thrombin time (seconds)	21	10–12
Fibrinogen (g/litre)	1.5	2–4
D-dimers (mg/litre)	8.48	0.0–0.3
Platelets (10^{-9}/litre)	26	150–400
Hb (g/dl)	7.8	13–18
WBC (10^{-9}/litre)	23.1	4–11
Neutrophils (10^{-9}/litre)	22.4	1.7–8.0
Lymphocytes (10^{-9}/litre)	0.7	1–4
Monocytes (10^{-9}/litre)	0.1	0.24–1.1
HCT	0.24	0.41–0.52
RBC (10^{-12}/litre)	2.91	4.5 –6.0
Urea (mmol/litre)	12.9	3–9
Creatinine (μmol/litre)	517	70–120 (male)
Creatine kinase (units/litre)	15571	30–210
Sensitive CRP (mg/litre)	244.8	0–10
Troponin T (ng/litre)	20	0–50

Q.1 Interpret Mr Williams' blood results and note the clinical significance of abnormal values. Consider which blood results are related to intrinsic activation and which are related to extrinsic activation of blood coagulation.

Q.2 Review which coagulation disorder is most likely to be associated with Mr Williams' symptoms, vital observations and blood results (e.g. HUS, DIC or other). Consider primary cause (e.g. sepsis, rhabdomyolysis) and how diagnosis may be confirmed.

Q.3 Three units of blood, cryoprecipitate, fresh frozen plasma and platelets are prescribed. Outline the rationale for these treatments and nursing approaches that can maximise their therapeutic benefits (e.g. specify methods, routes and order of administration, storage, temperature, minimising bleeding points and/or further fibrinolysis, evaluating effectiveness).

Part V

Respiratory

Chapter 27

Acute respiratory distress syndrome (ARDS)

Contents

Fundamental knowledge	269
Introduction	270
Ventilation	270
Reducing pulmonary hypertension	272
Fluid management	273
Psychological support	273
Implications for practice	273
Summary	273
Further reading	274
Clinical scenario	274

Fundamental knowledge

Respiratory anatomy and physiology – alveoli,
    pulmonary blood flow
V/Q mismatch; pulmonary shunting

Introduction

Acute respiratory distress syndrome (ARDS), the extreme form of acute lung injury (ALI), is a major cause and complication of ICU admission. It may be suspected if:

- there are increasing oxygen needs and difficulties ventilating;
- airway pressures rise and/or tidal volumes fall;
- there is new left ventricular failure;
- PaO_2/FiO_2 ratio is below 27 kPa (300 mmHg);
- bilateral infiltrates show on chest X-ray.

However, these may also be caused by other problems. Like most critical illnesses, the cost (mortality and financial) of ARDS is high, and evidence for benefits of specific management strategies is often limited and controversial. This chapter describes pathophysiology and likely medical interventions and treatments. Much nursing time is devoted to assisting doctors (monitoring, giving prescribed treatments) so nurses need to understand pathology and treatments. Prolonged stay and poor prognosis may increase psychological needs of ICU patients and families. Massive pulmonary emboli can be devastating and fatal, but are not discussed in this book as they are covered in Moore and Woodrow (2009).

ARDS is an inflammatory process. Early descriptions of ARDS usually identified two stages – exudative, followed by proliferative. These stages are now generally viewed as overlapping – exudation continuing throughout the disease. As water and protein accumulate in interstitial spaces, surfactant production declines, lung compliance is reduced, and fibrosis progresses (Jain and Belligan, 2007). This causes progressive decline in respiratory function, necessitating increasing FiO_2, PEEP and other ventilatory supports.

Mortality remains high – 35–65 per cent (Belligan, 2002; Hughes *et al.*, 2003). Many victims are young, with survivors often suffering poor quality of life, respiratory limitations (Orme *et al.*, 2003), muscle wasting and weakness (Herridge *et al.*, 2003) one year after discharge.

Ventilation

Severe lung injury is usually fatal without artificial ventilation, yet positive pressure ventilation can cause ventilator-associated lung injury (VALI). Large tidal volumes can cause 'volutrauma' (or 'volotrauma'). Smaller tidal volumes, and accepting abnormally high arterial carbon dioxide tensions (permissive hypercapnia) to limit peak airway pressure, can help alveoli recover (Putensen *et al.*, 2009). ARDSNet (2008) recommends initial tidal volumes of 8 ml/kg, reducing by 1 ml/kg at intervals of no more than two hours until tidal volume is 6ml/kg.

Permissive hypercapnia may create life-threatening respiratory acidosis, so should be used cautiously or avoided with:

- raised intracranial pressure;
- anoxic brain injury (e.g. following MI);
- severe ischaemic heart disease;
- hypotension;
- dysrhythmias.

So low tidal volume ventilation is not appropriate for every ARDS patient (Ricard *et al.*, 2003). Hypercapnia being a respiratory stimulant, neuromuscular blockage may be needed.

Mode of ventilation may affect outcome. As with other aspects of managing ARDS, options remain controversial, but spontaneous modes, such as airway pressure release ventilation (APRV), are more likely to reverse atelectasis (Yoshida *et al.*, 2009).

Debate persists about whether increasing *positive end expiratory pressure* (PEEP) improves outcome (Phoenix *et al.*, 2009; Caironi *et al.*, 2010), worsens it (Putensen *et al.*, 2009), or makes no difference (Briel *et al.*, 2010), but high PEEP often forms part of open lung strategies, which aim to maintain alveolar patency by preventing closure.

Inverse ratio ventilation (IRV) increases mean (but not peak) airway pressure: prolonging inspiratory time increases alveolar recruitment, while shorter expiratory phases prevent atelectasis. But IRV can cause air-trapping (auto-PEEP), and is usually distressing, requiring additional sedation, causing further hypotension.

Lung rest may limit or reverse damage (Gattinoni *et al.*, 1993); high-frequency oscillation (see Chapter 28) significantly reduces ARDS mortality (Derak *et al.*, 2002). Exogenous *surfactant* is ineffective for ARDS (Brackenbury *et al.*, 2001; Spragg *et al.*, 2003).

Prone positioning improves gases, and reduces rates of VAP (Abroug *et al.*, 2008), and may (Sud *et al.*, 2010a) or may not reduce mortality (Taccone *et al.*, 2009). It is labour-intensive, needing at least four nurses together with one doctor to manage the airway (Tidswell, 2001), and exposes patients to risks. Taccone *et al.* (2009) found it increased complication rates, although Abroug *et al.* (2008) claim it is safe, provided sufficient and appropriate staff are involved. Harcombe (2004) recommends:

- preoxygenation before turning;
- placing ECG electrodes on the back;
- supporting genitalia on a pillow.

Limbs should be placed in a 'swimmer's' position. Proning may reduce absorption, and so necessitate adjusting enteral feed rates (Seaton-Mills, 2000); angling the whole bed with the head up reduces reflux.

Complications of prone positioning are:

- pressure sores, especially on the thorax, head, iliac crest, breast and knee;
- benefits do not last;

- oesophageal reflux and vomiting;
- safety of limbs;
- extubation and line disconnection;
- need for more sedation;
- airway obstruction requiring suction;
- facial and orbital oedema;
- ocular damage ('ventilator eye');
- increased need for sedation and muscle relaxants;
- transient desaturation;
- hypotension;
- dysrhythmias;
- need for sufficient staff – up to six;
- difficulty in resuscitation.

Kinetic therapy can mobilise bronchial secretions (Welch 2002), and reduce extravascular lung water (Bein *et al.*, 2000) and VAP (Kennedy, 2004). Kinetic therapy needs to tilt at least 40° (Kennedy, 2004; Rance, 2005), and maybe 80–90° (McLean, 2001), for 18 hours/day (McLean, 2001; Kennedy, 2004). However, to prevent patients falling, most beds are limited to 20–30° (Morrell, 2010). Kinetic therapy can cause problems with:

- tachycardia;
- hypotension;
- desaturation;
- diarrhoea;
- discomfort and severe anxiety, necessitating sedation;
- claustrophobia;
- accommodating very large (height or weight) patients;
- wound *dehiscence*;
- need for heavy sedation to tolerate the movement;
- transportation (e.g. scanning).

(McLean, 2001; Welch, 2002; Kennedy, 2004)

Reducing pulmonary hypertension

Intra-alveolar damage increases pulmonary vascular resistance, causing pulmonary hypertension. Systemic vasodilators, such as glyceryl trinitrate (GTN) may cause problematic hypotension, but nebulised prostacyclin, such as epoprostenol or phosphodiesterase inhibitors (Sildenafil), dilate pulmonary vessels without significant systemic hypotension. However, coagulopathies, frequently complicating ARDS, may be aggravated by prostacyclin.

The rapid progression of ARDS, together with shortage of both donor organs and centres performing lung transplants, prevents lung transplantation being a viable option.

Fluid management

Fluid management in ARDS necessitates balancing problems from pulmonary oedema against perfusion needs. Measuring extravascular lung water (EVLW – see Chapter 20) has refined fluid assessment, but unfortunately optimum targets remain unclear – conservative fluid management reduces ventilator time but makes no difference to outcome (National Heart, Lung, and Blood Institute Acute Respiratory Distress Syndrome (ARDS) Clinical Trials Network, 2006).

Psychological support

Patients with ARDS may remain on the ICU for weeks, exposing them and their families to prolonged anxiety and stress, which may exhaust their coping mechanisms. One-fifth to one-third of patients with ARDS develop PTSD (Davydow *et al.*, 2008), with significant neurocognitive and emotional morbidity two years after hospital discharge (Hopkins *et al.*, 2005).

Prolonged stays can enable close rapport between families and staff, but can become stressful for both; both bedside nurses and nurse managers need to recognise distress. Families may seek hope where little exists, placing excessive trust, reliance and expectations on individual members of staff. As well as being a symptom of denial, this can be particularly stressful for staff.

Implications for practice

- ARDS is caused by inappropriate (excessive) inflammation in the lungs.
- ARDS may be suspected with increasing need for ventilatory support; other signs may include increasing airway pressure, new left ventricular failure and bilateral infiltrates on chest X-ray.
- Early recognition enables optimal treatment, so nurses should be able to recognise likely signs of developing ARDS, and report concerns.
- While increased ventilator support may benefit oxygenation, it may cause ventilator-associated lung-injury (VALI), so strategies such as permissive hypercapnia may be adopted.
- Prevention is better than treatment, and may be achieved by lung protection strategies – low tidal volume, lung rest/open lung strategies.
- Evidence supporting active treatments, such as steroids, surfactants and prone positioning, remains weak and controversial.
- After an initial fluid resuscitation, fluid restriction is probably beneficial.
- Cardiac output (flow) monitoring may be needed to guide fluid management.

Summary

ARDS, the extreme form of acute lung injury, is a relatively common complication of critical illness. Mortality remains high, and panaceas remain elusive. The mainstay of treatment is system support and attempting to prevent further lung injury. Prolonged ICU stays can place families, friends and nursing staff under considerable stress.

Further reading

Debate persists around most aspects, but meta-analyses such as Abroug *et al.* (2008) and Putensen *et al.* (2009) synthesise current evidence. The ARDSNet (2008) protocol provides evidence-based guidance for ventilation.

Clinical scenario

Ann O'Reilly, a 45-year-old mother of six children who weighs 104 kg, was admitted to hospital for elective ligation of fallopian tubes using fibreoptic surgery. Initially, Mrs O'Reilly was making a good recovery on the ward, but on the fourth post-operative day she presented with severe shortness of breath, fever and abdominal pains. Investigations revealed perforated bowel. Mrs O'Reilly became septic, developed ARDS and was transferred to the ICU for invasive ventilation and organ support.

In the ICU pressure-controlled inverse ratio ventilation was commenced:

PEEP 10 cmH$_2$O
Pressure control 30 cmH$_2$O
FiO$_2$ of 0.8
Rate 16 per minute
Tidal volumes 600 ml
I:E ratio of 2:1

Arterial blood gases on these settings were:

pH	7.25
PaO$_2$	6.53 kPa
PaCO$_2$	8.47 kPa
HCO$_3^-$	16 mmol/litre
Base excess	−5.8 mmol/litre

Q.1 List the physiological processes, investigations and signs that led to Mrs O'Reilly being diagnosed with ARDS.

Q.2 It is decided to place Mrs O'Reilly in the prone position in an effort to improve her alveolar gas exchange. Analyse the rationale underpinning this approach and resources required to implement this in your own clinical area.

Q.3 Mrs O'Reilly's gas exchange improves, allowing reduction in FiO$_2$ to 0.6. Appraise potential adverse effects of prone positioning with Mrs O'Reilly and propose nursing strategies to minimise or prevent occurrence (e.g. abdominal wound healing, pressure areas, breast-, eye- and mouthcare, and psychological effects on Mrs O'Reilly and her family).

Chapter 28

Alternative ventilatory modes

Contents

Fundamental knowledge	275
Introduction	276
Extracorporeal membrane oxygenation (ECMO)	276
Interventional lung assist (iLA)	277
High-frequency ventilation (HFV)	277
High-frequency oscillatory ventilation (HFOV)	278
High-frequency jet ventilation (HFJV)	278
Liquid ventilation	279
Hyperbaric oxygenation	279
Implications for practice	280
Summary	280
Further reading	281
Clinical scenario	281

Fundamental knowledge

Alveolar physiology, gas exchange and pulmonary
function
Surfactant production and physiology
V/Q mismatch

Introduction

Conventional ventilators remain the mainstay of ICU respiratory support, but significantly different methods of ventilation are occasionally used, usually as 'rescue therapies' when disease (usually ARDS) deteriorates despite optimal conventional ventilation. Although availability is often confined to specialist units, modes discussed in this chapter are:

■ extracorporeal membrane oxygenation (ECMO);
■ high-frequency ventilation (HFV), especially oscillatory (HFOV) and jet (HFJV);
■ interventional lung assist (iLA);
■ liquid ventilation (perfluorocarbon – PFC);
■ hyperbaric oxygenation.

Alveolar recovery is optimised if:

■ inflated sufficiently to prevent further atelectasis;
■ movement is minimised (low tidal volumes, to minimise volutrauma);
■ overdistension (high peak inflation pressures – barotrauma) is avoided.

Many modes discussed here achieve these aims, assisting alveolar recovery. Some modes are neither new nor established. Evidence on these is often sparse and dated, often from paediatric practice.

Most modes provide comparable oxygenation to conventional modes, but may provide lung protection. Many achieve better carbon dioxide clearance than conventional ventilation, so reducing respiratory drive, but potentially causing respiratory alkalosis.

Extracorporeal membrane oxygenation (ECMO)

ECMO, initially developed as 'bypass' for open-heart surgery (see Chapter 30), can replace or augment conventional ventilation. Like haemofiltration, ECMO pumps blood extracorporeally through semipermeable membranes. Concurrent lung ventilation is usually maintained during ECMO to prevent atelectasis, the efficient carbon dioxide removal by ECMO enabling use of lower tidal volume (lung protection) (Terragni et al., 2009). ECMO is an effective neonatal and paediatric treatment, but evidence for efficacy with adults is more controversial (Schuerer et al., 2008). As with most treatments, ECMO is more effective when used early (Brogan et al., 2009). However, the ethics of initiating controversial treatments early is debatable. Use currently therefore tends to be restricted to patients for whom conventional treatments have failed. Two recent studies report reasonable survival in patients for whom mortality would otherwise have been almost certain (ANZ ECMO Influenza Investigators, 2009; Peek et al., 2009), although Brogan et al. (2009) found mortality when used to treat severe acute respiratory failure was 50 per cent, a figure unchanged from older studies.

Complications of ECMO include:

- *bleeding*: circuits cause physical trauma to platelets (as with haemofiltration), compounding problems from anticoagulants and underlying pathologies (Gaffney *et al.*, 2010);
- *thrombosis*: blood surface interaction can cause thrombi, the other main complication of ECMO (Gaffney *et al.*, 2010);
- *cost*: from equipment, staff and extending life (or death) of very sick patients. Firmin and Killer (1999) suggest that 80 per cent of patient workload is from attending to circuits, compared to 20 per cent from nursing care of patients.

Interventional lung assist (iLA)

ECMO variants that have virtually fallen into disuse include extracorporeal carbon dioxide removal ($ECCO_2$-R) and intravenous oxygenation (IVOX). A recent development is the interventional lung assist (iLA) device, also called extracorporeal lung assist (ECLA). This uses a *shunt* in the femoral artery and, like other ECMO variants, achieves good carbon dioxide removal, but is less effective for oxygenation (Mallick *et al.*, 2008). NICE recommends that iLA should only be used with ARDS after conventional therapies have been exhausted (Mallick *et al.*, 2008).

High-frequency ventilation (HFV)

HFV includes various infrequently used modes, which have largely failed to establish a place in practice. Frequent but small tidal volumes prevent alveoli closure, so may prevent VALI (Carney *et al.*, 2005), although there is limited evidence to support their use (Wunsch and Mapstone, 2005). High-frequency jet ventilation (HFJV) and high-frequency oscillatory ventilation (HFOV) are used in some ICUs.

Complications of most high-frequency modes include:

- *Safety*: chest wall movement and air entry are barely perceptible and spirometry is impractical, and some ventilators have few alarms. Blood gas analysis and pulse oximetry are among the few remaining means of monitoring.
- *Variable tidal/minute volumes* are difficult to measure (Krishnan and Brower, 2000).
- *Gas trapping/shunting*.
- *Peak intra-alveolar pressures* are higher than measurable peak airway pressure. Excessive pressure may impair perfusion, so increasing mean airway pressure may exacerbate V/Q mismatch.
- *Noise*: like CPAP, high-frequency modes are usually noisy, provoking stress responses, inhibiting sleep, and contributing to sensory overload.

High-frequency oscillatory ventilation (HFOV)

Adding oscillation (5–10 *hertz* – Hz) to modified CPAP circuits or near-conventional ventilators achieves a form of high-frequency ventilation that can significantly reduce mortality from ARDS (Sud *et al.*, 2010b). Oscillation of alveolar air creates an active expiratory phase, reducing gas-trapping and improving carbon dioxide clearance. Carbon dioxide clearance can be increased either by increasing the power of the diaphragm or reducing the frequency. CPAP recruits alveoli and improves oxygenation. Both CPAP and fast respiratory rates (150–600 breaths each minute) keep alveoli open.

Usually a rescue therapy, FiO_2 is usually commenced at 1.0, with mean peak airway pressure slightly above the patient's previous setting (usually 3 cmH_2O) (Macintosh and Britto, 2000). As with other high-frequency modes, tidal volumes are small (10–15 ml), so only slight chest and abdominal wall movement ('wiggle') is seen. Amplitude of oscillation (delta P, ΔP) is increased until this movement reaches the groin or upper thighs (usual adult frequency 3–8 Hz). Mean pressure and oxygen are titrated down as oxygenation allows. Carbon dioxide removal can be increased by increasing amplitude, decreasing frequency, or creating a cuff leak – usually 5–7 cmH_2O (Higgins *et al.*, 2005).

Lungs should be auscultated, but low tidal volumes prevent clear air entry sounds. 'Wiggle' should be monitored – change indicating altered lung compliance or airway resistance. Suction causes alveolar deflation, and possible atelectasis, so should only be performed if specifically indicated, and if possible avoided completely for the first 12 hours. On chest X-rays, at most eight pairs of ribs should be visible; if more appear, lungs are overdistended.

Neonatal use has demonstrated alveolar recruitment and maximisation of alveolar lung volume (Bouchut *et al.*, 2004). It may increase risk of intraventricular haemorrhage (Keogh and Cordingley, 2002), although Bouchut *et al.* (2004) found no difference in cardiac output, organ perfusion, central venous pressure or cerebral perfusion between HFOV and conventional ventilation.

HFOV achieves higher mean airway pressures, which improves gas exchange, but may cause more barotrauma, pneumothoraxes and haemodynamic compromise (Chan *et al.*, 2007b). High mean airway pressures are also problematic with obstructive disease or asthma (Chan *et al.*, 2007b).

High-frequency jet ventilation (HFJV)

HFJV (or 'jet') uses tidal volumes of 1–5 ml/kg – with most adults, approximately the same volume as physiological dead space. Small tidal volumes may reduce lung injury, especially if patients have bronchopleural fistulae (Krishnan and Brower, 2000). Rates of 100–300 are usually used (Keogh and Cordingley, 2002). HFJV can be delivered through minitracheostomy (Allison, 1994), preventing many complications of intubation.

Carbon dioxide clearance is efficient. Pulmonary secretions are mobilised, presumably due to constant chest wall 'quivering' resembling physiotherapy, so increasing alveolar surface area and gas exchange. However, there is insufficient evidence of benefits for most units to justify costs of buying equipment and training staff for the small number of patients who might benefit (Krishnan and Brower, 2000).

Liquid ventilation

Perfluorocarbons (PFCs) are very efficient oxygen carriers, dissolving nearly 20 times more gases than water (Tremper, 2002). PFCs are also anti-inflammatory, creating fewer oxygen free radicals (Lange *et al.*, 2000; Haitsma and Lachmann, 2002). Although total liquid ventilation is possible, partial liquid ventilation – instilling PFC into lungs, then using conventional ventilation in the remaining lung fields – appeared attractive. However, while liquid ventilation improves oxygenation (Dernaika *et al.*, 2009), it also increases ventilator days and mortality (Kacmarek *et al.*, 2006), so cannot currently be recommended.

Hyperbaric oxygenation

Ratios between gases in air remain constant; if temperature remains constant, water content (volume) of humidified air also remains constant. So changes in atmospheric pressure alter the volume of each gas that can be dissolved in plasma. At sea level atmospheric pressure (approximately one bar), only small volumes of oxygen are dissolved in plasma (3 ml oxygen per 100 ml blood). If haemoglobin carriage is prevented (e.g. carbon monoxide poisoning), tissues rely on plasma carriage.

Twenty-one per cent oxygen at 2.8 bar (= 18 metres depth of water) increases oxygen pressure from 21 kPa to 284 kPa, providing sufficient plasma carriage to meet normal metabolism (Pitkin *et al.*, 1997). Hyperbaric oxygen of 3 bar reduces half-life of carbon monoxide from 320 minutes in room air and 74 minutes with 100 per cent oxygen to 23 minutes (Blumenthal, 2001), although benefits are controversial, and unless hyperbaric oxygen is readily available, its use for carbon monoxide poisoning cannot be supported (Juurlink *et al.*, 2005). Hyperbaric chambers can be single-patient, or rooms that staff and equipment can enter. Hyperbaric pressure can be discontinued once haemoglobin oxygen carriage is available (at most, usually a few hours).

Complications of hyperbaric oxygen include:

- *high atmospheric pressures*: causing barotrauma to ears and sinuses, oxygen toxicity, *tonic-clonic seizures* and visual problems such as myopia and cataracts (Wagstaff, 2009);
- *monitoring*: oxygen not being carried by haemoglobin, pulse oximetry value has no value;
- *infusions*: pressure may affect infusion pumps (Hopson and Greenstein, 2007), and tubing should be pressure-resistant (Bailey *et al.*, 2004);
- *access*: single-patient chambers may prevent equipment (including ventilators) being used, while transfer of equipment (e.g. emergency equipment)

between normal and hyperbaric pressures may be restricted or delayed; this may affect ventilation, inotropes and other infusions/mechanical support;

■ *scarcity*: few units have hyperbaric chambers, necessitating long-distance transfer of hypoxic patients.

Hyperbaric oxygen may provide support, enabling short-term survival; however, it does not reduce the incidence of neurological complications following carbon monoxide poisoning (Scheinkestel *et al.*, 1999).

Implications for practice

■ Modes discussed in this chapter are rarely seen outside specialist units; where used, staff should take every opportunity to become familiar with their use.

■ These modes are usually 'rescue therapies', so individual complications of each mode are compounded by complications of severe pathophysiologies; nursing care should be actively planned to optimise safety for each patient.

■ Visitors and patients may be anxious about use of rarer modes, or frightened by particular aspects (e.g. liquid ventilation = 'drowning'), so should be reassured.

■ Monitoring facilities are often limited with unconventional modes, so nurses should optimise remaining facilities (e.g. pulse oximetry, blood gases), which may need to be measured more frequently.

■ Highly invasive modes (e.g. ECMO) may cause haemorrhage; cannulae should (where possible) be easily visible.

■ Sensory disruption from noise should be minimised.

Summary

Modes discussed in this chapter are rarely used, but may offer significant benefits to some patients. ICUs not using these modes may transfer patients to units that do. This chapter provides an introduction to these modes for staff unfamiliar with them or new to units where they are used. More experienced users will wish to pursue supplementary material.

Whenever rarer modes/treatments are used, unidentified complications may occur. Therefore decisions to use (or suggest) alternative modes should be tempered by considerations of patient safety:

■ How will the patient benefit?
■ What are the known complications?
■ What is the likely risk from unidentified complications (research base)?
■ Are staff competent to use the mode safely?

Further reading

Brogan *et al.* (2009) and Peek *et al.* (2009) both report major recent ECMO trials, while Gaffney *et al.* (2010) provide a recent medical review. Mallick *et al.* (2008) provide some early evidence for iLA. Chan *et al.* (2007b) review HFOV. Carbon monoxide poisoning is reviewed by Weaver (2009).

Clinical scenario

Margaret Sheppard is a 60-year-old known asthmatic who was admitted to a respiratory ward with community-acquired pneumonia. Her respiratory function continued to deteriorate over nine days. She was then admitted to the ICU with a diagnosis of ARDS, intubated and commenced on high-frequency oscillatory ventilation (HFOV) to assist her breathing. The HFOV parameters were set as:

mPaw (mean airway pressure)	35.3 cmH$_2$O
FiO$_2$	1.0 (100% O$_2$)
Bias flow	20 litres/minute
Frequency	5 Hz
Amplitude (delta P)	82 cmH$_2$O
Inspiratory time	30%

Q.1 Explain the functions and settings used, and identify other respiratory observations/assessments required to be performed with patients receiving HFOV.

Q.2 Mrs Sheppard becomes increasingly hypercapnic (rising PaCO$_2$). Explain what parameters should be adjusted and explain the mechanism to reduce her CO$_2$ level.

Q.3 If the oscillator piston stops functioning, what actions should be taken? List the emergency equipment needed.

Q.4 Analyse potential complications of HFOV and strategies used to minimise these.

Q.5 Consider the criteria used to wean Mrs Sheppard and when the HFOV should be discontinued or changed to conventional ventilation.

Part VI

Cardiovascular

Chapter 29

Acute coronary syndromes

Contents

Fundamental knowledge	285
Introduction	286
Myocardial oxygen supply	286
Treatment	287
Cardiac markers	288
Thrombolysis	289
Some other drugs	289
Psychology	290
Health promotion	290
Implications for practice	290
Summary	291
Further reading	291
Clinical scenario	291

Fundamental knowledge

Coronary arteries – structure and location
Coagulation cascade
Renin-angiotensin mechanism
Reperfusion injury (Chapter 24)

Introduction

Cardiovascular disease (including strokes) remains the single main cause of death in western societies (Pottle, 2007). In cardiothoracic ICUs, interventions for coronary artery disease are usually the reason for admission (discussed further in Chapter 30). In general ICUs, coronary artery disease more often complicates other pathologies that have necessitated admission.

Coronary artery disease is an atherosclerotic process, with stable and unstable periods. During unstable periods, local inflammatory responses release vaso-active mediators that can cause *acute coronary syndromes* (Thygesen *et al.*, 2007):

- ST elevation (STE-ACS)
- non-ST elevation (NSTE-ACS)
- unstable angina (UA).

STE-ACS and NSTE-ACS are also called ST elevation myocardial infarction (STEMI) and non-ST elevation myocardial infarction (NSTEMI). If MI is suspected, or the person has chest pain that may be cardiac, a 12-lead ECG should be taken. Sedated patients may not show signs of chest pain, although most ICU monitors detect ST segment abnormalities. If the ECG shows ST elevation in two or more consecutive leads (2 mm in chest leads, 1 mm in limb leads) or a new left bundle branch block (i.e. not on the previous ECG), the patient has had a STE-ACS. If neither of these ECG abnormalities is present, troponin (or alternative cardiac markers) should be measured. Troponin positive indicates an NSTE-ACS. Negative troponin indicates UA, although troponin should be rechecked 10–12 hours after symptoms (NICE, 2010c). This diagnosis is summarised in Figure 29.1.

Myocardial oxygen supply

Myocytes have high metabolic rates, necessitating large quantities of oxygen. The right and left coronary arteries are the first arteries to leave the aorta, delivering one twentieth of cardiac output to the myocardium. The left artery divides into the *left anterior descending* and *circumflex* (see Figure 29.2). At rest, the myocardium normally extracts nearly all available oxygen, leaving little reserve for oxygen debt. In health, increased oxygen demand is met either through vasodilatation or tachycardia (or both). Unfortunately, coronary artery disease prevents significant vasodilatation. Critically ill patients typically already have compensatory tachycardias. Increasing tachycardia beyond 160 bpm reduces stroke volume (Hinds and Watson, 2008), making the myocardium work harder (increased oxygen demand) while further reducing oxygen supply.

Traditionally, high-concentration oxygen (15 litres via non-rebreathe mask, or pure oxygen if intubated) has been widely used with MI. The evidence for this is however controversial, and it is possible too much oxygen has caused more harm than good (Cabello *et al.*, 2010).

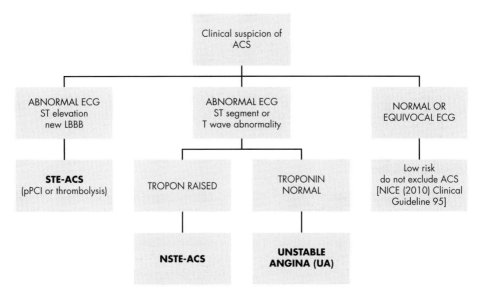

Figure 29.1 Acute coronary syndromes

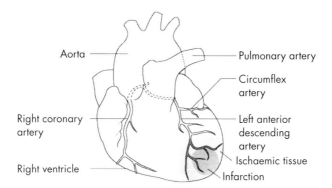

Figure 29.2 Coronary arteries, with anterior myocardial infarction

Treatment

STE-ACS should be treated either by primary percutaneous coronary intervention (pPCI – see Chapter 30) or thrombolysis (see page 289).

Task Force (2007) recommend managing NSTE-ACS and UA with:

- anti-ischaemic drugs (e.g. beta-blockers, nitrates, calcium channel blockers);
- anticoagulation (e.g. heparin);
- antiplatelet drugs (e.g. clopidogrel, aspirin);

and, increasingly:

■ coronary revascularisation (urgent angiography, early angioplasty).

Revascularisation for NSTE-ACS is controversial (Sharma and Kaddoura, 2005; Peters *et al.*, 2007), although the RCP (2010) recommends angiography with PCI if indicated within 96 hours for all patients at intermediate and high risk of cardiac events.

Cardiac markers

Injured cells release chemicals. Identifying and measuring these chemicals enables diagnosis of cell damage. The most useful chemical markers to identify cardiac damage are troponin (T or I) and B-type natiuretic peptide. Myoglobin is not sensitive or specific enough as a cardiac marker (Task Force, 2007). Creatine kinase (CK) and its isoenzymes, which are no longer widely used, can usefully assess skeletal muscle damage (e.g. with rhabdomyolysis).

Troponin ranges have been disputed, generally increasingly lower levels being recommended for diagnosing infarction. In the UK significant levels are considered to be > 50 nanograms/litre. Provided reasons for false positives can be excluded, higher levels indicate greater damage.

Troponin is elevated in many critically ill patients (Lim *et al.*, 2006), one-third of positive troponin results being for non-cardiac reasons (Blich *et al.*, 2008). Mild rises in blood troponin may be caused by:

■ kidney injury (Aviles *et al.*, 2002);
■ chronic heart failure and/or left ventricular failure (Wallace *et al.*, 2006);
■ pericarditis (Bonnefoy *et al.*, 2000);
■ pulmonary embolism (Konstantinides, 2008);
■ diabetes mellitus (Wallace *et al.*, 2006);

and any other damage to the myocardium.

B-type natiuretic peptide. Natiuretic peptides are hormones that increase renal sodium excretion ('natrium' = sodium) (Cuthbertson *et al.*, 2007). Originally isolated from the brain (hence 'B-type'), B-type natiuretic peptide is mainly secreted by ventricular myocardium in response to diastolic stretch (Saenger and Jaffe, 2007). Normal levels are < 25 picograms/ml (Rodseth, 2009), although being cleared by the kidney can normally be higher (< 100) in older people (Rodseth, 2009). Natiuretic peptides should not be used to diagnose acute coronary syndromes (NICE, 2010c).

Myoglobin (see Chapter 38) is released following muscle damage, including myocardial infarction. Normal serum myoglobin is < 85 ng/ml (Williams *et al.*, 2005).

Creatine kinase (CK) is also released from brain and skeletal muscle. There are three isoenzymes: MM (skeletal muscle), MB (heart), BB (brain). With availability of troponin tests, most laboratories no longer test isoenzymes.

Thrombolysis

STE-ACS, and arguably NSTE-ACS, should be treated by pPCI where possible. If pPCI is unavailable or impractical, urgent thrombolytics ('clot busters') should be given. Streptokinase (the oldest and cheapest) and t-PA/rt-PA (recombinant tissue plasminogen activator), both of which necessitate continuous infusions, have largely been replaced by third-generation thrombolytics that can be given by bolus, such as tenecteplase (Metalyse®). Urokinase, a weak thrombolytic, is useful for dissolving thrombi in vascular devices and shunts but not for treating MI.

Some other drugs

Many drugs are used in cardiology; the following are frequently seen in ICUs.

Nitrates (e.g. glyceryl trinitrate – GTN, isosorbide mono-/dinitrate) stimulate endogenous nitric oxide release, causing dilatation of coronary arteries, so increasing myocardial oxygen supply, limiting cell injury (Dezfulian *et al.*, 2009). Usually, GTN infusions are commenced. Isosorbide dinitrate can be given sublingually, enabling ready access and quick absorption. Surprisingly in view of their widespread usage, the Task Force (2008b) suggests there is no evidence that oral or transdermal nitrates improve prognosis.

Aspirin. A single dose of 300mg aspirin can reduce or prevent infarction. Optimal cardiac dose is 75–81 mg, with no clear benefit to doses above 100 mg (Steinhubl *et al.*, 2009). Like colleagues elsewhere, ICU nurses should ensure that patients and their families understand the prescribed dose – some patients self-medicate one 300 mg aspirin tablet each day.

Clopidogrel should be given to all acute coronary syndrome (ACS) patients: 300mg loading dose, then 75 mg daily (Chua and Ignaszewski, 2009).

Beta-blockers (drugs ending in -olol) inhibit beta stimulation of the heart, so reducing blood pressure (Chen *et al.*, 2010) and myocardial work.

ACE inhibitors inhibit *a*ngiotensin-*c*onverting *e*nzyme. Angiotensin is a more powerful vasoconstrictor than noradrenaline, so inhibiting the enzyme necessary for its activation prevents hypertension. This allows coronary artery 'remodelling'.

Calcium channel blockers (e.g. nifedipine, amlopidine, diltiazem, verapamil) regulate the calcium channel of action potential (see Chapter 22). This reduces myocardial excitability and vasodilates arteries.

Statins lower circulating lipid levels, so reversing the pathophysiology that causes atherosclerosis, significantly reducing coronary heart disease mortality (Cholesterol Treatment Triallists (CTT) Collaborators, 2008). Used for long-term treatment, they are unlikely to be commenced in ICUs, but patients already on statin therapy should resume their treatment as soon as practical. Most statins should be given at night (1800 or 2200 hours), as most cholesterol is synthesised overnight, although some statins are designed to be given earlier (e.g. artorvastatin). If in doubt about the timing of statin prescriptions, check with the unit pharmacist.

Psychology

Physical or psychological stress stimulates catecholamine release (see Chapter 1), which causes vasoconstriction, hypertension and other detrimental effects. While stress responses can be life-preserving for healthy people faced by physical danger in the community, negative emotions and the responses can be life-threatening to people with coronary heart disease (Todaro *et al.*, 2003). Patients with cardiac disease, and needing major cardiac interventions, appear more prone to long-term psychological ill health. Antidepressants do not affect long-term (18-month) physiological or psychological health (van Melle *et al.*, 2007).

Health promotion

Patients and families are often receptive to health information following infarction, and should be offered advice to reduce risks of further attacks. The British Heart Foundation produce a range of useful booklets that are available in most hospitals. Advice should be patient-specific, but is likely to include lifestyle changes such as:

- stopping smoking;
- exercise – walking or vigorous exercise is cardioprotective (Manson *et al.*, 2002), although exercise levels should be built up gradually to prevent acute ischaemia from sudden over-exertion;
- reducing alcohol – mild drinking appears to be cardioprotective (Lorgeril *et al.*, 2002), but heavy drinking contributes to atherosclerosis;
- reducing weight;
- healthy diet – reducing animal fats; fish oils and other sources of poly-unsaturated fatty acids (PUFAs) are cardioprotective (see *saturated fatty acids* in Glossary); dietician referral may be useful;
- good control of chronic co-morbidities (e.g. diabetes).

Implications for practice

- Hypoxic myocardium needs oxygen.
- Troponins are the best marker for myocardial infarction.
- New STE-ACS should be treated by primary percutaneous coronary intervention (pPCI).
- NSTE-ACS should be managed by angiography, possibly proceeding to percutaneous coronary interventions or open-heart surgery.
- Infarction risk is greatest between 0600–1000 hours, so avoid early morning strenuous stimulation (e.g. bedbaths) with all patients (unless requested by the patient).
- Pain relief is important both for humanitarian reasons and to prevent further stress responses; opioid analgesics are usually needed, and their efficacy should be assessed.

Summary

Coronary heart disease is endemic in western societies. Cardiovascular disease kills more people in the UK than any other single disease. Acute coronary syndromes may necessitate admission to the ICU (usually if there are other system complications), or occur in patients already on the unit. In addition to technical aspects, an important part of nursing care is health promotion.

Further reading

Jowett and Thompson (2007) is the key book on cardiac nursing. The European Society of Cardiology publishes various guidelines, both on its website and in the *European Heart Journal* (e.g. Task Force 2007, 2008b). Readers should be familiar with current UK Resuscitation Guidelines (currently, 2010).

Clinical scenario

Howard Gray is a 52-year-old insurance broker with a history of angina. He was admitted to the ICU four hours after he had woken up in the early morning with 'crushing' chest pain, unrelieved by sublingual nitroglycerine and with worsening dyspnoea.

His ECG shows wide Q waves (area of necrosis) in leads V_2–V_6, and ST elevation (area of injury) in leads I, aVL and V_2–V_6, with ST depression in II, III and aVF, no T wave inversion (peripheral area of ischaemia) noted.

HR 128 beats/minute
BP 80/45 mmHg (MAP 57 mmHg)
12-hour troponin T level 630 ng/litre

Q.1 Using a diagram of the surface of the heart and Mr Gray's ECG changes, identify which part of his myocardium is damaged and note the main coronary arteries that supply this area. List other cardiac markers used to assess myocardial damage.

Q.2 Mr Gray is given thrombolytic therapy. Review your role in administering and monitoring the effectiveness of this therapy (note frequency and type of investigation/assessment, identification of potential adverse effects).

Q.3 Evaluate the advice, information and follow-up services offered to patients like Mr Gray by your clinical practice area. What role does the ICU nurse have in relation to health promotion, advice and cardiac rehabilitation following myocardial infarction.

Chapter 30

Cardiac intervention and surgery

Contents

Fundamental knowledge   292
Introduction   293
Open-heart surgery   293
Percutaneous coronary intervention 294
Valve surgery   295
Coronary artery bypass grafts   296
Transplants   296
Post-operative nursing   296
Implications for practice   301
Summary   302
Further reading   302
Clinical scenario   302

Fundamental knowledge

Cardiac anatomy – arteries and valves
Coronary artery disease

Introduction

Coronary artery and valve disease (see Chapter 29) remain major causes of UK mortality, especially among older people. ST elevation myocardial infarction (STEMI, also called ST elevation acute coronary syndrome – STE-ACS) should be treated by urgent transfer for primary percutaneous coronary intervention (pPCI) (Antman *et al.*, 2008; di Mario *et al.*, 2008). With other cardiac disease, when drug therapies cannot support cardiac failure, percutaneous intervention or open-heart surgery may be needed either to repair or replace damaged tissue. Outcomes (survival and quality of life) for both are good, and have been for many years. Percutaneous and open surgery may be used to repair or bypass occluded coronary arteries or repair valves. This chapter also describes heart transplants. Intra-aortic balloon pumps and ventricular assist devices (means to support failing hearts) are described in Chapter 31. Immediate post-procedure nursing care largely follows from actual and potential problems created by procedures.

'Bypass' can variously mean the following:

1   *Blood pump oxygenators*, also called cardiopulmonary bypass (CPB), extra-corporeal membrane oxygenators (ECMO – see Chapter 28; more compact that other oxygenators) or heart–lung machines/devices, which oxygenate blood (replacing lungs) and pump the blood around the body (replacing the heart). These enable the heart to be bypassed, so it can be stopped with *cardioplegia* (see page 294) and operated on without movement from its beating.
2   *Surgery*, which grafts vessels to bypass occlusion in coronary arteries.

In this chapter, 'bypass' refers to grafts; in practice, contexts often clarify intended meanings.

Pump oxygenators can be:

- *disc* (blood exposed to oxygen-rich membrane);
- *bubble* (oxygen bubbled through blood);
- *membrane* (e.g. sheet and hollow-fibre membranes).

Membrane oxygenators are now usually used (Machin and Allsager, 2006).

Open-heart surgery

Open-heart surgery necessitates opening the thorax by sternotomy. Historically, this involved cross-clamping the aorta and venae cavae, using a blood pump oxygenator, arresting the heart with cardioplegia to enable surgery, and using moderate hypothermia to reduce metabolic oxygen demand. After completing surgery, the great vessels would then be reconnected, heartbeat restarted with DC shock, and hypothermia reversed. Some of these techniques are still used, but have been increasingly abandoned or replaced.

Pump oxygenators may cause or exacerbate:

- neurological complications, including strokes and delirium;
- respiratory failure, including atelectasis;
- inflammatory responses;
- kidney injury;
- blood cell damage.

Although pump oxygenator designs have improved, most open-heart surgery is now '*off-pump*' coronary artery bypass – OPCAB, often slowing the heart rate to about 40 bpm with beta-blockers. Off-pump surgery reduces:

- mortality (Demaria *et al.*, 2002);
- stroke (Douglas and Spaniol, 2009);
- post-operative atrial fibrillation (Møller *et al.*, 2008);
- hospital stay (Berson *et al.*, 2004).

However, Briffa (2008) claims there are no clear benefits to off-pump surgery, the technique is harder, and many surgeons are returning to pump oxygenators, while Shroyer *et al.* (2009) found one-year outcomes worse with OPCAB. Currently, off-pump surgery is impractical for valve repair/replacement, deep vessels and very small conduits, or patients who are very haemodynamically unstable or in cardiogenic shock. Four-fifths of operations still use pump oxygenators (Ailawadi and Zacour, 2009).

Cardioplegia, a potassium-rich crystalloid (Woods and Gray, 2009) used to arrest myocardium and so reduce metabolic oxygen demand, can cause post-operative dysrhythmias. Traditionally, cold cardioplegia (4–10°C) was used to reduce metabolism, but 'warm' (normothermic) cardioplegia is generally considered more cardioprotective, so is usually used.

Hypothermia (core temperature of 28–32°C) reduces metabolic oxygen demand and causes peripheral vasoconstriction (reducing venous capacity). Complications of hypothermia are identified in this chapter. Many centres have abandoned inducing perioperative hypothermia. To prevent hypervolaemia, two units of blood are usually removed for post-operative *autologous* transfusion. Post-operative rewarming causes vasodilatation, necessitating fluid monitoring and replacement.

Sternotomies are closed with permanent wire loops (usually five, visible on X-rays).

Percutaneous coronary intervention (PCI)

PCI is a generic term for procedures using catheters inserted into the vascular system and that enter the coronary circulation. PCI has increasingly replaced open-heart surgery. Among other interventions, procedures include:

- percutaneous transluminal coronary angioplasty (PTCA);
- coronary angiogram (diagnostic, although may proceed to PTCA);
- (increasingly) valve repair.

Originally usually inserted in the groin, whenever feasible a radial approach is now usually used. PCI tends to be preferred for single and two-vessel disease, while coronary artery bypass grafts (CABGs) remain standard care for triple-vessel disease (Serruys *et al.*, 2009). Angioplasty forces plaque back against the vessel wall and, unless vessels are especially tortuous, stents are inserted to maintain patency. Drug-eluting stents (DESs) reduce risk of restenosis (Brar *et al.*, 2009; James *et al.*, 2009), although Greenhalgh *et al.* (2010) suggest they do not reduce mortality and there is no evidence they are cost-effective.

Inevitably, many studies have compared outcomes between open and percutaneous repair. Long-term survival is similar (Hlatky *et al.*, 2009), although Bravata *et al.* (2007) suggest CABG relieves angina more effectively and reduces need for revascularisation, but stroke risk is increased (Serruys *et al.*, 2009).

Primary percutaneous coronary intervention (pPCI) (often referred to as primary angioplasty) is now recommended as the first-line treatment for MI, provided 'call to balloon' time does not exceed 120–150 minutes (DH, 2008a), although European guidelines suggest maximum time should be two hours (Task Force, 2010b). With therapeutic hypothermia used to reduce cerebral damage for out-of-hospital arrests, patients may be transferred significant distances to centres offering pPCI, with almost inevitable post-procedure admission to the ICU.

Valve surgery

Mitral valve disease, historically a late complication of rheumatic fever, has decreased in western countries, although incidence of age-related aortic stenosis is increasing (Blackburn and Bookless, 2002).

Diseased valves can be repaired or replaced. Replacement valves are either:

- biological (human cadaver, xenografts – porcine, bovine, baboon);
- prosthetic.

Biological valves are less thrombogenic, not requiring life-long anti-coagulation therapy, but are likely to need earlier replacement (Stasseno *et al.*, 2009). Most (> 85 per cent) mitral valve replacements in UK now use mechanical valves (Chikwe *et al.*, 2004).

Valve surgery is more complex than bypass grafts, so has higher mortality (Fisher *et al.*, 2002). Post-operative risks of valve surgery (open or percutaneous), include:

- tamponade
- infarction
- emboli
- dysrhythmias (from oedema and manipulation)
- chest pain.

(Lamerton and Albarran, 1997)

Valves can be replaced percutaneously (Coeytaux *et al.*, 2010), which enables post-operative recovery of uncomplicated cases in HDUs (Dewhurst and Rawlins, 2009). Mitral stenosis can be resolved by percutaneous balloon valvuloplasty (Chandrashekhar *et al.*, 2009).

Coronary artery bypass grafts

Occluded coronary arteries can be bypassed by grafts to restore myocardial blood supply. The saphenous vein, which is easy to remove, is often used, although arteries provide more effective grafts. The most commonly grafted arteries are the *internal mammary artery* (IMA, especially left – LIMA) (Tabata *et al.*, 2009), and increasingly the *radial artery* (Collins *et al.*, 2008). Arterial grafts can cause more pain, both from arterial spasm and from the graft site.

Transplants

Heart and heart/lung transplants can resolve endstage cardiac failure. Insufficient supply and preoperative mortality have encouraged interest in *xenografts* (including genetically engineered) and artificial alternatives, despite continuing problems with each alternative.

Post-operative nursing

In addition to the needs of any post-operative patient, cardiac surgery creates specialised needs. Complications vary, partly with procedures – normothermic and off-pump surgery avoid some problems. Common post-operative complications include:

- pain (including from sternal and saphenous wounds);
- respiratory failure and chest infection;
- neurological dysfunction;
- multiple and various dysrhythmias;
- hypothermia and hypervolaemia;
- initial polyuria causing hypokalaemia;
- haemodilution;
- anxiety.

Most patients undergoing cardiac surgery have only single-organ failure, so recovery is usually rapid, most patients being transferred to stepdown units the following day. Seeing and helping patients progress rapidly can be very rewarding for nurses. Emphasis should therefore focus on normalisation, promoting homeostasis and encouraging patients to resume normal activities of living.

Preparation

Any surgery is likely to be daunting for patients, but long-standing heart disease and traditional emotional connotations of the heart can heighten anxieties of patients undergoing cardiac surgery.

Ventilation

Extubation usually occurs at the end of surgery, or very soon after. *Hypoventilation* and *impaired cough* may be caused by:

- pain
- fear
- impaired respiratory centre function
- pleural effusion.

With adequate analgesia cover, patients should be encouraged to breathe deeply and cough. Good pain management and patient education can prevent many complications. Sternal instability, suffered by one-sixth of patients undergoing CABGs via median sternotomy (El-Ansary *et al.*, 2000), can cause 'clicking' sounds. Although not painful, external stabilisation with hands or a single-patient-use support, such as a 'cough lock', helps deep breathing and coughing. Incentive spirometry is often useful.

Exudative pleural effusions occur in half of patients (Light *et al.*, 2002). Brims *et al.* (2004) drained, on average, one litre of fluid from each patient, so improving oxygenation.

Hypertension/hypotension

Initial hypertension from hypothermic vasoconstriction may damage anastomoses, causing bleeding. Medical staff usually indicate upper limits for systolic pressure, frequently 100–120 mmHg, prescribing vasodilators (e.g. GTN) or inodilators (see Chapter 34). Persistent hypertension unresponsive to nitrates indicates neurological damage.

Hypotension is usually due to:

- hypovolaemia on rewarming;
- myocardial dysfunction.

Fluid is replaced to maintain CVP. Hypotension despite adequate CVP indicates myocardial dysfunction; inotropic support may be needed to maintain tissue perfusion.

Bleeding

Significant bleeding usually occurs from:

- anastomoses
- fibrinolysis and other coagulopathies (Pleym *et al.*, 2006).

Re-exploration for haemorrhage increases morbidity and mortality (Pleym *et al.*, 2006), so is avoided if possible.

Any sutures can prove incompetent, but aortic (from CPB) and myocardial sutures are exposed to high pressure and heartbeat/pulse movement. Arterial spasm with IMA grafts usually causes more bleeding. Pericardial bleeding may cause rapid *tamponade*. Two/three drains are inserted:

- pericardial
- mediastinal
- pleural (if pleura injured).

On arrival, volumes in each drain should be marked. Drainage, usually recorded hourly, should gradually reduce, becoming more serous. Sudden cessation may indicate thrombus obstruction, with likely tamponade; if patency of drains cannot be re-established, report this urgently, as emergency thoracotomy may be needed.

Coagulopathies are multifactorial (e.g. heparinsation using CPB), being monitored through full blood count and clotting studies. Haemostasis may require platelets/fresh frozen plasma (FFP) and/or other clotting factors.

Temperature

If hypothermic, gradual rewarming should bring central within 2°C of peripheral (pedal) temperature (avoid measuring pedal temperature on limbs from which saphenous veins are harvested). Warming hastens homeostasis and may prevent shivering (which increases metabolic rate, so increasing oxygen consumption).

Acid/base balance

Anaerobic metabolism from hypoperfusion causes metabolic acidosis. Although acidosis is closely monitored through blood gas analysis, it is not usually necessary to treat acidosis following cardiac surgery.

Dysrhythmias

Various dysrhythmias (often multifocal) often occur following cardiac (especially valve) surgery. Resolution is usually spontaneous and relatively quick. Causes include:

- chronic cardiomyopathy;
- oedema (from surgery, disrupting conduction pathways);
- acidosis;
- electrolyte imbalance;
- hypoxia/ischaemia;
- mechanical irritation (e.g. drain/pacing wire removal);
- hypothermia.

Only symptomatic and problematic dysrhythmias normally need treatment (drugs, pacing or resuscitation).

Atrial fibrillation occurs post-operatively in 20–40 per cent of patients (Cavolli *et al.*, 2008). As with other causes, amiodarone is usually effective (Kern, 2004), although Cavolli *et al.* (2008) found sodium nitroprusside useful.

Other post-operative dysrythmias include *bradycardias*, *blocks*, *junctional* and *tachydysrhythmias*. Persistent blocks often require pacing, hence perioperative placement of epicardial wires. Epicardial wires are unipolar, a negative pole being created by inserting a subcutaneous needle. Pacing wires usually remain in place until dysrhythmias become unlikely – usually 5–10 days.

Hypokalaemia necessitates frequent potassium supplements, usually diluted in small volumes of maintenance crystalloid fluid to maintain plasma concentrations of 4.0–4.5 mmol/litre.

Myocardial infarction may necessitate emergency thoracotomy/sternotomy and internal massage/defibrillation. Staff should therefore know where thoracotomy packs are situated. Internal defibrillation avoids transthoracic bioimpedance, so uses lower voltage (e.g. 20–50 *joules*).

Kidney function

Following initial polyuria, renal hypoperfusion may cause AKI, and reduce long-term survival (Hobson *et al.*, 2009). Maintaining adequate central venous pressure protects renal perfusion. Supplementary diuretics may be used, but some patients later require haemofiltration (see Chapter 39). Urinary catheters can normally be removed the day after surgery.

Pain control

Pain control is central to intensive care nursing; poor pain control may prolong recovery, circulating catecholamines impairing myocardial perfusion. Early post-operative pain usually needs opioid infusion.

Thoracic nociceptor innervation being relatively sparse, patients often experience relatively less pain from thoracic than saphenous incisions (Fisher *et al.*, 2002), although arterial graft spasm (e.g. IMA) can cause angina, and IMA harvest disrupts richly innervated tissue. Pain is individual, so should be individually assessed rather than stereotyped by operations performed. Nitrates (e.g. GTN) dilate arteries, reducing spasm pain and tension on newly grafted vessels.

Types of pain experienced following cardiac surgery include:

- bone pain (sharp/throbbing)
- visceral pain
- muscle pain (harvest site)
- cardiac/angina pain
- neurogenic pain
- psychogenic pain (anxiety)
- sudden pain/spasm.

Continuous analgesia may alleviate underlying/continuous pain (including anxiety-related pain), but nurses should observe for breakthrough (sudden/ spasm) pain, which may need bolus analgesia or nitrates. Once conscious, many patients benefit from patient-controlled analgesia (PCA).

Neurological complications

Up to two-fifths of patients admitted to ICUs after cardiac surgery have neurological deficits (Parnell and Massey, 2009), anxiety and depression often persisting long after ICU discharge (Gallagher and McKinley, 2009). Potentially fatal thrombi (and emboli) may be caused by:

- pump oxygenators;
- air emboli;
- thrombotic vegetations (chronic preoperative atrial fibrillation, infective endocarditis).

Neurological deficits can cause:

- impaired peripheral nerve function;
- cerebral/cognitive deficits;
- uncontrollable hypertension (injury to vital centres).

Cognitive function should therefore be assessed as soon as possible, and any deficits reported.

Psychological considerations

The heart, more than any other body organ, carries emotional connotations for most people – people 'love with their heart'. Both coronary artery disease and cardiac surgery increase incidence of depression (Wellwnius et al., 2008). Post-operatively, mood is often labile, euphoria (induced by opioids and survival) being followed (day 2–4) by reactive depression.

Stress provokes tachycardia, hypertension and hyperglycaemia (see Chapter 3), all impairing recovery in patients least able to tolerate such insults. Providing information, achieving optimum pain control, relieving anxieties and minimising sensory imbalance are therefore important aspects of holistic nursing care. Psychological distress, and sleep problems, may be reduced with off-pump surgery (Hedges and Redeker, 2008).

Skincare

Wound breakdown or skin ulceration may occur from poor perfusion, peri- or post-operative immobility and other factors. Pain and anxiety often make patients reluctant to move.

Wound dressings are usually removed within 24 hours; if clean and dry, wounds are then usually left exposed. Debilitation and poor cardiac output may delay wound healing. Sternal wound dehiscence is rare (3 per cent), but can prove fatal (Kuo and Butchart, 1995), especially following IMA grafts (which can reduce sternal blood supply by up to 90 per cent); complete sternal dehiscence necessitates surgical intervention.

Perfusion of graft sites (especially radial artery grafts; also arteriovenous shunts) should be protected, so pressure (e.g. blood pressure cuff, tourniquet) should be avoided.

Normalisation

Nurses can experience considerable satisfaction from assisting rapid post-operative recovery following cardiac surgery. Normalisation should be encouraged. Families and friends should be encouraged to visit, as they would on a surgical ward. The day following surgery, patients may enjoy breakfast before transfer. Early mobilisation should be encouraged.

Transplantation issues

Severing of sympathetic and parasympathetic pathways causes loss of vagal tone, resulting in resting heart rates of about 100 bpm. Denervation also (usually) prevents angina, increasing risk of silent infarction, but partial renervation does occur (Cox, 2002).

Loss of sympathetic tone impairs cardiac response to increased metabolic demands, making atropine ineffective.

Surgery preserves recipients' right atrium, which can cause two P waves (one intrinsic, one graft).

Implications for practice

■ Care of patients following cardiac surgery has much in common with care of other post-operative patients, but requires continuing full individual assessment.

■ Long-standing cardiovascular disease and acute responses to cardiac surgery necessitate close monitoring and system support – especially ECG and blood pressure.

■ Persistent problematic dysrhythmias may necessitate temporary pacing – epicardial wires are usually inserted perioperatively.

■ Cardiac drains should be measured on arrival, and excessive or sudden cessation of drainage reported.

■ Nurses should know where thoracotomy packs are kept, what they contain, and what will be expected of them in the event of emergency thoracotomy.

■ Patients should be encouraged to take deep breaths and cough periodically, especially following extubation.

■ Neurological events may prove fatal, so neurological state should be assessed as soon as possible after surgery, and any concerns reported.

- Physical and psychological pain cause various complications; patients should receive adequate analgesia, its effect being monitored by frequent assessment.
- Nursing care should focus on normalisation.
- Preoperative visits and information can significantly reduce stress, but psychological care of both patients and their families remains a nursing priority.
- Relatively rapid recovery requires nurses to spend much time on technical roles of assessing, observing, and administering drugs, but the human elements of care should be simultaneously maintained.
- Disease and interventions with the heart often cause greater anxiety than with other organs, so patients should be reassured and supported psychologically.

Summary

Most patients undergoing cardiac surgery are admitted to ICUs following treatment for single system failure, so usually recovery rapidly. This can be both rewarding and time-consuming for nurses. Many possible post-operative complications result from the necessities of intraoperative procedures; increasing percutaneous surgery may significantly reduce numbers of open-heart operations.

Further reading

The August 2009 (volume 89, issue 4) of *Surgical Clinics of America* was devoted to cardiac and vascular surgery. DH (2008a) and Antman *et al.* (2008) provide useful UK and USA perspectives, while the Task Force (2010b) provides European guidelines. There are many cardiac journals, and articles frequently appear elsewhere as well. Parnell and Massey (2009) provide a useful medical overview of care.

Clinical scenario

Johnny Doyle is a 57-year-old man with a history of angina, hypertension and insulin-dependent diabetes, and he weighs 110 kg. He was admitted to the ICU following two off-pump coronary artery bypass grafts (CABGs) using saphenous vein and left IMA to right ascending vein. Mr Doyle's blood sugar is 7.5 mmol/litre and managed by an intravenous infusion of 50% glucose at 20 ml/hour and insulin infusion running at 8 iu/hour.

Q.1 Describe Mr Doyle's preoperative preparation and explain its relevance to ICU care (e.g. type of investigations, patient information, pre-admission visits, diabetes control).

Q.2 Examine the nursing priorities and identify potential complications in the first 24 hours post-CABG surgery for Mr Doyle.

Q.3 Mr Doyle develops dehiscence of his sternal wound and can feel his sternum moving on deep breathing and coughing. Review causative factors for this complication and propose a plan of care to stabilise the sternum, and promote healing and recovery (evaluate various treatment approaches, pharmacological/surgical interventions, approaches used to stabilise sternum, blood sugar control).

Chapter 31

Shock

Contents

Fundamental knowledge   304
Introduction   305
Stages of shock   306
Perfusion failure   307
System failure   308
Types of shock   309
Supporting failing hearts   312
Implications for practice   314
Summary   314
Further reading   315
Clinical scenario   315

Fundamental knowledge

Cellular pathology (see Chapter 24)

Cardiac anatomy, including the mitral valve and pericardium

Autonomic nervous system – sympathetic and parasympathetic regulation, especially the vagus nerve

Baroreceptors and chemoreceptors

Renin-angiotensin-aldosterone mechanism

Normal inflammatory responses (increased capillary permeability, leucocyte migration, vasoactive mediators release)

Introduction

In health, normotension is maintained by matching blood volume to blood vessel capacity. This is achieved through autonomic reflexes and endocrine responses.

1 Hypotension is sensed by *baroreceptors* in major arteries, which activate the *hypothalamic-pituitary-adrenal* (HPA) *axis* (the stress response – fight or flight). More adrenocorticotrophic hormone (ACTH) is released by the pituitary gland, which stimulates adrenal production of adrenaline and noradrenaline, causing vasoconstriction. HPA axis activation also increases glucocorticoid secretion (O'Connor *et al.*, 2000).

2 Intrarenal hypotension initiates the *renin-angiotensin-aldosterone* mechanism:

renin (released by kidney)
activates angiotensinogen (in liver)

↓

angiotensin 1
mild vasoconstriction; changed by *angiotensin-converting enzyme* in (lungs) to:

↓

angiotensin 2
powerful vasoconstrictor – eight times more powerful than noradrenaline; also increases adrenal production of:

↓

aldosterone (adrenal gland)
increases renal sodium reabsorption

3 The pituitary gland releases more *antidiuretic hormone*, increasing renal water reabsorption.

So (1) reduces blood vessel capacity, (2) mainly reduces blood vessel capacity, while (3) together with increased aldosterone production (2) increases blood volume.

Adjusting these opposite responses enables the body to compensate for problems. Shock – inadequate blood flow to tissues or perfusion failure – occurs when compensatory mechanisms are exhausted or fail. Life-threatening hypotension may be caused by:

- loss of blood volume;
- increased blood vessel capacity; or
- both.

Because compensation usually occurs, hypotension is a relatively late sign. Earlier key signs, occurring during compensation, are:

- tachycardia
- tachypnoea.

Identifying these before hypotension occurs enables earlier intervention, and may prevent avoidable complications.

There are four types of shock:

- cardiogenic
- obstructive
- hypovolaemic
- distributive.

Some of these can be caused by different pathologies. This chapter provides an overview of the effects of shock, symptoms and main treatments. (Sepsis, septic shock and SIRS, the most common types of shock in ICUs, are discussed in the next chapter.) The first three types of shock (cardiogenic, obstructive and hypovolaemic) are then discussed. Some causes of distributive shock are discussed, but the main type seen in ICUs is septic shock and the *systemic inflammatory response syndrome* (SIRS) continuum, discussed in the next chapter. If other interventions fail, circulatory support with intra-aortic balloon pumps or ventricular assist devices are available in some centres; these are discussed near the end of the chapter.

Stages of shock

Shock is often classified into four stages, reflecting its progression and homeostatic responses:

- *Initial* (hypodynamic): poor cardiac output causes systemic hypoperfusion. Cells resort to anaerobic metabolism. Lactic acid begins to rise (> 1.7 mmol/ litre). Pulse oximetry may fail to detect a pulse.
- *Compensation* (hyperdynamic): neuroendocrine responses increase circulating catecholamine levels causing:

  - tachycardia;
  - increased stroke volume (palpitations);
  - tachypnoea;
  - oliguria.

  Other signs at this stage usually include:

  - dilated pupils, which are still responsive to light;
  - confusion, lethargy or agitation;
  - clammy/moist skin.

■ *Progression* (hypotensive): compensation fails (although tachycardia usually increases), causing hypotension. Arteriolar and precapillary sphincters constrict, trapping blood in capillaries. This activates inflammatory responses, including histamine release from mast cells, creating oedema. Signs include:

- hypotension;
- increasing tachycardia (> 150 bpm);
- hyperkalaemia (from cell damage – see Chapter 24);
- worsening metabolic acidosis;
- myocardia ischaemia (ECG changes);
- severely impaired consciousness;
- cold/cyanotic skin;
- progressive multi-organ failure.

Death often occurs at this stage, but shock may progress to a final stage:
■ *Refractory* (irreversible): symptomatic multi-organ failure, with no response to any treatments, death becoming inevitable within a few hours.

Early detection and appropriate treatment of shock may prevent progression, reduce complications, and improve outcome.

Perfusion failure

Perfusion may fail due to:

■ insufficient circulating volume;
■ inadequate cardiac output;
■ excessive peripheral vasodilatation.

However caused, perfusion failure deprives cells of glucose and oxygen. Tissue cells need energy – adenosine triphosphate (ATP), which is produced in their mitochondria. Without glucose and oxygen, mitochondria metabolise alternative energy sources (body stores – fat and muscle protein), and metabolism becomes anaerobic. Both anaerobic metabolism and metabolism of alternative energy sources are inefficient, producing relatively little energy and large amounts of waste, including lactate. Without perfusion, waste products of metabolism (carbon dioxide, water and metabolic acids) are not removed, creating an increasingly hostile, acidic internal and external environment, which, together with reduced energy production, progressively destroys cells. Shock therefore starves tissue cells of the oxygen and glucose they need for normal, healthy (aerobic) metabolism.

Anaerobic metabolism of alternative energy sources produces little energy but much waste, including metabolic acids (especially lactate, which forms lactic acid). Shock therefore causes metabolic acidosis:

■ pH < 7.35, with base excess < 2.0
■ lactate > 2 mmol/litre.

As cells progressively fail, intracellular contents progressively leak into blood. Normal intracellular and intravascular concentrations of many substances being very different (see Chapter 24), this causes many abnormalities, especially:

■ hyperkalaemia.

Progressive cell failure in organs causes progressive organ failure. Early symptoms of shock should therefore be aggressively treated with urgent micro-circulatory resuscitation (oxygen and fluids) to prevent organ failure.

System failure

Cardiovascular. In health, hypoperfusion triggers neuroendocrine compensatory responses (described on page 306):

■ hypothalamic-pituitary-adrenal (HPA) axis;
■ renin-angiotensin-aldosterone mechanism;
■ anti-diuretic hormone release.

Complex pathologies (most ICU patients) cause imbalance and failure of compensatory and autoregulation mechanisms. Reduced cardiac output reduces myocardial hypoxia, which usually triggers tachycardia. Tachycardia increases myocardial oxygen consumption, but reduces ventricular filling time and myocardial oxygenation time, so may make myocardium more ischaemic, provoking dysrhythmias and infarction.

Respiratory. Metabolic acidosis, from systemic hypoperfusion, stimulates tachypnoea. Pulmonary hypoperfusion increases pathological dead space and V/Q mismatch. Severe shock therefore increases work of breathing without improving tissue oxygenation. Ischaemic surfactant-producing cells in alveoli fail to produce surfactant, while increased capillary permeability causes pulmonary oedema, progressing to ARDS (once called 'shock lung').

Renal. Prolonged renal ischaemia (volume-responsive AKI) causes acute tubular necrosis (see Chapter 38), which increases toxic levels of active metabolites (e.g. urea contributes to confusion/coma).

Hepatic. The liver has a very high metabolic rate, so is particularly susceptible to ischaemic damage, although symptoms often appear later than with other major organs. The liver has many functions (metabolic, digestive, immune, homeostatic), so hepatic dysfunction causes many problems, including:

■ bilirubinaemia and (eventually) jaundice;
■ delayed clotting;
■ immunocompromise causing opportunistic infections, including sepsis.

Pancreas. Serum amylase and lipase become elevated. Pancreatic cell death releases myocardial depressant factor, further exacerbating shock.

Types of shock

Cardiogenic shock is caused by failure of the heart to pump sufficient blood. The most common cause of cardiogenic shock is myocardial infarction ('coronary cardiogenic shock'), occurring in about 8 per cent of myocardial infarctions (Babaev *et al.*, 2005). It can also occur following cardiac surgery (2–6 per cent) (Hausmann *et al.*, 2004). Other causes of cardiogenic shock include:

- valve disease, especially mitral regurgitation;
- congenital defects (e.g. ventricular septal defects);

and various other cardiac problems, collectively called 'non-coronary cardiogenic shock'.

Cardiogenic shock follows extensive left ventricular damage. Left ventricular dysfunction causes systemic hypotension, myocardial hypoperfusion and hypoxia, and pulmonary congestion (pulmonary oedema). Compensatory tachycardia may increase myocardial oxygen supply, but also increases consumption. Extensive left ventricular damage is rapidly fatal. The majority of people with cardiogenic shock will die (Power, 2009), usually fairly quickly. Survivors often develop congestive cardiac failure, necessitating cardiac surgery.

Treatment attempts to increase systemic perfusion pressure while limiting myocardial hypoxia. Inotropes may be necessary to increase cardiac output, but increase myocardial workload. As with sepsis (see page 318), increased nitric oxide production causes vasodilatation, so contributes to hypotension (Nicholls *et al.*, 2007). Van de Werf *et al.* (2003) recommend using intra-aortic balloon pumps (IABPs – see page 312) when cardiogenic shock complicates STEMI, although their efficacy has been challenged (Sjauw *et al.*, 2009).

Obstructive shock is caused by any obstruction to blood flow through the heart:

- raised intrathoracic pressure (positive pressure ventilation, PEEP);
- obstructed intrapulmonary flow (ARDS, pulmonary emboli, pneumo-/haemothorax);
- tamponade.

Tamponade is direct continuous compression of the heart, usually caused by pericardial haemorrhage. Accumulation forces myocardium inwards, reducing intraventricular space and stroke volume.

Tamponade can be slow or quick. Rapid tamponade (usually from cardiac surgery or trauma) is an emergency, usually causing imminent cardiac arrest once compensatory tachycardia and vasoconstriction fail. Tamponade should be suspected with sudden:

- CVP (or jugular venous pressure) increase;
- hypotension; and
- cessation of cardiac drainage.

309

These signs may be masked or absent because of hypovolaemia; other indications include:

- dysrhythmias and low voltage ECG trace;
- pulsus parodoxus;
- muffled apex heart sounds, due to transmission of the sounds through fluid;
- mediastinal widening (on X-ray);
- pericardial fluid accumulation (shown by echocardiography).

Rapid tamponade necessitates urgent needle aspiration of pericardial fluid, seldom allowing time for diagnostic tests, the needle usually remaining in place until drainage is < 50 ml/day (Spodick, 2003). Following pericardial aspiration, patients should be closely monitored for further accumulation (ECG, CVP, drainage).

Hypovolaemic (haemorrhagic) shock is caused by a rapid and large loss of blood volume, resulting in perfusion failure. Haemorrhagic shock causes more than half of deaths from trauma, and is the most common cause of shock in hospitalised patients. Hypovolaemia may be caused by:

- acute haemorrhage (trauma, surgery, gastrointestinal bleeding);
- other excessive fluid loss (e.g. diabetic ketoacidosis);
- insufficient fluid replacement if patients have difficulty drinking or are nil-by-mouth.

With compensation, people may survive loss of two-fifths of blood volume, but without compensation, losing one-fifth of blood volume over 30 minutes may be fatal (Guyton and Hall, 2005). When compensation fails, venous return falls (low CVP), inevitably reducing stroke volume. Compensatory tachycardia may restore blood pressure, but increased myocardial oxygen consumption can cause ischaemia, dysrhythmias and infarction.

Hypovolaemic shock should be treated, or (even better) prevented, by giving adequate fluid. When acute volume loss is uncomplicated by other disease, crystalloid fluid may be adequate. However, rapid infusion of crystalloids into critically ill patients usually provides only transient benefits, and can cause pulmonary and systemic oedema – see Chapter 33. To minimise risks from hypovolaemic shock, some ICUs routinely infuse gelatins before transferring patients by ambulance, as acceleration and deceleration during transport exaggerate blood pressure in hypovolaemia. Crystalloid or artificial colloid infusions dilute blood, and so clotting factors.

Distributive shock occurs when normal vasoregulation fails. Normally only one-quarter of capillaries are open at any one time (Deroy, 2000). Blood flow into capillaries is controlled by capillary sphincters. Excessive peripheral vasodilatation increases blood vessel capacity, so existing blood volume is maldistributed, excessive volume pooling in peripheral circulation at the expense of central blood volume and pressure.

The most frequent cause of distributive shock seen in ICUs is sepsis/SIRS, discussed in the next chapter. Other types of distributive shock include:

- neurogenic/spinal
- anaphylaxis
- toxic shock syndrome.

Neurogenic/spinal shock is caused when injury, oedema or disease of the spinal cord above the thorax interrupts autonomic sympathetic nerve control. Sympathetic tone, which increases heart rate and vasoconstriction, is impaired. Paradoxically, vagal (parasympathetic) regulation, which reduces both heart rate and vasoconstriction, usually remains intact. Problems above cervical vertebra 5 may cause respiratory failure, necessitating artificial ventilation.

Failure of autonomic response usually makes inotropes ineffective. Flow monitoring can identify whether vasopressures are effective. Volume replacement, mainly with colloids, can compensate for increased blood vessel capacity. Unresponsive sudden hypotension usually indicates a stroke, which, with critical illness, may prove fatal.

Anaphylactic shock is caused by T-lymphocytes (antibodies) recognising antigens, initiating an antigen-antibody reaction. This stimulates pro-inflammatory responses, releasing various chemical mediators from mast cells, which:

- vasodilate (e.g. interleukins, prostaglandins);
- increase capillary pore permeability (e.g. histamine);
- trigger clotting (e.g. platelet-activating factor).

Increasing capillary capacity together with increasing capillary leak (reduced blood volume) rapidly causes hypovolaemia, triggering tachycardia. Broncho-constriction causes respiratory distress.

Anaphylaxis typically occurs with second doses of drugs, but 'first doses' may not be danger-free – previous exposure to antigens (e.g. drug) may be unrecorded.

Anaphylactic shock is an emergency, treated with adrenaline to restore circulating blood pressure (Simons and Simons, 2010). Volume expanders, oxygen and other system supports may be needed.

Toxic shock syndrome is a rare form of sepsis, usually caused by *Staphylococcus aureus*, but can be caused by other organisms, such as A haemolytic *Streptococcus* (Nair *et al.*, 2006). There are very few cases each year in the UK – Nair *et al.* (2006) suggest about eighteen, although this is probably an underestimate due to under-reporting. Toxic shock syndrome is usually caused by poor tampon hygiene, but can be from any skin-surface *Staphylococci* invading the body, such as through wounds or dressings. Necrotising fasciitis (see Chapter 12) causes toxic shock syndrome. The rarity of toxic shock syndrome may delay recognition when it occurs, especially if unconscious women admitted to ICUs have tampons in place.

Supporting failing hearts

If other therapies fail, intra-aortic balloon pumps (IABPs) and ventricular assist devices (VADs) can support perfusion in heart failure, 'buying time' for transplantation (Shuhaiber *et al.*, 2010), PCI/surgery or recovery. Where available, IABPs are worth considering once inotropic support proves insufficient.

Balloon inflation in the upper descending aorta (see Figure 31.1) is synchronised with diastole, displacing 25–50 ml (Trost and Hills, 2006) (usually 40 ml) of blood both upwards (coronary and cerebral arteries, improving myocardial and cerebral perfusion) and downwards (increasing renal and systemic perfusion).

Increased systemic pressure is visible as augmented pressure waveforms on arterial blood pressure traces (see Figure 31.2).

Contraindications for IABPs include:

- aortic regurgitation (Trost and Hills, 2006);
- aortic aneurysm (Trost and Hills, 2006);
- severe calcific aorta-iliac disease or peripheral vascular disease.

The most common complication is limb ischaemia, so peripheral pulses should be assessed (Reid and Cottrell, 2005). Other complications include:

- bleeding at insertion site;
- thrombocytopaenia;

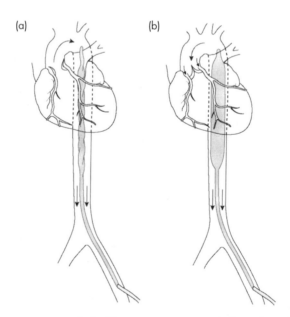

Figure 31.1 Intra-aortic balloon pump – (a) deflated and (b) inflated

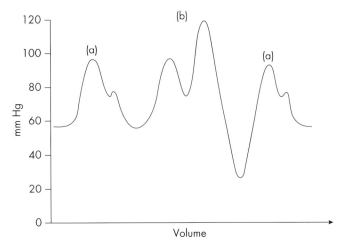

(a) Unassisted arterial pressure
(b) Augmented pressure with inflation increasing
    pressure after closure of the aortic valve creating
    a second pressure wave after the dicrotic notch

Figure 31.2 Arterial pressure trace, showing augmented pressure from use of an intra-aortic balloon pump

- infection;
- compartment syndrome (Reid and Cottrell, 2005).

Balloon rupture (rare) or gas diffusion through the balloon mixes gas used with aortic blood, so soluble gases (e.g. helium) are used. Helium causes rapid coagulation, so tubing should be frequently inspected for black flecks (clots). Gas cylinders maintain constant pressures to compensate for leaks. Alarms should sound before reserve gas in cylinders is exhausted, but nurses should still check cylinder volume and know how to replace them. While enabling survival, highly invasive devices expose severely immunocompromised patients to risks from infection and thromboembolism. If standby mode is used for prolonged periods (30 minutes), thrombi may have formed, so the IABP catheter should be changed. IABPs have high electrical consumption, which limits battery life during transfer.

In the event of cardiac arrest, the pressure trigger on IABPs augments compressions during cardiopulmonary resuscitation, and is vital for pulseless VT or PEA.

As the catheter is inserted into the femoral artery, clotting time should be checked before removal; this will usually be measured by activated clotting time (ACT; normal 120–150 seconds), a simple bedside test.

Ventricular assist devices (VADs – 'artificial hearts') may be biventricular (BiVADs – see Figure 31.3) or left ventricular assist devices (LVADs) (Task Force, 2010b). Percutaneously implantable devices have so far proved disappointing (Task Force, 2010b).

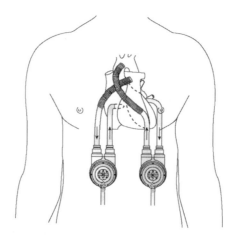

■ *Figure 31.3* Ventricular assist devices (left and right)

Implications for practice

■ Shock causes inadequate tissue perfusion at capillary (microcirculatory) level, so treatments should target microcirculatory resuscitation – primarily oxygen (aim SaO_2 > 94 per cent and fluid therapy (in ICU, usually colloids) to an adequate CVP – usually 10 cmH_2O (+PEEP).

■ Oxygen delivery can be assessed by comparing SaO_2 with $ScvO_2$ (see Chapter 20).

■ Once CVP is optimised, cardiac output can be increased with inotropes.

■ Unreversed shock will cause acute kidney injury (AKI). Volume-responsive AKI needs volume, and should not be treated with diuretics (Davenport and Stevens, 2008).

■ Sudden shock may be caused by tamponade, especially following cardiac surgery. If cardiac chest drains are present, patency should be restored. Otherwise, needle aspiration by medical staff may be necessary.

Summary

Many pathologies can cause shock. But however caused, shock results in inadequate perfusion to tissues, which, if not reversed, will cause progressive cell damage. Cells with high metabolic rates, such as cardiac and brain cells, are especially susceptible to perfusion failure. Once sufficient cells in an organ fail, the organ will fail to function adequately.

Priorities of care therefore focus on microcirculatory (capillary) resuscitation:

■ oxygen
■ fluids
■ system support.

Underlying causes of shock should, where possible, be treated.

Close monitoring and observation by ICU nurses, with an understanding of probable mechanisms of shock, enable prompt treatment.

Further reading

Shock is discussed in most nursing and medical texts. Garretson and Malberti (2007) provide a useful nursing review.

Clinical scenario

Reece Owen is a 71-year-old gentleman with COPD. He was originally admitted to hospital with acute exacerbation of COPD. Despite respiratory support and antibiotic therapy, his physical condition deteriorated. He became confused with a low GCS and unstable ECG, and was transferred to the ICU for flow monitoring, intubation and mechanical ventilation (PSIMV, PEEP of 8 cmH$_2$O, FiO$_2$ 0.4).

Observations on admission include:

Temperature	34.5°C
Heart rate	135 beats/minute
Rhythm	Sinus tachycardia with multifocal ventricular ectopics
BP	106/55 mmHg
CVP	24 mmHg
CO	4.72 litres/minute
CI	2.55 litres/minute/m^2
SV	35 ml
SVI	19 ml/beat/m^2
SVR	1000 dynes/second/cm^5
SVRI	1850 dynes/second/cm^5/m^2
ScvO2	68%
SVV	21%

Blood results are:

Haematology		Biochemistry		Arterial blood gases	
Hb	9.2 g/dl	CRP	129 mg/litre	pH	7.13
WBC	25.5 x 10^{-9}/litre	Na	142 mmol/litre	PaCO$_2$	7.13 kPa
Neutrophils	23.5 x 10^{-9}/litre	K	4.9 mmol/litre	PaO$_2$	14.67 kPa
Lymphocytes	0.2 x 10^{-9}/litre	Cl$^-$	110mmol/litre	HCO$_3^-$	16.3 mmol/litre

Blood results (cont.)

Haematology		Biochemistry		Arterial blood gases	
Platelets	334 x 10⁻⁹/litre	HCO₃⁻	18mmol/litre	Base excess	−10.1 mmol/litre
MCV	86 µm³	Glucose	10.5 mmol/litre	Lactate	1.5 mmol/litre
INR	1.5	Urea	14.2 mmol/litre		
APTT ratio	> 5.0	Creatinine	251 µmol/litre		
Thrombin time	> 100 secs	Albumin		11 g/litre	
		Troponin T	130 ng/litre		

Q.1 Identify the most likely cause and type of shock that Mr Owen may be experiencing. What other investigations might confirm this?

Q.2 Explain the physiology underlying Mr Owen's abnormal results. Comment on his organ and tissue perfusion.

Q.3 Consider interventions and devise a plan of care aimed at optimising cardiac index, tissue oxygenation and metabolic environment for Mr Owen.

The same patient is used in the clinical scenario for Chapter 32.

Chapter 32

Sepsis

Contents

Fundamental knowledge   317
Introduction   318
Sepsis   318
Systemic inflammation   319
Multi-organ dysfunction syndrome
  (MODS)   319
Treatments   320
Implications for practice   322
Summary   322
Further reading   323
Clinical scenario   323

Fundamental knowledge

Vascular anatomy – function of *tunica intima*
Cellular pathology (see Chapter 24), especially inflammatory
   response
Shock (see Chapter 31)
Immunity (see Chapter 25)

Introduction

Inflammatory responses usually complicate and accentuate critical illness, releasing many vasoactive and toxic chemicals, which, although designed to restore homeostasis, become pathological. They cause inflammation through the cardiovascular system, resulting in:

- vasodilatation
- capillary leak
- coagulopathies

and often progressive organ dysfunction. Although also seen with other pathologies, in ICUs this syndrome is seen most often with sepsis.

Sepsis-related conditions cause about one-tenth of ICU admissions, and remain the leading cause of death in critically ill patients (Hunter and Doddi, 2010). Infection can have many sources, although nearly half of cases are associated with central venous catheters (CVCs) (DH, 2007b).

The prevalence and problems of sepsis have prompted many searches for panaceas, which have remained largely elusive. Organ failure needs system supports – many of which have been discussed in previous chapters. This chapter therefore summarises progressive pathology, prognosis, and issues specific to sepsis.

Sepsis

Sepsis is an identified bloodstream infection. Severe sepsis occurs when sepsis causes organ failure. If infection provokes a balanced inflammatory response, recovery should follow. If responses are imbalanced, death is likely: inadequate inflammatory responses may cause death from the infection, while excessive responses may cause death from the effects of the response. This excessive response is sometimes called *systemic inflammatory response syndrome* (SIRS), where inflammatory responses throughout the cardiovascular system release a cascade of vasoactive and toxic chemicals (Hunter and Doddi, 2010). Inflammatory mediators vasodilate and increase capillary permeability ('capillary leak'); inappropriate and systemic release of these mediators causes distributive shock, hypovolaemia, profound hypotension and, if not reversed, progressive organ failure. If two or more organs fail, multi-organ dysfunction syndrome (MODS) exists. Each main organ/system failure carries approximately a 25 per cent mortality risk. Septic shock therefore forms part of the continuum:

sepsis → severe sepsis → SIRS → MODS.

Table 32.1 summarises the terminology.

Sepsis is usually caused by gram-negative organisms, although incidence of gram-positive sepsis, such as *MRSa*, has increased. Viruses or fungi, especially *Candida*, cause one-tenth of cases (Cohen *et al.*, 2004). Although SIRS is usually caused by sepsis, it can also be caused by non-infective triggers of systemic inflammation, such as severe pancreatitis, major burns and trauma.

Table 32.1 **Terminology of sepsis**

Term	Meaning
Sepsis	infection of bloodstream
Severe sepsis	sepsis with organ failure
Septic shock	sepsis with shock
SIRS	systemic inflammatory response syndrome
SSI	signs and symptoms of infection

Early identification of sepsis saves lives (Surviving Sepsis Campaign, 2007). Sepsis is diagnosed when patients have any two *signs and symptoms of infection* (SSI), together with a history suggesting a new infection. The SSI are:

- temperature > 38.3°C or < 36°C;
- heart rate > 90 bpm;
- respiratory rate > 20 bpm;
- white cell count > 12 or < 4 × 10^9/litre;
- acutely altered mental state;
- hyperglycaemia (> 6.6 mmol/litre) in the absence of diabetes.

(Surviving Sepsis Campaign, 2007)

Systemic inflammation

Tunica intima forms an active part of the cardiovascular system, releasing many vasoactive mediators, such as tumour necrosis factor (TNF), interleukins, nitric oxide, leukotrienes and platelet-activating factor (PAF). A balanced release of inflammatory mediators supports homeostasis, by local:

- vasodilatation
- increasing capillary pore permeability
- triggering clotting.

But excessive (systemic) response is pathological. The procoagulant state, combined with hypoperfusion, facilitates thrombus formation; disseminated intravascular coagulation (DIC) (see Chapter 26) complicates between one-quarter and a half of all cases (Zeeleder *et al.*, 2005). Neutrophil activation, by tunica intima, increases oxygen consumption, releasing superoxide radicals (Molnar *et al.*, 1999), which are negatively inotropic.

Multi-organ dysfunction syndrome (MODS)

Severe sepsis may progress to MODS; sometimes called 'multi-organ failure' – MOF). The sequence of organ failure varies, but often starts with respiratory failure, a major cause of ICU admission. Sepsis impairs respiratory muscle function (Lanone *et al.*, 2005). Cardiac dysfunction frequently follows. This is largely from vasodilatation and capillary leak (see page 250), but is compounded by sepsis reducing ejection fraction (Hunter and Doddi, 2010). If cardiac output is poor, dobutamine is the recommended inotrope (Hunter and Doddi, 2010). Cardiovascular failure typically causes AKI and low-grade liver failure. The liver is often the last main organ to show signs of failure.

There is no single treatment for MODS, but system support is attempted around each problem. A problem facing all systems is microcirculatory hypoperfusion, so tissue perfusion should be optimised, assessing needs through cardiac output study monitoring, and resuscitating with (colloid) fluids to deliver oxygen to tissues. However, once resuscitated, over-aggressive fluid therapy can cause pulmonary oedema (Durairaj and Schmidt, 2008). Capillary leak enables crystalloids to extravase rapidly, so many units prefer colloids, especially starches. Fluid therapy remains controversial.

Treatments

Human and financial costs of severe sepsis remain high, so much research has invested in finding solutions. Survival has improved, but remains poor, and solutions remain largely evasive. Treatment therefore focuses primarily on treating symptoms and preventing complications. The 'Sepsis Six' should be initiated as soon as sepsis is recognised, regardless of where patients are located, and completed within one hour. The Sepsis Six (initial bundle) are:

1   oxygen (100%)
2   blood cultures
3   antibiotics
4   fluids (20 ml/kg up to maximum 60 ml/kg)
5   lactate and Hb measurement
6   urinary catheter (aim > 0.5 ml/kg/minute).

(Surviving Sepsis Campaign, 2007)

A further bundle should be followed during the next six hours:

1   critical care
2   fluid resuscitation (as above)
3   CVC inserted
4   CVP: aim 8–12 mmHg
5   $ScvO_2$: aim ≥ 70%
6   Hb: aim > 7 g/dl
7   noradrenaline/dobutamine.

(Dellinger *et al.*, 2008)

Sepsis is caused by infection, so urgent antibiotics are fundamental to treatment. Survival is reduced by 7.6 per cent for each hour's delay in starting antibiotics (Kumar *et al.*, 2006), yet inappropriate initial antimicrobial therapy occurs in up to one-fifth of patients (Kumar *et al.*, 2009). Blood cultures should be taken before giving antibiotics. Effectiveness of antibiotics can be assessed by procalcitonin levels (Nobre *et al.*, 2008; Schuetz *et al.*, 2009; Stolz *et al.*, 2009; Bouadma *et al.*, 2010), enabling earlier changes from antibiotics than are ineffective.

Calcitonin is a hormone, or 'hormokine', which regulates calcium and phosphate in bone metabolism. Normal levels of its precursor, procalcitonin (PCT), are < 0.5 ng/ml; abnormal levels are listed in Table 32.2. Levels rise within hours of bacterial or fungal (but not viral) infection, peaking at six hours, allowing rapid evaluation of effectiveness of antimicrobial agents. Its half-life being less than 34 hours, levels should be monitored daily. Procalcitonin levels do not however predict outcome (Hillas *et al.*, 2010). Levels are not affected by steroid therapy.

Table 32.2 Significance of abnormal procalcitonin (PCT) levels

Level	Significance
< 0.5	normal
0.5	sepsis or surgery
2–10	severe sepsis
> 10	septic shock

However caused, shock results in tissue hypoperfusion. Shock creates a syndrome of microcirculatory hypoperfusion, creating an 'oxygen debt'. Reversing oxygen debt improves survival. Despite improvements in monitoring technology, oxygen debt (the difference between oxygen demand and oxygen delivery) cannot directly be measured. Where possible, causes are identified and treated and systems supported. Treatment should focus on early and aggressive resuscitation:

- CVP 8–12 mmHg
- mean arterial pressure ≥ 65 mmHg
- urine output ≥ 0.5 ml/kg/hour
- central venous saturation ≥ 70 per cent (or mixed venous saturation ≥ 65 per cent).

(Dellinger *et al.*, 2008)

Vasodilatory mediators and capillary leak cause profound hypotension. Aggressive fluid and inotrope therapy is often needed. Once adequately filled, noradrenaline can reverse inappropriate vasodilatation. Methylthioninium chloride (methylene blue) (Ghiassi *et al.*, 2004; Faber *et al.*, 2005) may be useful, but whether vasopressin/terlipressin is (Patel *et al.*, 2002) or is not (Russell *et al.*, 2008) is debated.

Steroids should theoretically reduce inflammatory responses. Views have varied, but most studies show no reduction in mortality from steroid therapy

(Sprung *et al.*, 2008; Annane *et al.*, 2009), so intravenous hydrocortisone should only be given if septic shock fails to respond to fluid resuscitation and vasopressors (e.g. noradrenaline) (Dellinger *et al.*, 2008).

High-flow haemofiltration (see Chapter 39), using rates of 35 ml/kg/hour, can remove many mediators of sepsis, but results have largely been disappointing, and the Surviving Sepsis Campaign does not support using haemofiltration in the absence of kidney injury (Dellinger *et al.*, 2008).

Early studies (e.g. Bernard *et al.*, 2001) suggested *activated protein C* (drotrecogin alfa; Xigris®) significantly reduced mortality from sepsis, but more recent evidence suggests it may be ineffective (Mackenzie, 2005; Kahil and Sun, 2008; Finfer *et al.*, 2008). The Surviving Sepsis Campaign (Dellinger *et al.*, 2008) recommends restricting use to patients at high risk of death – generally, this means APACHE ≥ 25 or with multiple organ failure.

Implications for practice

■ Sepsis, the most common pathology in most ICUs, causes inappropriate, systemic activation of inflammatory responses. This results in excessive vasodilatation, massive capillary leak, and coagulopathy.

■ Vasodilatation usually necessitates vasoconstriction (inotropes/vasopressors), and often flow monitoring (cardiac output studies).

■ Capillary leak necessitates aggressive fluid therapy, often with colloids, to maintain perfusion and prevent further organ dysfunction.

■ Multi-organ dysfunction syndrome (MODS) results from pathological processes initiated at cellular level, causing systemic inflammatory responses.

■ Mortality rates from MODS remain very high, increasing with each organ that fails, but early intervention to support failing systems (especially microcirculatory resuscitation) can improve survival.

■ Maintaining high standards of fundamental aspects of care, especially infection control, can reduce incidence and severity.

■ Mortality reflects the number of major organs failing; multidisciplinary teams should consider whether prognosis justifies continued treatment (is death being prolonged?); nurses should be actively involved in team decisions.

Summary

Sepsis often begins before ICU admission. The Sepsis Care Bundle has been widely promoted, and shown to improve outcome (El Solh *et al.*, 2008). Multi-organ dysfunction complicates many ICU admissions, incurring high human and financial costs. High incidence and paucity of curative (rather than supportive) treatment have encouraged a search for novel solutions. Such is the need that possible solutions are sometimes pursued with little (or even adverse) benefit. This chapter illustrates how progression from single to multi-organ failure remains the greatest challenge facing intensive care.

Further reading

SIRS remains the most frequent 'IGU pathology'. The Surviving Sepsis Campaign has published evidence-based international guidelines (Dellinger *et al.*, 2008). Aspects of management continue to be debated, researched and changed, so relatively frequent updates are likely to be issued. Garry *et al.* (2010) provides a recent overview.

Clinical scenario

Mr Reece Owen is a 71-year-old gentleman who was admitted to hospital with an acute exacerbation of COPD. His physical condition deteriorated, necessitating admission to the ICU for closer monitoring, flow monitoring, intubation and mechanical ventilation. By the second day, he remains sedated and ventilated (PSIMV, PEEP of 10 cmH$_2$O, FiO$_2$ 0.6). Mr Owen has multiple cannulation sites for haemodynamic monitoring and administration of drugs. He has a urinary catheter in situ draining < 30 ml/hour and a chest drain for an exudative pleural effusion.

Observations on the second day include:

Temperature	37.9°C
Heart rate	108 beats/minute
BP	110/60 mmHg
CVP	15 mmHg
CO	5.4 litres/minute
CI	2.92 litres/minute/m^2
SV	50 ml
SVI	27 ml/beat/m^2
SVR	750 dynes/second/cm^5
SVRI	1387 dynes/second/cm^5/m^2
ScvO$_2$	73%
DO$_2$I	420 ml/minute/m^2

Blood results are:

Haematology		Biochemistry		Arterial blood gases	
Hb	8.5 g/dl	CRP	135 mg/litre	pH	7.26
WBC	24 × 10^{-9}/litre	Na	141 mmol/litre	PaCO$_2$	8.08 kPa
Neutrophils	22.8 × 10^{-9}/litre	K	4.3 mmol/litre	PaO$_2$	12.2 kPa
Platelets	200 × 10^{-9}/litre	Cl$^-$	109 mmol/litre	HCO$_3^-$	18.4 mmol/litre
INR	1.5	HCO$_3^-$	20 mmol/litre	Base excess	−7.5 mmol/litre
APTT ratio	> 5.0	Glucose	9 mmol/litre	Lactate	1.5 mmol/litre
Thrombin time	> 100 secs	Urea	18.5 mmol/litre		
		Creatinine	326 μmol/litre		
		Albumin	10 g/litre		

Q.1 Using Mr Owen's results identify variables associated with tissue perfusion, organ function and potential survival. Outline the key interventions and optimal goals using perfusion variables that may improve his outcome.

Q.2 Review the inclusion and exclusion criteria for activated protein C (drotrecogin alfa, Xigris®). Consider how Mr Owen would benefit from this therapy and identify possible adverse effects.

Q.3 Justify using renal replacement therapy with Mr Owen. Analyse the evidence supporting this therapy and review potential risks versus benefits for patient with SIRS.

The same patient is used in the clinical scenario for Chapter 31.

Chapter 33

Fluid management

Contents

Introduction	326
Perfusion	327
Crystalloids	329
Colloids	330
Blood	330
Albumin	331
Other blood products	331
Gelatins	331
Dextrans	332
Starches	332
Oxygen-carrying fluids	333
Implications for practice	334
Summary	334
Further reading	335
Clinical scenario	335

Introduction

Most (60–80 per cent) of the body is water. Water is distributed unevenly between:

- extracellular
- intracellular

fluid, with potential 'third spaces' that normally contain no or insignificant volumes of fluid (e.g. 10–20 ml pericardial fluid), but which with disease can contain significantly more. Extracellular fluid is divided between the following compartments:

- intravascular
- interstitial.

In health, water distribution is approximately as shown in Figure 33.1.

Water moves across capillaries by pressure gradients; most water movement across cell membranes is actively controlled. In health, homeostasis maintains normal fluid balance. With ill health, gross and problematic fluid imbalance can occur.

In health, each day nearly five times total blood volume moves in and out of the cardiovascular system. Capillaries are semipermeable: thin, sqaumous (= scale-like) epithelium, with gaps between cells. Blood from arterioles has sufficient hydrostatic pressure to force water and small solutes through gaps between capillary cells. As capillary volume reduces, hydrostatic pressure falls, until extravasation ceases. Nearer the venule, large molecules (mainly plasma proteins, especially albumin) exert sufficient *osmotic* pressure to draw extravascular water back into capillaries. Osmotic pressure exerted within the bloodstream is called *colloid osmotic pressure* (COP). Colloid osmotic pressure is normally mainly created by plasma proteins, especially albumin. With critical

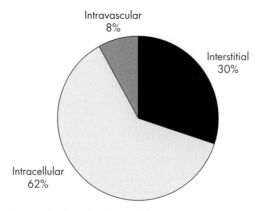

Figure 33.1 Normal distribution of body water

illness, inflammation often significantly increases capillary leak, while hypoalbu-minaemia reduces COP so less fluid returns to capillaries, resulting in both hypovolaemia and interstitial oedema.

Perfusion

Tissue perfusion is needed to supply nutrients to cells and remove waste products of metabolism. Tissue perfusion relies on pressure gradients across capillary walls. These gradients are the sum of:

- resistance in tissues
- (mean) arterial blood pressure (MAP)
- colloid osmotic pressure.

(See Figure 33.2.)

At the arteriolar end, intracapillary pressure (average: 35 mmHg (Guyton and Hall, 2005)) exceeds combined interstitial and COP, forcing fluid into tissues. As fluid extravases, intracapillary pressure progressively falls, (average: 15 mmHg by venule end (Guyton and Hall, 2005)), so interstitial and COP force most fluid to return into the capillary.

Capillary permeability varies greatly, ranging from the blood–brain barrier (least permeable) to renal glomerular capillaries (most permeable). Glomeruli may filter positively charged substances up to 70 *kiloDaltons* (kDa), although clearance rate reduces as molecular size increases.

All treatments, all drugs and all fluids have risks, so selection should depend on balancing risks and benefits in the context on each patient. Fluids used clinically have generally changed little in decades, but knowledge about their effects, benefits and problems has grown. Choice depends partly on whether the prime target is:

- maintenance;
- intravascular rehydration (resuscitation);
- whole-body rehdyration (especially intracellular).

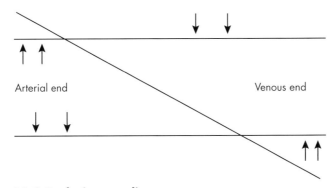

Figure 33.2 Perfusion gradients

Fluids for intravenous infusion are usually divided into two main groups: crystalloids and colloids. Crystalloids have small-molecule solutes, so extravase rapidly, hydrating mainly the extravascular compartment. Colloids have larger molecules, so remain longer in the bloodstream compartment. However, there are significant differences between different fluids in each group. Duration of fluids' effect, like drugs, is measured by *half-life*, although effect in critically ill people is often noticeably shorter. Table 33.1 summarises the main fluids.

Table 33.1 Summary of fluids (simplified)

Fluid	Half-life (hours)	kDa	Osmolarity (Osm/litre); COP	Benefits	(Some) disadvantages
Crystalloids	< ½	NaCl 58.5 Glucose 180	308 Osm/litre 252 Osm/litre	provide extravascular hydration	aggravate oedema; most are acidic
Blood	–	–	–	carries oxygen	limited supply; possible viral contamination (rare in UK); possible electrolyte imbalance
Albumin 4.5%	–	66.5	COP = 25 mmHg	no evidence of viral infection; hypoallergenic	limited supply; exogenous albumin effect only transient
Albumin 20%	–	66.5	COP = 75–100 mmHg	reduces oedema; free radical scavenger	limited supply; exogenous albumin effect only transient
Gelatins	2–3	20–40	274 mOsm/litre (Gelofusine®); 284 mOsm/litre (Volplex®)	cheap, stable during storage	short half-life (compared with other colloids)
Dextrans (almost obsolete)	4–6	40–70	274–301 mOsm/litre	promotes peripheral perfusion; prevents thromboembolism	coagulopathies; allergenic
Starches	12–24	200–450	308 mOsm/litre (Voluven®) COP = 280–1088 mmHg	prolonged effect; reduces oedema	expensive, prolonged clearance; prolonged clotting; allergenic
Oxygen-carrying fluids	6–48	–	–	can carry oxygen	novel therapy with multiple problems; vary between products; currently not licensed in UK

Note: normal plasma *osmolarity* = 275–300 Osm/litre.

Crystalloids

Most of the body is water; crystalloids are effective fluids for maintaining whole-body hydration, as they rapidly extravase, so quickly passing into extravascular (interstitial and intracellular) spaces, where most body water is. However, extravasation makes them poor resuscitation fluids: increases in blood volume are transitory, and oedema can rapidly develop (Norberg *et al.*, 2005), especially with ICU patients who usually have excessive inflammatory responses, and so excessive capillary leak. Most crystalloids are also acidic (see Table 33.1), and likely to exacerbate the acidosis that usually accompanies critical illness.

Sodium chloride: 0.9% sodium chloride ('normal saline') mostly extravases into interstitial spaces, where it largely remains, sodium being primarily an extracellular cation. Its 154 mmol/litre of chloride is approximately double normal plasma levels (95–108 mmol/litre); hyperchloraemia draws hydrogen ions from water, producing acid, so excessive saline infusion saline can cause hyperchloraemic metabolic acidosis (Surviving Sepsis Campaign, 2007; Ochola and Venkatesh, 2009). Hypotonic and hypertonic saline solutions (different percentages) are available, providing different osmotic 'pull', but currently are seldom used in most UK ICUs.

Glucose: 5% glucose is a little glucose (5 grams per 100 ml) and water. The water therefore moves freely, mainly into intracellular fluid, where most body water should normally be. Glucose solutions are therefore excellent intracellular rehydration solutions, but should be avoided with raised intracranial pressure as they will increase cerebral oedema (Ross and Eynon, 2005).

Compound sodium lactate (Hartmann's) contains similar electrolytes to plasma, so is often called a 'balanced solution'. It also reduces inflammation, endothelial activation, and kidney injury (Boldt *et al.*, 2009). Lactate is metabolised (by the liver) into bicarbonate – the main buffer in blood. So provided liver function is reasonable, lactate solutions buffer metabolic acidosis, hence their use during surgery or following trauma. Compound sodium lactate is usually the best choice for maintenance fluid therapy (Low and Milne, 2007; Powell-Tuck *et al.*, 2008), but should be avoided during diabetic ketoacidosis, as the liver may metabolise lactate into further glucose (the *Cori cycle*). Compound sodium lactate should also be avoided with:

- blood transfusion, as its calcium may cause coagulation (Cooper and Cramp, 2003);
- diabetic ketoacidosis, which impairs lactate metabolism (Low and Milne, 2007);
- liver disease, where glucosenesis can cause intracranial oedema (Low and Milne, 2007);
- lactic acidosis (Low and Milne, 2007);
- kidney failure (unless haemofiltered), as it contains potassium.

Colloids

Colloids have large molecules. They may be grouped as:

- blood and blood products
- gelatins
- dextrans
- starches.

Each group having advantages and disadvantages, choice (and availability) depend on required effect and the benefit/burden balance. This chapter also describes:

- oxygen carrying artificial fluids

which have little effect on COP, are not colloids, and are not yet currently licensed for UK use.

Blood

Blood for transfusion can be obtained from:

- donors
- recycling (usually perioperative) haemorrhage
- autotransfusion.

Problems/risks of transfusing blood and blood products include:

- limited supply;
- infection risk (low in UK);
- transfusion-related acute lung injury (TRALI) (Gajic *et al.*, 2007; Netzer *et al.*, 2007);
- reactions (usually mild, but can cause anaphylaxis).

TRALI occurs in 8 per cent of critically ill patients, and is more likely to occur with older blood (Benson *et al.*, 2009).

People can survive an 80 per cent loss of erythrocytes, but only a 30 per cent loss of blood volume. While higher haemoglobin increases oxygen-carrying capacity, increased viscosity reduces perfusion; survival from critical illness is highest if Hb is between 7–9 g/dl (Hebert *et al.*, 1999; McLellan *et al.*, 2003), although there is some evidence that older people benefit from slightly higher levels (NCEPOD, 2010b) – often assumed to be 8–10 g/dl.

Cell metabolism continues during storage. Hillman and Bishop (2004) suggest that after 35 days storage blood has:

- pH 6.98
- hydrogen ions 106.1 mmol/litre (normal 25.1)

- sodium 155 mmol/litre
- potassium 30 mmol/litre
- ATP reduced to 55 per cent of normal quantity
- 2,3 DPG none remaining.

Aboudara *et al.* (2008) found that (mean) transfusion of 11.2 units increased potassium from (mean) 3.6 to 5.2 mmol/litre. Later, hypokalaemia can occur as cell recovery draws serum potassium into cells (Isbister, 2009).

Recombinant erythropoietin reduces need for blood transfusion, but is expensive, can take four weeks to be fully effective, and its risks and benefits for critical illness are relatively unknown (McLellan *et al.*, 2003). It is not currently widely used in ICUs.

Albumin

Exogenous albumin is available as 4.5 per cent (isotonic, 100 ml and 400 ml) and 20 per cent (hypertonic/salt-poor, 100 ml). Hypertonic albumin has a high osmotic pressure, drawing extravascular water into the bloodstream. Although claimed benefits for albumin include:

- oxygen radical scavenging
- binding toxic substances
- anti-inflammatory action

evidence is mostly weak, and synthetic colloids offer cheaper, and often better, alternatives for maintaining intravascular volume (Boldt, 2010). There is some evidence it may cause kidney injury (Shortgen *et al.*, 2008). Boldt (2010) therefore recommends restricting albumin use.

Other blood products

Most blood components are available individually for transfusion, but most blood products (except albumin) carry potential for antigen-antibody reaction and virus infection, so are subject to similar cross-matching safeguards as blood, and are not given unless specifically indicated. Some of the most widely used blood products are fresh frozen plasma (FFP) and platelets, given to reverse haemorrhage. Platelets are usually transfused over 30–60 minutes, but infusion must be completed within four hours (Scottish National Blood Transfusion Service, 2007).

Gelatins

Gelatins (e.g. Gelofusine®, Volplex®) are relatively inexpensive and stable plasma substitutes, but have low mean molecular weights – typically 30,000–40,000. Being below renal threshold, this limits their half-life to about three hours (Low and Milne, 2007). Like most fluids, gelatins are iso-osmotic, only expanding blood by the volume infused.

They are hypoallergenic (Low and Milne, 2007). Gelatins are derived from beef extract, which raises ethical dilemmas of giving them to vegans. The *BNF* (2009) suggests cautious use of any plasma substitutes with:

■ cardiac disease
■ liver disease
■ renal impairment.

Traditionally, gelatins were suspended in 0.9% sodium chloride, such as those mentioned above. Some (e.g. Geloplasma®, Isoplex®) are now suspended in a Hartmann's-like solution.

Dextrans

Dextran 70 (number refers to molecular weight) is rarely used. Hypertonic saline dextran (HSD: 7.5% sodium chloride + 6% dextran 70) draws fluid from the extravascular spaces, increasing blood volume by four times the amount infused, and sustains intravascular volume for 3–6 hours. HSD also contains oxygen-free radical scavengers, which reduce inflammation (Bradley, 2001).

Starches

Starch is a large molecule, so starch solutions have high molecular weights, giving them a long half-life when infused. Properties are affected partly by percentage:

■ 3% = hypotonic
■ 6% = isotonic
■ 10% = hypertonic

partly by molar substitution:

■ low = 0.4–0.42
■ medium = 0.5
■ high = 0.62–0.7

and molecular weight:

■ low = 70 kDa
■ medium = 130–264
■ high = > 450.

Suffix numbers of starches (e.g. 130/0.4) represent the mean molecular weight, followed by the molar substitution. Lower molar substitution numbers indicate quicker clearance (Westphal *et al.*, 2009).

Although benefits and problems are disputed, problems caused by starches include:

- anaphylaxis;
- extravasation causing gross oedema from prolonged intravascular osmotic pressure;
- coagulopathies (Zaar *et al.*, 2009; Schramko *et al.*, 2010);
- hypervolaemia from overinfusion (most units limit to one litre per patient per day);
- circulatory overload in patients with impaired ventricular function;
- worsened AKI (Brunkhorst *et al.*, 2008; Wittlinger *et al.*, 2010).

Starches are also significantly more expensive than other artificial colloids.

There are significant differences between different starches (Westphal *et al.*, 2009), and much evidence frequently cited is based on earlier generations of starches (Hartog *et al.*, 2009). Current (third-generation) tetrastarches, such as 6% HES 130/0.4, have lower molar substitution to enhance degradation, and also cause less derangement of clotting, and seem to have less effect on renal function (Blasco *et al.*, 2008; Westphal *et al.*, 2009) and clotting (Kozek-Langenecker and Sibylle, 2005).

Benefits of starches include:

- long half-life (some starches remain clinically effective for 24 hours, although most third-generation starches are cleared more quickly);
- they do not extravase, so solely expand intravascular volume;
- some starches increase volume by double the infused amount, as osmotic pressure draws interstitial fluid into capillaries – e.g. 10% HES 200/0.5 increases volume by about 145 per cent (Westphal *et al.*, 2009);
- anti-inflammatory action (Wang *et al.*, 2010; Wittlinger *et al.*, 2010).

Oxygen-carrying fluids

Current plasma expanders increase blood volume without increasing oxygen-carry capacity, resulting in dilutional anaemia. Blood transfusion creates hazards, and supply and shelf-life are limited. Oxygen-carrying fluids attempt to resolve both these problems.

Oxygen-carrying fluids may be grouped as:

- haemoglobin derivatives;
- chemical (e.g. perfluorocarbon – see Chapter 28).

There are three types of haemoglobin derivatives:

- free haemoglobin (from expired human bank blood or bovine sources);
- recombinant haemoglobin (genetically engineered *E. coli*);
- modified haemoglobins (e.g. cross-linked haemoglobins).

While haemoglobin derivatives carry oxygen, absence of 2,3 DPG assists oxygen dissociation at tissue level. Haemoglobin being 'free' from erythrocytes, derivatives lack antigenic effects of blood, so cross-matching is unnecessary (Remy et al., 1999). Haemoglobin derivative half-life is 6–8 hours (Vlahakes, 2001). Free deoxyhaemoglobin is highly susceptible to oxidation, so causes oxidative damage, and releases oxygen radicals and other mediators (Creteur et al., 2000). Free haemoglobin also provides bacteria with a source of iron, so may cause immunocompromise (Creteur et al., 2000).

Oxygen-carrying fluids exert little colloidal osmotic pressure, so are not 'colloids'. Currently there are many problems with and limitations to both groups (e.g. short duration of action, limited oxygen carriage). Limited licences have been granted in the USA; Phase 3 trials show favourable results (Spahn et al., 2002; Sprung et al., 2002), so clinical use may be near.

Implications for practice

- Prescription of fluid remains a medical decision, but nurses are professionally responsible and accountable for all fluids they administer (so should be aware of efficacy and adverse effects) and their choice of route (e.g. central or peripheral).
- Crystalloids provide whole-body hydration.
- 0.9% sodium chloride mainly hydrates interstitial spaces; 5% glucose mainly hydrates cells; compound sodium lactate (Hartmann's) is generally the best crystalloid.
- Colloids have higher molecular weights, so remain longer in intravascular spaces and may reduce oedema formation (including pulmonary oedema).
- Increasing COP draws extravascular fluid into the intravascular compartment.

Summary

Critical illness usually predisposes to fluid imbalances, necessitating intravenous fluids, but also causes complications for many fluids. Fluids are traditionally divided between crystalloids, which extravase rapidly, and colloids. Choice of colloids falls into three groups. Blood and blood products are usually essential if specific components are needed, but most carry potential risks of viral transmission. Blood transfusion also creates further complications. Gelatins are useful for both their relative cheapness and stability, but have the shortest half-life of all colloids, so are of limited use for critically ill patients. Starch solutions, having the heaviest molecular weight of all colloids, are clinically the most useful for volume replacement, but expense and side effects limit their use. Oxygen-carrying solutions promise to be a useful development for the future, but are not yet licensed for UK use.

Further reading

Most textbooks include chapters on colloids and/or fluid replacement. *GIFTASUP* (Powell-Tuck *et al.*, 2008) is a comprehensive surgical review of fluids, while Low and Milne's (2007) medical review is also useful. Westphal *et al.* (2009) also provide a useful review of starches.

Addendum:
On 3 March 2011, *The Daily Telegraph* reported that allegations, including those of research fraud, had caused Joachim Boldt to be stripped of his professorship. There was the likelihood that some journals would retract his publications, and the *GISTASUP* guidelines had been withdrawn for rewriting. Whether evidence from Boldt, or that based on his work, is reliable is therefore currently unclear.

Clinical scenario

Kenneth McDowall is a 48-year-old known smoker, who had spent an afternoon drinking alcohol and watching sports with friends. While preparing an outdoor barbeque later that day, he collapsed on to the grill, which overturned dropping hot charcoal on to Mr McDowall. He sustained extensive burns down the right side of his head and body.

Mr McDowall was admitted unconscious, vasoconstricted, and diaphoretic with full-thickness burns. His ECG on admission revealed large left ventricular infracted area. Other results included tachycardia (130 beats/minute), BP 100/78 mmHg, CVP 10 mmHg, and tachypnoea (26 breaths/min). Arterial blood gases showed good oxygenation with uncompensated respiratory acidosis, Na^+ 148 mmol/litre, K^+ 4.5 mmol/litre, and blood glucose 12 mmol/litre. He is cannulated with one peripheral cannula and quad CVC in left jugular vein.

Q.1 Identify the signs that indicate Mr McDowall needs fluid management.

Q.2 Select an appropriate crystalloid and colloid to infuse. Justify this choice, the intravenous route and rate of infusion, and list expected effects (include benefits and limitations).

Q.3 Reflect on how fluid challenges are administered in your clinical area (type and volume of fluid, rate and route, use of dynamic indicators or a protocol).

Chapter 34

Inotropes and vasopressors

Contents

Fundamental knowledge	336
Introduction	337
Indications	337
Receptors	337
Safety	339
µg/kg/minute	340
Adrenaline (epinephrine)	341
Noradrenaline (norepinephrine)	341
Dobutamine	341
Dopexamine (hydrochloride)	342
Dopamine	342
Phosphodiesterase inhibitors (PDIs)	342
Some other drugs	343
Implications for practice	343
Summary	344
Further reading	344
Clinical scenario	344

Fundamental knowledge

Sympathetic nervous system
Negative feedback and parasympathetic effect
Renin-angiotensin-aldosterone mechanism

Introduction

Inotropes are frequently used to maintain adequate blood pressure in critically ill patients. Inotropes (*inos* = 'fibre' in Greek) alter stretch of cardiac and arteriole muscle fibres. Vasopressors (also called 'vasoconstrictors') stimulate vasoconstriction. These effects are mediated through stimulation of the sympathetic nervous system.

Some drugs and other chemicals are described as negative inotropes – e.g. digoxin, beta-blockers, tumour necrosis factor, possibly acidosis (especially pH < 7.2) – but 'inotrope' without any prefix usually presumes positive inotropes, drugs that increase muscle fibre stretch, so increasing cardiac stroke volume or systemic vascular resistance. This chapter discusses only positive inotropes. Blood pressure is the sum volume (cardiac output) multiplied by resistance (systemic vascular resistance, or 'afterload'). Cardiac output is the amount of blood ejected by the left ventricle each minute, so is heart rate multiplied by stroke volume. So:

$$BP = HR \times SV \times SVR$$

Provided other factors remain constant, increasing one factor necessarily increases blood pressure. Inotropes increase systemic blood pressure by increasing stroke volume (myocardial stretch) and/or systemic vascular resistance (vasoconstriction).

Positive inotropes may be divided into two main groups:

- adrenergic agonists (inoconstrictors);
- phosphodiesterase inhibitors (inodilators).

In ICUs adrenergic agonists are usually used.

Although the UK has now adopted international names for most drugs, it retains the traditional UK names for adrenaline (elsewhere, 'epinephrine') and noradrenaline (elsewhere, 'norepinephrine').

Indications

Inotropes and vasopressors are used to increase blood pressure. However, blood volume (CVP) should be optimised before using positive inotropes. Increasing cardiac work when there is insufficient circulating volume can cause myocardial ischaemia. Many patients are hypovolaemic on admission to ICUs.

Once circulating volume has been optimised, adrenaline is a first-line drug for cardiac arrest, increasing heart rate, stroke volume and systemic vascular resistance, the three factors that create blood pressure. Other than cardiac arrest, inotropes should only be used where patients can be safely monitored.

Receptors

The heart and blood vessels contain various types of receptors, many of which have subtypes. Inotropes primarily stimulate either alpha (α) or beta (β) receptors, although none is so pure to solely target only one.

Alpha receptors are located mainly in arterioles and veins, especially in peripheries. Alpha stimulation (e.g. with noradrenaline) causes arteriolar vasoconstriction, so increasing systemic vascular resistance. Alpha stimulation has little effect on cerebral, coronary and pulmonary blood flow, so maintaining perfusion to vital organs.

Alpha stimulation may adversely affect many major organs:

- heart (dysrhythmias, ischaemia, infarction);
- pancreas (reduced insulin secretion, causing hyperglycaemia);
- liver (accentuating immunocompromise and coagulopathies);
- kidneys (kidney injury);
- gut (translocation of gut bacteria);
- skin (peripheral blanching or cyanosis; extreme ischaemia may cause gangrene, necessitating amputation of digits).

Alpha stimulants are usually given to counter excessive vasodilatation, but excessive vasoconstriction may cause peripheral blanching/cyanosis and cold peripheries. Flow monitoring (cardiac output studies) can estimate systemic vascular resistance.

Beta (β) receptors are found primarily in the heart and lungs. Beta$_1$ receptors in pacemaker cells cause *chronotropic* effects, while in other myocardial cells they increase spontaneous muscle depolarisation (stretch). So, β_1 stimulation:

- increases contractility;
- improves atrioventricular conduction;
- hastens myocardial relaxation;
- increases stroke volume;
- increases heart rate (with potential dysrhythmias);

thus increasing cardiac output.

Beta$_2$ receptors are found mainly in bronchial smooth muscle, but a significant minority are also found in myocardium. Beta$_2$ stimulation is especially chronotropic, increasing myocardial workload and predisposing to dysrhythmias (hence tachycardic/dysrhythmic effects of bronchodilators such as salbutamol). Beta$_2$ receptors are also found in other smooth muscle, such as blood vessels and skeletal muscle. When stimulated, these β_2 receptors vasodilate arterioles and reduce systemic vascular resistance (afterload).

Beta$_3$ receptors are found in the heart, gall bladder, skeletal muscle and gut. Unlike β_1 and β_2 receptors, β_3 receptors are negatively inotropic when stimulated (Moniotte *et al.*, 2001). Beta$_3$ receptors are not significant for inotropic therapy in ICUs.

Prolonged β_1 (although not β_2) stimulation causes 'down regulation' (Moniotte *et al.*, 2001) or *tachyphylaxis* – progressive destruction of beta receptors, requiring progressively larger doses of inotropes to achieve the same effect. Destruction starts within minutes of exposure to stimulants, reaching clinically significant levels by 72 hours (Sherry and Barham, 1997). Beta receptors regrow once beta stimulation is removed (Sherry and Barham, 1997).

Main receptor sites targeted are summarised in Table 34.1, although no inotropes purely target only one receptor.

Safety

The half-life of most inotropes is very short – often 2–5 minutes, causing rapid changes to blood pressure. They should therefore only be used in areas where:

- blood pressure and ECG can be monitored continuously (or at least every 5 minutes);
- sufficient staff are available to observe monitors;
- staff have sufficient knowledge to understand significance of observations and know how to resolve excessive or insufficient effects.

Appropriate alarm limits should be set on monitors. Effectively, this usually limits inotrope use to ICUs and a few other designated specialist areas, such as CCUs and theatres.

Like most drugs, inotropes are heavier than the fluids they are diluted in, so if given through volumetric pumps may settle at bases of bags. Syringe drivers, almost invariably being horizontal, avoid this problem. When patients are dependent on large doses, interruptions when changing infusions, or syringe drivers taking up the 'slack' in the mechanism when a new syringe is inserted, can cause life-threatening hypotension. This risk can be reduced by:

- *double pumping* – commencing new infusions before switching off old ones, some units only switching off the old once blood pressure begins to increase;
- *quick change technique* – running new infusions before connecting to patients, then turning off old ones as the new are connected (Llewellyn, 2007).

While both methods are equally effective, a quick change technique is quicker, easier and more cost-effective, so double pumping is not recommended (de Barbieri *et al.*, 2009). If changing strength of infusions, dead space in lines contains a small volume of the previous concentration.

Table 34.1 Main target receptors for drugs

	α	β_1 (heart)	β_2 (mainly lungs)
Effect of stimulation	Vasoconstriction	Increased cardiac output	Bronchodilation
Adrenaline	✓	✓	✓
Noradrenaline	✓		
Dobutamine		✓	
Dopamine	(variable)	✓	

Some inotropes should be dissolved in 5% glucose. Most units dissolve all inotropes in glucose solutions, both reducing risks of error and enabling often limited venous access to be shared by more than one inotrope.

Although some inotropes can be infused peripherally, in practice they are usually given centrally, as poor peripheral circulation and possible alpha vasoconstriction may cause pooling of drugs in peripheries and extravasation into tissues. Lines should be clearly labelled, and no bolus or short-term drugs given through lines containing inotropes.

μg/kg/minute

Traditionally inotropes were measured in micrograms (*mcg* or *μg*) per kilogram per minute, or variants (e.g. micrograms per minute):

$$\mu\text{g/kg/minute} = \frac{\text{mg}}{\text{ml}} \times \frac{1000}{\text{patient's weight}} \times \frac{\text{infusion rate (ml/hour)}}{60}$$

This formula can be expressed in various other ways, for example:

$$\frac{\mu\text{g/kg/minute}}{1000} \times \frac{\text{ml}}{\text{mg}} \times \text{patient's weight} \times 60 = \text{infusion rate}$$

Some syringe drivers can calculate doses once patient and drug details are entered. Some units have replaced these potentially cumbersome calculations with simpler measurements (e.g. recording milligrams, as with most other drugs), titrating amounts given to achieve desired effects (e.g. mean arterial pressure). Adequate perfusion pressure being the desired goal, the benefit of investing nursing time in complex calculations is questionable, especially with calculations based on estimated weights, which necessitate recalculation when one guess is replaced by another.

Such calculations are however complex, and with drugs that have such short half-lives, and are titrated to a continuously monitored target, many units have adopted safer formulae. The variety of concentrations used does however create another risk, so the Intensive Care Society (ICS, 2010) recommends standard concentrations, which include:

Noradrenaline:

4 mg in 50 ml/8 mg in 100 ml	80 μg/ml
8 mg in 50 ml/16 mg in 100 ml	160 μg/ml
16 mg in 50 ml/32 mg in 100 ml	320 μg/ml

Dobutamine:

250 mg in 50 ml or 500 mg in 100 ml	5 mg/ml

Adrenaline (epinephrine)

Adrenaline, the main adrenal medullary hormone, stimulates alpha, β_1 and β_2 receptors, triggering the 'fight or flight' stress response via the sympathetic nervous system:

■ vasoconstriction (alpha receptors)
■ increased cardiac output (β_1, β_2)

therefore increasing blood pressure, and improving blood flow to coronary and cerebral arteries (Jowett and Thompson, 2007). This makes it valuable for resuscitation from cardiac arrest, where immediate short-term restoration of systemic blood pressure and circulation is essential. Its bronchodilatory qualities (β_2) make nebulised adrenaline useful during asthma crises, especially with children. Its use in ICUs varies, but it is the cheapest inotrope (Grebenik and Sinclair, 2003) and for many units the catecholamine of choice (Grebenik and Sinclair, 2003).

Adrenaline can cause gross tachycardia, ventricular dysrhythmias, hyperglycaemia, prekidney injury, increased lactate, hypokalaemia, hypophosphataemia and other metabolic complications, so although a first-line drug for resuscitation from MI, it is not widely used in most ICUs.

Noradrenaline (norepinephrine)

Noradrenaline, the most widely used inotrope in ICUs, primarily stimulates alpha receptors, causing intense arteriolar vasoconstriction, so normalises systemic vascular resistance in distributive shock (Martin *et al.*, 2000; Kellum and Pinsky, 2003), although Myburgh *et al.* (2008) found outcomes in critical illness were similar whether adrenaline or noradrenaline was used. Normalising afterload significantly improves coronary and renal perfusion (di Giantomasso *et al.*, 2002). Ideally, doses will be titrated to systemic vascular resistance measurements from flow monitoring; however, low diastolic blood pressure often provides an adequate indication of vascular resistance. Nurses should therefore observe peripheries for perfusion, and delayed capillary refill; pale/mottled skin or cold digits should be reported.

Noradrenaline appears to have fewer metabolic complications (e.g. lactate, glycaemia) than adrenaline. Extravasation of noradrenaline can cause necrosis and peripheral gangrene, so it must be given centrally.

Dobutamine

Dobutamine, a synthetic analogue of dopamine, is primarily a β_1 stimulant. It does have some β_2 and α effects, but is less chronotropic and dysrhythmic than most β_1 inotropes. It reduces systemic vascular resistance, so together with increased cardiac output, increases oxygen delivery to cells (Eliott, 2003). It is the first-line choice inotrope for ischaemic heart failure (Cooper *et al.*, 2006).

341

Dobutamine also increases diaphragm muscle contractility, so infusion might be useful for diaphragmatic failure (Smith-Blair *et al.*, 2003).

Dopexamine (hydrochloride)

Dopexamine, a synthetic dopamine derivative, primarily causes arterial vasodilatation (β_2 agonist) with weak β_1 and dopaminergic effects. Claimed renal and splanchnic benefits appear doubtful (Renton and Snowden, 2005), mortality is not reduced by its use (Gopal *et al.*, 2009), it causes hyperglycemia and lactic acidosis (Berendes *et al.*, 1997) and it is relatively expensive. It can be given peripherally, but being an irritant should be given through a large vein. Its half-life is 5–10 minutes.

Dopamine

Dopamine is an endogenous catecholamine and noradrenaline precursor. There are specific dopamine receptors (DA_1), but dopamine also stimulates alpha and beta receptors. Exogenous dopamine impairs immunity (van den Berghe and de Zegher, 1996; Grebenik and Sinclair, 2003) and gut motility (Dive *et al.*, 2000). As a vasopressor, it has similar mortality to noradrenaline, but is highly dysrhythmic, and is associated with more adverse events (de Backer *et al.*, 2010), and provides no protection against gut ischaemia (Azar *et al.*, 1996) or kidney injury (Australian and New Zealand Intensive Care Society Clinical Trials Group, 2000; Marik, 2002). It is therefore rarely used.

Insufficient brainstem production causes neurotransmission failure in Parkinson's disease, but dopamine cannot permeate mature blood–brain barriers (van den Berghe and de Zegher, 1996), so intravenous dopamine does not affect cerebral receptors.

Phosphodiesterase inhibitors (PDIs)

Phosphodiesterase is an intracellular enzyme that prolongs cardiac and coronary artery contraction. Inhibiting phosphodiasterase therefore:

- increases ventricular filling
- improves myocardial oxygenation
- vasodilates (reduces afterload).

Phosphodiesterase inhibitors combine mild inotropic effects with significant vasodilatation, so are called *inodilators*.

PDIs are protein-bound, giving them half-lives of about 45 minutes, but also usually necessitating loading doses. Half-life is increased by kidney injury. Unlike inotropes, they do not rely on receptor site stimulation, so down-regulation does not occur. Inodilators such as milrinone, enoximone or levosimendan are useful treatments for acute heart failure (Dickstein *et al.*, 2008), although dobutamine is as effective as levosemenden for treating acute decompensated heart failure (Mebazaa *et al.*, 2007).

Adverse effects of PDIs include:

- thrombocytopaenia
- gastrointestinal disturbances
- hepatic dysfunction/failure
- dysrhythmias
- hypotension.

Some other drugs

Some centres use various drugs to 'test' response to, or augment, noradrenaline:

- methylthioninium chloride (formerly called 'methylene blue' in the UK) (Ghiassi *et al.*, 2004);
- vasopressin (synthetic anti-diuretic hormone; synacthen) (Jolly *et al.*, 2005).

Vasopressin, with methylprednisolone and thyroxin (T3), is used during transplant retrieval to stabilise organs (Rosendale *et al.*, 2003).

Implications for practice

- Before commencing drugs to increase blood pressure, blood volume should be optimised, preferably with colloids, to achieve CVP of 10 mmHg (or higher with positive pressure ventilation, PEEP, or chronic heart failure).
- Most inotropes should be diluted in 5% glucose (to prevent oxidation) before preparation.
- Although some (not all) inotropes may be given peripherally, with hypo-perfusion (e.g. sepsis), central administration is usually safer, and is generally used in ICUs.
- Within prescribed limits, inotrope doses should be titrated to achieve desired effects, while minimising adverse effects.
- Noradrenaline increases systemic vascular resistance.
- Dobutamine increases cardiac output.
- Adrenaline increases both systemic vascular resistance and cardiac output.
- Methylthioninium chloride and vasopressin increase systemic vascular resistance.
- Most inotropes (but not phosphodiesterase inhibitors) have half-lives of only a very few minutes, so should only be used where continuous blood pressure and ECG monitoring is available, where there are sufficient staff to observe monitors, and where staff are familiar with using the drugs.
- With alpha stimulants (e.g. noradrenaline), monitor peripheral ischaemia. Ideally, measure systemic vascular resistance (flow monitoring), but visual and tactile observation of patients' peripheries is a useful adjunct.
- Many patients become highly dependent on inotropes, rapidly becoming hypotensive when infusions are changed; changes should therefore minimise risks (e.g. have a 'spare' syringe ready, and use a quick change technique).

■ Traditional practices of measuring inotropes by body weight and calcul-tions, rather than monitored effect, should be reconsidered.

Summary

Drugs and chemicals inhibiting myocardial contraction are labelled 'negative inotropes'; drugs increasing muscle contraction should be called 'positive inotropes', but practice usually limits the label 'inotropes' to positive inotropes.

Central blood pressure can be increased by increasing heart rate (chronotrope), increasing stroke volume (β_1 stimulation or phosphodiesterase inhibition) or increasing systemic vascular resistance (alpha stimulation). Beta$_1$ stimulation, the traditional mainstay of inotrope practice, creates problems of down-regulation, necessitating progressively higher doses.

For β_1 stimulation, most units rely on dobutamine or adrenaline. Alpha stimulation (from adrenaline or noradrenaline) can usefully raise central blood pressure by increasing systemic vascular resistance. Most ICUs use noradrenaline to counter inappropriate vasodilatation (sepsis) and dobutamine to increase cardiac output (cardiogenic shock).

Further reading

Other than studies of specific drugs, there have been very few articles about inotropes in recent years. Llewellyn's (2007) review of how to change infusions is worth reading.

Clinical scenario

Caroline Watson, 53 years old, is admitted post-laparotomy for faecal peritonitis. During induction she had a cardiac arrest and three cycles of CPR were performed. Mrs Watson has no previous cardiac history, is 1.6 m tall and weights 70 kg. She is six days post-op, and remains sedated and invasively ventilated with signs of septic shock. Arterial blood gases indicate severe metabolic acidosis with pH of 6.9.

Her haemodynamic results include:

Temperature	38.5°C
BP	135/72 mmHg (MAP 93 mmHg)
HR	100 beats/minute
CVP	16 mmHg
SV	52 ml
CO	5.4 ml/minute CI *to be calculated*
SVR	900 dynes/sec/m^{-5}
SVRI	1600 dynes/sec/m^{-5}/m^2
DO$_2$I	455 ml/minute/m^2

Mrs Watson has continuous infusions of noradrenaline (at 0.19 μg/kg/minute), hydrocortisone (10 mg/hour) and dopexamine (1 μg/kg/minute) in progress.

Q.1 Describe the therapeutic actions of Mrs Watson's vasoactive drug infusions. Explain their action on specific receptor sites and intended effects. Consider their effect on her haemodynamic values (increase or decrease SV, CO, SVR, DO_2I etc.).

Q.2 Identify other parameters that should be assessed and recorded when evaluating effectiveness (and monitoring for adverse effects) of Mrs Watson's treatment.

Q.3 Over the day, noradrenaline and dopexamine infusion rates are increased. A decision was taken to introduce milrinone and discontinue the dopexamine infusion. Justify the rationale for this change and review the approach used when introducing and discontinuing these specific drugs.

Chapter 35

Vascular surgery

Contents

Fundamental knowledge   346
Introduction   347
Aneurysms   347
Carotid artery disease   349
Nursing care   349
Implications for practice   351
Summary   351
Further reading   352
Clinical scenario   352

Fundamental knowledge

Pathology of atherosclerosis
Thrombolysis (see Chapter 29)
Sternotomy (see Chapter 30)
Anatomy and physiology of large arteries (including aorta, femoral, carotid, renal)
Pathology of connective tissue disease
How and where to assess pedal pulses

Introduction

Vascular disease is common, frequently needing medical or surgical intervention, only a few of which usually necessitate ICU admission:

- aneurysm repair
- carotid artery repair.

In addition to needs created by often prolonged and major operations, surgery on major arteries creates risks from:

- major bleeds;
- organ and tissue damage from perioperative ischaemia distal to the repair;
- thrombus/embolus formation (especially strokes);
- patients often having extensive vascular and other diseases that complicate recovery.

Traditionally, surgery involved grafting a synthetic prosthesis (aortic tube graft) into the vessel, but increasingly, major vessels are being repaired through endovascular insertion of fabric or metal stents, inserted through catheters similar to those used for angioplasty. Advantages of percutaneous approaches are:

- speed, and can be performed under light sedation (Latessa, 2002; Prinssen et al., 2004);
- lower risk of post-operative AKI (Wald et al., 2006);
- reduced morbidity and mortality (Peppelenbosch et al., 2005; Lettinga-van de Poll et al., 2007; Giles et al., 2009; McPhee et al., 2009; UK EVAR Trial Investigators, 2010).

However, endovascular aneurysm repair (EVAR) may increase risks of AKI (Abela et al., 2009). EVAR enables rapid recovery, seldom necessitating ICU admission, although overnight HDU admission is often needed. NCEPOD (2005) suggests that most patients undergoing open abdominal aortic aneurysm (AAA) repair can be extubated at the end of surgery and recovered overnight in level 2 facilities. Stenting may not be possible with tortuous, calcified vessels (Carrell and Wolfe, 2005).

Aneurysms

'Aneurysm' means 'widening' (Greek). Once believed to be simple stretching, aneurysms are now known to be caused by remodelling (Baxter, 2004), usually from atherosclerosis. Progressive deposits eventually separate the wall's layers, causing haemorrhage and rupture. Aneurysms are often asymptomatic (Irwin, 2007; Collin et al., 2009), pain often indicating impending rupture (Collin et al., 2009), so are usually found by chance – during investigations for other problems (Tambyraja and Chamlers, 2009); others present at critical stages, needing urgent surgery. Without surgery, rupture is usually fatal (Assar and Zarins, 2009; Collin *et al.*, 2009), and even with surgery mortality exceeds 40 per cent (Tambyraja and Chamlers, 2009). Aneurysms cause nearly 10,000 deaths each year in the UK, and incidence is increasing (Tambyraja and Chamlers, 2009). Vascular disease elsewhere typically creates significant co-morbidities, especially cardiac, lung and kidney disease (Puchakayala, 2006). Co-morbidities may necessitate ICU admission.

Atherosclerosis is an inflammatory process; vascular leak from inflammation frequently causes pleural effusions. Immediate treatment of aneurysms usually includes antihypertensives, such as beta-blockers, but earlier drug interventions may prevent or limit atherosclerosis. A minority of aneurysms are caused by trauma, bacterial or fungal infections, and other problems.

Aneurysms can, and do, occur in any vessels, but are usually most life-threatening when they occur in the aorta, carotid arteries or cerebral circulation. Cerebral aneurysms are not described in this chapter. Three-quarters of aortic aneurysms are abdominal (AAA or 'triple A'), but thoracic aneurysms may occur in the ascending or descending aorta. Surgery is usually only indicated if aortic aneurysms exceed 5 cm diameter (Schlösser *et al.*, 2010).

Renal compromise, both from the disease and surgery/repair, stimulates the renin-angiotensin-aldosterone cascade (Adembri *et al.*, 2004), exacerbating problems from hypertension. Open surgery necessitates cross-clamping the aorta. Most abdominal aneurysms occur below the renal artery, so clamps can normally be placed below the renal artery, preserving renal perfusion. But higher aneurysms necessitate clamping above the renal artery, which may cause acute tubular necrosis. With endovascular repair, intrarenal damage may be caused by obstruction from the endograft or nephrotoxic dyes, and so damage may accelerate after admission to the ICU. Acute kidney injury significantly increases post-operative mortality – possibly tenfold (Jacobs *et al.*, 2004).

Mortality and morbidity from ascending aortic repair is very high, partly because it precedes the carotid arteries, but also because it usually involves aortic valve disease, and so patients need simultaneous aortic valve replacement. For this reason, repair is usually undertaken in specialist centres by cardiothoracic, rather than vascular, surgeons. The ascending aorta stretches from the aortic valve to the carotid arteries, and is especially susceptible to aneurysm in people with *Marfan's syndrome* (Ranasinghe and Bonser, 2004) and other connective tissue disease. Surgery compromises cerebral perfusion, unless cardiopulmonary bypass is used, so few units outside cardiothoracic centres undertake this operation. Endovascular approaches may offer a viable alternative provided valve replacement is not needed, but may occlude the brachiocephalic, common carotid and subclavian arteries. '*Endoleak*' – blood flowing within the aneurysm sac but outside the graft – frequently occurs following surgical or endovascular repair (Veith *et al.*, 2002).

Although NICE (2008) cautiously recommended laparoscopic vascular surgery, including aortic repair, the technique is problematic and outcomes are not significantly different (Cau *et al.*, 2008), so few centres use this option.

Carotid artery disease

Atheromatous plaques frequently form in the carotid artery, especially in older people. About one-tenth of people aged over 80 have carotid artery stenosis (Carrell and Wolfe, 2005). Stenosis reduces cerebral blood flow, so may cause ischaemic strokes. Stenting carries greater risk of peri-procedure stroke, but endarterectomy carries greater risk of peri-procedure MI (Brott *et al.*, 2010); intermediate outcomes are similar between the two approaches (Meier *et al.*, 2010). Carotid endarterectomy is the treatment of choice (International Carotid Stenting Study Investigators, 2010).

Nursing care

In addition to system support, specific individual needs and standard post-operative care (such as observing wound site/dressings), patients with vascular disease are especially susceptible to complications from perfusion failure. Vascular surgery creates the problem of maintaining sufficient perfusion pressure (in patients who usually have extensive vascular disease), while preventing graft damage from excessive pressure – patients needing vascular surgery usually have a history of hypertension. The most common cause of post-operative death is MI, often from unidentified coronary artery disease (Carrell and Wolfe, 2005). Clonidine is useful for both its anxiolytic and anti-hypertensive properties (Schneemilch *et al.*, 2006). Extensive vascular disease often causes ischaemia and chronic pain. Immediate post-operative pain is usually managed with epidural analgesia.

To optimise post-operative perfusion, mean arterial pressure is maintained at MAP 80–100 mmHg (Puchakayala, 2006), with perfusion being monitored primarily through urine output (aim > 0.5 ml/kg/hour) and observing peripheries distal to the surgical site. Peripheries should be checked for perfusion and possible nerve damage by assessing:

- colour
- warmth
- pulses (one-tenth of people lack dorsalis pedis pulses)
- movement
- sensation.

Peripheral temperature monitoring can be useful. Aortic surgery (open or endovascular) may occlude the iliac artery, so flow will probably be assessed by Doppler. Doppler assessment may be undertaken by medical or nursing staff, depending on local policies, practice and skills.

Vascular surgery may cause bleeding from surrounding tissue, so drains should be clearly labelled or numbered, volume marked or measured on arrival, and drainage initially monitored hourly. If vacuum drains are used, vacuum should be checked hourly.

Endovascular repair, being less invasive, often avoids need for ICU admission unless there are specific concerns. When receiving patients, nurses should record on handover specific areas of concern. Endovascular surgery uses dye contrast, which may be nephrotoxic, or cause allergic reactions or other problems. So despite the less invasive nature of surgery, patients admitted to ICUs should be closely monitored, especially for renal function. Once stabilised (especially fluids optimised and clotting normalised) and extubated, recovery is usually quick.

Following abdominal aortic aneurysm repair, many patients develop SIRS (Norwood *et al.*, 2004), necessitating extensive system support. Patients with vascular disease are at high risk of developing pressure sores (Scott *et al.*, 2001), acute kidney injury (Puchakayala, 2006) and spinal cord injury (Puchakayala, 2006). Endovascular surgery has a high incidence of spinal cord ischaemia (Peppelenbosch *et al.*, 2005).

Blood pressure should be monitored and regulated to optimise perfusion while protecting grafts from damage. These, and other complications discussed earlier in the chapter, are listed in Table 35.1.

Although the carotid artery is relatively superficial, repair exposes patients to additional specific risks:

- neurological deficit from occlusion, thrombi or emboli;
- oedema, compressing the vagus nerve, causing bradycardia, hypotension, and possible heart blocks;
- displacement of the trachea.

Table 35.1 Common complications of open surgery to the aorta

System complications

- cardiac – infarction, left ventricular failure, coagulopathies, SIRS
- pulmonary – ventilatory failure, effusions
- acute kidney injury
- cerebrovascular (stroke)
- spinal cord (paraplegia)
- bowel ischaemia – paralysis, loss of appetite, nausea

Local – vascular

- haemorrhage (+ anaemia)
- graft complication
- graft infection
- endovascular leak
- thromboembolism
- renal artery obstruction
- arterial/graft obstruction

Local – non-vascular

- wound complications – pain
- iatrogenic bowel perforation
- pressure sores

Source: after Prinssen *et al.* (2004)

Nurses should therefore observe:

- neurological function, reporting any inappropriate or deteriorating responses;
- airway patency – tracheal shift will probably be detected on X-ray, but any respiratory problems in extubated patients should be reported;
- ECG, heart rate and blood pressure, setting appropriate alarms and reporting any signs of excessive vagal stimulation.

Drains used with carotid surgery are usually small, so are more likely to occlude and fill more quickly. Arterial flow to, and venous drainage from, the head should not be occluded. With possible oedema on the side of surgery, this necessitates avoiding interventions, such as feeling carotid pulse, on the opposite side of the neck.

Unlike most post-operative patients, anti-thrombotic stockings (TEDS™) are not usually used, as patients are at high risk of bleeding rather than clotting following vascular surgery, and pressure on any femoral incisions may occlude perfusion.

Implications for practice

- Pulses, colour and warmth should be monitored on limbs distal to surgery.
- Mean arterial pressure should be maintained > 70 mmHg.
- Urine output should be maintained > 0.5 ml/kg/hour.
- Pain should be assessed, together with side effects of epidurals or whatever analgesia is used (see Chapter 7).
- Following carotid artery repair, pressure to the opposite side of the neck should be avoided.
- Anticoagulant therapy is usually omitted post-operatively, and anti-thrombotic stockings (TEDS™) are usually not used.

Summary

Most vascular surgery does not necessitate ICU admission, unless patients develop complications or other problems. But following surgery on the aorta or carotid artery, patients usually are admitted to the ICU for observation. The main post-operative dangers are

- stroke
- graft/vessel occlusion
- kidney injury
- haemorrhage or bleeding from graft leak.

But patients with aortic or carotid artery disease often have extensive cardiovascular disease, underlying hypertension, and often other co-morbidities. Post-operative recovery centres on stabilisation, observation, symptom control and system support.

Endovascular treatments are quicker, less invasive, and so create fewer risks, but are not always possible with tortuous vessels. Developments in endovascular techniques may significantly reduce the numbers of patients admitted to ICUs following vascular surgery.

Further reading

Vascular surgical journals include the *Journal of Vascular Surgery*. Recent medical reviews include Assar and Zarins (2009), Collin *et al.* (2009) and Tambyraja and Chamlers (2009).

Clinical scenario

Owen Fowler is an 81-year-old gentleman with hypertension. He has been diagnosed with an abdominal aortic aneurysm (AAA) of 5.2 cm diameter. This was repaired under fluoroscopic guidance using digital subtraction angiography (DSA) to insert an endograft through his femoral arteries. During the endovascular repair, Mr Fowler lost 2 litres of blood and was transfused with 6 units of packed red cells. He was admitted to the ICU for further fluid and cardiovascular management, with Hb of 6.2 g/dl, a platelet count of 50×10^{-9}/litre and a BP of 110/58 mmHg. He has two vacuum drains located in the right and left groin incision wounds.

Q.1 Identify the potential complications for Mr Fowler following his endovascular repair. Explain why might occur and consider the effects of contrast dye, position and type of endograft etc.

Q.2 Analyse nursing interventions that monitor and enhance tissue perfusion for Mr Fowler (e.g. fluids, blood products, vasopressors, drain management, limb assessment, use of Doppler, antithrombolytic therapy, drugs versus anti-embolism stockings).

Q.3 Compare and contrast patients' selection, recovery and the long-term effects of AAA repair using endovascular repair and open surgical repair.

Part VII

Neurological

Chapter 36

Central nervous system injury

Contents

Fundamental knowledge 356
Introduction 356
Airway 357
Breathing 357
Circulation 357
Disability (neurological) 358
Traumatic brain injury (TBI) 359
Preventing raised intracranial pressure 359
Nutrition 360
Positioning 361
Pituitary damage 361
Epilepsy 361
Spinal cord injury (SCI) 362
Autonomic hyper-reflexia (dysreflexia) 364
Haemorrhage 365
Prognosis 365
Personality changes 366
Family care 366
Legal aspects 367
Implications for practice 367
Summary 368
Further reading 368
Clinical scenario 368

Introduction

Although neurology services are usually focused in regional centres, patients with acute neurological injuries and complications are admitted to general ICUs, sometimes for stabilisation before transfer. Traumatic brain or spinal injury can cause life-threatening respiratory and cardiovascular failure, necessitating urgent ICU admission. Some patients may later be transferred to regional centres, while others remain due to poor prognosis, injury being relatively minor, or lack of beds.

This chapter includes discussion of:

- traumatic brain injury (TBI)
- diabetes insipidus
- spinal cord injury (SCI)
- autonomic hyper-reflexia
- epilepsy
- intracranial haemorrhage.

There are some similarities, but also many differences, about complications from, and treatments for, this diverse group of pathologies. Patients with severe traumatic brain injury (TBI) or spinal cord injury (SCI) will usually be transferred to regional specialist centres. However, initial stabilisation may occur on general ICUs, which are not able to provide specialist interventions such as craniotomy or specialist monitoring such as intracranial pressure monitoring, and whose staff have less experience of neurology.

The 'golden hour' of trauma care applies to central nervous system (CNS) injury. Primary damage is largely irreversible, so focus of treatment should be on preventing secondary damage (Werner and Engelhard, 2007). Priorities are therefore system support (Hunningher and Smith, 2006), with early optimisation of:

- ventilation
- perfusion
- intracranial pressure (cerebral perfusion pressure).

Immediate priorities are preserving life:

- A – airway
- B – breathing

■ C – circulation
■ D – disability (neurological)

with special emphasis on neuroprotection: hypoxia and hypotension are the most likely causes of death.

Airway

Airway obstruction may be caused directly by trauma or impaired consciousness. Anyone with a GCS score of 8 or below may be unable to maintain their own airway, so should be intubated (Eynon and Menon, 2002).

Breathing

Without constant supplies of oxygen, brain cells die, so severe traumatic brain injury necessitates artificial ventilation. Diaphragmatic nerves normally leave the spinal cord at C3–C5, so spinal injuries involving or above these may cause apnoea, necessitating ventilation. Lower injuries may need initial respiratory support, but problems often resolve later (Ball, 2001). Even if able to self-ventilate, hypopnoea and weak cough reflexes expose patients to greater risk of chest infection. Other indications for artificial ventilation may include:

■ lung injury from multiple trauma – contusion, pneumothorax, fractured ribs;
■ hypercapnia – carbon dioxide vasodilates, so controlling levels (target 4.0–4.5 kPa) limits intracranial hypertension.

During crises, hyperventilation can rapidly reduce ICP (hypocapnia vasoconstricts) (Hickey, 2003b), but should be limited to a few minutes as it also reduces cerebral perfusion.

Sedation is usually needed, for humanitarian reasons, to facilitate effective ventilation, and to reduce brain activity (neuro-protection). Propofol, being short-acting, is usually the sedative of choice. Paralysing agents may be necessary to facilitate ventilation or reduce metabolism, especially to stop shivering, but do not reduce intracranial pressure, and may increase length of ICU stay and complications such as pneumonia and sepsis. Nurses should ensure patients are adequately sedated beneath paralysis, both from humanitarian reasons and because stress from being paralysed but not sedated will aggravate hypertension (see Chapter 6).

Increased intrathoracic pressure impairs cerebral venous drainage, so unnecessary coughing and straining at stool should be prevented if possible. Anti-tussive drugs and early tracheostomy may help prevent coughing. Constipation should be prevented through good bowel care, which usually necessitates laxatives (see Chapter 9).

Circulation

Spinal shock is the main life-threatening complication of spinal cord injury (SCI) (Harvey, 2008). Ninety per cent of autopsies show ischaemic damage (Moppett,

2007). Hypovolaemia causes cerebral vasospasm, further reducing perfusion. Fluid resuscitation should aim to maintain mean arterial pressure ≥ 80 mmHg (NICE, 2007b), thus maintaining cerebral perfusion pressure. Glucose solutions should be avoided, as they contain 'free water', which may cause cerebral oedema (Eynon and Menon, 2002; Cree, 2003). Low and Milne (2007) recommend 0.9% sodium chloride, as this has higher *osmolality* than Hartmann's. As with other pathologies, excessive crystalloid infusion can cause interstitial (and pulmonary) oedema, so 'filling' is usually with colloids, guided by CVP. Once adequately filled, blood pressure optimisation may necessitate inotropes.

Disability (neurological)

Traumatic brain injury (TBI), but not SCI, exposes patients to secondary dangers from intracranial hypertension. Medical imaging, such as computerised tomography (CT), may identify specific problems, such as haematoma or excessive cerebrospinal fluid (CSF) (usually from blockage), which may necessitate urgent drainage or surgery. Secondary brain damage may be prevented by:

- sedating (to reduce cerebral oxygen consumption – identified above);
- (sometimes) paralysing;
- (sometimes) inducing hypothermia;
- minimising intracranial pressure;

while identifying additional risks, such as:

- base of skill fracture;
- fitting.

Pyrexia increases cerebral oxygen consumption (Cooper *et al.*, 2006). Moderate hypothermia (32–33°C) reduces mortality and morbidity (Fukuda and Warner, 2007).

Cerebral *oedema* is traditionally removed with the osmotic diuretic mannitol (0.25–1 g/kg bolus), although supporting evidence for its use is poor (Moppett, 2007), Ichai *et al.* (2009) suggesting that a sodium lactate-based hyperosmolar solution is better. Mannitol is hypertonic, so should be given into a central (or large) vein. Fluid shifts from cells may cause hyperkalaemia. Steroids are not beneficial (Roberts *et al.*, 2004).

Cranial venous drainage should be optimised by *positioning* patients at angles of 30–45° (Wilson *et al.*, 2005; Hunninger and Smith, 2006), maintaining good neck alignment (Sullivan, 2000), ensuring endotracheal tube tapes do not restrict venous drainage (Odell, 1996), and avoiding hip flexion. Rigid neck collars may increase intracranial pressure, so should be removed as soon as injuries allow (Goh and Gupta, 2002). If the skull is fractured or has been surgically cut, pressure on any bone flaps should be avoided.

Base of skull fractures are not visually obvious, and may not have been diagnosed, but may still exist. With any cranial trauma, base of skull fracture should be suspected until excluded, and no equipment should be inserted nasally until excluded. Base of skull fractures may cause leakage of CSF from the nose (rhinorrhoea) or ear (otorrhoea). CSF stains on linen look yellow, often as rings around a bloodstain ('halo sign') (Hickey, 2003c). Rhinorrhoea and otorrhea usually seal spontaneously (Watkins, 2000).

Up to one-quarter of patients develop *fitting*. Likely causes (e.g. hypoxia) should be treated and, if fitting persists, antiepileptics are usually needed.

If the spine is uninjured but soft tissue injury is suspected, collars should be used for moving, and CT or magnetic resonance imaging (MRI) scans arranged when stable.

Traumatic brain injury (TBI)

TBI is the most common cause of death in younger people (Werner and Engelhard, 2007). Classification follows GCS scoring:

- mild = GCS 13–15
- moderate = GCS 9–13
- severe = GCS 3–8.

Trauma may cause externally visible fracture and bruising, but may also cause internal injuries, such as:

- *haematoma* (extradural, subdural);
- *contusion*;
- *contre-coup* (the brain hits the opposite side of the skull to the original injury);
- *rotation* (the brain rotates within the skull, wrenching away nerves and other brain tissue);
- *diffuse axonal injury*.

Victims of TBI often suffer multiple injuries to other parts of the body, so need multisystem support. Some injuries may not be immediately obvious, so nurses should continually assess all body systems and functions.

Following initial stabilisation, severely injured patients (GCS < 8) should be urgently transferred to specialist centres (NICE, 2007b; Andrews *et al.*, 2008b). Priorities of medical management are listed in Table 36.1.

Preventing raised intracranial pressure

In addition to the immediate care in Table 36.1, nurses have an important role in providing therapeutic care and environments for their patients, primarily by limiting stimuli that may increase intracranial pressure (ICP). Ideally, ICP should be maintained at 0–10 mmHg, with cerebral perfusion pressure (CPP)

Table 36.1 Possible main aspects of medical management of traumatic brain injury

- Diagnostic investigations (computerised tomography – CT, magnetic resonance imaging – MRI, lumbar puncture).
- Surgical (e.g. evacuation of haematoma, ventricular drainage to remove excess/blocked CSF).
- Artificial ventilation, keeping PaCO$_2$ 4.5–5.0 kPa; muscle relaxation sedation + short-term sedation (NICE, 2007b).
- Osmotic diuretics (mannitol) and/or barbiturates to reduce cerebral oedema and ICP fluid management.
- Stabilise electrolytes and blood glucose.
- ICP monitoring, maintaining ICP 0–10 and CPP > 70 mmHg.
- System support (e.g. vasoactive drugs to normalise blood pressure).
- Induced hypothermia.

50–70 mmHg (White and Venkatesh, 2008). ICP exceeding 15 mmHg should be treated, usually by draining CSF (Ghajar, 2000). However, not all general units have access to invasive monitoring.

Preventing pain has humanitarian and physiological benefits, as stress responses increase intracranial pressure. Codeine phosphate is less likely to mask neurological (diagnostic) signs than other opioids, but once diagnosis is established pain is usually controlled with standard opioids, such as fentanyl. Limbs should be kept in comfortable alignment. Skincare and pressure area care can help prevent pressure sore development, which both cause discomfort and expose patients to potential complications.

Visits from friends and family are usually comforting (Odell, 1996), but should be planned to allow sufficient rest between them. As with all patients, supporting the family should help reduce their distress, which benefits both the relatives and patients who sense distress among their loved ones.

Nutrition

Malnutrition increases risks of infection and delayed rehabilitation in all patients, but head injury significantly increases *catabolism* (Hunninger and Smith, 2006). Early and aggressive nutrition should be given, which may necessitate drugs (e.g. metoclopramide) to increase gut motility.

Electrolyte imbalances may occur from fluid shifts and loss. Levels should be checked and monitored, with supplements given as necessary.

Blood sugar is often labile following head injury, so should be monitored frequently (e.g. 2–4 hourly). Catecholamine-induced hyperglycaemia often occurs (Hunninger and Smith, 2006; Moppett, 2007), increasing intracellular osmotic pressure, so causing further cerebral ischaemia. Hypoglycaemia starves neurones of the main fuel used to produce energy. Outcome from severe TBI is improved with early tight glycaemic control (Jermitsky et al., 2005). Maintenance fluids should be saline solutions, not glucose (see page 329).

Positioning

Most ICU patients are at risk of developing pressure sores. Traumatic brain or spinal injury usually causes or necessitates immobility. However, pressure area care interventions should be planned against risks from stimulation. Aggressive manual handling can significantly increase intracranial pressure.

Severe spasticity is common (Iggulden, 2006), so assessment and care planning should include active consideration of:

- active/passive exercises;
- positioning;
- physiotherapy;
- removing any stimuli that reduce muscle tone (e.g. constipation).

Although these aspects will be the focus of later rehabilitation, neglect during the acute phase may prolong or limit rehabilitation.

Pituitary damage

Although rare, direct trauma from head injury, by CNS infection (meningitis) or by raised intracranial pressure can cause pituitary damage. The pituitary gland regulates the endocrine system, so damage can cause diverse problems, including diabetes insipidus, while damage to the adjacent hypothalamus may cause pryexia.

Diabetes insipidus is caused by insufficient antidiuretic hormone (ADH), a hormone produced by the pituitary gland. This is a common complication of severe TBI (Karali *et al.*, 2008). Damage might be permanent, but is more often transient, from oedema. Once oedema subsides, diabetes insipidus usually resolves. Until resolution, fluid balance should be carefully monitored, and adequate volume replacement prescribed.

Pyrexia frequently occurs following head injury and cerebral damage (Rossi *et al.*, 2001). The hypothalamus regulates body temperature, so hypothalamic damage disrupts thermoregulation. Autonomic nervous system dysfunction may cause inappropriate responses. Pyrexia increases cerebral oxygen consumption, potentially causing cerebral hypoxia, fitting and progressive cerebral damage. Temperature should therefore be closely monitored, and antipyretic drugs (e.g. paracetamol) prescribed prophylactically, or 'as required' for neuroprotection.

Epilepsy

Epilepsy is the most common serious neurological disease in the UK (Sisodiya and Duncan, 2004), but may occur in ICU patients from cerebral trauma, oedema or hypoxia. Seizures may be:

- *partial* – involving only one hemisphere of the brain;
- *generalised* – involving both hemispheres, and causing loss of consciousness;

with subclassifications of each group. Generalised seizures, usually more problematic, are described in terms of motor (muscle) symptoms:

- *tonic* – increased muscle tone;
- *clonic* – increased reflex activity;
- *atonic* – sudden loss of tone;
- *absence* – no motor symptoms.

Most generalised seizures are tonic-clonic seizures (previously called *grand mal*). Absence seizures (previously *petit mal*), typically causing a blank expression, are usually idiopathic, and occur mainly in children. *Status epilepticus* is prolonged fitting, often defined as lasting 30 minutes, although fitting that persists beyond 5 minutes is unlikely to self-resolve (Meierkord *et al.*, 2010).

Patient safety is a priority. If at risk of falling, patients may need to be repositioned. Pillows or other padding should be placed between patients and anything on which they may hurt themselves (e.g. cotsides). Tonic-clonic seizures almost invariably cause apnoea, so intubated patients should be fully ventilated and sedated. Facemask (Ambu-bag®) ventilation is usually necessary if patients are not intubated. If fitting persists, sedatives (e.g. lorazepam or other benzodiazepines, propofol) often control seizures (Meierkord *et al.*, 2010). If fitting persists, anti-epileptic drugs may be needed. Fits should be observed, and duration, appearance and effects recorded. Priorities of care are listed in Table 36.2.

Spinal cord injury (SCI)

Spinal cord injury may be:

- traumatic (e.g. road traffic accidents);
- non-traumatic (e.g. degeneration, tumours).

(Walker, 2009)

Recovery from spinal injury is highest if patients are treated at trauma centres (Macias *et al.*, 2009), but initial management and stabilisation in the ICU may be needed. Nearly all patients with complete SCI develop respiratory

Table 36.2 Priorities of care during fitting

- Summon help.
- Provide safety and privacy.
- Maintain clear airway (e.g. remove saliva/vomit, insert artificial airway).
- Give 100 per cent oxygen (intubation and artificial ventilation if apnoeic).
- Administer anti-epileptics.
- Reassure family.
- Observe fits – duration, which parts of the body are affected – and record observations.

complications (March, 2005). Even if not admitted with identified spinal injury, multiple trauma may have caused unidentified/unconfirmed injury, so should always be presumed present until excluded. The spinal cord forms the lowest part of the central nervous system, so damage affects function of all systems and organs regulated by nerves below the injury. Typically:

- injuries to cervical vertebra 1 (C1) to thoracic vertebra 1 (T1) cause tetraplegia;
- injuries to T2 to lumbar vertebra 1 (L1) cause paraplegia;
- injuries above T12 usually cause spasticity and hyper-reflexia;
- injuries above C3 cause complete paralysis, with loss of respiratory function.

(March, 2005)

Spinal injury necessitates supine positioning, and may require special ('spinal') beds. Controls for adjusting angles of the head or foot of the bed should be locked, if possible. If not possible, control panels should be clearly labelled to identify which controls may and may not be used (with most controls, only the vertical elevation control is safe to use).

Moving can cause further spinal injury, so spinal column alignment should be maintained. Specific instructions about positioning should be clearly visible in the bed area – for example, multiple trauma may involve the thoracic spine, necessitating maintenance of leg alignment as well. Most ICUs have guidelines for nursing and positioning patients with spinal injury. Sufficient staff should be gathered to safely log-roll patients. Before rolling, a team leader should be identified (normally the person holding the head), readiness of all staff involved should be identified, instructions clarified, and the destined angle specified. Additional staff may be required to manage specific injuries or equipment. Cervical and upper thoracic spine injury (C1 to T4) necessitates additional stabilisation of the head with a hard collar or head immobiliser, and one additional person holding just to maintain head alignment. Position changes, usually two hourly, should be recorded on observation charts.

Venous stasis causes high risk of thrombus formation. Within three months, more than one-third of patients develop DVTs (Anderson and Spencer, 2003), so thromboprophylaxis (TEDS™, subcutaneous heparin) should be prescribed unless contraindicated. Risk of intracranial bleed from thromboprophylaxis is small, and is usually outweighed by risks of developing DVTs (Hunningher and Smith, 2006).

Thermoregulation is impaired and labile due to:

- inappropriate cutaneous vasodilatation (hypothermia);
- inability to shiver (hypothermia);
- impaired sweating (hyperthermia).

Spinal injury care is often prolonged, benefiting from inclusion of various specialists. Neurophysiotherapists should be actively involved care of spinal injury patients, treating and advising about mobilisation, spasticity (Burchiel and Hsu, 2001), foot drop and other complications caused by loss of peripheral

363

nervous system control. Many patients develop severe pain and spasticity (Harvey, 2008), so pain control specialists should be consulted.

Acute SCI causes bowel flaccidity, necessitating manual evacuation (Thumbikat *et al.*, 2009). Complete lesions below T12/L1 affect bowels (Ash, 2005), causing permanent problems with elimination. For many patients, faecal incontinence is the most distressing aspect of their injury (Ash, 2005).

Autonomic hyper-reflexia (dysreflexia)

The autonomic nervous system regulates homeostasis, including vasodilatation/constriction and heart rate. Spinal injury causes loss of inhibitory neuro-transmitters, and so excessive sympathetic reflex responses (Harvey, 2008). Hypertensive crises may be fatal. Other symptoms include pounding headaches, profuse sweating, blurred vision, flushing of skin above lesions, with pallor below, nausea and nasal congestion.

Most spinal injuries above T6 cause autonomic hyper-reflexia (van Welzen and Carey, 2002) at least four weeks, and often six months following injury; it can occur with injuries above T10 (Keely, 1998). Until resolution (usually after a few years), blood pressure and pulse remain labile. Although usually occurring after transfer to spinal injuries units, ICU nurses may encounter it, especially with patients who have old SCI (Keely, 1998). Nurses should be able to recognise it should it occur in the ICU, and be able to provide appropriate information for patients and their families.

Most crises are caused by distended bladder or bowels (NPSA, 2004b; Cherian *et al.*, 2005; Furlan *et al.*, 2007). Other common causes are fractures, pressure ulcers and ingrowing toenails (Harvey, 2008). Unable either to sense stimuli or move, spinal reflexes occur without normal protective responses (e.g. changing position).

Treating crises requires urgent intervention – immediately elevating the bedhead to reduce intracranial hypertension and removing possible causes (e.g. straightening creased sheets). All acute hospitals treating patients with SCI should have bowel care protocols to prevent hyper-reflexic crises (NPSA, 2004b). Constipation may require manual evacuation (NPSA, 2004b) under topical anaesthetic (e.g. lidocaine) cover (Hickey, 2003d). Antihypertensives (e.g. hydralazine) may be used, but once sympathetic stimuli for hypertension are resolved, circulating drugs and bradycardia may cause excessive rebound hypotension.

Gentle bladder irrigation with 30 ml sterile water may be attempted (van Welzen and Carey, 2002), but blocked urinary catheters are usually replaced urgently (Hickey, 2003d).

As autonomic hyper-reflexia occurs during rehabilitation from spinal injury, patient and carer education become progressively important. Quadriplegia creates continuing dependency on carers for fundamental aspects of living, including movement. Pressure area care regimes are carefully staged to build skin tolerance until patients can remain in one position for prolonged periods, possibly all night, without developing sores or hyper-reflexic crises.

Carers should be increasingly involved in aspects of care, which they will have to perform following discharge (e.g. changing urinary catheters, performing manual evacuations). While later stages of rehabilitation are unlikely to be reached before transfer to spinal injury units, ICU nurses may initiate rehabilitation, and should therefore supply appropriate information to patients and carers, as well as being able to recognise and treat complications of autonomic hyper-reflexia.

Haemorrhage

Major intracranial haemorrhage is usually caused by severe TBI or spontaneous rupture of cerebral blood vessels, usually from aneurysms (Wilson *et al.*, 2005). Haemorrhage may be:

- subdural
- extradural
- subarachnoid (SAH).

SAH is often fatal. Haemorrhage is ideally treated by either surgical or endovascular coiling or neurosurgical clipping (Molyneux *et al.*, 2005), but these usually necessitate transfer to neurological centres, which may be impractical. Cerebral perfusion should be maintained, while maintaining arterial blood pressure below 160 mmHg (Wilson *et al.*, 2005). Gupta *et al.* (2010) recommend:

- head elevation
- sedation
- mannitol/hypertonic saline
- hyperventilation
- barbiturate coma.

Nimodipine can be useful to prevent vasospasm (Wilson *et al.*, 2005).

Prognosis

Prognosis of major CNS pathologies is often complex. Major intracranial bleeds are often fatal – mortality exceeds 40 per cent (Wilson *et al.*, 2005). Recovery from severe TBI or SCI is unpredictable, often prolonged or incomplete. Most (85 per cent) remain disabled one year after TBI; even with minor head injury less than half recover fully within one year (Watkins, 2000). Nearly half of survivors from subarachnoid haemorrhage suffer long-term cognitive impairment (Suarez *et al.*, 2006), and a significant minority develop major depressive disorders (Bombardier *et al.*, 2010). Rehabilitation can be a long and often frustrating process for both patients and their relatives, so planning for rehabilitation should begin early.

Many patients experience amnesia, often having no memory of events immediately before the injury (Watkins, 2000). This may be psychologically protective, but can also be psychologically distressing. Once their condition has stabilised, patients may be transferred to specialist rehabilitation centres.

Epilepsy carries a social stigma (Lanfear, 2002), which, although reduced through public education, has been reinforced by restrictions on driving, insurance policies and other restrictions on quality of life. Patients and their families may therefore be fearful of the label, or its potential effects on their lifestyle.

Personality changes

In addition to general psychological stressors from critical illness and ICU admission, central nervous system injury, prolonged recovery and fears about patients' futures can affect psychological function and cause depression (Bénony *et al.*, 2002). TBI can cause temporary or permanent changes in behaviour due to damage; on waking, patients may exhibit:

- lack of inhibition
- inflexible thinking
- memory deficits
- irritability.

(O'Neill and Carter, 1998)

Frontal lobe damage is especially likely to cause aggressiveness and loss of inhibition. Damage to other areas of the brain may cause other problems, such as dysphasia. Personality and mood changes are especially distressing for families (Powell, 2004), so they should be warned in advance about possible behavioural change. Victims of road traffic accidents or assault may be anxious about litigation or police involvement. Nurses should therefore assess psychological needs of both patients and families.

Family care

Prolonged, unpredictable and incomplete recovery exposes families to continuing distress. Families need help to enable them to cope (O'Neill and Carter, 1998). ICU staff can offer useful advice and support in the early stages. Social workers, support groups, counsellors or other social supports may be beneficial.

Family and friends often bring comfort, but might cause distress. Where visitors do cause undue distress, nurses may need to intervene to enable patients to rest, but visits that provide therapeutic benefits should be encouraged. Nursing documentation and handover should identify effects of visitors on patients.

While nurses' prime duty is to their patients, care of relatives is an important, albeit secondary, nursing role. Relatives usually appreciate being given appropriate information. They also need adequate rest themselves; they may feel obliged to stay by the bedside, exhausting both themselves and the patient, so planning care with the next of kin can prove beneficial to all. Providing somewhere to stay and access to catering facilities can greatly reduce the stress experienced by relatives.

Legal aspects

Admissions caused by road traffic accidents or other potentially criminal actions may involve the police. There are certain requirements in law for nurses to disclose information, but they are few in number, and often require a court order. In the absence of any specific legal requirement, nurses should remember their duty of confidentiality to patients (NMC, 2008a). If in doubt about whether the police or other authorities have a right to information or specimens, nurses should seek the advice of their line manager, and may need to consult their employer's legal department. Details of legal obligations can be found in Dimond (2008).

DLVA regulations forbid epileptics (with a few specified exceptions) from driving until they have been free from fitting for one year (Lanfear, 2002).

Implications for practice

- Complications and deaths of patients admitted with central nervous system injury are usually caused by hypoxia or cerebral ischaemia, so immediate priorities are:
  - airway and breathing – artificial ventilation;
  - circulation – fluid resuscitation, aiming for CPP 60 mmHg;
  - disability – neuroprotection (sedation, possible hypothermia, preventing intracranial hypertension).
- Following TBI, patients should be nursed at 15–30°, with head and neck alignment maintained, and nothing (e.g. endotracheal tapes) restricting venous drainage from the head.
- Spinal injury patients should be nursed supine, with their spine in alignment.
- Spinal injury patients should be turned at least two-hourly. Manual patient handling should always use log-rolls, with sufficient staff to safely turn the patient and manage equipment.
- Autonomic hyper-reflexia occurs with most spinal cord injuries above T6, so staff should observe for hypertensive crises and know how to manage them, and appropriate bowel care protocols should be available.
- Rehabilitation is often prolonged, and may remain incomplete. Patients and families often experience psychological distress, so nurses should assess both patients' and relatives' psychological needs, and refer to appropriate support agencies.
- There are a few instances where police or other authorities have rights to access confidential information; if in doubt, nurses should seek advice before disclosing anything.

Summary

Neurological admissions may be transferred to regional specialist centres, but early ICU care is more often managed on general units, significantly affecting outcome. When specialist centres consider they cannot offer additional care, patients remain on general units. Head injury can range from mild to severe, and skilled nursing care significantly contributes to survival and recovery. Prognosis is considerably worse with SCI, and very poor with subarachnoid haemorrhage. But with all CNS pathologies, priorities remain cerebral oxygenation and perfusion. Secondary deaths are often from complications, which should be prevented if possible. Additional aspects of nursing care include supporting fundamental activities of living, coordinating care and providing psychological support to patients and families.

Further reading

NICE (2007b) and Andrews *et al.* (2008a) provide comprehensive guidelines for TBI. Hickey (2003a) remains the key text on neurological nursing, although Iggulden's (2006) handbook is also useful. Harvey (2008) reviews autonomic hyper-reflexia. Walker (2009) reviews SCI. Meierkord *et al.* (2010) provide European guidelines for epilepsy.

Clinical scenario

Claire Healy is 56 years old and sustained a severe head injury after falling 10 feet from an attic. She experienced loss of consciousness for an unknown length of time. Mrs Healy was admitted to the ICU via A&E wearing a cervical collar with spinal immobilisation. The results from a neurological examination revealed the following:

GCS	7 (E: 2, V: 1, M: 4) which changed to GCS 3 (E: 1, V: 1, M: 1)
Pupil response	sluggish, equal response, size 3 mm diameter
	Cough and gag reflex present
	Blood discharging from both ears; active bleed in left ear; old dried blood in right ear

Other observations included:

Respiratory rate	29 breaths/minute
BP	150/96 mmHg (mean BP 114 mmHg)
HR	74 beats/minute
CVP	3 mmHg
Central temperature	36°C
Blood sugar	10.5 mmol/litre

A head CT scan confirmed fractures of basal skull, left occipital, left and right mastoid with a small left subdural haematoma.

Q.1 Interpret the significance of Mrs Healy's results in relation to her head injury and explore the physiological implications.

Q.2 The aim of ICU management is to anticipate, prevent and treat secondary physiological insults. Prioritise a plan of care that incorporates neuroprotection strategies, promotes cerebral perfusion pressure and is likely to improve Mrs Healy's outcome after traumatic brain injury.

Q.3 Reflect on how patients with head and spinal injuries are positioned and moved in your clinical area (e.g. equipment, personnel, other resources, specialists, guideline or protocol followed).

Chapter 37

Peripheral neurological pathologies

Contents

Fundamental knowledge	370
Introduction	371
ICU-acquired weakness	371
Guillain-Barré syndrome (GBS)	372
Implications for practice	373
Summary	373
Support groups	374
Further reading	374
Clinical scenario	374

Fundamental knowledge

Nerve anatomy and conduction – myelin, nodes of Ranvier

Introduction

Many patients in ICUs develop muscle weakness. This problem, which has been given various names, is increasingly called *ICU-acquired weakness*, a nebulous term reflecting problems around identifying its cause and making a clinical diagnosis. Peripheral neuropathy may also be a primary pathology. The primary pathology most frequently seen is ICUs is *Gullain Barré syndrome*.

Many of the problems, and some treatments, discussed in this chapter apply to other causes of peripheral neuropathy, such as *myasthenia gravis*. Myasthenia gravis is a relatively rare disease, so is not specifically discussed, but useful information is contained in the European guidelines for autoimmune neuro-muscular disorders (Skeie *et al.*, 2010).

Nursing patients with neurological complications can be labour-intensive and stressful. Patients need care and support with many activities of living, while minimising complications significantly improves recovery and survival. Nursing care is therefore especially valuable for patients with these conditions. Physiotherapy is beneficial for almost all critically ill patients (Schweickert *et al.*, 2009), but has an especially important role in rehabilitating patients with severe muscular weakness.

Management of both conditions centres on:

- attempts to remove underlying causes;
- prevention of complications;
- system support.

While there is some research evidence, practice varies between units; some approaches described below are anecdotal rather than evidence-based.

ICU-acquired weakness

Many ICU patients develop weakness that appears to be a complication of their disease and/or treatments. This weakness, which often delays weaning and recovery, has been nebulously termed 'critical illness neuropathy', among other variant names (e.g. polyneuropathy, myopathy). It probably encompasses a number of similar pathologies – Ricks (2007) suggests critical illness polyneuropathy involves axonal degeneration of both sensory and motor nerves, while critical illness myopathy causes degeneration of muscle fibres. Incidence is unclear – Patti *et al.*'s (2008) 25–85 per cent reflects conflicting evidence. It is more common among patients on ICUs for more than one week (Patti *et al.*, 2008).

Various causes have been speculated, but most dismissed. Treatment is largely supportive (Patti *et al.*, 2008; Dyer *et al.*, 2009), although direct stimulation of muscle fibres is recommended (Patti *et al.*, 2008), physiotherapy and passive exercises also help (Kennedy *et al.*, 2002), and intensive insulin therapy may help (Herman *et al.*, 2007; Dyer *et al.*, 2009) (dangers of intensive insulin therapy are discussed in Chapter 21).

Guillain-Barré syndrome (GBS)

GBS describes a group of similar pathologies that disrupt nerve conduction:

- acute inflammatory demyelinating polyneuropathy (AIDP);
- acute motor axonal neuropathy (AMAN);
- acute motor sensory axonal neuropathy (AMSAN);
- Fisher's syndrome.

(Hughes and Cornblath, 2005)

Chronic inflammatory demyelinating polyneuropathy (CIDP) is a similar, but longer-lasting, disease, once called 'chronic GBS'.

In Europe and North America the main cause of severe GBS is AIDP (Kuwabara *et al.*, 2002); Fisher's syndrome, although moderately frequent, is relatively benign (Hughes and Cornblath, 2005). GBS often follows minor viral respiratory or gut infections (Pritchard, 2008). Progressive loss of motor function ascends from peripheries; a quarter of patients develop respiratory failure (Dua and Banerjee, 2010).

Treatments are mainly supportive, although intravenous gamma globulin (IVIg) usually shortens duration of disease (Winer, 2008; Dua and Banerjee, 2010). Steroids are not beneficial (Winer, 2008).

Muscle weakness and autonomic dysfunction can cause the following:

- *Pain*. Pain is usually present (Dua and Banerjee, 2010), often severe and exacerbated by touch and anxiety. Analgesia (often opioids) is needed. Neuropathic analgesics, such as amitriptyline (Pritchard, 2008), gabapentin or carbamazepine (Hughes *et al.*, 2005; Kogos *et al.*, 2005) are useful. Pain contributes to depression (Kogos *et al.*, 2005).
- *Respiratory failure*. A quarter of GBS patients need artificial ventilation (Hughes and Cornblath, 2005). Non-invasive ventilation is usually attempted first, due to the high risk of VAP, but many patients later need intubation and invasive ventilation. Intensive physiotherapy may limit or prevent respiratory failure.
- *Hypotension*. This can result from extensive peripheral vasodilatation (poor sympathetic tone).
- *Hypertensive episodes*. These are caused by failure of normal negative feedback opposition to sympathetic stimuli.
- *Dysrhythmias*. Sinus tachycardia, bradycardia and asystole frequently occur.
- *Thrombosis*. DVTs especially can occur (Kogos *et al.*, 2005), from venous stasis (immobility) and hypoperfusion. Thromboprophylaxis (subcutaneous heparin) and thromboembolytic stockings (TEDS™) should be given.
- *Limb weakness*. This ascends from distal to proximal muscles, affecting hands, feet or both. Passive exercises may prevent contractures and promote venous return.
- *Hypersalivation*. Hypersalivation and loss of swallow from autonomic dysfunction necessitate oral suction for comfort and to prevent aspiration.

- *Bilateral facial muscle weakness.* This may cause dribbling of saliva and ophthalmoplegia, distressing both patients and relatives.
- *Sweating.* Sweating, from autonomic dysfunction, is often profuse, so frequent washes and changes of clothing help provide comfort.
- *Incontinence.* This is caused by bladder muscle weakness.
- *Psychological problems.* These arise from progressive and prolonged weakness. Mentally fit (often young) adults forced to rely on others to perform fundamental and intimate activities of living suffer distress, compounding environmental stressors of the ICU (see Chapter 3), and fears about prognosis (many GBS sufferers have extensive knowledge about their disease) often cause psychoses and acute depression (Kogos *et al.*, 2005). Most develop severe fatigue (Dua and Banerjee, 2010).
- *Immunocompromise.* This is multifactoral, aggravated by factors such as hepatic dysfunction, reduced functional residual capacity, sleep disturbance, stress responses and depression, as well as treatments such as intubation. Infection control and preventing opportunistic infection are therefore especially important.
- *Catabolism.* This necessitates aggressive (and early) nutrition to limit muscle wasting.

Depression reduces motivation, needed with protracted debility. Antidepressants are often useful, but should not become a substitute for active human contact and humane nursing (e.g. making environments as 'normal' as possible). Psychological support should be extended to family and friends.

ICU mortality from GBS is 5 per cent (Pritchard, 2008). ICU discharge typically occurs after two to four weeks (Hughes and Cornblath, 2005; Pritchard, 2008), although can take considerably longer (e.g. six months). Further rehabilitation is often slow, and sometimes incomplete (Kogos *et al.*, 2005; van Doorn, 2005; Hughes and Cornblath, 2005; Pritchard, 2008).

Patients with ICU-acquired weakness suffer similar psychological problems.

Implications for practice

- Prolonged admission makes nursing care an especially important factor in recovery for these patients.
- Holistic assessment enables many complications to be avoided.
- Depression and sensory imbalance can easily occur; psychological care should be optimised.
- Neurological deficits impair normal homeostatic mechanisms, so nurses should avoid interventions or lack of interventions that may provoke crises.
- Providing information to patients and families can help them cope and develop any skills they may need following discharge.

Summary

This chapter has described three neurological conditions that may be encountered with varying frequency on general ICUs. For nurses without specialist neurological training, these conditions can create very real challenges, but more than many pathological conditions, are largely resolved by nursing rather than medical interventions.

Support groups

Guillain-Barré helpline: 0800 374803
Guillain-Barré Syndrome Support Group: www.gbs.org.uk

Further reading

Hickey (2003a) remains the classic neurology nursing text. Useful medical articles on Guillain-Barré syndrome include Winer (2008) and Pritchard (2008). ICU-acquired weakness has been much discussed, although varying terminology complicates searches. Recent articles include Patti *et al.* (2008) and Dyer *et al.* (2009).

Clinical scenario

Donald McLean, 58 years old, presented with a ten-day history of dysphagia, progressive tachypnoea with increasing oxygen requirements, difficulty swallowing, weak cough, slurred speech, general fatigue, and deep tendon reflexes absent in all limbs, with numbness in both legs and tips of fingers in both hands. When examined the following results were noted:

Respiratory rate	42 breaths/minute
SpO$_2$	91% on 15 litres of oxygen
Vital capacity	380 ml
BP	150/100 mmHg
HR	80 beats/minute
Temperature	36°C

Chest X-ray revealed right middle and lower lobe pneumonia. Arterial blood gas analysis showed uncompensated respiratory acidosis with hypoxia.

In the previous month Mr McLean had flu-like symptoms and was recovering from an upper respiratory tract infection. Acute post-infective polyneuropathy or Guillain-Barré syndrome is suspected and Mr McLean was admitted to the ICU for respiratory support.

Q.1 Review the most suitable type of respiratory support for Mr McLean. Provide a rationale for your suggestion.

Q.2 Identify additional complications associated with polyneuropathy that Mr McLean may experience during his ICU stay. Propose specific nursing interventions to minimise these.

Q.3 Identify and reflect on a range of approaches that may support and strengthen the immune response in Mr McLean and promote an early recovery (e.g. immunonutrition, sleep, administration of IgIV, psychological support, mobilisation, pain management).

Part VIII

Abdominal

Chapter 38

Acute kidney injury

Contents

Fundamental knowledge   379
Introduction   380
Volume-responsive AKI   380
Intrinsic AKI   380
Postrenal AKI   381
Monitoring renal function   382
Urinalysis   382
Effects   384
Management   385
Diuretics   385
Rhabdomyolysis   386
Implications for practice   386
Summary   387
Further reading   387
Clinical scenario   387

Fundamental knowledge

Renal anatomy and physiology (including
   glomeruli and nephrons)
Urea and creatinine (see Chapter 21)

Introduction

Acute kidney injury (AKI) is a largely predictable and preventable complication of hypotension (Davenport and Stevens, 2008; NCEPOD, 2009). Insufficient perfusion of the kidney causes both ischaemia of kidney tissue and oliguria. Ischaemia causes:

- inflammation

and may progress to

- necrosis – especially *acute tubular necrosis* (ATN).

Oliguria causes:

- fluid retention;
- electrolyte imbalances (especially potassium);
- retention of toxins, and metabolites of drugs and hormones;
- metabolic acidosis.

Kidney injury therefore causes many problems and up to one-quarter of ICU patients develop AKI (Tillyard *et al.*, 2005; ICS, 2009b). This chapter describes AKI and rhabdomyolysis. Haemofiltration is discussed in Chapter 39.

Oliguria (< 0.5 ml/kg/hour) is often a sign of kidney disease, but functional failure can occur despite 'normal' or 'polyuric' urine volumes. Oliguria may be caused by:

- *volume-responsive* (previously *prerenal*) AKI;
- *intrinsic* (*intrarenal*) AKI;
- *postrenal* AKI.

Volume-responsive AKI

Volume-responsive AKI is caused by failure to perfuse kidneys; glomeruli and renal tubules remain undamaged. This is the most common cause of AKI (NCEPOD, 2009). Failure to treat volume-responsive AKI with early and adequate volume almost inevitably causes acute tubular necrosis (ATN) – intrinsic AKI.

Renal perfusion has often been compromised before arrival in the ICU. For example, AKI occurs in 10–23 per cent of surgical patients (Sykes and Cosgrove, 2007); perioperative haemodynamic optimisation can reduce AKI (Brienza *et al.*, 2009).

Intrinsic AKI

Intrinsic AKI is caused by damage to glomeruli and nephrons. Damage may be caused by:

- ischaemia
- inflammation
- nephrotoxicity.

Many drugs are nephrotoxic, including ACE inhibitors, gentamicin, and many radiocontrast dyes, but ATN remains the main cause of intrinsic AKI (Davenport and Stevens, 2008). Whereas volume-responsive AKI is immediately reversible, intrinsic AKI persists until tissue damage resolves, which often takes 7–21 days (Hussein *et al.*, 2009).

Acute tubular necrosis used to be attributed to death of renal tubule cells, but the pathology is more complex: while the problem is 'acute' and affects tubules, it is caused by ischaemia and oedema, rather than (necessarily) necrosis, of tubular cells. ATN, and most other types of intrinsic AKI, can be classified into three stages:

- initiation
- established or maintenance
- recovery or diuretic.

Initially, volume-responsive AKI causes ischaemia. Hypoxic damage causes intracellular oedema and, if unreversed, cell death (see Chapter 24). Oliguria usually occurs within two days of precipitating events and usually lasts up to two weeks, although can persist far longer. Prognosis worsens with prolonged oliguria. As renal function fails, urine volume falls, with serum urea and creatinine levels rising.

Cell damage releases vasoactive cytokines, provoking further intrarenal vasoconstriction. Preglomerular vasoconstriction reduces glomerular perfusion, and so glomerular filtration. Widespread tubule intracellular oedema physically compresses lumens, obstructing flow of what filtrate is produced. Oliguria, and often anuria, persists throughout the established phase. Medullary damage from intrinsic AKI reduces sodium reabsorption in the *loop of Henle*, so urinary sodium is high: > 40 mmol/litre. Hypernatraemia in the *macula densa* activates the renin-angiotensin-aldosterone cascade.

Tubular cells readily regenerate. When they do, the recovery phase begins. As damaged tubules begin to recover function and new (immature) tubule cells grow, filtration improves, but tubular reabsorption and solute exchange remain poor, causing large volumes of poor-quality urine; serum urea and creatinine remain elevated.

When tubular cells mature, normal function is recovered. Urea and creatinine levels fall, urine volumes return to normal, and electrolyte balance is restored.

Postrenal AKI

Postrenal AKI is usually caused by mechanical obstruction to the flow of urine – such as bladder tumours, renal/bladder calculi, strictures or enlarged prostate. Postrenal obstruction is the main cause of AKI in the community, but is unlikely to occur in ICUs unless already present on admission. Back pressure from obstruction can cause intrarenal damage (glomerulonephritis). Postrenal AKI is reversed by removing the obstruction, usually by surgery.

Monitoring renal function

There are many, but no ideal, ways to measure glomerular function, including:

- urinalysis (see below)
- urine volume
- plasma urea
- plasma creatinine
- creatinine clearance (24-hour urine collection).

However, probably the most useful measurement is:

- estimated glomerular filtration rate (eGFR).

Novel biomarkers include:

- neutrophil gelatinase-associated lipocalin (NGAL);
- copeptin (Meyer *et al.*, 2008).

Like most body systems, healthy kidneys have a large physiological reserve. Kidney injury occurs once three-quarters of nephrons are non-functional. Endstage renal failure occurs when 90 per cent of nephrons fail, leaving a relatively narrow margin between recoverable and terminal failure.

Urea and creatinine are described in Chapter 21. Blood creatinine, a waste product of muscle metabolism, varies throughout the day – renal clearance is highest during the afternoon. Therefore, 24-hour urine collections provide a more balanced indication of renal function than isolated blood samples. However, even creatinine only reflects function at the end of nephrons, and so provides a relatively late sign of problems. Estimated glomerular filtration rate (eGFR), largely calculated from creatinine, gives slightly earlier warnings of deterioration. Normal adult GFR is > 90 ml/minute (Murphy and Robinson, 2006).

Urinalysis

While reagent-strip urinalysis has limitations, it is a simple, non-invasive test that should be undertaken at an early stage for all acute hospital admissions (NCEPOD, 2009).

Blood/leucocytes

Like plasma proteins, blood cells are not normally filtered by the glomerulus. Inflammatory disease may allow cells to pass into urine, or trauma to the urinary tract (e.g. stones, cancers, catheterisation) may cause bleeding. If blood is present (haematuria), protein will inevitably also be detected. Leucocytes (white blood cells) are part of the immune system, and are usually only found in urine if infection is present (urinary tract infection – UTI).

Nitrite

Bacteria convert nitrate, which is normally in urine, to nitrite (Steggall, 2007), so nitrite will only be found if urine is infected. However, absence of nitrite cannot exclude UTI, as some bacteria do not convert nitrate (Steggall, 2007).

Urobilinogen/bilirubin

Bilirubinuria is only likely to occur if blood bilirubin levels are significantly raised. Bilirubin is a waste product of erythrocyte metabolism. Normally converted by the liver into bile, which flows to the gall bladder, gall bladder disease causes bilirubin loss in urine (Wilson, 2005). Bilirubinuria usually causes urine to look dark.

Protein

Protein is not normally filtered by the glomerulus, so proteinuria usually indicates an inflammatory response (disease, such as infection) in the kidney that has enabled it to pass through the glomerulus (Birn and Christensen, 2006; Steggall, 2007). Proteinuria is the single most important indicator of kidney injury (Barratt, 2007).

pH

Normal: 5–6.

Urine is made from blood. Blood pH is normally 7.4. A major factor in maintaining normal blood pH is excretion of excess hydrogen ions (an essential chemical for acids) into the renal tubule. Thus urinary pH varies according to physiological needs, but is almost always acidic. Provided renal function is reasonable, high pH may reflect alkalaemia, while low pH may reflect acidaemia.

Specific gravity

Normal: 1.002–1.035.

Urine is mainly water. The specific gravity of pure water is 1.0 (= low SG), so urine normally is just slightly more concentrated. High specific gravity suggests more water is being reabsorbed by the kidney, usually in response to dehydration – i.e. volume-responsive AKI. Specific gravity is often lower in older people as age-related decline in function reduces their ability to concentrate urine (Wilson,

2005). Low specific gravity (watery urine) often means excessive water in urine. Intrinsic and postrenal failure often cause low specific gravity, as damaged renal tubules lose their ability to concentrate urine (Barratt, 2007).

Ketones

Ketones are a waste product of fat metabolism. Blood sugar, not fat, is normally the main source of cell energy, so ketones in blood (and urine) indicate lack of availability of blood sugar. The two main reasons for this are:

- lack of insulin (diabetic ketoacidosis – see Chapter 33 – diabetic emergencies);
- starvation.

As well as indicating problems, ketones may form acids, hence the metabolic acidosis found with diabetic ketoacidosis.

Glucose

The kidney filters blood sugar, but normally reabsorbs it all provided blood sugar is below 10 mmol/litre. *Glycosuria* therefore usually indicates hyperglycaemia. Glucose has a high osmotic pressure and reduces water reabsorption, causing polyuria and dilute urine (low specific gravity). Diabetes is often initially detected from routine urinalysis. Acute illness and many drugs (especially cardiac) can cause transient hyperglycaemia.

Effects

Kidney disease disrupts homeostasis. The main complications to body systems that result from kidney disease are:

Cardiovascular:
- hyperkalaemia
- acidosis
- dysrhythmias
- anaemia.

Nervous system:
- confusion (from uraemia)
- twitching
- coma.

Respiratory:
- compensatory tachypnoea
- acidosis
- pulmonary oedema
- hiccough.

Gut:
- nausea
- diarrhoea
- vomiting.

Metabolic:
- electrolyte imbalances
- acidosis
- toxicity from active drug metabolites.

Potassium: most (90 per cent) potassium loss is in urine, so oliguria usually causes hyperkalaemia, while polyuria causes hypokalaemia.

Acid/base: normal renal function maintains acid/base balance by reabsorbing bicarbonate and excreting hydrogen atoms. Many hydrogen ions pass into *ultrafiltrate* in renal tubules, changing normal blood pH of 7.4 into normal urinary pH of 5–6. Kidney disease therefore causes metabolic acidosis.

Acidosis stimulates tachypnoea, normally compensating metabolic acidosis with respiratory alkalosis. But respiratory failure may limit effectiveness, causing excessive triggering without significant compensation.

Management

Poorly managed volume-responsive AKI usually progresses to intrinsic AKI. Kidney function can be protected by optimising perfusion with *fluids*. Once blood volume and pressure are optimised, a *fluid challenge* helps identify whether oliguria is volume responsive (urine volume increases) or caused by intrinsic injury (no significant increase in urine). Although much debated, choice between colloid and crystalloid for fluid challenges is probably less important than ensuring that glomerular beds receive sufficient volume to filter. Large volumes should be infused rapidly – at least 500 ml over no more than 30 minutes, preferably with CVP monitoring in case cardiac overload and pulmonary oedema occur.

If kidneys fail to respond to fluid challenges, medical options are mainly *drugs* and/or *continuous renal replacement therapy* (CRRT) (see Chapter 39). Renal replacement therapy buys time until recovery.

Diuretics

Furosemide, a loop diuretic, blocks sodium reabsorption in the ascending loop of Henle. Water reabsorption being passive, this increases urine volume. Furosemide is an effective way of treating fluid overload, but can compromise hypovolaemic patients – increasing mortality and development of chronic kidney disease of critically ill patients (Mehta *et al.*, 2002), so loop should not be routinely used to prevent AKI (Ho and Sheridan, 2006; Davenport and Stevens, 2008). Furosemide is ototoxic (Ho and Power, 2010), so intravenous administration should be slow (4 mg/minute). Large doses are therefore best given through a syringe driver or volumetric pump. Furosemide can cause hypokalaemia, so with large doses the ECG should be monitored and serum potassium levels checked.

Mannitol, an osmotic diuretic, is often used for treating cerebral oedema, but is seldom used for other problems, as it can cause pulmonary oedema (Davenport and Stevens, 2008).

Dopexamine, a synthetic analogue of dopamine, has been used for treating kidney disease, although benefit is doubtful (see Chapter 34).

Rhabdomyolysis

Extensive muscle damage, such as from crush injuries, major burns, severe infection/sepsis or prolonged immobilisation, can cause rhabdomyolysis, leading to AKI. Various speculated mechanisms of kidney disease from rhabdomyolysis include:

- blockage of tubules with myoglobin precipitate;
- myoglobin-induced vasoconstriction of renal arterioles;
- oxygen-free radical (mainly from iron-containing haem molecule) damage to renal tubules (Cooper *et al.*, 2006).

Hydrogen ion excretion by the kidney changes ultrafiltrate from alkali (normal pH 7.4) to acid (often reaching pH 5.0), creating the acid environment in which myoglobin can precipitate. As myoglobin contains iron, what little urine does filter through is stained a distinctively rusty colour. Rhabdomyolysis is diagnosed by clinical suspicion, but confirmed by elevated serum creatine kinase (CK – see Chapter 29) (Sharp *et al.*, 2004). A few centres can test for myoglobin.

Rhabdomyolysis is treated by rapid intravenous infusion to flush out myoglobin, often 10–12 litres over 24 hours (Hunter, 2002). To prevent cardiac overload, CVP monitoring is recommended. Diuretics, usually furosemide (mannitol has also been used), are given to maintain urine at 200–300 ml/hour (Meister and Reddy, 2002).

To reduce precipitation and free radical damage, urine may be alkalinised by bicarbonate infusions (Sever *et al.*, 2006), although Brown *et al.* (2004) question whether alkalinisation has benefits. Myoglobin may block urinary catheters, so urine flow should be observed closely. Obstructed catheters should be replaced rather than flushed, to prevent returning precipitate into the bladder. Extensive muscle cell damage may cause life-threatening hyperkalaemia (Hunter, 2002), which should be reversed.

Implications for practice

- Renal function should be determined by the ability of the kidneys to achieve and maintain homeostasis, not simply by the amount of urine produced.
- Creatinine, and its derivative eGFR (estimated glomerular filtration rate), is the most useful biochemical marker of kidney function.

■ Factors outside the kidneys (e.g. metabolism) may affect glomerular filtration of urea, so blood urea alone is not a reliable marker.

■ The most common cause of kidney disease in ICU patients is hypovolaemia, causing acute tubular necrosis.

■ Volume-responsive AKI can often be prevented if patients receive adequate fluids to maintain perfusion.

■ Diuretics can remove excess fluid, but can kill hypovolaemic patients.

■ Kidney disease prevents excretion of hydrogen ions from the body, so causes metabolic acidosis.

■ The many other metabolic functions of the kidney mean that kidney disease causes complications for all other major systems.

■ Diuretics may restore urine volumes, and are useful for offloading excess fluid, but should be avoided with hypovolaemia.

Summary

Acute kidney injury frequently complicates other pathologies in ICU patients. While mortality from primary kidney disease is encouragingly low, mortality from multi-organ dysfunction remains depressingly high. Mortality from AKI remains unchanged at about 50 per cent (Ympa *et al.*, 2005), so if the incidence of progression to AKI can be reduced, mortality and morbidity among ICU patients will significantly decrease.

Kidney disease causes failure of renal function, so causes fluid overload, electrolyte imbalances, acid/base balances, and other metabolic disturbances, these causing further complications. Nurses therefore need knowledge of physiology and effects to optimise prevention and provide holistic care.

Further reading

Most applied physiology texts include overviews of kidney disease, although recent changes in practice limit the value of older texts. UK guidelines (Davenport and Stevens, 2008) are comprehensive and valuable. Hussein *et al.* (2009) provide a useful medical overview of AKI. NCEPOD (2009) is useful, although not ICU-specific.

Clinical scenario

James Roger is 67 years old and has type 2 diabetes. He underwent an aortic valve replacement three months previously. He was found collapsed at home and was subsequently admitted to the ICU with abnormal clotting and diagnosed with sepsis secondary to endocarditis. Mr Roger had received high-dose intravenous antibiotics, including gentamicin, vancomycin, rifampicin and cefotaxime, and had been taking oral warfarin. His last recorded weight was 74 kg.

Mr Roger's blood investigations values include:

Urea	28.4 mmol/litre
Creatinine	255 µmol/litre
Creatine kinase	294 units/litre
Sodium	142 mmol/litre
Potassium	4 mmol/litre
Chloride	119 mmol/litre
Bicarbonate	17 mmol/litre
Base deficit	5.8 mmol/litre
Lactate	4.7 mmol/litre

Arterial blood gas results while invasively ventilated on FiO_2 of 0.5 were:

pH	7.2
$PaCO_2$	7.05 kPa
PaO_2	9.3 kPa
SaO_2	96.1%

Vital observations with a noradrenaline infusion at 0.5 µg/kg/minute were:

Temperature	36.2°C
Heart rate	107 beats/minute
Rhythm	atrial fibrillation
BP	76/46 mmHg
CI	3.1 litres/minute/m^2
CVP	11 mmHg
Urine	10, 5, 5, 0 ml/hour trend over 4 hours

Q.1 Examine Mr Roger's abnormal values and risk factors and give a rationale for developing volume-responsive, intrinsic, or postrenal acute kidney injury (AKI)?

Q.2 Compare Mr Roger's results to normal values. Estimate his GFR using the Cockroft-Gault formula (or refer to Chapter 21):

$$\frac{(140 - \text{age (years)}) \times \text{weight (kg)}}{\text{Serum creatinine } (\mu\text{mol/litre})} \times 1.25 \text{ for males, or } 1.03 \text{ for females}$$

Q.3 Consider the risk factors for developing AKI and for each factor explain the physiological processes resulting in AKI. Review the effects of hypoxaemia, hypercapnia, acid/base disturbances and mechanical ventilation on Mr Roger's sympathetic nervous system and ADH release. Formulate a plan of care that may enhance his renal blood flow and renal function.

The same patient is used in the clinical scenario for Chapter 39.

Haemofiltration

Contents

Fundamental knowledge	389
Introduction	390
Filtration	390
Preparation	392
Monitoring	393
Troubleshooting	395
Outcome	395
Implications for practice	396
Summary	396
Further reading	397
Clinical scenario	397

Fundamental knowledge

Normal renal anatomy and physiology
Acute kidney injury (see Chapter 38)

Introduction

About a quarter of critically ill patients develop acute kidney injury (AKI), usually from systemic hypotension (cardiovascular failure); about 4 per cent of ICU patients need renal replacement therapy (Uchino *et al.*, 2007). While renal units mainly use intermittent haemodialysis for renal replacement therapy, this is unsuitable for critically ill, hypotensive patients. Continuous renal replacement therapies (CRRTs) avoid aggressive reductions in blood pressure, so continuous venovenous haemofiltration/haemodiafiltration (CVVH/CVVHD) is the main CRRT used in ICUs.

Filtration

In the human kidney, glomerular capillaries filter large volumes of blood (minus blood cells and plasma proteins) to form *ultrafiltrate*. This ultrafiltrate is then concentrated into urine in the renal tubule, with active movement of solutes to conserve electrolytes and micronutrients, and remove waste. CVVH acts like a large glomerulus, the filter removing large volumes of ultrafiltrate. But unlike renal tubules, haemofilters cannot reabsorb either fluid or solutes. Provided they are smaller than pore size, solutes move across semipermeable membranes to form an equal concentration on either side (convection). Blood flowing through nephrons, or haemofilters, has a higher pressure than ultrafiltrate, so filtered solutes (and fluid) flow on through the system, making filtration a one-way process. Solutes exert an osmotic pressure, drawing water with them ('*solvent drag*'). In practice, *ultrafiltration* and *convection* are inseparable (see Figures 39.1 and 39.2). But whereas human renal tubules actively reabsorb water, electrolytes and micronutrients, haemofilters cannot do this. So replacement fluid aims to replace water and important electrolytes.

Continuous venovenous haemofiltration (CVVH) uses only ultrafiltration and convection. While this effectively removes volume, as solute concentration within the haemofilter increases, solute clearance is limited by the volume being removed. So CVVH is relatively inefficient in removing toxins.

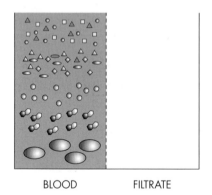
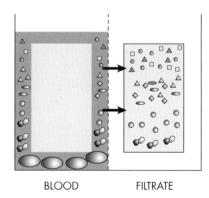

BLOOD   FILTRATE   BLOOD   FILTRATE

■ *Figure 39.1* **Ultrafiltration**

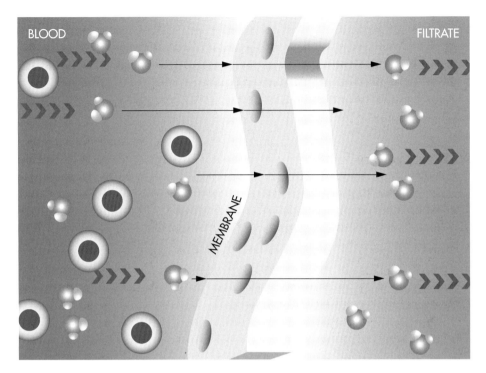

■ *Figure 39.2* **Convection**

CVVHD uses:

■ ultrafiltration
■ convection and
■ dialysis.

Dialysis is movement of solutes across a concentration gradient, so CVVHD adds *dialysate*, running in an opposite direction (counter-current) to the blood. This 'washes out' solutes, so enabling more to diffuse. To prevent electrolyte imbalances, dialysate fluid contains normal serum concentrations of many electrolytes (although little/no potassium). The main differences between CVVH and CVVHD are listed in Table 39.1. For this chapter, 'haemofiltration' refers to both CVVH and CVVHD, unless one of the abbreviations is specified.

Table 39.1 Main differences between CVVH and CVVHD

CVVH	CVVHD
Uses less fluid (less cost, less time). Effective fluid removal (ultrafiltration).	Better solute clearance.

Preparation

Haemofilters use high blood flow, so a large double-lumen cannula (e.g. Vaccath®) is inserted into a large vein – usually femoral or internal jugular. Blood is drawn from one side, normally coloured either red or brown and called *arterial* or *afferent*, into the circuit. Blood is returned to the patient through the other lumen, normally coloured blue and called *venous* or *efferent*. The terms 'arterial' and 'venous' derive from early haemofilters, which relied on arterial cannulation; however, with the pumped systems invariably now used all blood is venous.

Haemofilter pore size varies, but many have a similar pore size to human gomeruli – 65–70 kiloDaltons (kDa). Hollow-fibre haemofilters are usually used; these usually contain more than 20,000 fine capillary tubes, creating a large surface area for filtration while using small blood volumes.

Priming volumes are usually one litre (± heparin), to remove air emboli and potentially toxic chemicals used to protect filters during storage and transportation. Users should check local protocols and manufacturers' recommendations for priming. Heparin prime reduces initial platelet aggregation, enabling lower dose of subsequent anticoagulants, although some filters are manufactured to be primed without heparin.

Some units use *predilution* to reduce viscosity within filters, so reducing need for anticoagulants and prolonging filter life (Oudemans-van Straaten *et al.*, 2006; ICS, 2009b).

Anticoagulation helps reduce thrombus formation within filters, so prolonging their life. Thrombus formation is increased by slow blood flow. Signs of thrombus formation include:

- dark blood in circuits;
- kicking of lines;
- high *transmembrane pressure*.

Anticoagulation may be unnecessary with some filters or prolonged clotting. Anticoagulants are below filter threshold, but some inevitably reach patients, aggravating coagulopathies; reversal agents (e.g. protamine) can be added after the filter. The ICS (2009b) suggests avoiding anticoagulation with any of the following:

- INR > 2–2.5;
- APTT > 60 seconds;
- thrombocytopaenia (e.g. platelet count < 60×10^9/litre);
- high risk of bleeding;
- activated protein C.

Clotting times should be checked at least daily.

Heparin remains the most widely used anticoagulant, but *prostacyclin* (epoprostenol; prostaglandin I_2 – PGI_2) and citrate are also used. Prostacyclin inhibits platelet, and causes vasodilatation. Although much prostacyclin is removed by the filter, systemic vasodilatation does occur (Kanagasundaram, 2007). Prostacyclin is more expensive than heparin, so tends to be used if coagulopathies from heparin become problematic.

Citrate chelates calcium, a chemical used for clotting. Infusing citrate before the filter, together with calcium after the filter to maintain systemic levels of calcium, provides better anticoagulation than heparin (Monchi *et al.*, 2004), with less risk of bleeding (Palsson and Niles, 1999) and can prolong filter life (Monchi *et al.*, 2004). However, citrate infusion can cause:

■ metabolic alkalosis (citrate yields bicarbonate (Oudemans-van Straaten *et al.*, 2006));
■ metabolic acidosis (citrate is converted to citric acid) (Oudemans-van Straaten *et al.*, 2006);
■ hypernatraemia;
■ hypomagnesaemia.

It also relies on adequate hepatic function (Oudemans-van Straaten *et al.*, 2006). Few UK units use citrate, as it is complicated to use (Kanagasundaram, 2007), prevents use of standard bicarbonate or lactate bags, and exposes patients to the risks above (Sharman *et al.*, 2010). Units that use it often justify costs by prolonged filter life, but if this exceeds manufacturers' recommendations then users may become legally liable for any harm caused.

Extracorporeal circulation causes convention of heat, so may cause *hypothermia*, especially if circuits hold relatively large volumes of blood. Most manufacturers produce blood warmers for circuits.

Afferent pump speed should be commenced slowly (e.g. 100 ml/minute) as some patients develop acute hypotensive crises. If stable, speeds should usually be increased within 10 minutes, usually to the full target/prescribed speed, although readers should check local protocols.

Monitoring

Filtration relies on blood flow through filters and pressure gradients across the semipermeable membrane. While blood flow (blood pump) is adjustable, *pressure gradients* are created by settings for the blood pump, fluid removal, and resistance across the filter (transmembrane pressure – see page 394).

Blood flow is created by the blood pump speed. Because this draws blood into the circuit, it creates a negative pressure. If inadequate blood can be obtained from the cannulae, an alarm will sound. Likely reasons for blood pump alarms are:

■ occluded flow from patient position, especially with femoral cannulae;
■ afferent lumen against vessel wall;
■ thrombus in the catheter or at the tip.

So troubleshooting solutions include:

- position – change;
- lumen against vessel wall – swap afferent and efferent connections to catheter;
- thrombus – try aspirating, but this is unlikely to succeed; flushing is not recommended, as this may create an embolus; although the catheter may be saved with urokinase, by the time this works the haemofilter will probably clot.

Ultrafiltrate rate is regulated by the ultrafiltrate pump speed setting. Most units run ultrafiltrate at 20 ml/kg/hour, as faster speeds provide no benefit (VA/NIH Acute Kidney Injury Trial Network, 2008). Faster speeds remove more pro-inflammatory mediators; intermittent haemofiltration using 35 ml/kg/hour exchanges has been used to treat sepsis. The ICS (2009b) recommends using minimum exchanges of 35 ml/kg/hour. However, high-flow exchanges:

- increase costs (each treatment cycle necessitates a new circuit);
- increase workload;
- expose hypotensive patients to potentially greater haemodynamic instability.
  (Renal Replacement Therapy Investigators, 2009)

While overall mortality rates are similar, continuous modes provide better renal recovery than intermittent treatment (Bell *et al.*, 2007; VA/NIH Acute Kidney Injury Trial Network, 2008; Palevsky, 2009), so intermittent treatments are not recommended.

Transmembrane pressure (TMP – the pressure across the membrane inside the filter) gradients are created by:

- driving pressure
- resistance
- *oncotic*/osmotic pressure.

Maximum TMP should not exceed 100 mmHg. Rising pressure usually suggests significantly decreased filtration surface area from thrombus formation, and is usually an indication to discontinue filtration. High TMP can rupture ('blow', 'burst kidney') the filter, necessitating immediate cessation of filtration. Haemofilter rupture typically causes a sudden massive drop in TMP, blood may be seen in the filtrate, and usually machines will alarm and stop. If a filter ruptures no attempt should be made to return blood ('washback'), as fragments of membrane may be washed back with blood. Many machines also measure pressure drop.

Efficacy of haemofiltration is usually measured through daily bloods, such as serum creatinine levels If circuits fail to achieve aims (removal of volume and/or solutes), they are consuming nursing time and exposing patients to risks needlessly. Effectiveness should therefore be monitored through biochemistry.

Manufacturers' warranties usually limit circuit life to 72 hours; circuits primed but not used immediately should usually be changed before this time. Although circuits have been used for longer, they are major sources of infection, the majority of filters containing biofilm (Moore *et al.*, 2009). Exceeding manufacturers' warranties exposes nurses to risks of litigation.

Troubleshooting

While circuit volume is usually relatively small (often < 100 ml), nearly one-fifth of patients develop initial, usually transient, hypotension when commencing haemofiltration (Uchino *et al.*, 2007). Dysrhythmias can also occur (Uchino *et al.*, 2007). Likely causes include:

- hypovolaemia (bleeding on to circuit; crystalloid bolus replacing blood);
- prostacyclin infusion (vasodilates);
- cytokine release (as blood reacts with artificial circuit).

Although filters are biocompatible, to minimise cytokine release, biocompatibility is relative rather than absolute. If hypotension is problematic, most units give colloid, or if CVP remains adequate, increase inotropes.

Lactate-based dialysate reduces *metabolic acidosis* (Cole *et al.*, 2003), but relies on adequate hepatic function to convert lactate to bicarbonate (Kanagasundaram, 2007), so bicarbonate is the preferred buffer for haemofiltration (Davenport and Stevens, 2008). Provided liver function is adequate, the only undesirable effect of lactate is hyperglycaemia (Bollman *et al.*, 2004).

Drug clearance by haemofiltration is complex, requiring advice from unit pharmacists. Increased clearance may result in under-dosing, so whenever possible drugs should be titrated to desired effects. Any substance below filter pore size may be filtered; this invariably includes all electrolytes and micro-nutrients (e.g. magnesium, phosphate). It also includes gelatins (e.g. Gelofusine®); starch-based colloids are unlikely to be filtered.

Haemofiltration limits mobility, so pressure areas should be checked carefully.

Many, but not all, patients being haemofiltred are oliguric/anuric. In addition to the underlying kidney injury that is often the cause of filtration being needed, removal of fluid is likely to stimulate anti-diuretic hormone in an attempt to conserve body water. If urine is minimal or absent, it is usually wise to remove urinary catheters to reduce infection risks.

Haemofiltration machines are designed to be safe. They monitor many aspects of filtration, and have many alarms, many of which stop circuits. Problems should be resolved urgently, and if the circuit has been stopped, it should be restarted as soon as it is safe to do so, before the circuit clots.

Outcome

Haemofiltration in ICUs is largely used as a means for normalising blood chemistry while underlying diseases, such as sepsis, are resolved. Duration of haemofiltration is therefore usually limited to a few days. However, the risk of needing chronic dialysis is increased (Wald *et al.*, 2009), and hospital mortality exceeds 60 per cent (Uchino *et al.*, 2007). So, if intrarenal pathologies are suspected, ultrasound will usually be requested, and renal physicians involved.

Implications for practice

- Haemofilters resemble human nephrons, so although machines can appear daunting, follow through circuits comparing them with nephron function.
- When checking circuits, start from the beginning of the afferent line and work through the circuit until the end of the efferent line.
- Check the circuit and equipment at the start of each shift and whenever necessary.
- Large fluid balance errors can quickly accumulate; fluid balance should be kept as simple as possible; recheck calculations and running totals.
- 20 ml/kg/hour is probably the minimal optimal rate; some guidelines recommend 35 ml/kg/hour, although weight of evidence is increasingly shifting against this.
- Hypotension can occur quickly, especially when commencing filtration, so haemodynamic status should be closely monitored, and blood pumps commenced at 100 ml/hour.
- Most alarms halt circuits; identify and resolve problems urgently, restarting the system before coagulation blocks the filter.
- Small substances, including electrolytes and trace elements, are removed through haemofilters, so blood levels should be checked at least daily – especially sodium, potassium, magnesium, phosphate, bicarbonate and pH (many of these are measured with ABGs).
- Involve unit pharmacists to identify how therapeutic drugs are affected by filtration.
- Nurses who have not used haemofiltration equipment should take every opportunity to learn how to manage it before caring for patients being haemofiltered.
- If patients are anuric, urinary catheters should be removed.

Summary

Renal replacement in most ICUs is provided by haemofiltration/haemodiafiltration, although hospitals with renal units may use haemodialysis. Haemofiltration has proved to be a valuable medical adjunct to intensive care. While technology has made circuits and machines safer, haemofiltration is highly invasive, exposing patients to various complications and dangers. Kidney injury in ICU patients is usually secondary, so caring for patients receiving haemofiltration can create high nursing workloads. Care should be prioritised to ensure a safe environment. Nurses unfamiliar with using haemofiltration are encouraged to find out how to use it in practice before having to care on their own for patients receiving haemofiltration.

Further reading

Much relevant literature appears in renal journals, but the ICS (2009b) provides comprehensive guidelines. Medical reviews include Kanagasundaram (2007). Staff should familiarise themselves with handbooks for equipment used on their units. Most ICUs have local guidelines/protocols.

Clinical scenario

James Roger is 67 years old and developed acute kidney injury (AKI) from sepsis secondary to endocarditis. Mr Roger had received high-dose intravenous antibiotics, including gentamicin, vancomycin, rifampicin and cefotaxime, and had been taking oral warfarin prior to admission.

He was commenced on continuous venovenous haemofiltration (CVVH) with 3-litre fluid exchanges. The pump speed was recording 220–250 ml/minute; venous pressure was 97 mmHg and transmembrane pressures 60–70 mmHg. Mr Roger had deranged clotting, and infusions of heparin at 2500 iu/hour and epoprostenol (Flolan®) at 5 ng/hour are in progress.

Q.1 Reflect on the CVVH values and anticoagulation regime. Analyse how these drugs may affect Mr Roger's coagulation while on CVVH.

Q.2 The CVVH venous pressures increase over a three-hour period to 250 mmHg with transmembrane pressures of 150 mmHg. Analyse this change and review actions you would take.

Q.3 Appraise nursing interventions that help maintain effectiveness and patency of CVVH.

    (a) Explain the nurse's role in monitoring, troubleshooting and maintaining patency of filter and patient safety with circuit (e.g. blood flows, leaks, air, fluid and electrolyte management, patient position).

    (b) Justify other nursing approaches aimed at promoting renal recovery (e.g. drugs, temperature management, nutrition, psychological support, infection control, weaning CVVH, etc.).

    (c) Review approaches used for the disposal of ultrafiltrate, manual handling issues, filter changes, workload and resources, and nursing skills development.

The same patient is used in the clinical scenario for Chapter 38.

Chapter 40

Gastrointestinal bleeds

Contents

Fundamental knowledge	398
Introduction	399
Peptic ulcers	399
Helicobacter pylori	399
Stress ulceration	399
Variceal bleeding	400
Medical treatments	400
Nursing care	402
Lower GI bleeds	402
Implications for practice	403
Summary	403
Further reading	403
Clinical scenario	403

Fundamental knowledge

Gastrointestinal anatomy
Portal pressure

Introduction

Gut failure is increasingly recognised as a problem in critically ill patients. Being highly vascular, the gastrointestinal (GI) tract is prone to bleeding. Risk factors include:

- stress responses increasing gastric acid secretion;
- impaired gut perfusion;
- inflammatory responses impairing vascular endothelium function, which releases most extrinsic clotting factors;
- lack of enteral feeding;
- anticoagulation therapy, especially with thrombolytic therapy for acute coronary syndrome or pulmonary embolism;
- impaired liver function – intrinsic clotting factors are produced by the liver; alcoholic liver disease poses an especially high risk.

There are many other factors – for example, patients with arthritis are often prescribed non-steroidal anti-inflammatory drugs (NSAIDs), which impair clotting. Major haemorrhage may cause or complicate admission. While clotting is usually measured daily in most patients, and patients' histories may suggest risk factors, visible signs of ulceration are only likely to be seen once bleeding occurs. While the focus of critical care is usually on other major systems, gut function and integrity should be assessed, any signs of bruising noted, and all critically ill patients should be considered at risk.

Peptic ulcers

Although most upper GI bleeds are from peptic ulcers (Kokozides, 2006), these seldom necessitate ICU admission. Gastric mucosa maintains wide pH differences between gastric acid (or alkaline bile) and epithelium. While most ulcers stop bleeding spontaneously (Sung, 2010), a few necessitate endoscopic treatment, which may take place on the ICU.

Helicobacter pylori

Most duodenal ulcers in people not taking NSAIDs are caused by the bacterium *Helicobacter pylori* (Malfertheiner *et al.*, 2009). About half of adults are colonised by *H. pylori* (Fuccio *et al.*, 2008), colonisation usually beginning in childhood (McColl, 2010). To produce the alkaline environment they need to survive, *H. pylori* produce carbon dioxide; many tests for *H. pylori* measure gastric carbon dioxide. Ulcers usually heal quickly following eradication of *H. pylori* (Harris and Misiewicz, 2001), but treatment is prolonged, so is not usually commenced in the ICU.

Stress ulceration

Stress ulceration in critically ill patients rarely causes major bleeds (Ojiako *et al.*, 2008), although most (75–100 per cent) have endoscopically visible lesions within 24 hours of ICU admission (Spirt and Stanley, 2006). The ventilation care bundle includes stress ulcer prophylaxis (Marik, 2010). The most widely used groups of drugs used in ICUs to prevent ulceration are:

- H$_2$-blockers (e.g. ranitidine, cimetidine) (Quenot *et al.*, 2009);
- (increasingly) protein pump inhibitors (e.g. omeprazole, lansoprazole, esomeprazole) (Ojiako *et al.*, 2008).

Sucralfate used to be widely used. Quenot *et al.* (2009) suggest evidence for benefits of any particular drugs, or stress ulcer prophylaxis generally, is weak. H$_2$-blocker doses differ with oral and intravenous routes, and are usually reduced with renal impairment. Sucralfate, which is given enterally, can reduce absorption of other enteral drugs (Quenot *et al.*, 2009).

Variceal bleeding

One-tenth of upper GI bleeds are from varices (Park *et al.*, 2008). Varices are collateral vessels, typically surrounding the lower oesophagus and sometimes upper parts of the stomach, occurring when cirrhosis causes portal hypertension (Bosch and Abraldes, 2005; Toubia and Sanyal, 2008). Rupture causes massive haemorrhage, often fatal (Park *et al.*, 2008).

Urgent treatment should:

- stop haemorrhage;
- restore blood volume and haematocrit (fluid resuscitation);
- replace clotting factors.

Haemorrhage is usually stopped by endoscopy (banding and/or injection), but emergency stabilisation may also be achieved with *balloon tamponade*. Surgical intervention is occasionally needed. Once haemorrhage is stopped, anti-hypertensives will usually be needed.

Medical treatments

Endoscopy is the treatment of choice (Cappell and Friedel, 2008; Sung, 2010). Endoscopy therapies include:

- banding
- thermoregulation
- injection (sclerotherapy).

Injection alone is not recommended (Barkun *et al.*, 2010) as re-bleeds can occur (Park *et al.*, 2008), but it is a useful optional adjunct to banding or thermoregulation.

Vasopressin (antidiuretic hormone) and derivatives (desmopressin, terlipressin) cause splanchnic arterial vasoconstriction, so reducing portal hypertension.

Balloon tamponade (see Figure 40.1) is a 'first aid' intervention to stop bleeding, by placing direct pressure on varices. Tubes are often incorrectly called 'Sengstaken tubes'; Sengstaken tubes have only three lumens, and have virtually been replaced by the four-lumen 'Minnesota':

- oesophageal balloon (to stop bleeding);
- oesophageal aspiration port (omitted on three-port Sengstaken tubes);
- gastric balloon (to anchor tubes);
- gastric aspiration port.

Balloon tamponade controls most bleeds, but half re-bleed on balloon deflation (Therapondos and Hayes, 2002). Rigid tubes are easier to insert (Smith, 2000), so tubes should be stored in a fridge.

Oesophageal balloons should only be inflated if bleeding persists after inflation of the gastric balloon (Stanley and Hayes, 1997). Pressure should be sufficient to control haemorrhage; recommended pressures vary, up to 50–60 mmHg (Sung, 2009). External traction, which can further compress varices with the gastric balloon (Steele and Sabol, 2005), is controversial, as gastric varices, already compressed by the gastric balloon, should prevent flow to higher varices. If weights are used, lifting them should be avoided as this may dislodge clots. Periodic balloon deflation (e.g. for 30 minutes every 4–6 hours (Therapondos and Hayes, 2002)) is also controversial, as it reduces risk of ulceration, but may cause re-bleeding. Balloon tamponade should be limited to 12–24 hours.

Beta-blockers (e.g. propanolol) reduce cardiac output, and constrict mesenteric arteries, so reducing portal pressure. Beta-blockade or endoscopy are first-line treatments (Toubia and Sanyal, 2008). Beta-blockers or other anti-hypertensives also reduce risks of re-bleeding (Park *et al.*, 2008).

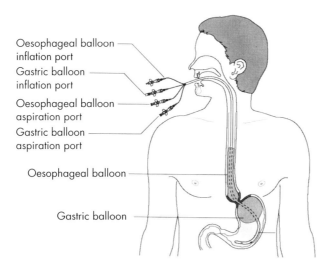

Oesophageal balloon inflation port
Gastric balloon inflation port
Oesophageal balloon aspiration port
Gastric balloon aspiration port
Oesophageal balloon
Gastric balloon

Figure 40.1 Tamponade ('Minnesota') tube

Transjugular intrahepatic portosystemic shunt (TIPSS) reduces portal hypertension (Toubia and Sanyal, 2008). A percutaneous angioplasty-type catheter creates a fistula between the portal and hepatic veins, which is then kept open with expandable metal stents (usually 8–12 mm diameter) (Therapondos and Hayes, 2002). Shunted blood bypasses the liver without being detoxified, so may cause encephalopathy (Smith, 2000).

Gastric irrigation to remove blood may also prolong or restart haemorrhage. Cold water may also cause vagal stimulation, increasing gastric motility and irritation to ulcers.

Surgical oesophageal transection or implantation of portocaval shunts effectively controls bleeding, but without improvement in long-term survival (Sung, 2009).

Nursing care

While nursing care largely follows from medical interventions, and many specific aspects to these interventions are included above, as with any emergency, ABCDE assessment facilitates prompt and appropriate care:

- A (airway) – is the airway patent? If not protected by an endotracheal tube or tracheostomy, patients may need to be placed in the recovery position until intubated; if a Ryles or balloon tamponade tube is in place, gastric aspiration can be performed. Is cuff pressure sufficient to prevent aspiration?
- B (breathing) – has the patient aspirated? If so, ventilator support may need increasing.
- C (circulation) – monitor vital signs, especially heart rate, blood pressure and CVP. Is Hb satisfactory?
- D (disability) – if neurological state is acutely altered, reasons for this should be assessed. With vascular disease, possibility of strokes should be considered.
- E (exposure) – seeing blood or blood-stains can distress patients and/or relatives, so if reasonably possible soiled bedding should be quickly replaced, and relatives warned of the possibility of seeing blood.

Lower GI bleeds

One-fifth of gastrointestinal bleeds are from the lower tract (Fearnhead, 2007), but these are rarely acutely life-threatening. Most stop spontaneously, seldom necessitating ICU admission. But many ICU patients have coagulopathies, so may bleed from the highly vascular lower GI tract.

Stools should be observed for frank blood; occult bleeding can be confirmed by testing. Observations should be recorded and reported; samples may be required for testing. Bleeding may be fresh (red; usually lower GI bleeds) or old (black, tarry; usually upper GI bleeds).

Most bleeds are small, but if large bleeds do not resolve spontaneously, early surgery (e.g. hemicolectomy) may be needed.

Implications for practice

- The gut is highly vascular, so is prone to bleeding.
- All critically ill patients are at risk of gut dysfunction, and many have legions visible on endoscopy.
- Upper GI haemorrhage can be massive and life-threatening, requiring urgent fluid resuscitation and close haemodynamic monitoring.
- With major bleeds, follow ABCDE assessment; fluid resuscitation forms a major aspect of management.
- Endoscopy is the preferred treatment for major upper GI bleeds.
- Balloon tamponade quickly stops bleeding from oesophageal varices, but is only a temporary measure, and removal often restarts bleeding.
- Lower gut bleeds are more often insidious, and can increase morbidity, but are seldom life-threatening; the first sign of lower gut bleeds may be frank blood in stools, or melaena (black, tarry stools).
- Stress ulcer prophylaxis is part of ventilator care bundles, although evidence for routine prophylaxis has been questioned.
- Seeing blood can make patients and families especially anxious; psychological support/care can help them cope and warn them about possibly seeing/smelling blood; if possible, remove soiled linen.
- Signs of significant bleeding should be recorded and reported.

Summary

Many factors can contribute to coagulopathies and bleeds in critical illness, but major haemorrhage may also cause ICU admission. Immediately life-threatening situations necessitate urgent resuscitation, but predisposing factors may be prevented by nursing assessment and observation of risks – for example, ensuring that all patients receive stress ulcer prophylaxis (unless contraindicated). While lower gut bleeds are not usually life-threatening, they may be detected by melaena.

Further reading

Barkun *et al.* (2010) is the international consensus for non-variceal bleeding. Sung (2010) and Malfertheiner *et al.* (2009) provide recent medical reviews.

Clinical scenario

Victor Newton is a 51-year-old known alcoholic who was admitted to the ICU via A&E with a three-week history of melaena, recent large-volume haematemesis that morning and severe epigastric pain. He had previous episodes of melaena and haematemesis over the Christmas holiday season and was awaiting an outpatient endoscopy appointment.

Q.1 List the nursing priorities when preparing for and admitting a patient with an emergency GI bleed. Include resources needed such as equipment, drugs, investigations, specialists.

An emergency endoscopy is performed which confirms three bleeding oesophageal varices that were banded. Mr Newton then re-bled. A balloon tamponade tube was inserted to exert direct pressure on the ruptured and bleeding vessels. His current medications include intravenous infusion of omeprazole at 8 mg/hour and oral sucralfate (antepsin®) suspension of 2 grams every six hours.

Q.2 Analyse nursing interventions following balloon tamponade tube insertion that monitor effect and minimise potential complications (e.g. checking tube placement, type of traction methods, free drainage or not, sputum clearance, saliva removal, aspiration pneumonia, tissue pressure necrosis, melaena, metabolic effects of blood in lower GI tract).

Q.3 It is decided to remove the balloon tamponade tube at 24 hours. Consider how this process should be managed to minimise the risk of re-bleeding.

Q.4 Mr Newton's experience of haematemesis and emergency intervention have made him very anxious. Review possible causes of his ruptured varices and the risk of reoccurrence. Specify the liver function investigations he may undergo.

Q.5 Design a plan of care for Mr Newton that focuses on reducing his anxiety and the risk of re-bleeding in the ICU, following transfer to the ward and after discharge from hospital care.

Advice should include the reasons for and practical strategies regarding:

- avoiding vigorous coughing and sneezing;
- recognition of early signs and symptoms of re-bleeding;
- relaxation techniques;
- drug action affected by his condition and hepatic impairment (e.g. benzodiazepines, aspirin, paracetamol, some antibiotics, alcohol, cigarettes/nicotine);
- lifestyle changes;
- use of specialist nurses or referral groups.

Chapter 41

Liver failure

Contents

Fundamental knowledge	405
Introduction	406
Acute failure	406
Chronic failure	407
Liver function tests	408
Decompensation	409
Intra-abdominal pressure	411
Artificial livers	412
Prognosis	412
Implications for practice	412
Summary	413
Further reading	413
Clinical scenario	413

Fundamental knowledge

Hepatic anatomy and physiology
Kupffer cell function

Introduction

The liver has more, and more diverse, functions than any other major organ, including:

■ nutrition (synthesis of plasma proteins, glucogenesis);
■ immunity;
■ heat production;
■ synthesis of homeostatic controls (most intrinsic clotting factors, angiotensin 1);
■ detoxification (ammonia, drugs).

Thus, hepatic failure affects most other major systems. However, symptoms of liver dysfunction are less immediately apparent than respiratory, cardiac or renal dysfunction, and usually occur with co-morbidities from other systems. Except in specialist liver centres, liver failure or poor function more often complicates than causes ICU admission.

Liver failure may be acute or chronic, and compensated or decompensated. ICU treatment (whatever the permutation) largely focuses on supporting failing systems, and preventing complications. Like most systems, compensation for liver failure can maintain apparent health for a considerable time. But because it has so many functions, once decompensated liver failure develops, many other systems are likely to be compromised. This chapter describes pathophysiologies, major complications and treatments, focusing on acute failure. Main liver function tests are identified, but because liver function is so diverse, no single test exists to identify liver failure. Severe hepatic failure may necessitate referral to specialist centres.

Acute failure

The term *fulminant hepatic failure* (extensive hepatocyte necrosis together with encephalopathy occurring within eight weeks of onset) has largely been replaced by:

■ *hyperacute*: jaundice occurs < 7 days before encephalopathy;
■ *acute*: jaundice occurs 8–28 days before encephalopathy;
■ *subacute*: jaundice occurs 4–12 weeks before encephalopathy.

The main complications of acute liver failure are:

■ hepatocellular dysfunction (failure to detoxify drugs and hormones – e.g. aldosterone causes sodium retention and potassium loss);
■ disruption of blood flow through the liver (portal hypertension, contributing to *ascites* and GI bleeds – see Chapter 40);
■ cerebral oedema.

(McKinley, 2009)

Overwhelming failure is usually fatal, unless liver transplantation can be performed (Fontana, 2008; McConnell and Cressey, 2008; Bernal *et al.*, 2010). Death from acute liver failure is usually caused by cerebral oedema, sepsis and multiple organ failure (McConnell and Cressey, 2008). Until transfer, priorities are:

- cardiovascular (optimal filling, then inotropes);
- coagulopathy (give clotting factors);
- neurological (treat cerebral oedema, treat pyrexia);
- sepsis;
- kidney injury;
- respiratory/airway management;
- nutrition.

(McConnell and Cressey, 2008)

Acute hepatic failure may be caused by:

- paracetamol (see Chapter 46)
- other drugs
- chemicals
- viruses
- unknown causes.

In addition to system support, for paracetamol overdose acetylcysteine (Parvolex®) (Bateman, 2007) should be prescribed.

In the UK, unlike most other countries, paracetamol overdose remains the main cause of liver failure (Bateman, 2007). Many other therapeutic drugs (e.g. isoniazid and other anti-TB drugs, chlorpromazine) can also provoke failure (Rashid *et al.*, 2004).

Chronic failure

Chronic liver disease is usually caused by:

- alcohol;
- non-alcoholic steatohepatitis (NASH);
- hepatitis B or C (HBV, HCV);
- primary hepatocellular carcinoma.

However, it can develop from acute failure, and sometimes causes are unknown. Chlordiazepoxide is useful for alcohol withdrawal.

Alcohol remains the main chemical cause of chronic liver failure; UK alcohol-related mortality is increasing (Forrest, 2009), with significant increases in ICU admissions for alcoholic liver disease (O'Brien *et al.*, 2007; Welch *et al.*, 2008). Liver failure can (rarely) be caused by industrial solvents, such as carbon tetrachloride (CCl_4, widely used, including for dry cleaning) and mushroom poisoning (usually *Amanita phalloides* – 'death cap'); NASH usually occurs with obesity and insulin resistance (Lucey *et al.*, 2009). Hepatitis can be caused by many viruses, although in the UK the main viral causes are HBV and increasingly HCV. In the developing world, liver failure is usually viral (Bernal *et al.*, 2010).

Chronic failure may cause:

- hyperdynamic circulation;
- portal hypertension;
- oesophageal varices and bleeding.

While some of these problems may necessitate ICU admission, acute failure and hypofunction more often complicate other diseases in ICUs, so this chapter focuses on acute rather than chronic aspects.

Liver function tests

The liver metabolises toxins in blood, so with liver failure levels of many solutes increase. The most useful indicators of liver function are usually:

- clotting (especially INR)
- bilirubin
- albumin; total protein
- transaminases.

(See Table 41.1.)

With severe acute failure, *INR* rises rapidly, potentially exceeding 10. Clotting is discussed in Chapter 21.

Bilirubin, a waste product of erythrocyte metabolism, is normally metabolised by the liver into bile. If flow through the liver is obstructed, for example by cirrhosis, then bilirubin metabolism will not occur, causing bilirubinaemia. Serum bilirubin above 50 micromols causes jaundice. Critical illness may cause obstruction through inflammation.

Table 41.1 Main liver function tests

Liver function tests	Normal range
Bilirubin (Bil)	1–20 μmol/litre
Alkaline phosphatase (Alk phos/ALP)	< 100 iu/litre
Aspartate aminotransferase (AST)	< 40 iu/litre
Alanine aminotransferase (ALT)	< 40 iu/litre
Gamma glutamyl transpeptidase (GGT)	10–48 iu/litre
Albumin	30–52 g/litre
Total protein (TP)	60–80 g/litre

The liver metabolises dietary *proteins* into plasma proteins, so liver hypo-function contributes to low plasma protein levels. Albumin forms more than half of plasma proteins, so is used as a marker of illness/recovery. However, other factors contribute to low albumin/plasma protein levels in critical illness (see Chapter 21), and with a half-life of nearly three weeks, albumin levels are unlikely to significantly rise until many days after recovery begins.

Transaminases are intracellular enzymes and chemicals released by hepatocyte damage, just as myocyte damage is detectable by the biomarker troponin. The main transaminases are:

- alkaline phosphatase (alk phos/ALP);
- aspartate aminotransferase (AST);
- alanine aminotransferase (ALT);
- gamma glutamyl transpeptidase (GGT).

Unfortunately, transaminases are not liver-specific, although ALT is slightly more specific than AST (Agarwai and Cottam, 2009). Alkaline phosphatase is found in bone, so leeches with bedrest, making ICU patients prone to raised levels. Although indicating necrosis, levels do not correlate with extent of damage, so cannot be used to predict outcome.

As the liver detoxifies ammonia into urea, urea levels are also raised.

Decompensation

Progressive liver failure causes failure of homeostasis, especially:

- encephalopathy
- gross ascites
- hypotension
- haemorrhage (especially gastrointestinal – see Chapter 40).

Increased permeability of the blood–brain barrier, together with failure of liver metabolism, exposes the brain to excessive amounts of ammonia and other toxins, causing hepatic *encephalopathy*. Cerebral irritation from oedema may cause fitting, which may be subclinical. The normal sleeping pattern may be reversed, patients remaining awake overnight. Increased muscle tone may cause decerebrate postures (Hawker, 2003). Encephalopathy reduces patients' ability to understand, often making them more agitated and distressing relatives.

Cerebral oedema may be prevented by keeping the head aligned (to facilitate venous drainage), treating underlying infections, and reducing gut bacterial production of ammonia with lactulose or neomycin, aiming for two to four soft stools each day (Saggs, 2000). It can be reversed with mannitol, an osmotic diuretic. Psychological care should include:

- frequent, simple explanations;
- calm, low voice;

- avoiding/minimising conflict;
- supporting relatives.

Specialist units may use intracranial pressure monitoring (see Chapter 23) to guide management, but this is not often available in general ICUs. Jugular venous saturation monitoring may be a useful alternative.

Ascites compresses the liver, lungs and other major organs, as well as contributing to hypovolaemia, If large, it is usually drained through ascitic tap or paracentesis. Ascites is albumin-rich, so aggressive fluid replacement, usually including albumin, is needed, to both restore plasma volume and create an osmotic pull from remaining ascites into the bloodstream. Intra-abdominal pressure measurement (see page 411) is useful to prevent liver damage from mechanical compression.

Cardiac output increases, but hypovolaemia causes *hypotension*, mainly due to:

- vasodilatation and increased capillary permeability (inflammatory responses);
- hypoalbuminaemia;
- bleeding (most intrinsic clotting factors are produced in the liver).

Angiotensinogen, the precursor of angiotensin (see Chapter 31), is produced in the liver, so hepatic failure causes failure of the renin-angiotensin-aldosterone mechanism, contributing to vasodilatation.

Prolonged hypotension results in tissue hypoxia, anaerobic metabolism, widespread cell dysfunction and death, and eventually multi-organ dysfunction. Hypotension should therefore be treated with aggressive fluid resuscitation. Relatively prolonged effects from liver dysfunction and increased capillary permeability make colloids preferable to crystalloids.

The liver synthesises most clotting factors, so bleeding may be an early symptom of acute hepatic failure. Activated clotting factors are not broken down, so disseminated intravascular coagulation (DIC – see Chapter 26) may occur (Krumberger, 2002). Gastrointestinal and respiratory, although not cerebral, *bleeds* frequently occur (Hawker, 2003). ICU nurses should therefore minimise trauma and observe for bleeding during endotracheal suction or from nasogastric tubes. Oozing around cannulae, or healing of sites after removal, may also cause problems. Cannulae, especially arterial, should remain visible whenever possible.

The liver contributes significantly to immunity through:

- producing complements;
- Kupffer cells – phagocytotic cells in the liver that destroy bacteria from the gut.

Liver dysfunction therefore causes *immunocompromise*. Most patients with liver failure develop infection (Fontana, 2008), often progressing to sepsis (O'Brien *et al.*, 2007; Forrest, 2009).

Acute kidney injury (AKI) usually occurs with acute liver failure (McKinnell and Holt, 2007), often from hypotension, so should be prevented by optimising perfusion with fluid management.

The liver has over 500 metabolic functions, so hepatic failure causes complex disorders. Many *electrolyte* abnormalities occur, including *hypokalaemia* and *hypocalcaemia* from *hyperaldosteronism* (Saggs, 2000). Magnesium and phosphate deficiencies also frequently occur.

Metabolic acidosis occurs in any tissue relying on hypoxic metabolism; but the liver is the main organ that metabolises lactate, so lactate accumulation with hepatic failure inevitably results in metabolic acidosis. Concurrent kidney injury aggravates acidosis. Acidosis being negatively inotropic, cardiac output is reduced.

Hypoglycaemia frequently occurs (Rylah and Vercueil, 2010) due to depleted glycogen stored in the liver and elevated circulating insulin levels. Blood sugar levels should therefore be frequently monitored (2–3 hourly), with glucose supplements being given accordingly. Crystalloid fluids should be glucose-based, to both avoid sodium (ascites) and provide glucose, although glucose solutions should be avoided if encephalopathy is present.

Jaundice occurs once serum bilirubin reaches 40 mmol/litre (Saggs, 2000). It is both a symptom and a problem, often causing *pruritis*. Skincare and dressings should be selected to minimise irritation. If pruritis occurs, drugs such as antihistamines may be useful.

Intra-abdominal pressure

Pressure in the abdomen affects perfusion and function of abdominal and other organs, including lungs, liver, kidneys and gut. Normal intra-abdominal pressure (IAP) is 5–7 mmHg, rising in obese people to 9–14 (de Keulenaer *et al.*, 2009). Increasing positive ventilator pressures increases IAP (Ashraf *et al.*, 2008). Pressure below 15 mmHg seldom causes problems. *Abdominal compartment syndrome* is IAP ≥ 20 mmHg with an organ failure that was not previously present. This significantly increases risk of organ failure (Malbrain *et al.*, 2005; de Laet and Malbrain, 2007). As tissue perfusion determines whether organ damage occurs, abdominal perfusion pressure may be defined as mean arterial pressure (MAP) minus IAP (Cheatham *et al.*, 2007); pressures below 60 mmHg place organs at risk. Typically caused by fractures, especially of a leg or forearm (Mar *et al.*, 2009), abdominal compartment syndrome has high mortality (> 2/3) (Brush, 2007).

If intra-abdominal hypertension is identified, the following (depending on the cause) can preserve organ function:

- early decompressive laparotomy (possibly with 'open abdomen' – covered only by a dressing, but without the incision being closed, to allow relief of pressure);
- paracentesis;
- reducing ventilator pressure;

- maintaining negative fluid balance;
- flatus tube;
- intravascular volume resuscitation.

Various devices are marketed to measure intra-abdominal pressure, but bladder devices, usually as part of urinary catheter systems, are used most (de Keulenaer *et al.*, 2009). Ideally, measurement should be taken supine – angles of 30° increase IAP by 4 mmHg, while 45° increases IAP by 9 mmHg (de Keulenaer *et al.*, 2009), although Shuster *et al.* (2010) recommend measuring at 30°. IAP should be measured at the end of expiration (de Laet and Malbrain, 2007). PEEP may increase IAP (de Keulenaer *et al.*, 2009).

Artificial livers

Various 'artificial livers' have been developed, ranging from extracorporeal circulation through cadaver and animal livers to semi- and fully synthetic machines, but they are still essentially experimental (Murphy, 2006). Technological improvements, such as the Molecular Adsorbent Recirculating System (MARS), enable people with endstage chronic liver to survive until transplantation (Rylah and Vercueil, 2010), although they are probably not beneficial in centres unable to perform transplantation. Technology will doubtless further improve, perhaps to permanently implantable devices.

Prognosis

When liver failure necessitates ICU admission, there are often life-threatening co-morbidities as well as life-threatening complications. Outcome is therefore often poor, although not hopeless. Intensive Care National Audit and Research Centre (ICNARC) data from 2008 (Welch *et al.*) suggests two-thirds of patients admitted to ICU with acute liver failure will not survive.

Implications for practice

- Most ICU patients suffer hepatic dysfunction, usually due to hypoperfusion; nurses should actively assess liver function (e.g. clotting, consciousness), documenting their observations.
- Assess neurological state. Deterioration may indicate encephalopathy.
- Maintain head in alignment and at 15–30° to facilitate venous drainage.
- Gross ascites should be drained.
- Intravenous volume should be aggressively restored, especially with colloids.
- If clotting is prolonged, reassess traumatic aspects of nursing care (e.g. shaving, mouthcare); vitamin K and/or folic acid supplements may be needed.
- Hepatic dysfunction impairs immunity, so infection control is essential to maintain a safe environment.

- Monitor blood sugars initially two- to three-hourly and maintain normoglycaemia.
- Electrolytes should be monitored and supplements given – potassium, calcium, magnesium and phosphate imbalances often occur.
- Early nutrition facilitates recovery.
- Intra-abdominal pressure measurement facilitates early identification of, and treatment for, hepatic compromise.
- Patients are often forgetful, confused and agitated, needing simple and frequently repeated explanations. Conflict should be avoided. Relatives should be reassured that altered personality is caused by the disease, and that patience is needed.

Summary

The liver can be the forgotten vital organ in ICUs; other than transplantation centres, few units specialise in hepatic failure, but it frequently complicates most pathologies seen in ICUs. Liver function affects many other organs and systems, so care of patients with liver dysfunction requires a range of knowledge and skills. Extracorporeal liver devices are currently largely experimental and confined to specialist liver centres. Once liver failure becomes apparent, prognosis is poor, so ICU nurses should assess liver function to try and prevent/minimise potential complications.

Further reading

A number of journals specialise in hepatic and gastrointestinal medicine, but articles of use to ICU nurses are more likely to be found in general medical journals, such as de Keulenaer *et al.* (2009), Forrest (2009), Lucey *et al.* (2009) and Bernal *et al.* (2010). *Medical Clinics of North America* often devotes issues to hepatology; July 2009 (volume 93, issue 4) covers cirrhosis, while July 2008 (volume 92, issue 4) covers hepatic emergencies. Nursing articles are fewer, especially in the UK. McKinley (2009) is a recent article from the USA.

Clinical scenario

Julia Smith is 60 years old with a past medical history of alcoholic liver disease and remains alcohol dependent. She was admitted to the ICU with respiratory compromise associated with gross ascites, bacterial peritonitis and thrombocytopaenia. A peritoneal drain was inserted; 16 litres were drained initially with 3 litres on second drainage.

An insulin infusion is administered at 10 iu/h and her blood glucose is 8.3 mmol/litre.

413

Blood results include:

INR	2.9
Hb	9.5 g/dl
Platelets	35 x 10^{-9}/litre
WBC	30.6 x 10^{-9}/litre
Neutrophils	29.7 x 10^{-9}/litre
Lymphocytes	0.5 x 10^{-9}/litre
Monocytes	0.5 x 10^{-9}/litre)
Urea	22.3 mmol/litre
Bilirubin	223 μmol/litre
ALT	34 iu/litre
Alkaline phosphatase	89 iu/litre
Gamma GT	65 iu/litre)
Albumin	28 g/litre
Lactate	4.9 mmol/litre

Arterial blood gas results while mechanically ventilated on FiO$_2$ of 0.5 were:

pH	7.25
PaCO$_2$	5.8 kPa
PaO$_2$	12.2 kPa
SaO$_2$	94.8%

Q.1 Examine the results and their significance in terms of Miss Smith's liver function and liver damage.

Q.2 Seven litres of albumin 4.5% are administered to replace ascetic loss. What are the alternative therapies to the use of albumin with Miss Smith?

Q.3 Consider other treatment strategies Miss Smith may require. Is she a candidate for transplantation? Justify the rationale for transplantation in her case.

Chapter 42

Obstetric emergencies

Contents

Fundamental knowledge	415
Introduction	416
Normal pregnancy	416
Hypertensive disorders of pregnancy	418
Haemorrhage	418
Thromboembolism	418
Amniotic fluid embolus	419
HELLP syndrome	419
Brain death incubation	420
Drugs and pregnancy	420
Psychology	420
Implications for practice	421
Summary	421
Support groups	421
Further reading	421
Clinical scenario	422

Fundamental knowledge

Normal pregnancy, including normal physiological changes

Introduction

Most deliveries are 'normal', ICU admission only being needed in 2 per cent of cases in the UK, although incidence is higher elsewhere (Price *et al.*, 2009). However, numbers of older mothers, and rates of complications, are increasing (DH, 2010a), resulting in increasing ICU admissions. Overall maternal mortality is extremely low (12 per 100,000 maternities (Lewis, 2007)), but obstetric patients can be among the sickest patients in ICUs, one-third of maternal mortalities occurring in ICUs (Germain *et al.*, 2006). This, together with limited literature in ICU texts and journals, and few ICU staff being qualified midwives, can provoke special anxieties among staff.

Antenatal emergencies usually necessitate early delivery or termination of pregnancy, rarely being admitted to the ICU. Antenatal ICU admissions are more likely to occur for non-obstetric conditions, such as road traffic accident. Specific obstetric care, if any, depends on foetal age and condition. Antenatal care should optimise conditions for both mother and foetus. Foetal mortality may occur in addition to, or independently of, maternal mortality.

ICU obstetric admissions are usually postnatal. The four main causes of obstetric critical illness are:

- pregnancy-specific reasons (e.g. pre-eclampsia);
- increased susceptibility due to pregnancy (e.g. thromboembolism);
- underlying medical conditions (e.g. congenital heart disease);
- unrelated coincidence (e.g. pneumonia).

(Germain *et al.*, 2006)

Many critically ill obstetric patients have co-morbidities (such as diabetes, obesity or ischaemic heart disease), or other health problems (such as drug dependency or alcohol abuse) (Lewis, 2007).

Medical/nursing care centres on complications, medical treatments supporting failing systems (e.g. ventilation) and the human care familiar to ICU staff. For example, genital tract sepsis is increasing (Lewis, 2007), but managed in the same way as sepsis from any other cause (see Chapter 32), so is not discussed further in this chapter. ICU nurses do not need midwifery expertise to care for these admissions; midwives should actively be involved in multidisciplinary teams, to provide both psychological reassurance and practical care, such as expressing breast milk, assessing and monitoring uterine contractions, monitoring vaginal discharge, and checking need for anti-rhesus D injections. Midwives also provide valuable links between mother and child while the mother is in the ICU.

Normal pregnancy

Most crises result from physiological changes of pregnancy. Normal physiological changes during pregnancy favour foetal growth but place stress on the mother's body, altering many 'normal' biochemical/haematological values from non-pregnant levels.

From the first *trimester* (weeks 1–12) the *cardiovascular* system becomes hyperdynamic; by the second trimester cardiac output is about 150 per cent of pre-pregnant levels (Price *et al.*, 2009). If cardiac reserve is limited, increased cardiac work may precipitate cardiac failure. Patients should not be nursed supine, as aortocaval compression may cause hypotension, and so foetal distress. Increase in erythrocyte numbers does not match increase in blood volume, so causes dilutional *anaemia*, which improves capillary flow.

Onset of labour accelerates cardiovascular changes. In first-stage labour, pain and anxiety increase circulating catecholamines, increasing cardiac output by nearly half. Second-stage labour (contractions and delivery) creates a Valsalva effect, reducing both venous return and cardiac output. Uterine contraction during the third stage of labour (delivery of placenta) returns 300–400 ml of blood to systemic circulation, potentially precipitating hypertensive crises.

Maternal hearts are usually robust enough to cope with demands of pregnancy, but increased demands may precipitate crises. Cardiac death is currently the single main cause of UK maternal mortality (Lewis, 2007).

Respiratory changes occur for many reasons. Foetal growth reduces functional residual capacity (Price *et al.*, 2009). Increased maternal oxygen demand (one-third during pregnancy, a further two-thirds during labour) increases respiratory and cardiovascular workload. Minute volume increases by about half, mainly from larger tidal volumes, increasing PaO_2 and decreasing $PaCO_2$. Renal function normally compensates for respiratory alkalosis to maintain normal pH. Artificial ventilation should mimic this respiratory alkalosis by maintaining $PaCO_2$ at 4 kPa (Dhond and Dob, 2000).

Reduced colloid osmotic pressure (dilution), hypertension and vasoconstriction encourage *oedema* formation, including:

- pulmonary oedema (impairing gas exchange);
- airway oedema (obstructing airways);
- cerebral oedema (increasing intracranial pressure).

Airway mucosa becomes more vascular and oedematous, necessitating smaller endotracheal tubes while increasing airway resistance and pressures.

Neurological changes are not normally seen, but cerebral oedema and hypoxia can cause fitting from eclampsia (see page 418).

Gastrointestinal motility is reduced, contributing to nausea/vomiting, malnutrition and potential acid aspiration ('Mendelson's syndrome'). Liver disease occurs in less than 1 per cent of pregnancies, but up to 5 per cent may have abnormal liver function tests (Sillender, 2002). Hypertension can cause liver dysfunction, resulting in potential hypoglycaemia, immunocompromise, jaundice, coagulopathies, encephalopathy and other neurological complications. However, gestational hyperglycaemia is more common due to increased insulin resistance. Hyperglycaemia may facilitate foetal supply, but maternal blood sugar levels should be monitored regularly as insulin supplements may be needed. Normal hepatic function resumes postnatally.

Glomerular filtration increases by half (McNabb, 2004), so drug clearance may be increased. Increased urine output and antenatal bladder compression from the foetus cause urgency.

Impaired *immunity* during the third trimester prevents foetal rejection, but increases risk of viral infections.

Hypertensive disorders of pregnancy

Hypertension occurs in 5–7 per cent of pregnancies (Soydemir and Kenny, 2006). Pre-eclampsia and haemorrhage are the main obstetric causes of ICU admission (Germain *et al.*, 2006; Martin and Foley, 2006). *Pre-eclampsia* (hypertension and proteinuria, with or without oedema) is the single main underlying cause of maternal deaths (Soydemir and Kenny, 2006; Schutte *et al.*, 2010).

Systemic thromboplastin release in severe pre-eclampsia (probably from damaged placental tissue) causes intense arteriolar vasoconstriction and DIC (Bewley, 2004), compounding hypertension and coagulopathies.

Eclampsia is convulsions occurring in a woman with pre-eclampsia (Watson *et al.*, 2010). Eclamptic deaths often occur after only one fit, so convulsions should be controlled (Bewley, 2004). Delivery is essential to resolve eclampsia, usually necessitating Caesarean section or termination of pregnancy. Eclampsia should be controlled with magnesium (Price *et al.*, 2009).

Acute fatty liver is a rare variant of pre-eclampsia, affecting one in 10,000 pregnancies (Germain *et al.*, 2006) and causing gross microvascular fatty infiltration, without hepatic necrosis or inflammation.

Haemorrhage

With pre-eclampsia, haemorrhage is the main obstetric cause of ICU admission (Germain *et al.*, 2006; Martin and Foley, 2006). Bleeding from normal third-stage labour is reduced by arterial constriction and development of a fibrin mesh over the placental site, placental circulation, about 600 ml/minute at term (Lindsay, 2004) being autotransfused by uterine contraction. Incomplete contraction therefore causes major haemorrhage. Bleeding can also occur from genital tract lacerations and coagulopathies. Disseminated intravascular coagulation (DIC – see Chapter 26) may be triggered by pregnancy or its complications.

Postpartum haemorrhage volume is often underestimated (e.g. from loss on sheets) (RCOG, 2009). Prophylactic oxytocics should already have been routinely given (RCOG, 2009), but it is worth checking they have not been forgotten. Transfer to the ICU is usually for fluid resuscitation and monitoring – especially CVP and arterial line insertion.

Thromboembolism

Pregnancy causes a *procoagulant* state, increasing thromboembolism risks tenfold (RCOG, 2007). Thromboembolism remains the single main direct cause of obstetric deaths, most of these being from pulmonary emboli (Lewis, 2007). Antenatally, oral anticoagulants are contraindicated because they cross the placenta and may cause placental/foetal haemorrhage. All patients should receive venous thromboembolism (VTE) prophylaxis (Price *et al.*, 2009).

Amniotic fluid embolus

This rare condition, sometimes called 'anaphylactoid syndrome of pregnancy', occurs when amniotic fluid, foetal cells, hair or other debris enter maternal circulation (Dedhia and Mushambi, 2007), causing vascular obstruction (especially pulmonary artery) and anaphylactoid release of vasodilatory mediators (Tufnell and Hamilton, 2008). These typically progress to seizures, DIC and pulmonary oedema (Price *et al.*, 2009). It usually occurs in older women with higher *parity*, progressing rapidly, and is usually diagnosed post-mortem (Lewis, 2007). Mortality is high – up to 30 per cent of mothers and up to 44 per cent of foetuses/newborns (Tufnell and Hamilton, 2008; Conde-Agudelo and Romero, 2009).

Delivery should be rapid (Tufnell and Hamilton, 2008), after which treatment is largely supportive:

- oxygen;
- supporting blood pressure and cardiac output (fluids, inotropes);
- reversing coagulopathy.

(Conde-Agudelo and Romero, 2009)

Other treatments sometimes used include:

- selective pulmonary vasodilators, such as nitric oxide, prostacyclin or sildenafil.

(Conde-Agudelo and Romero, 2009)

Most survivors (mothers and children) have neurological symptoms (Dedhia and Mushambi, 2007).

HELLP syndrome

HELLP stands for:

- Haemolysis
- Elevated Liver enzymes and
- Low Platelets.

This syndrome causes severe hypertension, coagulopathies and grossly disordered liver function. It is more likely to occur following pre-eclampsia (Lefkou and Hunt, 2008; Kulungowski *et al.*, 2009), and usually necessitates ICU admission.

Early symptoms are often vague, so HELLP may become life-threatening before it is diagnosed. HELLP can cause:

- *abruptio placentae*;
- disseminated intravascular coagulation (DIC);
- acute kidney injury (AKI);

and other life-threatening problems (Steegers *et al.*, 2010). Fitting commonly occurs (Zeeman *et al.*, 2004).

Treatments include urgent delivery of the foetus (induction, Caesarean section) (Kulungowski *et al.*, 2009) and system support (e.g. ventilation). Steroids are not useful (Fonseca *et al.*, 2005).

Brain death incubation

Technology can support body systems following brain death, enabling foetal growth despite maternal death (Powner and Bernstein, 2003). Although rare, admission of brain-dead mothers creates stress for families and places nurses in a similar (but more prolonged) situation to caring for organ donors (see Chapter 43).

Drugs and pregnancy

Additional considerations when giving drugs during pregnancy include:

- Will they cross the placenta?
- Are they expressed in breast milk (if breastfeeding)?
- Foetal/newborn drug clearance.

Being professionally accountable for each drug given, nurses should withhold drugs and seek advice from their pharmacist if unsure of likely effects. Pharmacists should be actively involved in multidisciplinary teams.

Psychology

Most babies are wanted, so obstetric emergencies can be especially devastating. Miscarriages or abortions may create guilt. Other children, usually young, may experience various emotional traumas. Psychological support and care for the mother, partner and family is therefore especially important. Support may be gained from family and friends, chaplains, counselling services or various support groups.

Bereavement is traumatic, but photographs can become treasured mementoes, which parents may not think to ask for, or take, at the time.

Obstetric emergencies can be psychologically traumatic for staff, most nurses being female, of a similar age, and possibly planning or raising families of their own.

Implications for practice

- ICU admission will usually be to provide respiratory and/or cardiovascular support, so care should follow from problems necessitating admission.
- Do not nurse supine; aortocaval compression occludes circulation.
- Electrolyte imbalances and coagulopathies are common, so urgent blood screens should be sent, and appropriate treatments instigated.
- Pregnancy causes immunocompromise, so minimise infection risks.
- After the hopes of pregnancy, critical illness can cause devastating stress to patients, partners and families, so psychological needs should be assessed and support provided.
- Midwives are valuable members of the team, providing specialist care and advice.
- Antenatally, the mother's body should provide an optimal environment for foetal development.
- Postnatal obstetric observations should include vaginal examination (amount and type of discharge) and uterine contraction.
- Mothers wishing, but currently unable, to breastfeed should be offered opportunities to express breast milk (breast pump); this also relieves breast pain.
- Bereavement counselling and care may be needed.

Summary

Pregnancy is a normal physiological function, and most pregnancies occur without serious complications. However, life-threatening complications can and do occur, sometimes necessitating ICU admission, usually for cardiovascular or respiratory failure. Antenatal admissions should consider foetal health, but most admissions are postnatal; the precipitating cause (foetus/placenta) being delivered, system support may be all that is required until homeostasis is restored, although some problems require more aggressive treatments. Interventions used will be familiar to most ICU nurses, but terminology and pathophysiology may differ.

Support groups

Pre-Eclamptic Toxaemia Society (PETS): 01286 880057
Miscarriage Association: 01924 200799 (Scotland: 0131 354 8883)
Stillbirth and Neonatal Death Society (SANDS): 020 7436 7940; helpline@ uk-sands.org

Further reading

Triennial reports of maternal mortality provide valuable information and advice, and include a chapter specifically on Critical/Intensive Care; at the time of writing, the current report is Lewis (2007). The Royal College of Obstetricians and Gynaecologists publish 'Green Top Guidelines' on many topics, which can be downloaded from their website. The main midwifery textbook is Mayes (Henderson and Macdonald, 2004). There are a number of midwifery journals, which rarely contain articles of critical illness; critical care nursing journals occasionally contain articles on obstetrics. Medical journal reviews include Germain *et al.* (2006), Price *et al.* (2009), Steegers *et al.* (2010) and Watson *et al.* (2010).

Clinical scenario

Susan Jackson, a 27-year-old *primigravida* with recently diagnosed pre-eclampsia, is admitted to the ICU following an emergency Caesarean delivery at 34 weeks' gestation. Mrs Jackson was progressively hypertensive, oedematous with proteinuria, and experienced visual disturbances and epigastric pain. Mrs Jackson is mechanically ventilated with intravenous infusions of magnesium and hydralazine. She is cold with tachycardia of 125 beats/minute, BP of 160/110 mmHg, oliguria and hypoalbuminaemia.

Q.1   Explain the potential causes of Mrs Jackson's oliguria, including the significance of her proteinuria and hypoalbuminaemia. Formulate a plan for her fluid management and renal support.

Q.2   What other investigations should be performed to check for complications associated with pre-eclampsia (e.g. HELLP syndrome, DIC).

Q.3   Appraise the role of others within the interdisciplinary team, including the midwife, in planning collaborative care for Mrs Jackson while she is mechanically ventilated.

Chapter 43

Transplants

Contents

Fundamental knowledge	423
Introduction	424
Death	424
Nursing care	425
Ethical issues	427
Living donors	427
Post-operative care of recipients	428
Graft versus host disease (GvHD)	428
Immunosupression	429
Implications for practice	429
Summary	430
Useful contacts	430
Further reading	430
Clinical scenario	430

Fundamental knowledge

Brainstem and cranial nerve function
Immune response

Introduction

While organ transplantation (e.g. kidneys, heart, lungs, liver) can be life-saving, increasingly many tissues (e.g. eyes, skin, bone, heart valves) can be retrieved to improve recipients' quality of life. Up to 50 people may now be helped by a single donor. For more than a decade, numbers of donors and donated organs have been essentially static, while numbers living and dying on waiting lists for organs have continued to increase. Numbers of patients needing transplants in the UK are expected to continue to rise (Long and Sque, 2007). The UK has the lowest transplant rate in Europe (DH, 2008b), so each UK Trust now has a Senior Nurse Organ Donation (SNOD) and Clinical Lead Organ Donation (CLOD), with the aim of increasing organ donation by 50 per cent by 2013 (DH, 2008b). There is also the national 'Organ Donation Tsar' – currently (2011), Chris Rudge. This chapter focuses on organ donation; tissue donation is discussed in more detail in Moore and Woodrow (2009).

Death

Historically, death was synonymous with cessation of breathing and/or heartbeat. Development of technologies to replace breathing (ventilators) and heartbeat (pacing) coincided with transfer of organ donation from science fiction to science fact, necessitating revision of concepts of death.

For organ retrieval to occur the patient must be dead, but organs cannot have suffered significant ischaemic time. There are therefore two possible classifications for donors:

- brainstem
- donation following cardiac death (DCD – previously called non-heart-beating).

The brainstem contains the vital centres that enable life (respiratory, cardiac, hypothalamus, pituitary gland), so if the brainstem is dead the person cannot survive. Brainstem death, first described in 1959, is established in the UK through the Department of Health's *Code of Practice* (1998).

Any medical conditions that could prevent brainstem function must be excluded (see Table 43.1) before testing for brainstem death. Reflexes and responses of each cranial nerve are then tested (individually or in combination). Brainstem death tests should establish absence of:

- pupil reaction to light;
- corneal reflex;
- oculo-vestibular reflex;
- motor response to central stimulation;
- gag reflex;
- cough reflex;
- respiratory effort.

424

If higher centre responses are absent, brainstem death may be diagnosed. The legal time of death is the first test, although death is not pronounced until confirmed by the second test (DH, 1998). Any response from higher centres, however abnormal or limited, prohibits brainstem death diagnosis. Spinal reflex responses ('Lazarus' signs) are not significant, but may be misinterpreted by relatives or other witnesses as signs of life, so causing anxiety. One study, reported by Voelker (2000), found 39 per cent of patients diagnosed as brainstem dead exhibited such movements.

Tests should be carried out by two doctors, both of whom have been qualified more than five years, and at least one of whom is a consultant, usually the patient's own. Neither doctor making the test should be a member of the transplant team. Tests should follow all criteria in the *Code of Practice*.

If brainstem death cannot be diagnosed, DCD can occur. In theatre, supporting treatments are withdrawn, followed by a 'stand-off' time, usually at least five minutes. Provided death occurs, organs may then be retrieved.

The *Human Tissue Act 1961* established that after death the body becomes the property of the next of kin, giving next of kin the right to refuse donation. Technically, the *Human Tissue Act 2004* makes wishes of patients paramount, although the practice of requesting relatives' consent remains, and is unlikely to be legally challenged in the foreseeable future.

Nursing care

All patients from whom care is withdrawn should be considered as potential donors. Previous exclusion criteria are frequently extended, as 'marginal' organs/tissues prove life-saving (Anderson *et al.*, 2008). Each Trust should have a SNOD who can advise on likely organs and/or tissues that might be retrieved, and can offer advice and information to staff and patients' families. Out of hours a regional SNOD carries a pager for the region. The NHS Organ Donor Register enables people to record their willingness to be organ donors, and can be accessed by NHS staff to check whether patients are on the register. However, as with a donor card, while the majority of the UK population approve of

Table 43.1 Brainstem death: preconditions

- There should be no doubt that the patient's condition is due to irremediable brain damage of known aetiology.
- The patient is deeply unconscious.
- There should be no evidence that this state is due to depressant drugs.
- Primary hypothermia as a cause of unconsciousness must be excluded.
- Potentially reversible circulatory, metabolic and endocrine disturbances must be excluded as a cause of the continuation of unconsciousness.
- The patient is being maintained on a ventilator because spontaneous respiration has been inadequate or has ceased altogether.

Source: DH (1998)

donation, only a minority are on the register or carry cards. So while being on the donor register indicates patients' wishes, absence from the register should not be interpreted as not wishing to donate.

Donation is now coordinated nationally by NHS Blood and Transplant (NHSBT). Staff making referrals out of hours will need:

- name, date of birth, address, hospital number (not direct line to a unit);
- patient GP details;
- date and time of death, and provisional cause;
- next-of-kin details, including a contact number;
- brief medical history, including any recent infection, trauma and medication;
- height and weight of patient;
- results of any blood samples.

Caring for donors and their families can be psychologically stressful. Nurses will usually be involved in discussions with families. Typically, a senior doctor will break the bad news, and suggest donation. If the next of kin agrees to donation, a SNOD will then describe the process, and obtain consent, using a proforma from NHSBT. This is designed to ensure next of kin are informed about the process and anticipated outcome, while risk factors that might make organs or tissues unsuitable are identified. Detailed, often probing, questions at a time of distress and mourning can be difficult. Nurses will usually accompany the SNOD, both as a witness and to support relatives if needed.

Unlike other terminal care, where (hopefully) peaceful death is followed by last offices, diagnosis of brainstem death is followed by optimising organ function for retrieval. For example, brainstem dysfunction can cause diabetes insipidus, resulting in hypovolaemia, poor organ perfusion, and electrolyte imbalance (Bugge, 2009). Aggressive donor management can significantly reduce the number of potential donors who are lost due to circulatory collapse (Bugge, 2009). While logical, this focus on supporting body systems in someone who is diagnosed as dead potentially conflicts with nursing values, whereby actions should be in patients' best interests. However, facilitating patients' wishes to donate *is* in their best interests. With death already diagnosed, following retrieval the body is normally transferred to the mortuary; last offices ('letting go') are performed elsewhere.

Relatives facing bereavement should be allowed to grieve; they may also gain comfort from knowing their loved one's organs will help others to live. Relatives' responses vary. SNODs are experienced at comforting relatives and may prove a valuable resource, although some relatives prefer to speak with staff with whom they have already developed rapport and trust.

Once transferred, the SNOD coordinates nursing care, including last offices. If possible, in the UK, available donor organs are matched and allocated to UK patients; where this is not possible, they are offered to other European organ-sharing organisations. Family, and staff involved in donation, are thanked in writing by the SNOD, and informed of how organs are used, but identification of recipients is avoided.

Ethical issues

Transplantation has always maintained a high public profile, ensuring widespread discussion of ethical issues. Organ donation relies on public goodwill, so healthcare staff should encourage public awareness.

Organ donation can literally be life-saving; *moral duty* to facilitate transplantation creates dilemmas between whether the onus of duty falls on society or individuals. Some nations (e.g. France, Belgium, Austria, Sweden, Norway, Switzerland, Spain) operate systems of presumed consent: people have to actively opt out if they do not wish to donate. The UK, like most countries, has an opt-in system, donation becoming a gift, but there have been calls to change to an opt-out system from the BMA in 1999 and the Chief Medical Officer in 2006.

Organs and tissues are only considered if the offer is *unconditional*. So any condition that organs should not be given to recipients with particular diseases or from various social/religious/cultural/ethnic groups will result in transplant services refusing the donation.

Publicity significantly influences donor supply: positive publicity (e.g. transplant games) encourages donation, while negative publicity increases refusal rates.

Except for Rastafarians, no major *religions* oppose organ donation (Randhawa, 1997), although some ministers (e.g. some Jewish rabbis (Levine, 1997)) may discourage donation, believing the body should remain unmutilated. As with all patients and families, cultural beliefs and values should be respected. NHSBT produces various information leaflets for major religions, which can valuably be made available in relatives' rooms. The SNOD, and ministers of religions, can also often provide useful cultural-specific information and support.

Distressed *relatives*, facing inevitable and usually sudden bereavement, may not think to ask about donation. Ormrod *et al.*'s (2005) small study found no relatives regretted agreeing to organ donation, but some who refused donation later regretted their decision. Offering donation therefore should be viewed as offering relatives a choice; not offering donation denies them that choice. Some relatives may decline donation due to not wishing to 'sacrifice' the body (Sque *et al.*, 2008), although the majority of relatives asked will give consent (NICE, 2010d).

Living donors

Limited supply of cadaver organs has encouraged use of living donors (Ikegamin *et al.*, 2008). About 20 per cent of renal transplants are from living donors, usually related. Sections from the liver, lung and (occasionally) small bowel can also be transplanted from living donors. Combined heart and lung transplants can also be performed from living donors if the recipient's heart is sufficiently healthy to transplant into the donor; there are many combinations of such 'domino' transplants.

Post-operative care of recipients

Post-operative care of transplant recipients includes aspects needed for any patient who has undergone major surgery, with the addition of complications created both for supporting the grafted organ to function effectively, while preventing infection in patients receiving strong immunosuppressive drugs. Early extubation is therefore a priority (Glaspole and Williams, 1999). Transplant recipients should be monitored closely for signs of:

- rejection
- electrolyte imbalance
- infection.

Non-function. Transplanted organs may fail ever to function. Organ-specific function should be monitored, and if *primary non-function* occurs, urgent further transplantation is usually organised, if possible. Rejection is classified as follows:

- *Hyperacute rejection* occurs within minutes of anastomosis, pre-existing mediators provoking thrombotic occlusion of graft vasculature and irreversible ischaemia. It is relatively rare.
- *Acute rejection* is more common, causing necrosis of individual cells.
- *Chronic rejection*, which only begins weeks to years after transplantation, is caused by fibrosis.

Various interventions may support the failing organ, but rejection usually necessitates retransplantation.

Electrolytes. Storage and cooling of organs for transportation usually causes electrolyte imbalance and metabolic acidosis, so homeostasis should be restored. Imbalances, acidosis and reperfusion injury may all cause dysrhythmias. If biochemistry does not stabilise over the first post-operative day, graft failure should be suspected.

Infection. Immunosuppressant drugs and multiple invasive lines make patients particularly susceptible to opportunist infection. Patients should be monitored for signs of infection.

Pain. Pain varies both between individuals and in the nature of surgery, but epidural analgesia often provides the most effective cover for patients (Glaspole and Williams, 1999).

Additional organ-specific care may also be needed.

Graft versus host disease (GvHD)

When foreign tissue, such as a tissue transplant, enters the body, the immune system initiates a host reaction. Severe cases may cause organ failure or death (Ferrara *et al.*, 2009). GvHD causes fibrosis, and necrosis in skin, liver and gut epithelium. Incidence increases with older donors, older recipients, or those with human leucocyte antigen (HLA) mismatch.

Symptoms include:

■ skin rashes (typically, face, palms, soles, ears)
■ jaundice
■ diarrhoea.

Treatments include corticosteroids and chemotherapy, often with system support.

Immunosuppression

Healthy immunity would reject transplanted tissue, so donor recipients (except for corneas) are given immunosuppresents to prevent rejection.

Until the introduction of *ciclosporin* (Neoral®, Sandimmune®) in 1979, transplant surgery was very limited. *Tacrolimus* (and sirolimus) provide better graft function (Ciancio, 2006) and so have largely replaced ciclosporin (Grimm *et al.*, 2006). Oral tacrolimus is usually commenced the day after surgery. Tacrolimus often interacts with other drugs binding to plasma proteins, such NSAIDs, oral anticoagulants and oral hypoglycaemics. It has many adverse effects, the main, and earliest, one usually being fitting; others include nephro-toxicity (Mihatsch *et al.*, 1998) and diabetes mellitus (Knoll, 1999). Tacrolimus levels should be monitored.

Both ciclosporin and tacrolimus can cause hirsuitism, gum hypertrophy, hypertension, renal impairment, hypercholesterolaemia, hypomagnesaemia and central nervous system symptoms (e.g. tremor, headaches, fits) (Glaspole and Williams, 1999). Immunosuppression can cause opportunist infection, so prophylactic antibiotics (often for 48 hours) and antifungal agents (e.g. acyclovir) are usually given to prevent herpes simplex.

Implications for practice

■ Donation should routinely be considered when withdrawing active treatment.
■ Donation offers families the opportunity to salvage something positive from bereavement.
■ SNODs can offer useful support and information at all stages of donation, so should be alerted and involved early.
■ Any medical conditions that may affect brainstem function must be excluded before brainstem death tests.
■ Spinal reflexes may occur despite absence of brainstem function; staff and relatives should be warned about these – they are not a sign of life.
■ In addition to general ICU care, nurses should monitor transplant recipients for signs of:

● rejection;
● infection (immunosupression);
● side effects of immunosupressants and other drugs, especially fitting.

Summary

Transplantation of organs and tissues can offer possible cures and improved quality of life to people with endstage and life-threatening pathologies, but continuing donor shortage often causes long waiting lists, many patients dying before suitable organs are found. Most organs being retrieved from patients already in the ICU, ICU nurses should promote (without coercion) awareness about transplantation. The (usually) close rapport with families enables nurses to offer valuable support during crises and discussion.

Nurses are normally present during brainstem death testing, so should be aware of the *Code of Practice* (DH, 1998) and its requirements.

Useful contacts

NHSBT Tissue Donation: 0800 432 0559
NHSBT Tissue Services, Colindale Avenue, Colindale NW9 5BG:
0208 258 2700

Further reading

Department of Health (2008, 2009) policy documents provide useful overviews together with likely futures. Forthcoming NICE guidelines for improving donor identification and consent rates are likely to be similarly useful. Sque *et al.*'s (2008) research examines relative refusal, while Millson (2009) provides a recent medical review. Rudge (2010) describes recent UK changes.

Clinical scenario

Irene Wallace is 50 years old and suffered an out-of-hospital VF arrest. She was successfully resuscitated at the scene, but en route to hospital required further resuscitation and seven defibrillation shocks. She was admitted to the ICU for mechanical ventilation prior to transfer to CT scan the following day. This head scan revealed extensive and diffuse cerebral damage. Her GCS is E1, V_t, M1.

Q.1 Identify features from Mrs Wallace's history that would allow her to be considered as a potential organ donor. What other information and actions are required?

Q.2 Review how permission for Mrs Wallace's organ donation might be obtained.

Q.3 Analyse interventions that can optimise Mrs Wallace's organ function. Consider the beneficial and adverse effects of such interventions on Mrs Wallace, her family and the staff on the ICU.

Q.4 Following brainstem death confirmation, should Mrs Wallace be resuscitated in the event she has a cardiopulmonary arrest? Discuss this with medical colleagues.

Part IX

Metabolic

Chapter 44

Severe acute pancreatitis

Contents

Fundamental knowledge	433
Introduction	434
Pathology	434
Complications	435
Symptoms	436
Medical treatments	437
Implications for practice	438
Summary	438
Further reading	438
Clinical scenario	438

Fundamental knowledge

Pancreatic anatomy and physiology – endocrine
and exocrine functions, Sphincter of Oddi,
Ampulla of Vater

Introduction

Pancreatitis is a relatively common disease affecting people of all ages, usually caused by:

- alcoholism (usually in men under 40);
- biliary obstruction (usually in older women; usually caused by gallstones);

although only a minority of alcoholics or people with gallstones develop pancreatitis. Rarer causes include:

- drugs, such as NSAIDs, thiazides, contraceptives (Hughes, 2004);
- animal venoms (rarely seen in the UK);
- idiopathic causes, such as endoscopy.

Alcohol causes protein in pancreatic enzymes to precipitate, obstructing pancreatic ductules (Hughes, 2004). UK incidence has doubled in the last 30 years (Siva and Pereira, 2007).

Pancreatitis may be acute or chronic. Patients with chronic pancreatitis are seldom admitted to ICUs, so this chapter describes acute pancreatitis. Acute pancreatitis is usually mild, not needing ICU admission, but mild pancreatitis can rapidly (within hours) become severe, causing progressive organ failure. Acute severe pancreatitis typically progresses rapidly (also within hours), causing:

- severe continuous abdominal pain;
- shallow, rapid breathing;
- massive hypovolaemia, hypotension and shock;
- other resulting symptoms, such as oliguria and pyrexia.

Overall mortality for pancreatitis is about 7 per cent (Rickes and Uhle, 2009), but about one-fifth progress to severe disease (Hayden and Wyncoll, 2008; Rickes and Uhle, 2009), which has a mortality of about 30 per cent (Hayden and Wyncoll, 2008). Mortality remains unchanged since the 1970s, with no major innovations in treatment (Goldacre and Roberts, 2004). Medical and nursing management focuses on system support to minimise/limit complications (Williams and Williamson, 2010). Priorities of nursing care are listed in Table 44.1.

Pathology

Pancreatic juice, secreted by reflex vagal responses to acidic chyme, enters the duodenum at the Sphincter of Oddi. It is strongly alkaline (pH about 8.0) and contains phospholipidase A, a powerful protein-digesting enzyme. Obstruction to the Ampulla of Vater prevents acidic chyme being neutralised, so stimulating continuing release of pancreatic juice. Congestion eventually ruptures pancreatic ductules, releasing pancreatic juice directly into the gland. Autodigestion causes

***Table 44.1* Priorities of nursing care for pancreatitis**

▪ Haemodynamic monitoring (ECG, BP, CVP, flow monitoring) – dysrhythmias and hypovolaemia likely.
▪ Monitor and support ventilation – probable pulmonary oedema/effusions; diaphragmatic splinting.
▪ Pain management – morphine usually needed.
▪ Restore normovolaemia – massive fluid shifts; monitor CVP; give precribed 'filling' (mainly colloids).
▪ Monitor and resolve electrolyte imbalances.
▪ Early nutrition – monitor absorption.
▪ Thermoregulation – monitor temperature; blood cultures if infection suspected; antipyretics.
▪ Monitor urine output – CRRT may be needed.
▪ Normoglycaemia – frequent blood glucose monitoring; insulin regime.

oedema, necrosis and haemorrhage (Sargent, 2006). If fistulas form, pancreatic juice also digests peripancreatic fat.

Damage to cell membranes triggers inflammatory responses:

▪ vasodilatation and hypotension;
▪ microvascular thromboses;
▪ further release of cytokines and other mediators;

while adrenal (cortisol) insufficiency impairs anti-inflammatory response (de Waele *et al.*, 2007).

Biomarkers. Serum amylase (normal 30–100 iu/litre) is the most widely used biomarker, often rising to 1000 iu/litre within a few hours. Amylase levels do not correlate with severity (Hayden and Wyncoll, 2008). Sargent (2006) suggests lipase (normal 0–160 units/litre) is a more sensitive marker than amylase, as it is only found in the pancreas. However, lipase tends to rise slightly later than amylase, taking 24–48 hours (Nydegger *et al.*, 2007), and its sensitivity can be reduced by late presentation, hypertriglyceridaemia, and chronic alcoholism (Matull *et al.*, 2006). Procalcitonin and interleukin 6 allow earlier prediction, at 12–24 hours (Matull *et al.*, 2006).

Complications

Acute fluid collections can develop in or near the pancreas (Valencia, 2000). These fluid collections lack a wall of granulation of fibrous tissue (Valencia, 2000).

Acute oedematous pancreatitis may progress to *pancreatic necrosis*, creating an ideal environment for bacterial growth. Infection is usually from colon bacteria. Mortality from infected severe pancreatitis can exceed 50 per cent (Pickworth, 2003).

Pancreatic pseudocysts are collections of pancreatic juice enclosed by a wall of fibrous or granulation tissue (Murphy *et al.*, 2002). Pseudocysts frequently occur, and usually resolve spontaneously, but until resolution surrounding tissues can be compressed, and fistulae into surrounding tissue can develop, causing haemorrhage (especially liver or spleen) or infection (especially with bowel fistulae).

Pancreatic abscesses are circumscribed intra-abdominal collections of pus (Murphy *et al.*, 2002). Mortality is 40 per cent (Larvin, 1999). Once confirmed by CT scan, abscesses should be drained.

Symptoms

Oedema and distension of the pancreatic capsule, biliary tree obstruction or chemical peritoneal burning (phospholipidase A) cause severe acute abdominal *pain*, requiring opioid analgesia such as morphine.

Hypermetabolism is the main cause of *pyrexia*, although infections often occur. Temperature should be monitored. If high, blood cultures should be taken and antipyretics may be needed (see Chapter 8).

Infection occurs in one-tenth of patients with acute pancreatitis. About half of patients develop infection within three weeks. Early antibiotic therapy reduces infection rates to one-third (Uhl *et al.*, 1998), so preventing infection is currently the 'most promising . . . treatment' (Uhl *et al.*, 1999: 103).

Common *electrolyte imbalances* include:

- *hyperglycaemia* (from impaired insulin secretion, increased glucagon release, circulating antagonists such as catecholamines, and glucose in parenteral feeds); blood sugars should be closely monitored; sliding scales of insulin may be prescribed;
- *hypocalcaemia*, which is mainly caused by extravasation of albumin (to which calcium is bound) (Hale *et al.*, 2000);
- *hypomagnesaemia*, which is common, especially with alcohol-related pancreatitis.

Respiratory failure, the main cause of death with acute pancreatitis, and often requiring artificial ventilation, may be caused by:

- pleural effusions, from autodigestion of lung tissue, especially on the left side; .
- atelectasis and ARDS from phospholipidase A impairing surfactant production (Hale *et al.*, 2000);
- pulmonary oedema caused by inflammatory mediators (Pastor *et al.*, 2003) and inappropriate fluid management, especially excessive crystalloid infusion or low molecular weight colloids;
- reduced lung volume from diaphragmatic splinting, caused by ascites and the grossly distended pancreas.

Cardiovascular instability is caused by systemic inflammatory responses (SIRS) to autodigestion. Gross inflammatory responses cause excessive vasodilatation and capillary leak. Fluid shifts aggravate electrolyte imbalances.

Aggressive fluid resuscitation and inotropes are usually needed, often necessitating flow monitoring (see Chapter 20).

Four-fifths of people with severe pancreatitis develop intra-abdominal hypertension (Hayden and Wyncoll, 2008), which can cause organ failure (see Chapter 41). Hypotension and/or intra-abdominal hypertension often cause *acute kidney injury* (AKI), often necessitating haemofiltration.

Direct *gastrointestinal damage* can cause:

- peptic ulceration
- gastritis
- translocation of gut bacteria
- bowel infarction
- paralytic ileus.

Hypermetabolism increases energy expenditure, necessitating additional nutritional support.

Enteral nutrition is usually possible, and preferable, with pancreatitis (UK Working Party on Acute Pancreatitis, 2005; Meier *et al.*, 2006; Petrov *et al.*, 2008; Al-Omran *et al.*, 2010). If gastric ileus occurs, jejunal feeding should be attempted (Nathens *et al.*, 2004). If enteral feeding is not possible, parenteral nutrition is necessary.

Intra-abdominal haemorrhage often causes bruising or other skin discolouration, such as '*Grey Turner's sign*' (bluish-purple discolouration of flanks) or '*Cullen's sign*' (irregular, bluish-purple discolouration around the umbilicus).

Medical treatments

Historically, the treatment of choice was surgery, which is why pancreatitics are usually admitted under surgeons. However, almost the only remaining indication for surgery is necrotic tissue, which needs urgent surgical debridement. Many drug treatments have been attempted, but cures remain evasive. Treatment, discussed in Table 44.1, is largely supporting systems and minimising complications:

- artificial ventilation
- fluids
- (early) antibiotics
- inotropes
- renal replacement therapy
- analgesia
- nutrition
- supplements (insulin, electrolytes, trace elements and micro-nutrients.

Gallstones should be removed with early endoscopic retrograde cholangiopancreatography (ERCP) (van Santvoort *et al.*, 2009). Infected pancreatic necrosis needs early surgical debridement, but if sterile, surgery should be avoided (Nathens *et al.*, 2004; Malangoni and Martin, 2005).

Implications for practice

- Pain is severe; analgesia (usually opioid) should be provided and its effectiveness assessed.
- Large fluids shifts can rapidly cause oedema (including ascites and pulmonary oedema) and hypovolaemia; aggressive fluid resuscitation, mainly with colloids, may prevent organ failure. Arterial blood pressure and fluid balance charts give little indication of intravascular volume.
- Respiratory failure is the main cause of death with acute pancreatitis. Respiratory function should be monitored closely, and atelectasis and pleural effusions treated. Severe respiratory failure often progresses to ARDS.
- Fluid shifts/loss can cause various electrolyte imbalances. Biochemistry should be monitored, and major imbalances rectified.
- Blood sugars should be monitored regularly, and insulin regimes followed.
- Nurses should ensure nutrition is optimised; if possible, use enteral routes, including jejunostomy.

Summary

Pancreatitis can cause rapid and severe complications in most other major systems. Severe pancreatitis, seen in ICUs, continues to cause high mortality. Current treatment is largely system support to prevent further complications, pain control being a particularly important nursing role.

Further reading

National guidelines by the UK Working Party on Acute Pancreatitis (2005) are comprehensive. Articles frequently appear in medical, and especially surgical, journals; Rickes and Uhle (2009) and Williams and Williamson (2010) provide recent reviews. Sargent (2006) provides a nursing review.

Clinical scenario

Myla Vegas is 56 years old and was admitted to the ICU with sudden acute abdominal pain. The pain radiated towards her back and was accompanied by nausea and vomiting. Two years ago she had an ultrasound, which detected gallstones. She is 1.6 metres tall and weighs 74 kg. On admission her abdomen was distended.

Other abnormal results from admission assessment include:

Vital signs		Blood serum	
Temperature	38.4°C	Glucose	12 mmol/litre
Respiration	32 per minute	WBC	19.3×10^{-9}/litre
SpO$_2$	88% on FiO$_2$ of 0.6	CRP	151 mg/litre
Heart rate	145 bpm	Amylase	1 543 iu/litre
3-lead ECG	sinus rhythm, ST elevation	Alkaline phosphate	250 iu/litre
BP	110/60 mmHg	Potassium	3.4 mmol/litre
MAP	77 mmHg	Calcium	1.8 mmol/litre
CVP	8 mmHg	Magnesium	0.78 mmol/litre

Q.1 With reference to physiology, explain Miss Vegas's results (e.g. why has her temperature and respiratory rate increased, why does she have low potassium with presenting symptoms and diagnosis?).

A CT scan reveals bilateral pleural effusions, basal consolidation, diffuse pancreatic enlargement with peri-pancreatic fluid and a small amount of fluid around the liver and spleen.

Q.2 Consider the implications of the CT scan results for Miss Vegas's condition, and note other complications that may occur. Discuss how these should be managed.

Q.3 Review pain management strategies for Miss Vegas's abdominal pain and discomfort caused by nursing, medical and surgical interventions.

Chapter 45

Diabetic crises

Contents

Fundamental knowledge   440
Introduction   441
Type 1 diabetes   442
Type 2 diabetes   442
Ketones   442
Metabolic syndrome   442
Hyperglycaemia   443
Severe hypoglycaemia   443
Diabetic ketoacidosis (DKA)   443
Hyperosmolar hyperglycaemic
    state (HHS)   444
Implications for practice   444
Summary   445
Useful contact   445
Further reading   445
Clinical scenario   445

Fundamental knowledge

Pancreatic anatomy and physiology, especially production
    of insulin

Introduction

'Diabetes' is taken from the Greek word for 'siphon', used to describe the classic symptoms of *polyuria* and *polydipsia*. *Diabetes mellitus* is caused by lack of, or antagonism to, insulin, causing hyperglycaemia, glycosuria (mellitus = 'honey', from the time when urinalysis was performed by taste), and so osmotic diuresis. *Diabetes insipidus*, from lack of anti-diuretic hormone, causes polyuria from lack of renal reabsorption of water. This chapter follows the convention of 'diabetes' implying diabetes mellitus.

Diabetes mellitus affects more than two million people in the UK (DH, 2010b), with many diabetics remaining undiagnosed until a crisis occurs (Audit Commission, 2001). Ageing populations and endemic obesity cause continuing increases in incidence (González *et al.*, 2009; DH, 2010b). Diabetes may cause or complicate ICU admission.

Insulin, produced by pancreatic beta (β) cells, transports glucose into cells. Lack therefore deprives cells of their main energy sources. Hyperglycaemia causes acute complications, including:

- polyuria (if glucose exceeds the renal reabsorption threshold – blood glucose exceeds 10 mmol/litre) and so hypovolaemia;
- immunocompromise (reduced oxygen dissociation from haemoglobin, impaired leucocyte migration and increased blood viscosity);
- inflammatory responses from vascular endothelium.

Poorly controlled diabetes can cause many diseases, outlined in this chapter. The *metabolic syndrome* is also discussed. Many patients are diabetic, or develop short-term hyperglycaemia in response to stressors of critical illness. But diabetes can also cause crises that necessitate ICU admission. This chapter discusses:

- severe hypoglycaemia;
- diabetic ketoacidosis (DKA);
- hyperosmolar hyperglycaemic state (HHS); sometimes called 'hyperosmolar non-ketotic state' (HONKS): hyperglycaemia, minimal ketosis, coma.

Incidence of severe hypoglycaemia and DKA is increasing (DH, 2010b).
Diabetes causes many complications, including:

- hypertension (Gallego *et al.*, 2008);
- strokes (Jeerakathil *et al.*, 2007);
- chronic kidney disease (NICE, 2009b);
- ischaemic heart disease (NICE, 2009b);
- retinopathy and blindness (Gallego *et al.*, 2008);
- peripheral neuropathy, leg ulcers and amputation (Jeffacote and Harding, 2003);
- depression (Pouwer *et al.*, 2010).

Even if not acutely life-threatening, complications such as ulcers need nursing care, and as ulcers are often chronic, advice from specialists such as tissue viability nurses is valuable.

There are two different types of diabetes mellitus: type 1 and type 2.

Type 1 diabetes

Previously called 'insulin-dependent diabetes mellitus' (IDDM), this is an autoimmune disease (Walltmahmed, 2006), which destroys pancreatic beta cells, but leaves other pancreatic cells unharmed, so glucagon (which releases sugar stores into blood) is produced (Devendra *et al.*, 2004). This disease typically develops in childhood, the almost total destruction of beta cells usually necessitating life-long insulin therapy. Most type 1 diabetics suffer complications relatively early in life.

Type 2 diabetes

Previously called 'non-insulin-dependent diabetes mellitus' (NIDDM) or 'late-onset', this accounts for most diabetes (90 per cent (Nolan, 2002)). Typically, this develops in later life (65–74 years (DH, 2002)) partly from age-related pancreatic decline, and often aggravated by obesity (DH, 2010b) – fat causes insulin resistance (Jefrey, 2003). But incidence in children is increasing (Haines *et al.*, 2007). Type 2 is less severe than type 1, as the pancreas has significant remaining function, but not sufficient to cope with the demands placed upon it.

Ketones

Glucose is normally the main energy source for cell mitochondria to produce adenosine triphosphate (ATP). Glucose needs insulin to transport it across cell membrane. Therefore insulin lack deprives cells of their normal main energy source, forcing cells to resort to metabolism of alternative energy sources, mainly free fatty acids (lyposis). Alternative energy source metabolism is relatively inefficient, producing limited energy but much waste, including ketones. Ketones are filtered by the kidneys, so can be detected on urinalysis. Excessive ketones, and other metabolic acids, cause:

- acidosis;
- nausea and vomiting (Jerreat, 2010);
- '*Kussmaul respiration*' – deep, rapid and sighing breaths (Jerreat, 2010);
- osmotic diuresis;
- a distinctive sickly-sweet smell to breath (in unintubated patients).

Metabolic syndrome

A syndrome of various interrelated metabolic problems can be caused when type 2 diabetics accumulate risk factors, such as chronic hyperglycaemia, obesity, hypertension, dyslipidaemia and work-related stress (Chandola *et al.*, 2006; Kahn, 2007). Although other authorities sometimes given slightly different criteria, National Cholesterol Education Program Adult Treatment Panel III (ATP III) criteria for diagnosis (cited in Tonkin, 2004) are three or more of:

- fasting plasma glucose ≥ 6.1 mmol/litre;
- abdominal obesity (e.g. waist circumference > 102 cm in men, > 88 cm in women);
- triglyceride level ≥ 1.7 mmol/litre;
- high-density lipoprotein cholesterol (HDL-C) < 1 mmol/litre in men, 1.3 mmol/litre in women;
- BP ≥ 130/85 mmHg.

Widespread inflammatory vascular disease can cause atherosclerosis and myocardial infarction (Reilly and Rader, 2003; Wilson and Grundy, 2003; Malik *et al.*, 2004; Marik and Raghaven, 2004; Sasso *et al.*, 2004).

Hyperglycaemia

Critical illness usually causes transient hyperglycaemia (van den Berghe *et al.*, 2001; Cely *et al.*, 2004) by increasing insulin resistance. Drugs, such as adrenaline or steroids, also increase insulin resistance. Such transient hyperglycaemia usually resolves with recovery or once treatment is reduced/removed.

Severe hypoglycaemia

This may occur if type 1 diabetics either receive an insulin overdose or have not eaten adequately, but recent years have seen deaths caused by aggressive insulin therapy to achieve tight glucose control, but inadequate monitoring of blood glucose (see Chapter 21). Blood glucose < 2 mmol/litre creates a medical emergency (Keays, 2009), as brain cells rely on constant supplies to survive. Severe hypoglycaemia is treated by giving intravenous glucose, stabilising acid/base and electrolyte balances, and frequent monitoring. Stanisstreet *et al.* (2010) recommend using 10% or 20% glucose, rather than the more widely used 50%. Severe hypoglycaemia is usually managed in Accident and Emergency or acute admission wards, but could occur on ICUs, especially if feeds are stopped but insulin infusion continues.

Diabetic ketoacidosis (DKA)

DKA typically occurs when type 1 diabetics fail to receive insulin, although it is often precipitated by infection (Park, 2007), usually necessitating ICU admission. DKA causes:

- hyperglycaemia
- ketosis
- metabolic acidosis.

Patients may be comatose or acutely confused. Osmotic diuresis from both glycosuria and ketonuria usually causes hypovolaemic shock. Venous statis and hyperosmolality can cause thromboembolism, epilepsy and strokes.

Priorities are to:

- reduce blood ketones by 0.5 mmol/litre/hour;
- increase venous bicarbonate by 3 mmol/litre/hour;
- reduce capillary blood glucose by 3 mmol/litre/hour;
- maintain potassium between 4–5 mmol/litre.

(Joint British Diabetes Societies Inpatient Care Group, 2010)

This necessitates close monitoring of vital signs, blood sugars, fluid balance, electrolytes and neurological state. Rapid reduction in blood glucose may cause cerebral oedema, so target reduction is often < 5 mmol/hour, although evidence for this is lacking (Park, 2007). Once blood glucose is < 14 mmol/litre, fluids should be changed to 10% glucose (Park, 2007; Joint British Diabetes Societies Inpatient Care Group, 2010). Severe acidosis (pH < 7.1) may necessitate bicarbonate infusion, but less severe acidosis usually resolves with recovery.

Hyperosmolar hyperglycaemic state (HHS)

Also called hyperosmolar non-ketotic state (HONKS), this rare condition is most likely to occur with type 2 diabetics, and resembles diabetic ketoacidosis, except that it develops more slowly, and ketosis does not occur. Hyperglycaemia causes osmotic diuresis and electrolyte imbalance; as HHS often develops over some days, dehydration is often more severe (Keays, 2009). Dehydration increases serum osmolality, which causes neurological complications, including tonic-clonic seizures. Type 2 diabetics are usually more sensitive to insulin (Charalambous *et al.*, 1999), so it should be infused more cautiously and monitored more frequently. Otherwise HHS is managed as DKA.

Implications for practice

- Diabetes can cause widespread complications and problems throughout the body, so patients should be assessed and treated holistically.
- Insulin management should be adjusted with changes in feeding regimes, especially when feeds are stopped.
- Recent practices of tight glycaemic control have caused avoidable mortality from severe hypoglycaemia.
- UK guidelines for managing diabetic ketoacidosis (Joint British Diabetes Societies Inpatient Care Group, 2010) have moved from focusing primarily on hyperglycaemic management to controlling ketoacidosis.
- Diabetic ketoacidosis and HHS should also be treated with aggressive fluid replacement.

Summary

Diabetes affects people of all ages, and incidence is increasing. It may cause or complicate ICU admission. Most diabetics are type 2, although diabetic crises more commonly occur with type 1. Diabetics frequently have co-morbidities and complications.

Useful contact

Diabetes UK, 10 Queen Anne Street, London W1G 9LH: 020 7323 1531; info@diabetes.org.uk; www.diabetes.org.uk

Further reading

Many books and journals (such as *Diabetic Medicine*) focus on diabetes, while articles frequently appear in general nursing and medical journals. Less literature focuses on critical care issues, but Jerreat (2010) reviews diabetic ketoacidosis. NHS Diabetes (www.diabetes.nhs.uk) publishes resources, such as Stanisstreet *et al.* (2010) and Joint British Diabetes Societies Inpatient Care Group (2010).

Clinical scenario

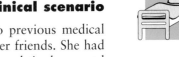

Rosemary Davies, a 34-year-old accountant with no previous medical history, was found unconscious and incontinent by her friends. She had been recovering from flu, complaining of fever, thirst and tiredness, and feeling confused.

Mrs Davies was admitted to the ICU self-ventilating at 32 breaths/minute, HR 120 bpm, BP 80/60 mmHg, CVP 0–1 mmHg, and hypothermic 35.5°C. Blood investigation revealed blood sugar of 40 mmol/litre, Na^+ 150 mmol/litre, K 4.8 mmol/litre, HCO_3^- 19 mmol/litre with metabolic acidosis. A diagnosis of hyperosmolar hyperglycaemic state (HHS) was made.

Q.1 Mrs Davies is extremely hyperglycaemic. Identify the effects of hyperglycaemia that resulted in her admission (hyperglycaemia causes tachycardia, hypothermia, unconsciousness etc. by which physiological process?).

Q.2 An intravenous insulin infusion is commenced. Select and give the rationale for infusion rate in units/hour to correct Mrs Davies's hyperglycaemia. What other factors should be considered in correction of hyperglycaemia?

Q.3 Reflect on patients' blood glucose management in your clinical area, and consider the benefits and limitations of this strategy (e.g. use of sliding scale insulin prescription versus insulin protocols, equipment required, type of insulin, route and rate of administration, life of infusion, dose adjustments, minimum and maximum dose, methods and frequency of blood glucose assessment, inclusion of 10% glucose and potassium supplementation).

Chapter 46

Self-poisoning

Contents

Fundamental knowledge	446
Introduction	447
Antidepressants	447
Paracetamol	448
Illicit drugs	448
Symptoms	450
Airway/breathing	450
Cardiovascular	451
Disability (neurological)	451
Health promotion	452
Implications for practice	453
Summary	453
Support groups	453
Further reading	454
Clinical scenario	454

Fundamental knowledge

Neurotransmission synapse
Cell metabolism

Introduction

Deliberate self-harm (DSH) causes about 140,000 hospital admissions each year in the UK (Bennewith *et al.*, 2002), usually from drug overdose (Boyce *et al.*, 2001). Although only a minority of these need ICU admission, drugs can precipitate crises. Care focuses on:

- physiological support;
- preventing recurrence of self-harming behaviour (psychiatry);
- dealing with underlying psychopathology.

This chapter focuses on physiological support, as specialist psychological care usually follows ICU discharge. However, potential wishes to self-harm during ICU stays should be remembered, and risk factors minimised.

Accidental overdose of therapeutic drugs seldom causes critical illness, so is not specifically discussed. However, critical illness can be caused by self-poisoning with 'street drugs', taken with the intention of achieving pleasure rather than deliberate self-harm. This chapter will therefore discuss some of the more commonly encountered therapeutic and illicit drugs that cause critical illness, their main effects, and medical and nursing care.

Many drugs and chemicals have potentially harmful/fatal effects if taken in sufficient quantity. The drugs that cause most ill health are nicotine (and the hundreds of other toxins in cigarettes) and alcohol (Fogarty and Lingford-Hughes, 2004). However, these are relatively socially acceptable drugs, and usually cause insidious rather than sudden changes in health. Deliberate overdoses are usually impulsive, so easily accessed drugs such as mild analgesics or prescribed antidepressants are used. Although accidental overdose could occur with any drug, life-threatening problems necessitating ICU admission are more likely to occur with illicit ('street') drugs. This chapter focuses on drugs that more often precipitate crises:

- tricyclic antidepressants
- paracetamol
- cocaine
- 'Ecstasy' (MDMA).

Individual drugs are briefly described, followed by discussion of common physiological effects. Self-poisoning with drugs not described often causes similar problems, which will be managed similarly. Many wider issues of nursing care discussed in this chapter can be applied to self-poisoning from other drugs, although readers should check applicability before transferring specific aspects.

Antidepressants

People being treated for depression often have access to, or accumulate, large numbers of antidepressant tablets (such as amitriptyline), while suffering from

447

depression places them at high risk of attempting suicide. Tricyclic antide-pressants are the most common cause of acute poison-related ICU admission in the UK (Greene *et al.*, 2005).

Doses above 10 mg/kg are toxic, and 20–30 mg/kg is potentially lethal (Greene *et al.*, 2005). Symptoms usually begin within an hour of ingestion, and include:

- tachycardia
- sedation
- fitting.

(Greene *et al.*, 2005)

Death usually occurs within 4–6 hours (Finnell and Harris, 2000).

Paracetamol

Paracetamol (= acetaminophen in USA) remains the most common drug used for self-poisoning in the UK, causing nearly half of all poison admissions to hospitals, and 100–200 deaths each year (Wallace *et al.*, 2003). It is the main cause of hyperacute liver failure (McKinley, 2009), and often also causes acute kidney injury (AKI) (Gunning, 2009). It is treated with acetylcysteine (Parvolex®) (Bateman, 2007) or methionine, and system support.

Paracetamol is rapidly absorbed, plasma levels peaking within 1–2 hours of ingestion (Smith, D.H., 2007). The toxic threshold for liver damage is 150 mg/kg in adults; as little as 10–15 grams in 24 hours can cause severe hepatocellular necrosis (Bateman, 2007) because metabolism varies greatly between individuals. Plasma levels exceeding 200 mg/litre at 4 hours or 50 mg/litre at 12 hours usually progress to hepatic failure (Wyncoll, 2009), although severe symptoms may be delayed for two to three days, appearing only after significant, possibly fatal, damage.

Paracetamol overdose is usually impulsive (Turvill *et al.*, 2000; Hawton *et al.*, 2001), so guilt and remorse are likely to become problems for both patients and their families and friends.

Illicit drugs

Paracetamol and antidepressants are usually obtained legally, but 'recreational' or 'street' drugs are obtained, and often produced, illegally. Purity and strength of recreational drugs are often very variable, whether from deliberate dilution (to reduce cost) or chance contamination during non-aseptic illegal manufacture. Different tablets may have dissimilar strengths (Schifano *et al.*, 2006), so even users with previous experience of drugs cannot be sure how each dose will affect them. Accidental 'overdose' occurs easily; individual metabolism and tolerance further influence effects.

Drug use among adolescents is declining, although use of 'club drugs' has increased (Koesters *et al.*, 2002). Cannabis is probably the most widely used recreational drug in the UK (Patton *et al.*, 2002; Fogarty and Lingford-Hughes, 2004), but seldom necessitates ICU admission, so is not included here.

Many recreational drugs (such as cocaine and Ecstasy) are taken to achieve desired effects or mood, not with intent to self-harm. Usually, the desired effect will be pleasure, through either:

- calming/suppressing/reducing or
- stimulating/increasing

central nervous system function. Drugs that stimulate more often cause acute life-threatening emergencies.

Many drugs taken for pleasure become addictive. They replace endogenous neurotransmitters (especially dopamine), causing a 'high' – euphoria, increased libido, and energy. The attractions of many drugs may be seen in clubs; the miseries are more often seen in ICUs. After a few hours the benefits fade, leaving insufficient endogenous neurotransmitters, so causing a 'low' (depression). Drug users often respond by taking further, often larger, doses, becoming progressively addicted or dependent.

Chemical changes in brain tissue cause permanent neurological damage, while effects on other organs often cause acute and sometimes permanent damage. Drugs are also frequently mixed with alcohol, tobacco and other recreational drugs.

Illicit drugs are often transported in body cavities ('body packing'), using plastic bags or condoms, swallowed or inserted into the rectum. The gut is highly vascular, so if bags break drugs are efficiently absorbed. Drug traffickers may be admitted with accidental self-poisoning and, understandably, may be reluctant to admit their continuing rectal drug infusion. Attempts to remove bags may cause further internal spillage (Bulstrode *et al.*, 2002). If drugs have not yet been absorbed, activated charcoal slurry washout may limit absorption within two hours of ingestion (Schofield *et al.*, 1997). Bags may obstruct the gut, causing abdominal pain, distension, vomiting and constipation (Bulstrode *et al.*, 2002). Progress of intact bags can be monitored with abdominal X-rays and CT scans.

Patients may be drug pushers, regular users or novices experimenting with the drug. Patients may be in police custody while in hospital, and know they face prison when they recover. Whatever their personal views, nurses caring for victims have the same professional duty of care as for other patients (NMC, 2008a), so should:

- maintain safe environments;
- treat with unconditional positive regard;
- adopt non-judgemental attitudes.

Cocaine ('coke') has long been used as a therapeutic analgesic, but also has a long history as a recreational drug. It is the most commonly used class A drug in England and Wales (Treadwell and Robinson, 2007) and use is increasing

(Galvin *et al.*, 2010). Mortality is very high – 60 per cent in Galvin *et al.*'s study, although death is usually from long-term use rather than overdose (Albarran and Cox, 2008). *Crack* is modified cocaine and causes similar symptoms.

Amphetamine sulphate ('speed') has similar effects to cocaine, except they usually last far longer. The amphetamine derivative 3–4 methylenedioxy-methamphetamine (MDMA, usually called 'Ecstasy' or 'E') is discussed below, but other amphetamines have similar effects. Amphetamines are hepatotoxic (Mokhlesi *et al.*, 2004).

MDMA ('Ecstasy') is not a new drug, but widespread illicit use is a recent phenomenon. Up to two million tablets are consumed each week (Hall and Henry, 2006). Mortality appears to bear little relation to the number of tablets taken, some people surviving considerable numbers, while single tablets prove fatal to others.

Ketamine ('special K'), used therapeutically as an anaesthetic, is often taken as a cheap alternative to amphetamines. It induces hallucinations, often nightmare-like (Shehabi and Innes, 2002), and can cause nausea, disrupt coordination and provoke schizophrenia. Because psychedelic effects usually disappear after one hour, many users take sequential doses (Ricaurte and McCann, 2005).

Many other street drugs are used, and fashion frequently changes. Effects of different drugs vary; for example, *nitrites* ('poppers') vasodilate (Ricaurte and McCann, 2005).

Symptoms

Gross sympathetic system stimulation is especially likely to precipitate cardiovascular crises (e.g. hypertension, myocardial infarction), and so necessitate admission. But problems may be complicated by impurities in the mixture, mixing with alcohol or other drugs, and the conditions in which the drugs are used – for example, 'clubbing' activities may include vigorous dancing, while costs of drinks may contribute to dehydration and electrolyte imbalances. Care is often complicated by psychological and social problems (Chummun *et al.*, 2010).

If the drug remains in the gut, activated charcoal is usually given. Toxic blood levels may be treated with haemofiltration. If there is an antidote to the drug, that will be started. Otherwise, priorities are system support and psychological care.

Airway/breathing

Many inhaled drugs are smoked, the smoke being far hotter than from cigarettes. Therefore, like burns victims, drug smokers can develop severe laryngeal oedema, necessitating prophylactic intubation. If consciousness is impaired, they may have aspirated. Respiratory failure frequently occurs. Multisystem complications often necessitate intubation and artificial ventilation. Cocaine can cause status asthmaticus, upper airway obstruction, pulmonary hypertension, barotrauma and pulmonary oedema (Mokhlesi *et al.*, 2004). Many drugs cause fluid and electrolyte imbalances and trigger inflammatory responses, causing pulmonary oedema (Welsch *et al.*, 2001). Hypercalcaemia may cause trismus (tightening of jaw muscles – 'lockjaw') and bruxism (jaw-clenching) (Koesters *et al.*, 2002), which may make oral intubation difficult.

Cardiovascular

Sympathetic nervous system stimulation often causes extreme hypertension and tachycardia. Illicit drug self-poisoning victims are usually young, but may have congenital or drug-induced cardiac disease (Ghuran and Nolan, 2000). Intravenous drug abuse ('mainlining') and heavy smoking may have accelerated vascular damage.

Electrolytes and metabolites are often grossly deranged on arrival, including:

- hyperkalaemia;
- hyper-/hyponatraemia (Ricaurte and McCann, 2005; Hall and Henry, 2006; Campbell and Rosner, 2008);
- hypercalcaemia (Brotto and Lee, 2007);
- hypoglycaemia.

Muscle contraction and hypercapnia often cause lactic acidosis (Brotto and Lee, 2007).

Hypermetabolism and 'serotonin syndrome' often induce malignant hyperpyrexia (Crandall *et al.*, 2002; Ricaurte and McCann, 2005; Hall and Henry, 2006), the cause of most Ecstasy-related deaths (Wake, 1995). Malignant hyperthermia should be actively reversed with dantrolene sodium. Ischaemia and rhabdomyolysis may cause AKI (Campbell and Rosner, 2008) – see Chapter 38. Kidneys should be protected with aggressive fluid therapy, but haemofiltration is often needed. Kidney injury exacerbates hyperkalaemia.

Disability (neurological)

Immediate neurological complications are likely to be caused by:

- cerebral vasospasm;
- intracranial hypertension, causing intracranial bleeding, subarachnoid haemorrhage and strokes (Welsch *et al.*, 2001; Treadwell and Robinson, 2007);
- hyponatraemic encephalopathy (Hartung *et al.*, 2002);
- seizures.

Cerebral perfusion and oxygenation should be optimised; antiepileptics may be needed – usually benzodiazepines, although these can exacerbate cardiac instability. Major tranquillisers (such as chlorpromazine) should be avoided as they lower seizure threshold, aggravate hypotension and provoke dysrhythmias (MacConnachie, 1997). Treatment for cerebral oedema is discussed in Chapter 36.

Small-scale studies indicate that long-term use causes chronic neurological and psychiatric problems (Semple *et al.*, 1999; Reneman *et al.*, 2001), including permanent cognitive impairment (Parrott *et al.*, 1998).

The 'low' usually causes generalised fatigue, muscle ache, limited concentration, confusion, anxiety, hypersomnia or insomnia, bizarre and unpleasant dreams, and depression (Chychula and Sciamanna, 2002; Koesters *et al.*, 2002). Survivors often experience frequent and persistent panic attacks ('bad trips'), believing death to be imminent (McGuire *et al.*, 1994).

Patients, relatives and friends often experience guilt about drug use and fear about prosecution. Parents may have been unaware their children were taking drugs. Drug levels in blood and other specimens will be tested for therapeutic purposes, but there may be legal requirements about saving samples or releasing results to the police or other authorities. Staff should check what samples/information police have a right to demand. Passwords will usually be used for telephone calls from the police, and often for family members. Many patients, families and friends are likely to fear what staff will tell the authorities.

Healthcare professionals have a duty of care to all patients. But negative attitudes to patients considered as 'time-wasters', 'bed-blockers', immature or 'mad' or 'sad', may both impair quality of care given, and cause further psychological distress to patients and families. Nurses need to be aware not only of their own attitudes, but attitudes of others, promoting a team approach of unconditional positive regard.

The young age of many illicit drug victims can create uncomfortable reminders for nurses of their own mortality.

Psychiatric referral will often be made following recovery.

Health promotion

With recovery, health promotion for the patient and other significant people, who may be family or friends, can prevent future crises. With accidental overdose of prescribed medicines, prescriptions should be reviewed and patients should understand the correct dose and any symptoms of over- or under-dose. Those who have deliberately self-harmed should be referred for psychiatric support. Users of illicit drugs may also benefit from referral to psychiatric or other support services. Health education can raise awareness of dangers and suggest safer ways to take drugs, so users can make their own informed decisions. Friends and families may need support from specialist agencies, such as support groups or counsellors. When providing information to families and friends, nurses should remember their duty of confidentiality to their patients.

Realisation that drugs are not as safe as they previously thought may make patients and friends receptive to health education, so ICU nurses can provide useful information and contacts. However, users often have greater knowledge about recreational drugs than nurses, and may have different values and beliefs;

adopting moralistic/righteous attitudes may cause alienation. ICU nurses should assess individual needs and offer what support they can. However, they will usually not possess the specialist knowledge of drugs involved, and should therefore work within their limitations, using specialist services that are available locally.

Implications for practice

- Self-poisoning from drugs can affect all major body systems; vital signs should be closely monitored.
- Medical management centres around reversing/removing drugs if possible and supporting failing systems.
- Toxbase and the National Poisons Information Service can provide practical information for healthcare staff about drugs causing ICU admission.
- Peak effects often occur within hours of ingestion, although wide variations occur, partly depending on dose and individual tolerance and metabolism.
- Suicide attempts may cause guilt and/or anger among families and friends. Nurses should encourage families to express their needs and emotions, but may need to involve counselling or other services. Listening is often more useful (cathartic) than replying to guilt or anger.
- Friends and victims are often reluctant to share information with staff, and often experience guilt and fears.
- Nurses, and other healthcare professionals, have a duty of care to patients, regardless of the cause of illness.
- Nurses should maintain their duty of confidentiality (unless specifically exempted by statute law).
- ICU nurses may be able to offer health information about drugs or support groups.
- Psychiatric support should be offered to those who self-harm.

Summary

Self-harm may necessitate ICU admission. Immediate care necessarily focuses on resuscitation and system support. As well as multisystem physiological problems, not usual for younger people, users (and friends) often experience anxiety or guilt. Care therefore needs to integrate urgent multisystem physiological support with skilful psychological care. Caring for such patients is challenging and can cause distress, but holistic nursing care can contribute significantly to every aspect of recovery.

Support groups

Families Anonymous: 0845 1200 660
Drugline Ltd, Drug Advisory Bureau: 0208 692 4975
Turning Point, Grove Park, Camberwell, London SE5 8LG: 0207 274 4883

Further reading

Articles on individual drugs periodically appear in medical, and sometimes nursing, journals; those referenced in the relevant sections of this chapter are likely to be useful for nurses wanting to know more about individual drugs. Brotto and Lee (2007) and Chummun *et al.* (2010) provide useful nursing perspectives, while Ricaurte and McCann (2005) and Greene *et al.* (2005) provide the medical aspects. Betts *et al.* (1999), written by the parents of probably the most famous victim of Ecstasy, provide valuable psychosocial insights. Galvin *et al.* (2010) researched outcome of cocaine victims in ICUs.

Clinical scenario

Lisa Young is 25 years old and was admitted to the ICU ten hours after ingesting 75 amitriptyline (50 mg) tablets. A plasma toxicology screen tested positive for heroin and methadone. Miss Young's urine also tested positive for opioids, benzodiazepine, cocaine and cannabis. Paracetamol and salicylate were not detected. Miss Young is not receiving any sedation, and she is agitated and non-compliant with care. She has a urinary catheter, but has removed her central venous and arterial cannulae.

Other results are:

Glasgow Coma Scale (GCS) 6   (E1, V1, M5)
All limbs flexing spontaneously without any stimuli
Both pupils are equal size at 2 mm and increasingly dilated with a brisk response
    to light

Respiration rate	34 bpm
SpO_2	97% on FiO_2 of 0.6
Temperature	38.1°C
HR	135 sinus bpm
BP	127/68 mmHg
Capillary refill	< 1 seconds with warm peripheries

Skin feels hot and dry, mouth and tongue are dry
Blood glucose   6.1 mmol/litre
Urine output over previous 4 hours was 1650ml, 500ml, 680 ml, 250ml

---

Q.1 Explain the effects of an amitriptyline overdose on Miss Young's cardiovascular system and identify the most common associated arrhythmias. What is the likely cause and significance of her urine output and temperature?

Q.2 Consider interventions to reduce Miss Young's risk of seizures and dysrhythmias and justify appropriate fluid management. Discuss other strategies used to monitor and minimise other complications.

Q.3 Review the long-term effects and outcome of this type of overdose. Evaluate the advice and support offered to patients like Miss Young in your clinical area, including availability of specialist referrals and support groups.

Part X

Professional

Chapter 47

Professional perspectives

Contents

Fundamental knowledge	457
Introduction	458
Accountability	458
Limits of accountability	460
Conflicts of accountability	460
Accountability in practice	460
Record keeping	461
Implications for practice	462
Summary	462
Further reading	462
Clinical questions	462

Fundamental knowledge

Nursing and Midwifery Council (NMC) publications:

■ *The Code*
■ *Standards for Medicines Management*

Local hospital and unit policies, guidelines and patient group directions

Introduction

Every nurse is accountable for their own practice (NMC, 2008a), but ICUs often heighten problems due to:

- critical conditions of patients;
- differing roles of ICU nurses (see Chapter 1);
- increased technology.

Nurses are often trusted to perform specialised tasks. But enthusiasm to develop skills should be tempered by considerations of safety. Unsafe clinical practice was the largest single category of complaints made to the Healthcare Commission in 2004–2006 (Tingle, 2007). This chapter explores issues of what professional practice means, accountability of nurses, professional standards and the civil law of negligence, issues affecting all registered nurses.

Professionalism necessitates accepting:

- autonomy
- accountability
- responsibility.

Nursing care should be in patients' best interests. Humans are fallible, so mistakes are inevitable. But risk management seeks to minimise mistakes by altering situations that contribute to error. Nurses should therefore report concerns about actual or potential risks. Where patients are endangered, a clinical incident form should be completed, which will be reviewed by the Trust's Clinical Risk department.

In law, as in life, we are accountable both for what we do (acts) and for what we do not do (omissions). So conscious or unconscious decisions not to act may be called to account.

Professionals are individually accountable for their own practice (NMC, 2008a), so should continue to develop professionally, updating skills and knowledge. Unfortunately, many employers underinvest in their nursing staff's development, forcing nurses to invest in themselves (Joshua-Amadi, 2002).

Accountability

Dimond (2008) identifies four arenas of professional accountability and adds that accountability between these arenas may conflict:

- criminal law
- civil law
- employer's contract
- professional body (NMC).

For civil actions of *negligence* to succeed, three conditions must be met:

- a duty of care must exist;
- that duty of care must have been breached;
- resulting harm must have been reasonably foreseeable.

Civil cases failing to establish any one condition on the 'balance of probabilities' cannot make a conviction. 'Negligence' in different contexts, such as industrial tribunals or the NMC's Professional Conduct Committee, need not carry these same conditions.

While all four of Dimond's arenas can apply to nurses, conflicts with criminal law are rare. Few laws specifically mention nurses or nursing, so legal account-ability and rights of nurses are usually the same as for any other citizen. Any individual suffering harm from another may sue that person through civil law; negligence and assault with battery are the charges most frequently brought against healthcare staff. Negligence is briefly outlined later; assault is covered in Chapter 3 (under 'Safety') and Chapter 25 (under 'Ethical and health issues'); nursing accountability through civil law is comprehensively covered in Dimond (2008).

A *duty of care* clearly exists to patients allocated to nurses' care. Breach of that duty will usually form the basis of any case. So any case reaching court almost certainly fulfils the first criterion for negligence. The condition least likely to be established is the third. There are two parts to this third condition:

- breach of care must directly cause *harm*;
- harm suffered must have been *reasonably foreseeable*.

If the harm may reasonably have been caused by other factors (judged by the balance of probabilities), links to breach of duty of care cannot be clearly established. Even where harm can be linked to breach of care, it may not be reasonably foreseeable: all drugs and treatments have adverse effects, and nurses should be aware of common effects of whatever they give, and of recorded allergies of patients, but cannot reasonably know, or be held accountable for, every possible effect. However, as professional practitioners, nurses are expected to act with reasonable autonomy, so decision-making should be underpinned by sufficient knowledge to evaluate relative benefits and risks from possible actions and omissions ('reasonable' and 'sufficient' might be evaluated by the '*Bolam test*' – see Glossary). This places an onus on both individual nurses and their employers to maintain relevant knowledge and skills.

The primary, and implicitly primarily important, clause of *The Code* (NMC, 2008a) states: 'make the care of people your first concern'. However, employers pay salaries; nurses failing to satisfy employers' requirements may find them-selves unemployed. Pragmatically, resisting instructions of employers, managers or senior staff can prove difficult.

Employment contracts and expectations vary; breach of contract can lead to litigation, or more often dismissal. Although this chapter focuses on pro-fessional accountability (through the NMC), readers should remember their concurrent accountability to other arenas.

Accountability raises two main questions:

■ What are the limits of accountability?
■ How can conflicts of accountability be reconciled?

Limits of accountability

Individual accountability and professional autonomy may seem desirable ideals, but quality healthcare also relies on multidisciplinary teamwork (Mullally, 2001). Responsibility is inevitably partly shared between disciplines and members of the same discipline. Delegation of particular tasks varies between units, and may vary within each unit depending on whoever is best able to perform that task at that time: endotracheal suction may be performed by anaesthetists intubating patients, and later by physiotherapists and nurses.

While only individuals on a professional register have professional account-ability (i.e. can be removed from the professional register), in law each mentally competent adult remains legally accountable for their actions. Civil law precedent (*Nettleship* v *Weston*, 1971) establishes learner/student accountability, despite their inexperience or lack of knowledge (Dimond, 2008). Learners and junior staff may be individually sued if they cause harm, hence the importance of professional indemnity.

Local, national and international guidelines are widely available, including via the internet. Individual and local factors may affect applicability and appropriateness of guidelines to individual patient care, but where guidelines are generally reliable, such as those from the National Institute for Health and Clinical Excellence (NICE), failure to follow them could result in legal action (Samanta and Samanta, 2004). However, apparent authoritative guidelines can be legally overruled, as shown by *Burke* v *GMC*, 2004, which overruled the 2002 BMA guidelines on withdrawing treatment. Each nurse must individually decide whether (and if so, how) they should perform tasks.

Conflicts of accountability

Few tasks are ascribed by law to particular professions (Cox, 2010), and the DH (2006) encourages extension of nursing practice.

In civil law, standards of care expected from qualified nurses are those of the ordinary skilled nurse ('Bolam test'). Failure to meet professional standards may also cause removal from the professional register. However, where nursing roles are expanded to work previously performed by other professions (e.g. junior doctors), the standards expected are those of the other professions (Caplin-Davies, 1999). So nurses have a professional duty to ensure they have adequate knowledge and skills to perform tasks they undertake.

Accountability in practice

Patient group directions (PGDs) are legally recognised prescriptions (DH, 2000c), but made for patient groups rather than individual patients. They are agreed locally by relevant professions – usually doctors, nurses and pharmacists. Where both patients and nursing staff fulfil agreed criteria for each direction, nurses can give specified drugs. This facilitates prompt administration, and may prevent complications caused by delay. Kingston *et al.* (2002) describe a PGD for haemofiltration.

Complaints are a familiar aspect of contemporary healthcare. They highlight deficiencies in services provided, provide a conduit for public accountability, and may diffuse concerns that would otherwise end in litigation. However, they have unfortunately encouraged defensive nursing. A significant number of complaints result from failures of communication (Tingle, 2007); ironically, those least ill often complain most, so encouraging diversion of time away from those needing it most. Nurses have a professional duty to prioritise care (acts and omissions) so that actions can be justified.

Litigation consumes millions of the NHS budget – in 2008–2009 the NHS Litigation Authority paid £807 million in damages, and an additional £8.8 million in out-of-court settlements. Fear of litigation sometimes fosters an ethos of secrecy that conflicts with political rhetoric and professional philosophies of empowerment through providing information. Minimising litigation risks effectively creates substantial income generation, but has the added human value of fostering trust between nurses and patients. Vicarious liability (employers being legally liable for actions of their employees, provided employees follow employers' policies (Cox, 2010)) has been made more robust through the Clinical Negligence Scheme for Trusts (CNST).

ICU nurses spend much time administering medicines, so should be familiar with the *Standards for Medicines Management* (NMC, 2008b). Although the whole document is professionally binding for all nurses, some of its most significant clauses for ICU practice include:

- You must know the therapeutic uses of the medicine to be administered, its normal dosage, side effects, precautions and contraindications (part of standard 8).
- Registrants must not prepare substances for injection in advance of their immediate use or administer medication drawn into a syringe or container by another practitioner when not in their presence (standard 14).

Record keeping

In addition to recording observations, nursing records should be detailed enough both to provide a basis for immediate care, and to provide information in the event of future enquiries. Records should be factual, as under the Freedom of Information Act 2001 individuals have the right to copies of records about them. Unfortunately, nursing documentation is often poor (Saranto and Kinnunen, 2009). Like any written records, nursing documentation may be used in a court of law; this does not make them a 'legal document'; however, unlike informal notes, nursing records require clear identification of date, time, patient and nurse. If care is not recorded, courts may assume that it was not given.

Implications for practice

- ■ Concerns should be reported. Where patient safety is compromised, clinical incident forms should be completed.
- ■ Guidelines are useful resources, but are not infallible, and do not replace individual accountability.
- ■ Each nurse remains individually accountable for their actions.
- ■ Nurses should only undertake tasks if competent to do so, refusing any task they do not consider they can safely complete.
- ■ Nursing care should be prioritised by patients' best interests.
- ■ Each nurse is responsible for ensuring adequate and current knowledge for their own practice.
- ■ Nurses should be familiar with local policies, procedures, guidelines and standards.

Summary

Society's demands, and pace of change, are both likely to continue to increase. ICU nurses often respond positively to challenging and changing work, but enthusiasm should be tempered by considerations of safe practice, and how far care meets the holistic needs of each patient. The human and financial costs of professional malpractice can be high for each nurse, employer and patient.

Further reading

Readers should be familiar with NMC publications. Dimond (2008) is the key text on nursing and the law, while Cox (2010) provides a useful summary of the issue.

Clinical questions

Q.1 Identify areas of accountability and responsibility within the ICU. Reflect on the main areas of accountability in your practice while supervising novice ICU nurses.

Q.2 A colleague has failed to attend consecutive mandatory training sessions (resuscitation skills, moving and handling, drug administration, drug calculations, medical devices) for over three years, despite being rostered and given study leave. Identify who is accountable when this nurse makes an error in practice. How should this situation be managed to ensure professional accountability and vicarious liability?

Q.3 You administer a new trial drug that is currently unlicensed in the UK. The patient suffers associated adverse effects and dies. Who is accountable for the patient's death? Examine the extent of nurse accountability in this situation (nurse's knowledge of drug administration, awareness of adverse effects, appropriateness of drug etc.).

Chapter 48

Transferring critically ill patients

Contents

Fundamental knowledge	463
Introduction	464
Planning	464
Airway	465
Breathing	465
Circulation	466
Disability	466
Exposure	466
During transport	466
Implications for practice	467
Summary	467
Further reading	467
Clinical scenario	468

Fundamental knowledge

Local transfer guidelines
Local transfer equipment

Introduction

Critically ill patients may be transferred for clinical (to specialist centres) and non-clinical (bed shortage) reasons. Between 1994 and 2004 interhospital transfers doubled, at least 5 per cent of adult ICU patients being transferred (Smith *et al.*, 2004). Numbers transferred continue to increase (Fried *et al.*, 2010). While some of these are to meet patient needs, numbers of non-clinical transfers have not significantly changed (Critical Care Stakeholder Forum, 2005). Interhospital transfer of critically ill patients creates many risks; Beckmann *et al.* (2004) found serious adverse events occurred in nearly one-third of transfers. So transfers should be managed by experienced and reliable nursing and medical staff. Dedicated transfer teams improve outcomes (Andrews *et al.*, 2008b), but these are not generally available at present. Most ICU nurses will therefore assist with transfers moderately frequently during their careers. This chapter provides an overview of how nurses can prepare for safer journeys. It therefore uses the ABCDE approach.

Transfers within hospitals (e.g. to CT scanning) should create fewer risks, but are sometimes given less priority and foresight than external transfers; this chapter largely focuses on external transfers, although many principles apply to internal transfers as well, which should be planned just as carefully.

This chapter focuses on ambulance transfer of level 3 patients, but many principles apply to transfer by other means (helicopter, air ambulance) and level 2 patients. Staff involved in aircraft transfer should seek advice on any special issues and requirements before leaving– for example, plane transfers are usually over longer distances, so are more likely to be at higher altitudes, where differences in atmospheric pressure are more likely to affect equipment. Less equipment and monitoring may be needed for level 2 patients, although risks should not be underestimated.

Planning

Once outside the ICU doors, staff have to rely on whatever and whoever is at hand or readily contactable. So while every possible eventuality cannot be predicted, risks should be assessed and safety maintained. Most units have guidelines and equipment for transfer, but it is the individual nurse's responsibility to ensure safety. Allow for the unexpected – ambulances and lifts can break down.

Intubated patients should be accompanied by a nurse and doctor; unintubated patients are usually accompanied only by a nurse. The nurse should have previous experience of transfers (unless gaining the experience by shadowing another). Many Trusts provide programmes to prepare staff for transfers, and usually require that only nurses who have completed the programme accompany transfers. The accompanying doctor should be an anaesthetist, in case airway problems occur, but should also have sufficient experience of intensive care to be able to manage other problems safely.

Problems and clinical incidents are often caused by equipment failure, or failure to secure equipment (Everest and Munford, 2009; Fried *et al.*, 2010).

Both equipment and medicines should be rationalised so there is sufficient, without excess. Unnecessary equipment may delay transfers, and access to what is needed. Infusions should be minimised (usually limited to sedatives and inotropes). Emergency drugs and equipment should be taken. Many units have transfer bags, containing resuscitation drugs, endotracheal tubes and suction equipment, but the transferring nurse should check equipment before leaving the unit. If the patient is ventilated, a portable ventilator is necessary. If possible, this should be attached about an hour before transfer, so that blood gases can be checked in time for any necessary changes to be made, enabling stabilisation of the patient on the ventilator before leaving the unit.

With internal transfers, porters are often asked to fetch patients about a quarter of an hour before the time of booked procedures. Monitoring will be needed; this should be rationalised so that it is sufficient for safety without being excessive. For some procedures, there may be specific limitations on equipment (e.g. some MRI scanners cannot be used with any metal – including ECG electrodes). Appropriate (usually narrow) alarm limits should be set, as in hospital corridors it may not always be possible to see all equipment con- tinuously, and for radiographical and some other procedures staff usually have to leave the patient, with only a distant view through a window.

Spare drugs may be needed, and the doctor may request specific drugs for transfer. Equipment should be secured safely; many units have a transfer trolley. Spares should be taken of anything that may be removed (e.g. ECG electrodes in some MRI scanners). For external transfer, patients are often deeply sedated, and sometimes paralysed, so their body should be appropriately protected.

Transfer ambulances are usually well equipped, but the ambulance will usually be an unfamiliar environment to both the nurse and the doctor, so a member of the ambulance crew should accompany the patient to access whatever is needed.

Family will not usually be able to accompany patients in the ambulance, but if possible parents should accompany children (Davies *et al.*, 2005).

Often with limited time to prepare, ABCDE assessment is useful.

Airway

- Check the patient's airway is secure and safe.
- Check transfer kits contain spare intubation and suction equipment in appropriate sizes.

Breathing

- Check the portable ventilator.
- Establish the patient on the portable ventilator about an hour before transfer, giving time to check blood gases and make appropriate adjustments to settings.
- Take spare batteries and sufficient oxygen.

- Monitor saturation and end-tidal carbon dioxide (etCO$_2$) (ICS, 2002).
- Set appropriate alarm limits.
- Observe respiratory rate and depth.
- If patients are ventilated, oxygen supply, inspired oxygen concentration, ventilator settings and airway pressure should be monitored (ICS, 2002).

Circulation

- Ambulance transfer, and moreso aircraft transfer, can negatively affect body function. For example, acceleration exaggerates hypertension and deceleration exaggerates hypotension, so vascular filling should be optimised before leaving the unit (ICS, 2002).
- Patients should have at least two large-bore cannulae (ICS, 2002).
- Ensure sufficient inotropes are prepared.
- Check resuscitation drugs (usually in a transfer kit).
- ECG, blood pressure (preferably invasive) and temperature should be monitored during transfer (ICS, 2002).
- With some transfers, other equipment (e.g. intra-aortic balloon pump), monitoring and infusions may be indicated.

Disability

- Ensure desired levels of analgesia, sedation and paralysis are achieved before leaving the unit.
- Ensure sufficient analgesics, sedatives and paralysing agents are prepared.

Exposure

- Check lines and limbs are safe on transfer to the transport trolley.
- Protect any vulnerable parts of the patient's body (e.g. eyes may need a protective cover to prevent corneal abrasions).
- Ensure access is available to any cannulae, infusions or other equipment likely to be needed during transfer.

During transport

The law requires that all passengers wear seatbelts; as this includes doctors and nurses, any interventions that necessitate leaving seats also necessitate stopping the vehicle. Before the vehicle starts, ensure monitoring and infusions are visible, and that appropriate access is possible. Each critical care network should have its own documentation for transfer, including observation charts. Frequency and type of observations will usually be at the discretion of the nurse, but should be complete enough for early detection of problems, and to withstand scrutiny should actions be brought before the court or professional bodies.

Ambulances should have a mobile telephone so the source or destination hospital can be contacted (ICS, 2002). Should problems, such as breakdown, necessitate leaving the ambulance, high-visibility clothing should be worn. Within hospital buildings, in the event of crisis in the corridor, generally it is best to seek help from the nearest ward/department, but avoid non-essential delays in reaching the destination. In the event of cardiac arrest, 2222 is the national number (remember to state which hospital).

Ambulances normally return staff to their hospital, but in case ambulances are diverted, it is wise to have means of paying for public transport, and to know your own hospital's telephone number.

Implications for practice

- Prepare carefully, ensuring adequate supplies without excess.
- Be familiar with local equipment, guidelines and documentation.
- Assess risks and needs, using an ABCDE approach.
- Check all equipment and supplies (including emergency drugs, spare airways and suction) before leaving the unit.
- If using a portable ventilator, commence it early enough to check arterial blood gases before leaving the unit.
- Minimise infusions, but take sufficient spare syringes/vials of essential drugs.
- If patient is hypovolaemic, ensure adequate filling before leaving the unit.
- During transfer, maintain essential observations.
- If you have any concerns, alert the doctor, ambulance crew or any other appropriate staff.

Summary

Transfers occur for clinical (patient need) and non-clinical (bed shortage) reasons. All staff will almost inevitably transfer patients, so skills should be developed through accompanying more experienced colleagues on transfer if possible, and attending any local development programmes. Transfer exposes patients to potential risks, but these can be minimised through careful planning. Take sufficient, but not excessive, equipment for the transfer, and ensure sufficient supplies of batteries and oxygen for the journey.

Further reading

The Intensive Care Society (ICS, 2002) provides clear guidance for transporting critically ill (level 3) patients, much of which is also applicable to level 2 patients. Staff transferring patients should be familiar with local protocols and guidance.

Clinical scenario

Richard Jones is 54 years old and was admitted eight days ago with community-acquired pneumonia, which failed to respond to any of the antibiotics prescribed during his admission. He has progressively deteriorated, and has now developed ARDS and AKI. He is fully ventilated, on 100 per cent oxygen, PEEP 20 cmH$_2$O, and reverse ratio ventilation (1:1). Drugs infusions include morphine 10 mg/hour, midazolam 10 mg/hour, atracurium 25 mg/hour, and noradrenaline 0.5 μg/kg/minute. Prone positioning has been unsuccessfully attempted, and his gases continue to deteriorate. Currently they are:

pH	7.210
PaCO$_2$	8.75
PaO$_2$	7.15
HCO$_3^-$	16.2
SBE	−8.3

Mr Jones is to be transferred to the regional unit for extracorporeal membrane oxygenation (ECMO). Transfer time is estimated to be about one hour by emergency ambulance. You will accompany him during transfer.

Q.1 List the equipment, drugs and personnel that you consider will be needed for safe transfer. Include specific details (e.g. quantities of drugs, qualifications of personnel). Do you know where to locate all of the equipment on your unit?

Q.2 Review the transfer proformas/documentation used on your unit. Which parts are and are not applicable to Mr Jones's transfer? What observations would you want to undertake during transfer, and how often would you take these?

Q.3 From reading this chapter, what do you think are the six complications that are most likely to occur during transfer? How would you prepare to minimise these risks?

Q.4 Reflect on transfers you have experienced, and those you have heard colleagues talk about. What problems occurred? How could you avoid similar problems in future transfers?

Chapter 49

Managing the ICU

Contents

Introduction   470
Starting to manage   470
Time out 1   470
Morale   473
Time out 2   474
Staffing levels   475
During the shift   475
Time out 3   476
Implications for practice   476
Summary   477
Further reading   477
Clinical questions   477

Introduction

Staff who have gained necessary bedside nursing experience, and any required educational developments or qualifications, may plan managerial experience as part of their professional development, or find one day they are the most senior person on duty (possibly due to sickness of senior staff) and are therefore expected to manage the unit for that shift. This chapter provides a trouble-shooting introduction for staff not normally in charge of their units (hence the direct address to readers).

There is noticeably little literature in ICU nursing journals advising staff how to develop management skills. As many staff are unlikely to resource management journals unless undertaking management courses, this consigns development of management skills to the 'sitting with Nellie' ethos so antithetical to evidence-based nursing. Evidence and theory for nurse management is often, as here, either drawn from management outside healthcare, or is about senior healthcare management, such as lead nurse and team leader roles. When specifically discussing the shiftleader of the shift, this chapter uses 'shiftleader', reserving 'manager' either for more senior managers, or for evidence about senior roles that may also be applicable to shiftleaders.

Much has been written about management, mostly from industrial perspectives, although there is a growing body of literature on health service management. Many principles of industrial management or managing other healthcare areas are applicable to ICUs.

Starting to manage

Each unit functions slightly differently, depending on its size, location, skill mix, patient groups, local traditions and other factors. Traditions, and so expectations of staff, can help guide shiftleaders, who should not be afraid of drawing on experience and views of others. Shiftleaders should also draw on any previous experiences (professional or social) that are transferable to managing the ICU.

Staff may look to the shiftleader (nurse in charge) for direction. Shiftleaders therefore need sufficient knowledge to provide information. Some information may be factual, some may be local requirements and expectations, but much will be sharing experience and ideas to help others make clinical decisions. There are often no right or wrong answers, just different ways of doing things.

Time out 1

Compare previous experience of management (professional or social) with how you have seen others manage the ICU where you work. Note down significant differences. Reflect on why these differences may be necessary. Note what you would do differently, and why.

This chapter therefore raises issues that different readers may disagree about. Options, rather than answers, are usually provided; these issues serve their purpose if they help readers clarify their own values.

Vaughan and Pillmoor (1989) suggest that management is getting the work done through people. A good shiftleader is a good team leader (Firth-Cozens, 2001), enabling other people to do their work. Drucker (1974) identifies five roles for managers:

- setting objectives;
- organising;
- motivating and communicating;
- measuring targets;
- developing people, including themselves.

The shiftleader should establish constructive working conditions at the start of each shift, enabling development of staff's individual strengths and skills, while recognising individual needs and limitations. Managers should individually assess and proactively plan and respond to needs for each shift, rather than seek to impose their own agendas on staff.

You may remember most patients from your previous shift; if not, briefly assess patients before taking handover. You may need to walk through your unit to take handover, but, if not, a brief look at the unit can suggest both the number and dependency of patients. Many units have data sheets providing brief synopses of patients.

Managers rely on their staff to achieve the work, so staff are the shiftleader's most important resource. Staff numbers are important – are there enough staff for patients already on the unit and expected/potential admissions? Staffing levels were discussed in Chapter 1, although the ratios 1:1 for level 3 patients and 1:2 for level 2 patients reflect medical condition more than nursing care. But abilities and qualities of staff are also important. 'Skill mix' is more than simply counting numbers of staff at each grade. Some staff need more support than others; each has different experience, knowledge and skills to draw on. Most staff will probably be known to you, so scanning the off-duty roster helps your planning; with new or unfamiliar staff (e.g. temporary), you may gain insight into their qualities by asking about their experience and what they feel able and not able to do.

Allocating staff may be guided by managerial structures, such as teams. Specific allocation should consider:

- maintaining patient safety;
- optimising patient treatment;
- developing and supporting staff.

Safety during break cover should also be considered: two junior nurses may safely manage adjacent patients when both are present, but become unsafe if caring for two patients through covering each other's breaks. Nurse managers remain accountable for their actions; unsafe allocation breaches *The Code* (NMC, 2008a).

The Health and Safety at Work Act 1974 places specific requirements on managers (and employees) to ensure workplaces are safe; the shiftleader also has wider moral responsibilities for health and safety of their staff and patients. Fire exits should remain clear and accessible at all times and safety and emergency equipment should be complete and in working order. Emergency equipment varies between units, but may include the resuscitation trolley, intubation trolley and (on cardiothoracic units) thoracotomy pack. Any environmental hazards should be minimised and, where possible, removed.

The shiftleader is responsible for all patients on their unit, even if some responsibilities are devolved to team/area subleaders. Following handover, the shiftleader should visit each patient to make their own assessment, identify the needs of each bedside nurse, and pass on any relevant additional information or expectations. Allow sufficient time for bedside nurses to take individual handovers, complete their own safety checks, and make their own patient assessments; seeking information before bedside nurses can fully assimilate it creates stress for the nurse without providing information for shiftleaders. Looking through each patient's notes gives bedside nurses time to complete initial assessments and checks, while giving shiftleaders information that may have been missed in handover. Relevant aspects should then be passed on to the bedside nurse.

The shiftleader should ensure imminent shifts are adequately covered: check staff numbers and initiate booking of any additional staff required. Numbers of staff needed for each shift may vary with:

- number, location and dependency of patients;
- skill mix of other staff;
- anticipated specific needs, such as transfer or procedures.

Other services (e.g. equipment suppliers/repair) may also need to be contacted.

The shiftleader may have to assume direct patient care, but this causes role conflict between responsibility to the whole unit as shiftleader and individual responsibility to your patient, and limits your availability to other members of staff. The experience of many nurses in charge who also assume direct patient care is that their patient tends to get neglected. The BACCN standards (Bray *et al.*, 2009) state that units with more than six beds require a supernumerary clinical coordinator. Instead, it may be reasonable to allocate two patients to one member of staff; the appropriateness or otherwise of assuming direct patient care necessarily remains an individual decision, based on resources available, and remembering that you remain accountable for whatever decision you make.

Endacott (1999) identifies four key aspects of shift leadership:

- presence (availability);
- information gathering (from bedside nurses);

■ supportive involvement (e.g. fetching equipment, checking drugs, reassuring staff);

■ direct involvement (taking over from bedside nurses when they are away or unable to cope).

Shiftleaders may also coordinate services, contacting other people or departments, or liaising with staff on the unit. Shiftleaders should be present during ward rounds so that they are aware of current plans, and can contribute to discussion, support staff and coordinate activity. Shiftleaders need to maintain clinical skills and credibility; with career progression and increasing management duties, staff may need to identify shifts when they assume direct patient care without unit management responsibilities.

The shiftleader role can therefore be very demanding. The busy-ness of most units, together with limited staffing resources, may mean that ideals are not always met; crisis management is often unavoidable. Like bedside nurses, shiftleaders should therefore prioritise their workload, aiming to achieve as much as they reasonably can in the time given. Shiftleaders, like bedside nurses, often work unpaid overtime to complete their work. While the motivation for this is understandable, it is morally questionable, and arguably provides an unhealthy example for other staff. Shiftleaders should therefore aim to ensure they, and their staff, leave the unit as near to the end of paid time as reasonably possible.

Morale

Shiftleaders are responsible for enabling others to achieve their work, so should motivate and communicate (Drucker, 1974). Nursing demands high levels of cognitive, affective and psychomotor skills, so the ability of staff to realise their potential is affected by morale. Maintaining staff and unit morale is therefore a management priority (Joshua-Amadi, 2002; Erlen, 2004) – loyal staff are more likely to support shiftleaders during crises.

Management theory often identifies styles of leadership as authoritarian, laissez-faire and democratic. Democratic or authoritarian leaders use their power and authority to achieve goals and objectives (Firth-Cozens and Mowbray, 2001). The traditional authoritarian ethos of healthcare has arguably been increasingly replaced by promoting democratic involvement and autonomy. For example, the 'blame' culture should be replaced by one of 'safety' (DH, 2000b), which recognises that errors will occur and that, if errors are reported, we can learn from our mistakes (NPSA, 2008b) and change practice.

An alternative approach to management is 'transformational' leadership, which seeks to transform the culture of care through:

■ staff empowerment
■ practice development
■ developing other workplace characteristics.

(Manley, 2004)

Time out 2

Reflect on the different styles of management you have witnessed and experienced. Make one list of benefits of each style, and another of problems each did or could have caused.

Empowering staff through resources, support and information improves nurses' practice (Manojilovich, 2005).

Different styles of management may be appropriate in different situations. For example, authoritarianism is usually the most useful way to manage a cardiac arrest.

People respond to the way they are treated, and this applies as much to staff as to patients. Shiftleaders therefore need good interpersonal skills and respect for their staff. They should seek to empower and value their staff. Staff who are actively involved are likely to provide better care, so negotiation is a core management skill. But shiftleaders also have a professional duty to maintain standards. If they observe unsatisfactory practices, they should approach staff constructively, identifying why staff are acting that way (rationale, knowledge base), and treating incidents as developmental learning opportunities rather than belittling and humiliating experiences for the junior nurse (or possibly shiftleaders). If patient safety is compromised, shiftleaders may need to act before discussion.

Breaks from work provide a psychological coping mechanism. European working time regulations are prescriptive, including the right to 20-minute breaks every six hours. Delayed, compromised or missed breaks often cause dissatisfaction, so ensuring smooth (and safe) organisation of breaks for staff is an important managerial duty. Organising break relief varies between units and shifts; where units have a system that works and is familiar to staff, this should be followed. Shiftleaders may need to assume some direct patient responsibilities to cover breaks; this can also provide shiftleaders with valuable opportunities to assess patients, and the nurse's skills and needs. Possible conflicts with managerial duties (above) should be considered, especially if relieving for breaks in inaccessible areas (e.g. side rooms). Shiftleaders should also ensure they have breaks themselves, as (like their staff) they are less likely to be able to function effectively without reasonable breaks.

Ideally, staff should take breaks away from their workspace, but busy shifts may sometimes prevent this. If full breaks cannot be taken, providing refreshments within the clinical area (this task could be delegated) may help staff function safely and maintain morale. Staff needing breaks are likely to function inefficiently, give less empathy to others, and be more difficult to motivate.

When situations are particularly stressful, shiftleaders may be able to support staff by offering additional 'stress breaks', making themselves (and other experienced staff) available when necessary, and by acknowledging the stress of the situation.

474

ICU work is unpredictable; workload will sometimes exceed resources, so shiftleaders and staff should identify priorities, accepting that some lesser priorities are not always achieved. Shiftleaders unable to offer ideal support to staff can still build team rapport and loyalty by acknowledging others' stress.

Staffing levels

Staff levels should be individualised to patient and unit needs, although there are recommended minimum staffing levels – see Chapter 1. If shiftleaders consider unit, patient or staff safety is compromised through inadequate staff (or any other problem they are unable to resolve), they should inform senior managers, who have (higher) responsibility for the unit.

During the shift

Shiftleaders who have established mechanisms for staff to work effectively have achieved their most important role, but throughout the remainder of the shift, shiftleaders should ensure the unit continues to run smoothly, solving problems as they occur and providing a resource (knowledge, experience) for, and support to, more junior staff.

Staff need to feel confidence in their shiftleader. While shiftleaders usually have more experience and knowledge than their staff, each member of staff has potential to contribute knowledge, experience or values, and shiftleaders should be prepared to learn from, as well as guide and teach, their staff. Like all nurses, shiftleaders should acknowledge the limits of their own knowledge and competence (NMC, 2008a).

Staff need to feel confident that they can approach their shiftleader, so shiftleaders should show positive attitudes and remain accessible, including spending most of their time in the main patient-care area.

The shiftleader is a link between unit nurses and other hospital staff, facilitating active involvement of bedside nurses in ward rounds (Manias and Street, 2001). If medical review of patients does not involve bedside nurses, shiftleaders often become links between medical and nursing staff. Similarly, information to/from other hospital departments, or telephone messages from family members, are often siphoned through the nurse-in-charge.

Shiftleaders may be pressurised to accept patients because there is an empty bed, there appear to be enough staff, or because patients need ICU admission. Rationing is an unfortunate reality of healthcare, and when an 'ultimate' area such as ICU is involved, pressures cannot always be relieved by admission to other wards. While medical staff must decide whether patients require ICU admission, shiftleaders must decide whether patients can be safely nursed on the unit. This decision includes:

- imminent shifts;
- dependency of patients already on the unit;
- skills of staff available.

The shiftleader is professionally accountable for decisions about managing nursing on the unit, but faced with coercion or moral blackmail may need considerable assertiveness skills.

Good shiftleaders may inspire loyalty in their staff, but being in charge can isolate shiftleaders from other support mechanisms. Shiftleaders also need their breaks: a stressed shiftleader is less likely to be able to support their staff.

Devolvement of budgets has inevitably led to shiftleaders having both financial authority and responsibilities. At early stages of management experience, these are likely to be deferred to more senior staff, but as you develop your management skills these will increasingly become part of your role. It is therefore valuable to discuss these with your nurse manager or mentor.

Time out 3

Using the cues below, jot down plans for your professional development over the next six months. Aims may be clinical, educational and professional. Be realistic, setting sufficient aims to help you develop, but not too many to achieve (six aims is often a reasonable target, but the number and scope vary between individuals). You may wish to share all or part of this with your manager, mentor or colleagues, or retain this as a private document in your professional profile. You may wish to divide aims between short term (a few weeks), medium term (up to six months) and long term (after six months), or cover all aims together. Long-term aims will not be achieved fully by your six-month review, but you may have partially progressed towards them. You will probably find setting target dates for achieving aims helpful.

- Over the next six months I would like to achieve (include target times):
- I would like to achieve these because:
- To achieve these I will need (include people and resources):
- I will now have achieved these aims because (i.e. evaluation):
- Possible problems I anticipate for myself/others:
- Ways to minimise these problems:

Implications for practice

- Staff who have met minimum criteria to manage their unit should plan a structure to develop their skills before they find themselves unexpectedly in charge.
- Shiftleaders should enable their staff to work safely, efficiently and effectively.

■ Shiftleaders rely on their staff, so should encourage morale and meet the needs of their staff (professional development, support, breaks).
■ Shiftleaders should coordinate unit activity, so participate in decision-making, both during and between ward rounds.
■ Shiftleaders should recognise potential role conflicts and priorities.
■ Nurse shiftleaders, like all qualified nurses, are professionally accountable for their decisions and actions.

Summary

This chapter has considered some of the practical issues for ICU nurses who are beginning to develop their management skills. Much has been written elsewhere on wider management issues and theory; nurses developing management careers may need to develop this knowledge further, but should first gain practical management skills through structured experiential programmes. The shiftleader is morally and professionally responsible and accountable for their managerial decisions.

Further reading

Shiftleaders should be familiar with local policies and guidelines. Practising being in charge is probably more valuable than reading about it, especially as little literature on management is written by nurses, and rarely specifically about healthcare. Drucker (e.g. 1974) is an influential management theorist. Literature on nursing management is rarely ICU-specific, but McCormack and Manley (2004) include many valuable chapters.

Clinical questions

Q.1 Describe the responsibilities of the shiftleader within your own clinical practice area (e.g. specify responsibilities towards resource management, people management, monitoring standards and quality).

Q.2 Review the range of management style(s) used within your own ICU. Are there differences in styles and behaviours used between different shiftleaders? Analyse any perceived differences in terms of leadership, relationship, personality and change theories.

Q.3 Formulate a training programme to prepare ICU nurses for shift and unit management. Propose and justify the selection criteria, basic nurse competencies required for managing the ICU, resources needed for training and the evaluation and feedback strategy.

Chapter 50

Cost of intensive care

 Contents

Introduction	479
Spending on health	479
Scoring critical illness	480
Mortality	481
Morbidity	481
Nursing	482
Implications for practice	482
Summary	483
Further reading	483
Clinical questions	483

Introduction

Critical illness is costly. Mortality and morbidity are higher than with less advanced disease; emotional costs to patients, relatives and staff are also significant. But in a world of finite resources, and increasing financial pressures, financial costs affect care. In 2004, costs per patient day were £1,328 in ICUs, compared with £195 for wards (Ridley and Morris, 2006). Inevitably, the high financial costs of ICUs invite scrutiny. The introduction of tariffs into the UK's National Health Service is intended to improve quality and productivity (DH, 2009a). Increasing financial pressures are paralleled by increasingly higher public and political expectations. Nurses must therefore assert the financial value of ICU care in the marketplace of healthcare. While financial costs may have some objectivity, subjectivity surrounds human costs. Having reached the end of this book, nurses developing their ICU careers should be grappling with the questions:

- What price intensive care?
- Are the costs of treating critical illness justifiable from financial, humanitarian, and/or moral and ethical perspectives?
- Are the costs of nurses and nursing justifiable?

Spending on health

Workforce costs account for over half of the NHS budget (DH, 2005), and nurses are the largest single group of workers in health services (Büscher *et al.*, 2009). ICUs are labour-intensive and expensive. Successful cures of simpler pathologies (e.g. single-organ failure) have created more complex pathologies (e.g. MODS), which increase both cost per patient day, and length of stay. Increasingly complex and expensive technology and drugs further strain budgets. But ICU budgets may subsidise other departments by providing support services, such as Outreach, and programmes for high-dependency care. Financial stringencies often encourage budget holders to reduce staff. But this may prove a short-term financial saving with long-term costs. Reducing ICU nurse:patient ratios:

- delays weaning from ventilation;
- increases nosocomial infection;
- increases readmission to ICUs;
- increases medication errors;
- increases length of ICU patient episodes.

(EfCCNa, 2007)

Treating patients who do not survive costs more than treating patients who do (Vedio *et al.*, 2000), and prolonging dying is cruel. Predicting survival could therefore reduce humanitarian and financial burdens in ICUs, but raises ethical concerns about reliability and 'playing God'.

479

Costs and performance of units, and of their staff, are scrutinised closely. Poor-quality critical care may increase financial costs, morbidity and mortality (Davoudian and Blunt, 2009). While external scrutiny is almost inevitable, internal scrutiny can help improve efficiency and effectiveness. There are many ways units can review their effectiveness, including:

■ audit
■ mortality and morbidity meetings (Ksouri *et al.*, 2010)
■ case review.

Whatever means is used, multidisciplinary involvement is beneficial.

Scoring critical illness

There are various scoring systems, mostly developed for medical audit. Audit can help staff learn from experience, and inappropriate admission to ICUs can cause excessive and unnecessary human suffering, but applying retrospective audit tools to prospective prediction may create dilemmas. While these tools measure survival in different patient groups, they are poor predictors of outcomes for individual patients, and they often fail to measure morbidity (Ethics Committee of the Society of Critical Care Medicine, 1997; Davoudian and Blunt, 2009). This echoes nursing debate around quality against quantity of life.

The Acute Physiology and Chronic Health Evaluation (*APACHE*) is the most widely used scoring system in ICUs; APACHE II is the version generally used, although a fourth version (Zimmermann *et al.*, 2006) has now been developed. It aims to measure and predict mortality. Its design is not too dissimilar to that of the Waterlow pressure scoring system. Other scoring systems used include:

■ Simplified Acute Physiology Score (SAPS II);
■ Health-related Quality of Life (HRQL);
■ Quality-adjusted Life Years (QALYs) system;
■ Intensive Care National Audit and Research Centre (ICNARC) model.

SAPS II also aims to predict mortality, but Khwannimit and Bhurayanontachai (2009) found customised APACHE II more reliable than customised SAPS II. QALYs is a system for calculating outcome in financial terms, and therefore investing limited financial resources in the best 'value for money' interventions. QALYs measure benefit against cost, and are considered by NICE (2009a) to be the ideal measurement for economic evaluation. Not surprisingly, ICU costs per QALY are high – Ridley and Morris (2007) suggest £7,010; nevertheless they suggest adult ICUs represent value for money. Although HRQL scores can measure single-disease states, they are probably more useful for longer-term assessment, and have limited value when used during critical illness (Ramsay *et al.*, 2008). Harrison and Rowan (2008) suggest the ICNARC model is better than other options.

Mortality

ICU mortality rates vary, depending on speciality and local factors, but Vincent *et al.*'s (2009) figure of nearly one-fifth reflects most reports and probably most units. However, statistics are often measured to ICU discharge. NICE (2009a) suggests that three-quarters of ICU patients survive to discharge home, which means one-quarter do not.

Recent reductions in mortality rates (Hutchins *et al.*, 2009) may reflect improvements in treatments and practice, but may also reflect increasing numbers of patients admitted for level 2 care. Mortality is, however, higher in patients admitted overnight (Pilcher *et al.*, 2007), so timely admission to the ICU, often facilitated through Critical Care Outreach, can be life-saving. More than half of adverse events occurring within 72 hours of ICU discharge are preventable, involving problems such as poor fluid management (McLaughlin *et al.*, 2007). Improving communication for handover can therefore help reduce morbidity and mortality.

While admission to ICUs should be limited to patients who can potentially benefit from them – critically ill patients who have potentially reversible conditions, treatment is not always successful, which risks prolonging death rather than life. When it seems unlikely conditions can reasonably be reversed, treatment is usually withdrawn to enable dignified death. Most deaths in ICUs follow withdrawal of treatment (Meissner *et al.*, 2010), although incidence and practice vary greatly (Azoulay *et al.*, 2009). Experience may suggest interventions are futile, but predictions are based on balancing probabilities rather than absolute certainties; many staff have occasionally seen 'miracle' recoveries, but prolonging suffering for many for the benefit of a small minority is ethically dubious. Decisions to withdraw should therefore be team decisions.

Morbidity

Quality of life is widely cited, but interpreting quality is subjective. Most ICU patients suffer significant psychological problems months after discharge. Post-traumatic stress disorder (PTSD) appears more widespread than previously suspected (see Chapter 3), and only a minority resume normal work (Garner and Sibthorpe, 2002; NICE, 2009a). While antipsychotic drugs may be useful, nurses should also consider all the non-pharmacological approaches (e.g. reducing sensory imbalance – see Chapter 3) that can reduce or prevent post-discharge psychosis.

Prolonged ICU stays (> 48 hours) result in higher mortality (Laupland *et al.*, 2006) and morbidity in survivors (Hofhuis *et al.*, 2008b; Unroe *et al.*, 2010). Prompt ICU discharge therefore appears beneficial. But discharge during the night increases mortality and morbidity, presumably because discharge is more likely to be premature (Goldfrad and Rowan, 2000). If nurses are to be advocates for their patients, they should voice concerns whenever they consider discharge to be premature.

Handover, and especially handover documentation, from ICU to ward staff can reduce adverse events following ICU discharge (Chaboyer *et al.*, 2008). Chaboyer *et al.* found the three main adverse events were:

- healthcare-associated infection/sepsis;
- accident or injury;
- other complications (e.g. deep vein thrombosis, pulmonary oedema, myocardial infarction).

While critical illness incurs some mortality and morbidity, avoidable mortality and morbidity does occur, and can be reduced by multidisciplinary review, audit and case conferences (Ksouri *et al.*, 2010), which provide an opportunity to learn from experience and change practices.

Nursing

Within the relatively few decades that ICUs have existed, nursing and nursing roles have changed dramatically. Nurses have adopted increasingly complex technical skills, especially in areas such as ICUs. New roles have developed, such as that of the advanced practitioner. While such roles emerge from aims to reduce costs while improving quality (WHO, 2009), and individual motivation may be more important than formal roles or titles for improving quality of nursing care, new roles do provide opportunities for nurses to develop nursing practice, and to justify the costs of nursing. Individually, nurses should proactively constantly seek to improve their own practice. Collectively, nurses should seek to advance the value of nursing within their own area of practice. Continuing expansion of roles is likely, and probably desirable, although this must be tempered if it risks compromising individuals' health (e.g. sickness, 'burnout') and quality of care.

Implications for practice

- Costs involve both financial and human aspects; human costs are subjective, including debatable issues such as quality of life, but are fundamentally central to nursing values.
- Medical outcome scoring systems are available, but predictive reliability for individuals is debated, so rationing by scoring systems is ethically questionable.
- Post-discharge follow-up can reduce psychological costs for patients and identify areas of nursing practice needing development. Critical Care Outreach teams can often provide units with valuable insights from former patients.
- Multidisciplinary case conferences, audit and/or mortality and morbidity meetings provide a valuable means to learn from avoidable mortality and morbidity, and to change practices.
- Nurses and nursing are valuable within ICUs; quality nursing can reduce financial, emotional, mortality and morbidity costs of critical illness.

Summary

This final chapter has revisited issues raised at the start of this book:

- What fundamentally are we doing for our patients?
- What should we be doing?
- How should we be doing it?

There are many possible answers to these questions; discussion in other chapters should have developed readers' awareness of these in everyday practice. As professionals, ICU nurses need to evaluate both financial and humanitarian costs of intensive care to determine its ultimate value. In the UK's chronically grossly underfunded and bureaucratic NHS, enthusiasm to cut costs can lead to false economies. Cheapest is not always best, and nurse advocacy may include resisting inappropriate and dangerous decisions at all levels. Attempts to equate financial with humanitarian (morbidity) costs may help nurses justify their value, but also create the danger that (to adapt Oscar Wilde) we know the price of everything but the value of nothing.

Further reading

NICE (2009a) provides valuable insights into and guidance about rehabilitation after critical illness. The Department of Health's *End of Life Care Strategy* (2008c and subsequent publications), although not ICU-specific, has promoted humane perspectives, including the Liverpool Care Pathway. Professional groups such as the Intensive Care Society and the British Association of Critical Care Nurses occasionally publish relevant documents about ICU economics.

Clinical questions

Q.1 List the positive benefits of the critical care process and categorise these into:

(a) benefits to patients;
(b) benefits to friends and family;
(c) benefits to health practitioners;
(d) benefits to society and the public.

Q.2 Analyse the cost per day of a typical patient in your own clinical area; break this down into staff costs, treatments, disposables, resources. Include also the recruitment costs incurred over the last 12 months, replacement costs for study leave or mandatory training, and temporary staff.

483

Q.3 Review practical strategies that can be implemented by ICU nurses, which can impact on the long-term survival of ICU patients once discharged home. Consider ICU nurses' role in community health, feasibility of specialist community link nurses, advice booklets, and follow-up/discharge clinics.

Glossary

Abdominal compartment syndrome   IAP ≥ 20 mmHg with organ failure not previously present.

Abruptio placentae   Premature separation of the placenta from the wall of the uterus before the baby is born.

Albumin   A protein made by the liver.

Anabolism   The process by which organisms make complex molecules and substances from less complex components.

Anacrotic notch   Abnormal notch occurring on arterial blood pressure traces before the main pressure peak.

Anaphylaxis   An allergic, potentially fatal, reaction to a substance that the body perceives as a threat (also called 'anaphylactic shock').

Anion   A negatively charged ion

Anxiolysis   Removing ('breakdown' of) anxiety.

Ascites   An accumulation of fluid in the peritoneal cavity, causing abdominal swelling.

Atelectasis   Collapse of alveoli.

Autologous   From the same individual (e.g. autologous blood = patients' own blood).

Balloon tamponade   Inflation of balloon-tipped catheters (e.g. Minnesota tube), which places direct pressure on bleeding points, so can stop internal bleeding in the same way nurses use digital pressure to stop bleeding after arterial lines are removed.

Barotrauma   Damage to alveoli from excessively high (peak) airway pressure.

Blepharitis   Inflammation of eyelash follicles and sebaceous glands.

Böhr effect   Carbon dioxide and hydrogen reduce affinity of oxygen for haemoglobin, so acidosis increases dissociation.

Bolam test Case law precedent establishing that practitioners are not guilty of negligence if their practice conforms to that of a reasonable body of opinion held by practitioners skilled in the area of question.

Bradycardia Heart rate below 60 beats per minute.

Calorie (cal, c) Amount of heat needed to raise one gram of water 1°C at atmospheric pressure (= small calorie) (*see also* Kilocalorie).

Capillary occlusion pressure The pressure at which capillary flow will be prevented, resulting in ischaemia, anaerobic metabolism and (eventually) infarction of tissue (e.g. pressure sore formation).

Catabolism Breakdown of complex molecules to form simpler ones, often resulting in release of energy.

Cation A positively charged ion.

Chronotrope (*Chronos* = time) affecting heart rate. Positive chronotropes (e.g. atropine) increase heart rate. Negative chronotropes (e.g. beta-blockers) reduce heart rate. Inotropes are usually also chronotropic.

Circadian rhythm The 'body clock', an endogenous rhythm around the day. Normal circadian rhythm lasts about 24 hours, but abnormal rhythms can take longer or shorter. Circadian rhythm affects various endogenous hormone levels, so disturbed circadian rhythm results in various abnormal body responses (e.g. wakefulness at night).

Citric acid cycle *see* Krebs' cycle.

Coagulopathies Disorders (pathologies) of clotting, such as DIC and sickle cell anaemia.

Colloid osmotic pressure The osmotic pressure created by large molecules (e.g. proteins) that retain plasma in the intravascular space. Fluids with high colloid osmotic pressures therefore assist return of extravascular fluid (oedema) into the bloodstream.

Commensal bacteria Endogenous bacteria helping normal human functions.

Complements Plasma proteins (produced in the liver) that facilitate phagocytosis.

Coning *see* Tentorial herniation.

Convection *see* Solvent drag.

Cori cycle Glycolysis in contracting muscles produces lactate, which the liver converts back into glucose, enabling further glycolysis-induced lactate. Therefore, lactate solutions are best avoided with uncontrolled hyperglycaemic diabetes mellitus.

Cullen's sign Irregular, bluish-purple discolouration around the umbilicus, which is an indication of intraperitoneal haemorrhage, especially in a ruptured ectopic pregnancy.

Cytokines Chemical mediators of inflammatory and immune processes, including tumour necrosis factor alpha (TNFα) and interleukins.

Daltons (Da) *see* KiloDaltons.

D-dimer A fibrinolysis product used to measure clotting.

Dead space The space between air/gas mix and alveoli; physiological adult dead space is about 150 ml; on ventilators dead space extends from the Y connector to alveoli.

Dehiscence Of a wound, gaping or bursting open.

Depolarisation Reduction of membrane potential to a less negative value.

Dialysate A fluid used for dialysis.

Dialysis Movement of solutes through semipermeable membranes by a concentration gradient, so greater differences in concentrations result in faster movement.

Dicrotic notch The notch normally seen on downstrokes of arterial waveforms, representing closure of the aortic valve, which causes transient slight increases in pressure.

Diffuse axonal injury Widespread injury caused by shearing forces, usually from rotational acceleration (e.g. road traffic accidents).

Diffusion Movement of molecules from an area of higher concentration to an area of lower concentration.

Diuresis Increased or excessive passing of urine.

E. coli *Escherichia coli*, a species of gram negative bacteria, one of the major gut commensals; presence of *E. coli* in the blood (or wounds) is an infection.

Ejection fraction Stroke volume as a fraction of ventricular blood volume. Normal ejection fraction is 0.6–0.75 (60–70 per cent), but dysfunctional ventricles (e.g. myocardial infarction) eject less. Figures inversely indicate extent of myocardial damage.

Endogenous From inside the person.

Endoleak Continued bloodflow through an aneurysm sac around a repair/stent.

Erythropoiesis Production of erythrocytes (red blood cells).

Exogenous From outside the person

Extravasation Letting/forcing out a fluid from a vessel that normally contains it.

Flow monitoring Monitoring of cardiovascular flow, previously called 'cardiac output studies'.

Free radicals Molecules with one or more unpaired electron in their outer orbit; which makes them inherently unstable, so they react readily with other molecules to pair the free electron.

Glycolysis Breakdown of glucose.

Glycosides Carbohydrates that, when hydrolysed, produce a sugar and a non-sugar. Digoxin is a cardiac glycoside.

Glycosuria Sugar in urine; blood sugar is filtered by the kidney, but normally is all reabsorbed. When blood sugar exceeds 10 mmol/litre, renal tubules are unable to reabsorb all the sugar. As glucose creates high osmotic pressure, the tubules also reabsorb less water, resulting in polyuria.

Grey Turner's sign Bluish-purple discolouration of flanks, indicating acute haemorrhagic pancreatitis.

Haldane effect Observed when a rise in oxyhaemoglobin shifts the carbon dioxide dissociation curve to the right.

Half-life Time taken by a chemical to lose half of its active effect.

Hertz (Hz) SI unit of frequency, equal to one cycle per second.

Hyper- High.

Hyperalderostonism Where the adrenal gland releases too much of the hormone aldosterone, which can lead to low levels of potassium and calcium.

Hyper-/hypocalcaemia High/low serum calcium (normal whole blood level = 2.25–2.75 mmol/litre; normal ionised level = 1.0–1.5 mmol/litre).

Hyper-/hypocapnia An increased/decreased concentration of carbon dioxide in the blood.

Hyper-/hypochloraemia High/low blood chloride (normal = 98–108 mmol/litre).

Hyper-/hypoglycaemia High/low serum glucose (normal = 4–8 mmol/litre).

Hyper-/hypokalaemia High/low serum potassium (normal = 3.5–4.5 mmol/litre).

Hyper-/hyponatraemia High/low serum sodium (normal = 135–145 mmol/litre).

Hyper-/hypotension High/low blood pressure.

Hyper-/hypovolaemia Increased/decreased volume of circulating blood.

Hypo- Low.

Immunocompromised Less able to battle infections because the immune system has been impaired by disease or treatment.

Interleukins Naturally occurring proteins, produced by white blood cells and regulating immune responses.

Ionised calcium The portion of calcium present as free ions. It is biologically active and plays a crucial role in muscular contraction, cardiac function and blood clotting.

Ischaemia Inadequate blood supply to a part of the body, expecially heart muscles.

Isothermic saturation boundary Where 100 per cent relative humidity is reached at 37°C; normally (in adults) just below the carina.

Joule A unit to measure energy (= 10^7 ergs or 1 watt second).

Keratitis Inflammation of the cornea.

Keratopathy Non-inflammatory corneal disease.

Kilocalorie (kcal, C) Amount of heat needed to raise one kilogram of water 1°C at atmospheric pressure (= large calorie).

KiloDaltons (kDa) A unit of molecular weight (1000 daltons (Da) = 1 kDa).

Krebs' cycle A chain of intracellular chemical reactions to metabolise fat for energy. Krebs' cycle is efficient at energy (adenosine triphosphate) production, but produces metabolic wastes (acids, ketones, carbon dioxide, water). (Also called 'citric acid cycle'.)

Kussmaul respiration Deep, rapid, sighing type of breath, caused by ketones, so associated with diabetic ketoacidosis.

Leukotrienes Mediators released by leucocytes; they increase capillary 'leak'.

Loop of Henle A long, U-shaped portion of the tubule that conducts urine within each nephron of the kidney.

Macula densa A zone of heavily nucleated cells in the distal renal tubule.

Marfan's syndrome A hereditary connective tissue disorder; symptoms include elongation of limbs and aortic aneurysms.

Metabolic acidosis Acid/base imbalance where there is an accumulation of too much acid in the body and not enough bicarbonate to neutralise its effects.

Microcirculation Capillaries.

Millimole (mmol) A unit for measuring chemicals; 1 mole = relative atomic mass in grams of each element.

Mitochondria Organelles within cytoplasm that produce cell energy by glycolysis (combustion of glucose with oxygen); often called the 'power-house' of the cell. (Single: mitochondrion.)

Monro-Kellie hypothesis The pressure:volume relationship between intracranial pressure, volume of cerebrospinal fluid, brain tissue and cerebral perfussion pressure.

Myocytes Cardiac muscle cells.

Neuromuscular blockade (Chemical) paralysis.

Nitric oxide An endogenous vasodilator.

Non-invasive transcranial Doppler   An ultrasound technique.

Nosocomial infection   An infection acquired in hospital (technically, at least 22 hours following admission).

Oedema   A build-up of excess fluid in the body tissues.

Oncotic pressure   Osmotic pressure of colloids in solution.

Osmolality   Number of dissolved particles per kilogram of solvent.

Osmolarity   Number of dissolved particles per litre of solution.

Osmosis   Movement of a pure solute (e.g. water) through a semipermeable membrane (the membrane being impermeable to the solute, but permeable to the solvent), from an area of low to an area of high solute concentration, to form a concentration equilibrium on both sides (osmotic = of osmosis).

Ototoxic   Toxic to the ear (*oto* = ear); damage is caused to the eighth cranial nerve or the organs of hearing and balance. Many drugs (e.g. gentamicin, furosemide) can be ototoxic.

Parity   Number of pregnancies (including stillbirths/abortions/miscarriages) reaching 20 weeks' gestation.

Paroxysmal   Sudden; paroxysmal atrial tachycardia is atrial tachycardia that appears (and often disappears) suddenly.

Permissive hypercapnia   Tolerating abnormally high arterial carbon dioxide tensions (pCO_2) to enable smaller tidal volumes, and so limiting/avoiding barotrauma and volutrauma.

Plethysmograph (pleth)   An instrument for measuring changes in blood volume.

Polydipsia   Excessive thirst.

Polyunsaturated fatty acids   *see* Saturated fatty acids.

Polyuria   Excessive urination.

Primagravida   Woman undergoing her first pregnancy.

Prostacyclin (PGI2)   An active arachidonic acid metabolite; it inhibits angiotensin-mediated vasoconstriction, stimulates renin release, and inhibits platelet aggregation (so is used for anticoagulation).

Pruritis   Itching.

Radicals   Molecules with an unpaired electron (*see* Free radicals).

Repolarisation   Restoration of a cell to its resting potential.

Saturated fatty acids   Fats with univalent bonds joining all atoms; valency determines hydrogen-binding capacity of molecules, so saturated fatty acids contribute to hypercholestrolaemia and cardiovascular (especially coronary) disease. Most animal fats are saturated.

Serotonin Tryptophan derivative found in platelets and cells of brain and intestine; a vasopressor and neurotransmitter.

Shunt An abnormal conduit directly joining an artery to a vein, such as an arteriovenous shunt used for haemodialysis access, or a drain inserted to remove excess fluid (e.g. an intraventricular shunt to drain CSF from the ventricles of the brain, and so relieve intracranial hypertension).

Shunting Describes a conduit between two body compartments. In respiratory medicine this usually describes movement of blood from venous to arterial circulation without effective ventilation, typically from intrapulmonary problems, such as ARDS, but it can also be caused by an atrial-septal defect allowing blood to pass between the atria without entering the pulmonary circulation.

Solvent drag Movement of fluid by osmotic pressure from solutes moving across a semipermeable membrane. (Also called 'convection'.)

Tachycardia A fast or irregular heart rhythm, usually more than 100 beats per minute.

Tachypnoea Rapid breathing.

Tamponade Compression of the heart caused by a build-up of fluid in the pericardial sac.

Tentorial herniation Brainstem forced into the spinal column by raised intracranial pressure.

Thromboelastography A method of testing the efficiency of coagulation in the blood.

Tonic-clonic seizures Generalised fitting.

Transmembrane pressure The pressure across a membrane. Where artificial technologies replicate capillary function, such as the 'artificial kidneys' used for haemofiltration, excessive pressure may rupture the necessarily delicate membrane. Being artificial, damage is permanent and irreparable. As the surface area of the filter becomes progressively engorged with clots, filtrate is forced through a smaller area, increasing transmembrane pressure. Therefore measuring the transmembrane pressure should identify impending rupture of the artificial kidney. Stopping filters before maximum transmembrane pressure is reached enables blood in the circuit to be safely returned to the patient. See manufacturers' instructions for maximum transmembrane pressures of individual models.

Trimester Pregnancy is divided into three trimesters: trimester 1 = up to week 12; trimester 2 = weeks 13–28; trimester 3 = week 29 to delivery.

Tunica intima The inner layer of a blood vessel wall.

Ultrafiltrate A solution that has passed through a semipermeable membrane with very small pores.

Ultrafiltration Removal of fluid through a membrane under pressure.

Volutrauma Damage from alveolar distension (excessive volume); high lung volumes (in relation to space available) can cause sheering damage to lung tissue; the concept is similar to barotrauma. (It is sometimes spelled 'volotrauma'.)

References

Abbas, A.K., Lichtman, A.H. and Pober, J.S. (1994) *Cellular and Molecular Immunology*, 2nd edition. Philadelphia: W.B. Saunders.

Abela. R., Ivanova, S., Lidder, S., Morris, R. and Hamilton, G. (2009) An analysis comparing open surgical and endovascular treatment of atherosclerotic renal artery stenosis. *European Journal of Vascular and Endovascular Surgery*, 38 (6): 666–675.

Aboudara, M.C., Hurst, F.P., Abbott, K.C. and Perkins, R.M. (2008) Hyperkalaemia after packed red blood cell transfusion in trauma patients. *Journal of Trauma*, 64 (2): S86–S91.

Abraham, E., Gallagher, T.J. and Fink, S. (1996) Clinical evaluation of multiparameter intraarterial blood-gas sensor. *Intensive Care Medicine*, 22 (5): 507–513.

Abroug, F., Ouanes-Besbes, L., Elatrous, S. and Brochard, L. (2008) The effect of prone positioning in acute respiratory distress syndrome or acute lung injury: a meta-analysis. Areas of uncertainty and recommendations for research. *Intensive Care Medicine*, 34 (6): 1002–1011.

Adam, S.K. and Osborne, S. (2009) *Oxford Handbook of Critical Care Nursing*. Oxford: Oxford University Press.

Adembri, C., Kastamoniti, E., Bertolozzi, I., Vanni, S., Dorigo, W., Coppo, M., Pratesi, C., de Gaudio, A.R., Gensini, G.F. and Modesti, P.A. (2004) Pulmonary injury follows systemic inflammatory reaction in infrarenal aortic surgery. *Critical Care Medicine*, 32 (5): 1170–1177.

Adhikari, N.K.J., Fowler, R.A., Bhagwanjee, S. and Rubenfeld, G.D. (2010) Critical care and the global burden of critical illness in adults. *Lancet*, 376 (9749): 1339–1346.

Afshari, A., Wettersley, J., Brok, J. and Moller, A. (2007) Antithrombin III in critically ill patients: systematic review with meta-analysis and trial sequential analysis. *British Medical Journal*, 335 (7632): 1248–1251.

Agarwai, M. and Cottam, S. (2009) Laboratory tests in hepatic failure. *Anaesthesia and Intensive Care Medicine*, 10 (7): 326–327.

Ahlers, S.M., van der Veen, A., van Dijk, M., Tibboel, D. and Knibbe, C.A.J. (2010) The use of the Behaviour Pain Scale to assess pain in conscious sedated patients. *Anesthesia & Analgesia*, 110 (1): 127–133.

Ailawadi, G. and Zacour, R.K. (2009) Cardiopulmonary bypass/extracorporeal membrane oxygenation/left heart bypass: indications, techniques and complications. *Surgical Clinics of America*, 89 (4): 781–796.

Akansel, N. and Kaymakçi, Ş. (2008) Effects of intensive care unit noise on patients: a study on coronary artery bypass graft surgery patients. *Journal of Clinical Nursing*, 17 (12): 1581–1590.

Akça, O., Doufas, A.G., Morioka, N., Iscoe, S., Fisher, J. and Sessler, D.I. (2002) Hypercapnia improves tissue oxygenation. *Anesthesiology*, 97 (4): 801–806.

Åkerman, E., Granberg-Axéll, A., Ersson, A., Fridlund, B. and Bergbom, I. (2010) Use and practice of patient diaries in Swedish intensive care units: a national survey. *Nursing in Critical Care*, 15 (1): 26–33.

Albarran, J. and Cox, H. (2008) Assessing and managing the patient with chest pain due to cardiac syndrome X, cocaine misuse and herpes zoster, in Albarran, J. and Tagney, J. (eds) *Chest Pain: Advanced assessment and management skills*. Oxford: Wiley-Blackwell, pp. 234–255.

Allen, S. (2005) Prevention and control of infection in the ICU. *Current Anaesthesia & Critical Care*, 16 (5): 191–199.

Allison, A. (1994) High frequency jet ventilation – where are we now? *Care of the Critically Ill*, 10 (3): 122–124.

Almerud, S., Alapack, R.J., Fridlund, B. and Ekebergh, M. (2007) Of vigilance and invisibility – being a patient in technologically intense environments. *Nursing in Critical Care*, 12 (3): 151–158.

Al-Omran, M., Al-Balawi, Z.H., Tashkandi, M.F. and Al-Ansary, L.A. (2010) Enteral versus parenteral nutrition for acute pancreatitis. *Cochrane Database of Systematic Reviews*, issue 1, art. no. CD002837; doi: 10.1002/14651858.CD002837.pub2.

Amirlak, I. and Amirlak, B. (2006) Haemolytic uraemic syndrome: an overview. *Nephrology*, 11 (3): 213–218.

Anderson, C.D., Vachharajani, N., Doyle, M., Lowell, J.A., Wellen, J.R., Shenoy, S., Lisker-Melman, M., Korenblat, K., Crippin, J. and Chapman, W.C. (2008) Advanced donor age alone does not affect patient graft survival after liver transplantation. *Journal of the American College of Surgeons*, 207 (6): 847–852.

Anderson, F.A. and Spencer, F.A. (2003) Risk factors for venous thromboembolism. *Circulation*, 23 (supplement): I9–I16.

Andrew, C.M. (1998) Optimizing the human experience: nursing the families of people who die in intensive care. *Intensive and Critical Care Nursing*, 14 (2): 59–65.

Andrews, P.J.D., Citero, G., Longhi, L., Polderman, K., Sahuquillo and J., Vajkoczy, P., Neuro-Intensive Care and Emergency Medicine (NICEM) Section of the European Society of Intensive Care Medicine (2008a) Intensive care of aneurismal subarachnoid hemorrhage: an international survey. *Intensive Care Medicine*, 34 (8): 1362–1370.

Andrews, S., Catlin, S., Lamb, N. and Christensen, M. (2008b) A dedicated retrieval and transfer service: The QUARTS Project. *Nursing in Critical Care*, 13 (3): 162–168.

Angoules, A.G., Kontakis, G., Drafoulakis, E., Vrentzos, G., Granik, M.S. and Giannoudis, P.V. (2007) Necrotising fasciitis of upper and lower limb: a systematic review. *Injury*, 38 (supplement 5): S19–S26.

Annane, D., Bellisant, E., Bollaert, P.-E., Briegel, J., Confalonieri, M., de Gaudio, R., Keh, D., Kupfer, Y., Oppert, M. and Meduri, G.U. (2009) Corticosteroids in the treatment of severe sepsis and septic shock in adults. *JAMA*, 301 (12): 2362–2375.

Ansen, T.C., van Bommel, J., Mulder, P.G., Lima, A.P., van der Hoven, B., Rommes, J.H., Snellen, F.T.F. and Bakker, J. (2009) Prognostic value of blood lactate levels: does the clinical diagnosis at admission matter? *Trauma*, 66 (2): 377–385.

Anthony, D., Parboteeah, S., Salen, M. and Papnikolaou, P. (2008) Norton, Waterlow and Braden scores: a review of the literature and a comparison between the scores and clinical judgement. *Journal of Clinical Nursing*, 17 (5): 646–653.

Antman, E.M., Hand, M., Armstrong, P.W., Bates, E.R., Green, L.A., Halasyamani, L.K., Hochman, J.S., Krumholz, H.M., Lamas, G.A., Mullany, C.J., Peale, D.L., Sloan, M.A. and Smith, S.C. Jr (2008) 2007 focused update on the ACC/AHA 2004 guidelines for the management of patients with ST-elevation myocardial infarction: a report of the American College of Cardiology/American Heart Association Task Force on Practice Guidelines. *Journal of the American College of Cardiology*, 151 (2): 210–247.

ANZ ECMO (Australia and New Zealand Extracorporeal Membrane Oxygenation) Influenza Investigators (2009) Extracorporeal membrane oxygenation for 2009 influenza A (H1N1) acute respiratory distress syndrome. *JAMA*, 302 (17): 1888–1895.

Arbour, R. (2000) Mastering neuromuscular blockade. *Dimensions of Critical Care Nursing*, 19 (5): 4–20.

——, Waterhouse, J., Seckel, M.A. and Bucher, L. (2009) Correlation between the Sedation-Agitation Scale and Bispectral Index in ventilated patients in the intensive care unit. *Heart & Lung*, 38 (4): 336–345.

ARDSNet (2008) *NIH NHLBI ARDS Clinical Network Mechanical Ventilation Protocol Summary*. Available online at www.ardsnet.org/system/files/6mlcardsmall_2008update_final_JULY2008.pdf (accessed 29 December 2010)

Arroyo-Novoa, C.M., Figueroa-Ramos, M.I., Puntillo, K.A., Stanuk-Hutt, J., Thompson, C.L., White, C. and Wild, L.R. (2008) Pain related to tracheal suctioning in awake acutely and critically ill adults: a descriptive study. *Intensive and Critical Care Nursing*, 24 (1): 20–27.

Artinian, V., Krayem, H. and DiGiovine, B. (2006) Effects of early enteral feeding on the outcome of critically ill mechanically ventilated medical patients. *Chest*, 129 (4): 960–967.

Ascione, R., Rogers, C.A., Rajakaruna, C. and Angelini, G.D. (2008) Inadequate blood glucose control is associated with in-hospital mortality and morbidity in diabetic and nondiabetic patients undergoing cardiac surgery. *Circulation*, 118 (2): 113–123.

Ash, D. (2005) Sustaining safe and acceptable bowel care in spinal cord injured patients. *Nursing Standard*, 20 (8): 55–64.

Ashraf, A., Conil, J.M., Georges, B., Gonzalez, H., Cougot, P. and Samii, K. (2008) Relation between ventilatory pressures and intra-abdominal pressure. *Critical Care*, 12 (supplement 2): P324.

Ashworth, P. (1980) *Care to Communicate*, London: Royal College of Nursing.

Ässaoui, Y., Zeggwagh, A.A., Zekraoui, A., Abidi, K. and Abouqal, R. (2005) Validation of a Behavioral Pain Scale in critically ill, sedated, and mechanically ventilated patients. *Anesthesia & Analgesia*, 101 (5): 1470–1476.

Assar, A.N. and Zarins, C.K. (2009) Ruptured abdominal aortic aneurysm: a surgical emergency with many clinical implications. *Postgraduate Medical Journal*, 85 (1003): 268–273.

Astle, S.M. (2005) Restoring electrolyte balance. *RN*, 68 (5): 34–39.

Atherton, J.C. (2003) Acid-base balance: maintenance of plasma pH. *Anaesthesia and Intensive Care Medicine*, 4 (12): 419–422.

Audit Commission (2001) *Testing Times*. London: Audit Commission.

Ault, M.L. and Stock, M.C. (2004) Respiratory monitoring. *International Anaesthesiology Clinics*, 42 (1): 97–112.

Australian and New Zealand Intensive Care Society Clinical Trials Group (2000) Low-dose dopamine in patients with early renal dysfunction: a placebo-controlled randomised trial. *Lancet*, 356 (9248): 2139–2143.

Avidan, M.S., Zhang, L., Burnside, B.A., Finkel, K.J., Searleman, A.C., Selvidge, J.A., Saager, L., Turner, M.S., Rao, S., Bottros, M., Hantler, C., Jacobsohn, E. and Evers, A.S. (2008) Anesthesia awareness and the Bispectral Index. *New England Journal of Medicine*, 358 (11): 1097–1108.

Aviles, R.J., Askari, A.T., Lindahl, B., Wallentin, L., Jia, G., Ohman, E.M., Mahaffey, K.W., Newby, L.K., Califf, R.M., Simoons, M.L., Topol, E.J. and Lauer, M.S. (2002) Troponin T levels in patients with acute coronary syndromes, with or without renal dysfunction. *New England Journal of Medicine*, 346 (226): 2047–2052.

Ayello, E. and Braden, B. (2002) How and why do pressure ulcer risk assessment. *Advances in Skin & Wound Care*, 15 (3): 125–131.

Ayliffe, G.A.J., Babb, J.R. and Taylor, L.J. (2001) *Hospital-acquired Infection: Principles and prevention*, 3rd edition. London: Arnold.

Azar, G., Love, R., Choe, E., Flint L. and Steinberg, S. (1996) Neither dopamine nor dobutamine reverses the depression in mesenteric blood flow caused by positive end-expiratory pressure. *Journal of Trauma*, 40 (5): 679–685.

Azoulay, E., Chevret, S., Leleu, G., Pochard, F., Barboteu, M., Adrie, C., Canoui, P., Le Gall, J.R. and Schlemmer, B. (2000) Half the families of intensive care unit patients experience inadequate communication with physicians. *Critical Care Medicine*, 28 (8): 3044–3049.

——, Metnitz, B., Sprung, C.L., Timsit, J.-F., Lemaire, F., Bauer, P., Schlemmer, B., Moreno, R. and Metnitz, P., SAPS 3 Investigators (2009) End-of-life practices in 282 intensive care units: data from the SAPS 3 database. *Intensive Care Medicine*, 35 (4): 623–630.

——, Pochard, F., Chevret, S., Arich, C., Brivet, F., Brun, F., Charles, P.-E., Desmettre, T., Dubois, D., Galliot, R., Garrouste-Orgeas, M., Goldgran-Toledano, D., Herbecq, P., Joly, L.-M., Jourdain, M., Kaidomar, M., Lepape, A., Letellier, N., Marie, O., Page, B., Parrot, A., Rodie-Talbere, P.-A., Sermet, A., Tenaillon, A., Thuong, A., Thuong, M., Tulasne, P., Le Gall, J.-R. and Schlemner, B., French Famirea Group (2003) Family participation in care to the critically ill: opinions of families and staff. *Intensive Care Medicine*, 29 (9): 1498–1504.

——, Pochard, F., Kentish-Barnes, N., Chevret, S., Aboab, J., Adrie, C., Annane, D., Bleichner, G., Bollaert, P.E., Darmon, M., Fassier, T., Galliot, R., Garrouste-Orgeas, M., Goulenok, C., Goldgran-Toledano, D., Hayon, J., Jourdain, M., Kaidomar, M., Laplace, C., Larché, J., Liotier, J., Papazian, L., Poisson, C., Reignier, J., Saidi, F., Schlemmer, B. (2005) Risk of post-traumatic stress symptoms in family members of intensive care unit patients. *American Journal of Respiratory and Critical Care Medicine*, 171 (9): 987–994.

Babaev, A., Frederick, P.D., Pasta, D.J., Every, N., Sichrovsky, T. and Hochman, J.S., NRMI Investigators (2005) Trends in management and outcomes of patients with acute myocardial infarction complicated by cardiogenic shock. *JAMA*, 294: 448–454.

Badacsony, A., Goldhill, A., Waldmann, C. and Goldhill, D.R. (2007) A prospective observational study of ICU patient position and frequency of turning. *Journal of the Intensive Society*, 8 (2): 26.

Baglin, T.P., Keeling, D.M. and Watson, H.G., British Committee for Standards in Haematology (2006) Guidelines on oral anticoagulation (warfarin), 3rd edition, 2005 update. *British Journal of Haematology*, 132 (3): 277–285.

Bahouth, M.N. and Yarbrough, K.L. (2005) Patient management: nervous system, in Morton, P.G., Fontaine, D.K., Hudak, C.M. and Gallo, B.M. (eds) *Critical Care Nursing: A holistic approach*, 8th edition. Philadelphia, PA: Lippincott Williams & Wilkins, pp. 775–795.

Baid, H. (2009) A critical review of auscultating bowel sounds. *British Journal of Nursing*, 18 (18): 1125–1129.

Bailey, A., Leditschke, I., Ranse, J. and Grove, K. (2008) Impact of a pandemic triage tool on intensive care admission. *Critical Care*, 12 (supplement 2): P349.

Bailey, D., Jackson, L. and White, D. (2004) HBO therapy: beyond the bends. *RN*, 27 (9): 31–35.

Ball, P.A. (2001) Critical care of spinal cord injury. *Spine*, 26 (24S): S27–S30.

Ballantyne, J.C., McKenna, J.M. and Ryder, E. (2003) Epidural analgesia – experience of 5628 patients in a large teaching hospital derived through audit. *Acute Pain*, 4 (3–4): 89–97.

Barbier, F., Coquet, I., Legrief, S., Pavie, J., Darmon, M., Mayaux, J., Molina, J.-M., Schlemmer, B. and Azoulay, E. (2009) Etiologies and outcome of acute respiratory failure in HIV-infected patients. *Intensive Care Medicine*, 35 (10): 1678–1686.

Barkun, A.N., Bardou, M., Kulpers, E.J., Sung, J., Hunt, R.H., Martel, M. and Sinclair, P., International Consensus Upper Gastrointestinal Bleeding Conference Group (2010) International consensus recommendations on the management of patients with nonvariceal upper gastrointestinal bleeding. *Annals of Internal Medicine*, 152 (2): 101–113.

Barratt, J. (2007) What to do with patients with abnormal dipstick urinalysis. *Medicine*, 35 (7): 365–367.

Barrett, K.E., Barman, S.M., Boitano, S. and Brooks, H.L. (2010) *Ganong's Review of Medical Physiology*, 23rd edition. New York: McGraw Hill Lange.

Barrett, S.P. (1999) Control of the spread of multi-resistant Gram-positive organisms. *Current Anaesthesia and Critical Care*, 10 (1): 27–31.

Bateman, D.N. (2007) Poisoning: focus on paracetamol. *Journal of the Royal College of Physicians of Edinburgh*, 37 (4): 332–334.

Baxter, B.T. (2004) Could medical intervention work for aortic aneurysms? *American Journal of Surgery*, 188 (6): 628–632.

Baylis, C. and Till, C. (2009) Interpretation of arterial blood gases. *Surgery*, 27 (11): 470–474.

Beale, R.J., Hollenberg, S.M., Vincent, J.-L. and Paiillo, J.E. (2004) Vasopressor and inotropic support in septic shock: an evidence-based review. *Critical Care Medicine*, 32 (11): S455–S465.

Beckmann, U., Gillies, D., Berenholtz, S., Wu, A. and Provenvost, P. (2004) Incidents relating to the inter-hospital transfer of critically ill patients: an analysis of the reports submitted to the Australian Incident Monitoring Study in Intensive Care. *Intensive Care Medicine*, 30 (8): 1579–1585.

Behrendt, C.E. (2000) Acute respiratory failure in the United States. *Chest*, 118 (4): 1100–1105.

Bein, T., Reber, A., Ploner, F., Taeger, K. and Jauch, K.-W. (2000) Continuous axial rotation and pulmonary fluid balance in acute lung injury. *Clinical Intensive Care*, 11 (6): 307–310.

Bell, M., SWING, Granath, F., Schön, S., Ekbom, A. and Martling, C.-R. (2007) Continuous renal replacement therapy is associated with less chronic renal failure than intermittent haemodialysis after acute renal failure. *Intensive Care Medicine*, 33 (5): 773–780.

Belligan, G.J. (2002) Resolution of inflammation and repair, in Evans, T.W., Griffiths, M.J.D. and Keogh, B.F. (eds) *ARDS*. Sheffield: European Respiratory Society Journals, pp. 70–82.

Benner, P., Sutphen, M., Leonard-Kahn, V. and Day, L. (2008) Formation and everyday ethical comportment. *American Journal of Critical Care*, 17 (5): 473–476.

Bennett, C. and Baker, K. (2001) HIV and AIDS: an overview. *Nursing Standard*, 15 (24): 45–52.

Bennewith, O., Stocks, N., Gunnell, D., Peters, T.J., Evans, M.O. and Sharp, D.J. (2002) General practice based intervention to prevent repeat episodes of deliberate self harm: cluster randomised controlled trial. *British Medical Journal*, 324 (7348): 1254–1557.

Bénony, H., Daloz, L., Bungener, C., Chahraoui, K., Frenay, C. and Auvin, J. (2002) Emotional factors and subjective quality of life in subjects with spinal cord injuries. *American Journal of Physical Medicine and Rehabilitation*, 81 (6): 437–445.

Benson, A.B., Moss, M. and Silliman, C.C. (2009) Transfusion-related acute lung injury (TRALI): a clinical review with emphasis on the critically ill. *British Journal of Haematology*, 147 (4): 431–443.

Berendes, E., Mollhoff, T., van Aken, H., Schmidt, C., Erren, M., Deng, M. Weyand, M. and Loick, H.M. (1997) Effects of dopexamine on creatinine clearance, systemic inflammation, and splanchnic oxygenation in patients undergoing coronary artery bypass grafting. *Anesthesia and Analgesia*, 84 (5): 950–957.

Bergbom, I. and Askwall, A. (2000) The nearest and dearest: a lifeline for ICU patients. *Intensive and Critical Care Nursing*, 16 (6): 384–395.

Bergstrom, N., Braden, B.J., Laguzza, A. and Holman, V. (1987) The Braden Scale for Predicting Pressure Sore Risk. *Nursing Research*, 36 (4): 205–210.

Bernal, W., Auzinger, G., Dhawan, A. and Wendon, J. (2010) Acute liver failure. *Lancet*, 376 (9736): 190–201.

Bernard, G.R., Vincent, J.-L., Laterre, P.-F. LaRosa, S.P., Dhainaut, J.-F., Lopez-Rodriguez, A., Steingrub, J.S., Garber, G.E., Helterbrand, J.D., Ely, E.W. and Fischer, C.J. (2001) Efficacy and safety of recombinant human activated protein C for severe sepsis. *New England Journal of Medicine*, 344 (10): 699–709.

Bernard, S.A. and Buist, M. (2003) Induced hypothermia in critical care medicine: a review. *Critical Care Medicine*, 31 (7): 2041–2051.

Berry, A.M., Davidson, P.M., Masters and J., Rolls, K. (2007) Systematic literature review of oral hygiene practices for intensive care patients receiving mechanical ventilation. *American Journal of Critical Care*, 16 (5): 552–562.

Berson, A.J., Smith, J.M., Woods, S.E., Hasselfeld, K.A. and Hiratzka, L.F. (2004) Off-pump versus on-pump coronary artery bypass surgery: does the pump influence outcome? *Journal of the American College of Surgeons*, 199 (1): 102–108.

Bertrand, X., Thouverez, M., Talon, D., Boillot, A., Capellier, G., Floriot, C. and Helias, J.P. (2001) Endemicity, molecular diversity and colonisation routes of *Pseudomonas aeruginosa* in intensive care units. *Intensive Care Medicine*, 27 (8): 1263–1268.

Bethel, J. (2008) *Paediatric Minor Emergencies*. Keswick: M&K Update.

Betts, J., Betts, P. and Sage, I. (1999) *Leah Betts: The legacy of Ecstasy*. London: Robson Books.

Bewley, C. (2004) Hypertensive disorders of pregnancy, in Henderson, C. and Macdonald, S. (eds) *Mayes' Midwifery: A textbook for midwives*, 13th edition. Edinburgh: Baillière Tindall, pp. 780–792.

Bigatello, L.M., Davignon, K.R. and Stelfox, H.T. (2005) Respiratory mechanics and ventilator waveforms in the patient with acute lung injury. *Respiratory Care*, 50 (2): 235–244.

Bilotta, F., Caramia, R., Paoloni, F.P., Delfini, R. and Rosa, G. (2009) Safety and efficacy of intensive insulin therapy in critical neurosurgical patients. *Anesthesiology*, 110 (3): 456–458.

Bird, J. (2003) Selection of pain measurement tools. *Nursing Standard*, 18 (13): 33–39.

Birn, H. and Christensen, E. (2006) Renal albumin absorption in physiology and pathology. *Kidney International*, 69 (3): 440–449.

Bisson, J. and Younker, J. (2006) Correcting arterial blood gases for temperature: (when) is it clinically significant? *Nursing in Critical Care*, 11 (5): 232–238.

Blackburn, F. and Bookless, B. (2002) Valve disorders, in Hatchett, R. and Thompson, D. (eds) *Cardiac Nursing: A comprehensive guide*. Edinburgh: Churchill Livingstone, pp. 260–286.

Blackwood, B. (1999) Normal saline instillation with endotracheal suctioning: primum non nocere (first do no harm). *Journal of Advanced Nursing*, 29 (4): 928–934.

Blackwood, B., Wilson-Barnett, J. and Trinder, J. (2004) Protocolized weaning from mechanical ventilation: ICU physicians' views. *Journal of Advanced Nursing*, 48 (1): 26–34.

Blasco, V., Leone, M., Antonini, F., Geissler, A., Albanèse, J. and Martin, C. (2008) Comparison of the novel hydroxyethyl starch 130/0.4 and hydroxyethyl starch 200/0.6 in brain-dead donor resuscitation on renal function after transplantation. *British Journal of Anaesthesia*, 100 (4): 504–508.

Bleeker-Rovers, V., van der Meer, J.W.M. and Beechning, N.J. (2009) Fever. *Medicine*, 37 (1): 28–34.

Blenkharn, A., Faughnan, S. and Morgan, A. (2002) Developing a pain assessment tool for use by nurses in an adult intensive care unit. *Intensive and Critical Care Nursing*, 18 (6): 332–341.

Blich, M., Sebbag, A., Attias, J., Aronson, D. and Markiewicz, W. (2008) Cardiac troponin I elevation in hospitalized patients without acute coronary syndromes. *American Journal of Cardiology*, 101 (10): 1384–1388.

Blot, F., Similowski, T., Trouillet, J.-L., Chardon, P., Korach, J.-M., Costa, M.-A., Journois, D., Thiéry, G., Fartoukh, M., Pipien, I., Bruder, N., Orlikowski, D., Tankere, F., Durand-Zaleski, I., Auboyer, C., Nitenberg, G., Holzapfel, L., Tenailon, A., Chastre, J., Laplanche, A. (2008) Early tracheostomy versus prolonged endotracheal intubation in unselected severely ill ICU patients. *Intensive Care Medicine*, 34 (10): 1779–1787.

Blot, S.I., Serra, M.L., Koulenti, D., Lisboa, T., Deja, M., Myrianthefs, P., Manno, E., Diaz, E., Topeli, A., Martin-Loeches, I. and Rello, J., EU-VAP/CAP Study Group (2011) Patient to nurse ratio and risk of ventilator-associated pneumonia in critically ill patients. *American Journal of Critical Care*, 20 (1): e1–e9. Available online at http://ajcc.aacnjournals.org/content/19/6.toc; doi:10.4037/ajcc2011555 (accessed 2 January 2011).

498

Blumenthal, I. (2001) Carbon monoxide poisoning. *Journal of the Royal Society of Medicine*, 94 (6): 270–272.

BNF (British National Formulary) (2009) *British National Formulary 58. September 2009*. London: BMJ Group/RPS Publishing.

Board, M. (1995) Comparison of disposable and glass mercury thermometers. *Nursing Times*, 91 (33): 36–37.

Boldt, J. (2010) Use of albumin: an update. *British Journal of Anaesthesia*, 104 (3): 276–284.

——, Suttner, S., Brosch, C., Lehmann, A., Röhm, K. and Mengistu, A. (2009) The influence of a balanced volume replacement concept on inflammation, endothelial activation, and kidney integrity in elderly cardiac surgery patients. *Intensive Care Medicine*, 35 (3): 462–470.

Boles, J.-M., Bion, J., Connors, A., Herridge, M., Marsh, B., Melot, C., Pearl, R., Silverman, H., Stanchina, M., Vieillard-Baron, A. and Welte, T. (2007) Weaning from mechanical ventilation. *European Respiratory Journal*, 29 (5): 1033–1055.

Bollman, M.-D., Revelly, J.-P., Tappy, L., Berger, M.M., Schaller, M.-D., Cayeux, M.-C., Martinez, A. and Chioléro, R.-L. (2004) Effect of bicarbonate and lactate buffer on glucose and lactate metabolism during hemofiltration in patients with multiple organ failure. *Intensive Care Medicine*, 30 (6): 1103–1110.

Bombardier, C.H., Fann, J.R., Temkin, N.R., Esselman, P.C., Barber, J. and Dikmen, S.S. (2010) Rates of major depressive disorder and clinical outcomes following traumatic brain injury. *JAMA*, 303 (19): 1938–1945.

Bonnefoy, E., Godon, P., Kirkorian, G., Fatemi, M., Chevalier, P. and Touboul, P. (2000) Serum cardiac troponin I and ST-segment elevation in patients with acute pericarditis. *European Heart Journal*, 21 (10): 832–836.

Boralessa, H., Goldhill, D. and Boralessa, H. (2003) Blood and the critically ill. *Care of the Critically Ill*, 19 (1): 15–17.

Borthwick, M., Bourne, R., Craig, M., Egan, A. and Oxley, J. (2006) *Detection, Prevention and Treatment of Delirium in Critically Ill Patients*. London: United Kingdom Clinical Pharmacy Association.

Bosch, J. and Abraldes, J.G. (2005) Variceal bleeding: pharmacological therapy. *Digestive Diseases*, 23 (1): 18–29.

Bouadma, L., Luyt, C.-E., Tubach, F., Cracco, C., Alvarez, A., Schwebel, C., Shortgen, F., Lasocki, S., Veber, B., Dehoux, M., Bernard, M., Pasquet, B., Régnier, B., Brun-Buisson, C., Chastre, J. and Wolff, M., PRORATA trial group (2010) Use of procalcitonin to reduce patients' exposure to antibiotics in intensive care units (PRORATA trial): a multicentre randomised controlled trial. *Lancet*, 375 (9713): 463–474.

Bouchut, J-C., Godard, J. and Claris, O. (2004) High-frequency oscillatory ventilation. *Anesthesiology*, 100 (4): 7–12.

Bougnoux, M.-E., Kac, G., Aegerter, P., d'Enfert, C. and Fagon, J.-Y., CandiRea Study Group (2007) Candidemia and candiduria in critically ill patients admitted to intensive care units in France: incidence, molecular diversity, management and outcome. *Intensive Care Medicine*, 34 (2): 292–299.

Boumendil, A., Maury, E., Reinhard, I., Luquel, L., Offenstadt, G. and Guidet, B. (2004) Prognosis of patients aged 80 years and over admitted in medical intensive care units. *Intensive Care Medicine*, 30 (4): 647–654.

Bourdages, M., Bigras, J.-L., Farrell, C.A., Hutchison, J.S. and Lacroix, J. (2010) Cardiac arrhythmias associated with severe traumatic brain injury and hypothermia therapy. *Pediatric Critical Care Medicine*, 11 (3): 439–441.

Bowling, T.E. (2004) Enteral nutrition. *Hospital Medicine*, 65 (12): 712–716.

Bowsher, J., Boyle, S. and Griffiths, J. (1999) Oral care. *Nursing Standard*, 13 (37): 31.

Boyce, P., Oakley-Browne, M. and Hatcher, S. (2001) The problem of deliberate self-harm. *Current Opinion in Psychiatry*, 14 (2): 107–111.

Brackenbury, A.M., Puligandla, P.S., McCaig, L.A., Nikore, V., Yao, L.-J., Veldhuizen, R.A.W. and Lewis, J.F. (2001) Evaluation of exogenous surfactant in HCl-induced lung injury. *American Journal of Respiratory and Critical Care Medicine*, 163 (5): 1135–1145.

Bradley, C. (2001) Crystalloid, colloid or small volume resuscitation? *Intensive and Critical Care Nursing*, 17 (5): 304–306.

Brady, J.E., Sun, L.S., Rosenberg, H. and Li, G. (2009) Prevalence of malignant hyperthermia due to anesthesia in New York State, 2001–2005. *Anesthesia & Analgesia*, 109 (4): 1162–1166.

Branson, R.D. (2005) The role of ventilator graphs when setting dual-control modes. *Respiratory Care*, 50 (2): 187–201.

Brar, S., Leon, M.B., Stone, G.W., Mehran, R., Moses, J.W., Brar, S.K. and Dangas, G. (2009) Use of drug-eluding stents in acute myocardial infarction. *Journal of the American College of Cardiology*, 53 (18): 1677–1689.

Brauser, D. (2010) Critically ill patients with H1N1 often have acute kidney injury, failure. *National Kidney Foundation (NKF) 2010 Spring Clinical Meetings*: Abstract 31, presented 14 April 2010.

Bravata, D.M., Gienger, A.L., McDonald, K.M., Sundaram, V., Perez, M.V., Varghese, R., Kapoor, J.R., Ardehall, R., Owens, D.K. and Hlatky, M.A. (2007) The comparative effectiveness of percutaneous coronary interventions and coronary artery bypass graft surgery. *Annals of Internal Medicine*, 147 (10): 703–716

Bray, K., Hill, K., Robson, W., Leaver, G., Walker, N., O'Leary, M., Delaney, T., Walsh, D., Gager, M. and Waterhouse, C. (2004) British Association of Critical Care Nurses position statement on the use of restraint in adult critical care units. *Nursing in Critical Care*, 9 (5): 199–211.

——, Wren, I., Baldwin, A., St Ledger, U., Gibson, V., Goodman, S. and Walsh, D. (2009) *BACCN Standards for Staffing in Critical Care*. Newcastle-upon-Tyne: BACCN.

Brenner, B., Corbridge, T. and Kazzi, A. (2009) Intubation and mechanical ventilation of the asthmatic patient in respiratory failure. *Proceedings of the American Thoracic Society*, 6 (4): 371–379.

Brenner, Z.R. (2002) Lessons for the critical care nurse on caring for the dying. *Critical Care Nurse*, 22 (1): 11–12.

Briel, M., Meade, M., Mercat, A., Brower, R.G., Talmor, D., Walter, S.D., Slutsky, A.S., Pullenayegum, E., Zhou, Q., Cook, D., Brochard, L., Richard, J.-C.M., Lamontagne, F., Bhatnagar, N., Stewart, T.E. and Guyatt, G. (2010) Higher vs lower positive end-expiratory pressure in patients with acute lung injury and acute respiratory distress syndrome: systematic review and meta-analysis. *JAMA*, 303 (9): 865–873.

Brienza, N., Giglio, M.T., Marucci, M. and Fiore, T. (2009) Does perioperative hemodynamic optimization protect renal function in surgical patients? A meta-analytic study. *Critical Care Medicine*, 37 (6): 2079–2090.

Briffa, N. (2008) Off-pump coronary artery bypass: a passing fad or ready for prime time? *European Heart Journal*, 29 (11): 1346–1349.

Brignall, K.A. and Davidson, A.C. (2009) Weaning from mechanical ventilation: art or science? *Care of the Critically Ill*, 25 (1): 22–28.

Brims, F.J.H., Davies, M.G., Elia, A. and Griffiths, M.J.D. (2004) The effects of pleural fluid drainage on oxygenation in mechanically ventilated patients after cardiac surgery. *Thorax*, 59: ii40: S129.

British Society for Standards in Haematology, Blood Transfusion Task Force (2003) Guidelines for the use of platelet transfusions. *British Journal of Haematology*, 122 (1): 10–23.

Brogan, T.V., Thiagarajan, R.R., Rycus, P.T., Bartlett, R.H. and Bratton, S.L. (2009) Extra-corporeal membrane oxygenation in adults with severe respiratory failure: a multi-center database. *Intensive Care Medicine*, 35 (12): 2105–2114.

Broomhead, R. (2002) Percutaneous tracheostomy. *Anaesthesia & Critical Care*, 3 (6): 210–212.

Brott, T.G., Hobson, R.W., Howard, G., Roubin, G.S., Clark, W.M., Brooks, W., Mackey, A., Hill, M.D., Leimgruber, P.P., Sheffet, A.J., Howard, V.J., Moore, W.S., Voeks, J.H., Hopkins, L.N., Cutlip, D.E., Cohen, D.J., Popma, J.J., Ferguson, R.D., Cohen, S.N., Blackshear, J.L., Silver, F.L., Mohr, J.P., Lal, B.K. and Meschia, J.F., CREST Investigators (2010) Stenting versus endarterectomy for treatment of carotid-artery stenosis. *New England Journal of Medicine*, 363 (1): 11–23.

Brotto, V. and Lee, G. (2007) Substance abuse and its implications for the critical care nurse. *Intensive & Critical Care Nursing*, 23 (2): 64–70.

Brown, C.V., Rhee, P., Chan, L., Evans, K., Demetriades, D. and Velmahos, G.C. (2004) Preventing renal failure in patients with rhabdomyolysis: do bicarbonate and mannitol make a difference? *Journal of Trauma*, 56 (6): 1191–1996.

Brundage, S.I., Kirilcuk, N.N., Lam, J.C., Spain, D.A. and Zautke, N.A. (2008) Insulin increases the release of proinflammatory mediators. *Journal of Trauma*, 65 (2): 367–372.

Brunkhorst, F.M., Engel, C., Bloos, F., Meier-Hellmann, A., Ragaller, M., Weiler, N., Moerer, O., Gruendling, M., Oppert, M., Grond, S., Olthoff, D., Jaschinski, U., John, S., Rossaint, R., Welte, T., Schaefer, M., Kern, P., Kuhnt, E., Kiehntopf, M., Hartog, C., Natanson, C., Loeffler, M. and Reinhart, K., German Competence Network Sepsis (SepNet) (2008) Intensive insulin therapy and pentastarch resuscitation in severe sepsis. *New England Journal of Medicine*, 358 (2): 125–139.

Brush, K.A. (2007) Abdominal compartment syndrome. *Nursing2007*, 37 (7): 37–40.

BTS (British Thoracic Society) (2002) Non-invasive ventilation in acute respiratory failure. *Thorax*, 57 (3): 192–211.

—— (2003) British Thoracic Society guidelines for the management of suspected acute pulmonary embolism. *Thorax*, 58 (6): 470–484.

—— (2008) BTS guideline for emergency oxygen use in adult patients. *Thorax*, 63 (supplement VI): vi1–68.

Buchan, J. (2002) Global nursing shortages. *British Medical Journal*, 324 (7340): 751–752.

Bugge, J.F. (2009) Brain death and its implications for management of the potential organ donor. *Acta Anaesthesiologica Scandinavia*, 53 (10): 1239–1250.

Bulstrode, N., Banks, F. and Shrotria, S. (2002) The outcome of drug smuggling by 'body packers' – the British experience. *Annals of the Royal College of Surgeons of England*, 84 (1): 35–38.

Burchiel, K.J. and Hsu, F.P. (2001) Pain and spasticity after spinal cord injury: mechanisms and treatment. *Spine*, 26 (24S): S146–S160.

Burke, A.P. and Virmani, R. (2007) Pathophysiology of acute myocardial infarction. *Medical Clinics of North America*, 91 (4): 553–572.

Burns, K.E.A., Adhikari, N.K.J., Keenan, S.P. and Meade, M. (2009) Use of non-invasive ventilation to wean critically ill adults off invasive ventilation: meta-analysis and systematic review. *British Medical Journal*, 339 (7706): 1305–1308.

Burr, G. (1998) Contextualising critical care family needs through triangulation: an Australian study. *Intensive and Critical Care Nursing*, 14 (4): 161–169.

Büscher, A., Sivertsen, B. and White, J. (2009) *Nurses and Midwives: A force for health*. Copenhagen: WHO Regional Office for Europe.

Cabello, J.B., Burls, A., Emparanza, J.I., Bayliss, S. and Quinn, T. (2010) Oxygen therapy for acute myocardial infarction. *Cochrane Database of Systematic Reviews 2010*, issue 6, art. no. CD007160; doi: 10.1002/14651858.CD007160.pub2.

Cade, C. (2008) Clinical tools for the assessment of pain in sedated critically ill adults. *Nursing in Critical Care*, 13 (6): 288–297.

Cahill, N.E., Dhaliwal, R., Day, A.G., Jiang, X. and Heyland, D.K. (2010) Nutrition therapy in the critical care setting: what is 'best achievable' practice? An international multicenter observational study. *Critical Care Medicine*, 38 (2): 395–401.

Caironi, P., Cressoni, P., Chiumello, D., Ranieri, M., Quintel, M., Russo, S.G., Cornejo, R., Bugedo, G., Carlesso, E., Russo, R., Caspani, L. and Gattinoni, L. (2010) Lung opening and closing during ventilation of acute respiratory distress syndrome. *American Journal of Respiratory and Critical Care Medicine*, 181 (6): 578–586.

Callaway, D.W., Shapiro, N.I., Donnino, M.W., Baker, C. and Rosen, C.L. (2009) Serum lactate and base deficit as predictors of mortality in normotensive elderly blunt trauma patients. *Journal of Trauma*, 66 (4): 1040–1044.

Calzia, E. and Stahl, W. (2004) The place of helium in the management of severe acute respiratory failure. *International Journal of Intensive Care*, 11 (2): 65–69.

Camargo, L.F.A., Marra, A.R., Büchele, G.L., Sogayar, A.M.C., Cal, R.G.R., de Sousa, J.M.A., Silva, E., Knobel, E. and Edmond, M.B. (2009) Double-lumen central venous catheters impregnated with chlorhexidine and silver sulfadiazine to prevent catheter colonisation in the intensive care unit setting: a prospective randomised study. *Journal of Hospital Infection*, 72 (3): 227–233.

Campbell, G.A. and Rosner, M.H. (2008) The agony of ecstasy: MDMA (3,4-methylenedioxy-methamphetamine) and the kidney. *Clinical Journal of the American Society of Nephrology*, 3 (6): 1852–1860.

Caplin-Davies, P.J. (1999) Doctor-nurse substitution: the workforce equation. *Journal of Nursing Management*, 7 (2): 71–79.

Cappell, M.S. and Friedel, D. (2008) Initial management of acute upper gastrointestinal bleeding: from initial evaluation up to gastrointestinal endoscopy. *Medical Clinics of North America*, 92 (3): 491–509.

Carney, D., DiRocco, J. and Nieman, G. (2005) Dynamic alveolar mechanics and ventilator-induced lung injury. *Critical Care Medicine*, 33 (3 supplement): S122–S128.

Carrell, T.W.G. and Wolfe, J.H.N. (2005) Non-cardiac vascular disease. *Heart*, 91 (2): 265–270.

Carter, S. (2009) Renewing pride in teaching: using theory to advance nursing scholarship. *Nurse Education in Practice*, 9 (2): 119–126.

Casey, G. (2002) Physiology of skin. *Nursing Standard*, 16 (34): 47–51.

Cason, C.L., Tyner, T., Saunders, S. and Broome, L. (2007) Nurses' implementation of guidelines for ventilator-associated pneumonia from the centers for disease control and prevention. *American Journal of Critical Care*, 16 (1): 28–37.

Catalano, G., Houston, S.H., Catalano, M.C., Butera, A.S., Jennings, S.M., Hakala, S.M., Burrows, S.L., Hickey, M.G., Duss, C.V., Skelton, D.N. and Laliotis, G.J. (2003) Anxiety and depression in hospitalized patients in resistant organism isolation. *Southern Medical Journal*, 96 (2): 141–145.

Cau, J., Ricco, J.B. and Corpataux, J.M. (2008) Laparoscopic aortic surgery: techniques and results. *Journal of Vascular Surgery*, 48: 37S–44S.

Cavaliere, F., Antonelli, M., Arcangeli, A., Conti, G., Pennisi, M.A. and Proietti, R. (2002) Effects of acid-base abnormalities on blood capacity of transporting CO_2: adverse effect of metabolic acidosis. *Intensive Care Medicine*, 28 (5): 609–615.

Cavolli, R., Kaya, K., Aslan, A., Emiroglu, O., Erturk, S., Korkmaz, O., Oguz, M., Tasoz, R. and Ozyurda, U. (2008) Does sodium nitroprusside decrease the incidence of atrial fibrillation after myocardial revascularisation? *Circulation*, 118 (5): 476–481.

Cayley, W.E. (2007) Preventing deep vein thrombosis in hospital patients. *British Medical Journal*, 335 (7611): 147–151.

Cely, C.M., Arora, P., Quartrin, A.A., Kett, D.H. and Schein, R.M.H. (2004) Relationship of baseline glucose homeostasis to hyperglycaemia during medical critical illness. *Chest*, 126 (3): 879–887.

Cepeda, J.A., Cooper, B., Hails, J., Kwaku, F., Taylor, L., Hayman, S., Cookson, B., Shaw, S., Kibbler, C., Singer, M., Belligan, G. and Wilson, A.P.R. (2005) Isolation of patients in single rooms or cohorts to reduce spread of *MRSa* in intensive-care units: prospective two-centre study. *Lancet*, 365 (9456): 295–304.

Chaboyer, W., Thalib, L., Foster, M., Ball, C. and Richards, B. (2008) Predictors of adverse events in patients after discharge from the intensive care unit. *American Journal of Critical Care*, 17 (3): 255–263.

Chadda, K., Louis, B., Benaïssa, L., Annane, D., Gajdos, P., Raphaël, J.C. and Lofaso, F. (2002) Physiological effects of decannulation in tracheostomized patients. *Intensive Care Medicine*, 28 (12): 1761–1767.

Chan, E.Y., Ruest, A., O'Meade, M. and Cook, D.J. (2007a) Oral decontamination for prevention of pneumonia in mechanically ventilated adults: systematic review and meta-analysis. *British Medical Journal*, 10 (7599): 889.

Chan, K.P.W., Stewart, T.E., Mehta, S. (2007b) High-frequency oscillatory ventilation for adults with ARDS. *Chest*, 131 (6): 1907–1916.

Chandler, B. and Hunter, J. (2009) Ventilator-associated pneumonia: a concise review. *Journal of the Intensive Care Society*, 10 (1): 29–33.

Chandola, T., Brunner, E. and Marmot, M. (2006) Chronic stress at work and the metabolic syndrome: prospective study. *British Medical Journal*, 332 (7540): 521–524.

Chandrashekhar, Y., Westaby, S. and Narula, J. (2009) Mitral stenosis. *Lancet*, 374 (9697): 1213–1300.

Chaney, J.C. and Derdak, S. (2002) Minimally invasive hemodynamic monitoring for the intensivist: current and emerging technology. *Critical Care Medicine*, 30 (10): 2338–2345.

Chang, L.-Y., Wang, K.-W.K. and Chao, Y.-F. (2008) Influence of physical restraint on unplanned extubation of adult intensive care patients: a case-control study. *American Journal of Critical Care*, 17 (5): 408–415.

Chanques, G., Payen, J.-F., Mercier, G., Lattre, S. de, Viel, E., Jung, B.C., Lefrant, J.-Y. and Jaber, S. (2009) Assessing pain in non-intubated critically ill patients unable to self-report: an adaptation of the Behavioral Pain Scale. *Intensive Care Medicine*, 35 (12): 2060–2067.

Chao, Y.-F.C., Chen, Y.-Y., Wang, K.-W.K., Lee, R.-P. and Tsai, H. (2009) Removal of oral secretions prior to position change can reduce the incidence of ventilator-associated pneumonia for adult ICU patients. *Journal of Clinical Nursing*, 18 (1): 22–28.

Charalambous, C., Schofield, I. and Malik, R. (1999) Acute diabetic emergencies and their management. *Care of the Critically Ill*, 15 (4): 132–135.

Chassard, D. and Bruguerolle, B. (2004) Chronobiology and anesthesia. *Anesthesiology*, 100 (2): 413–427.

Cheatham, M.L., Malbrain, M.L.N.G., Kirkpatrick, A., Sugrue, M., Parr, M., de Waele, J., Balogh, Z., Leppäniemi, A., Olvera, C., Ivatury, R., D'Amours, S., Wendon, J., Hillman, K. and Wilmer, A. (2007) Results from the International Conference of Experts on Intra-abdominal Hypertension and Abdominal Compartment Syndrome. II. Recommendations. *Intensive Care Medicine*, 33 (6): 951–962.

Chen, J.M.H., Heran, B.S., Perez, M.I. and Wright, J.M. (2010) Blood pressure lowering efficacy of beta-blockers as second-line therapy for primary hypertension. *Cochrane Database of Systematic Reviews*, issue 1, art. no: CD007185; doi: 10.1002/14651858.CD007185.pub2.

Cherian, J., Thwaini, A., Rao, A., Arya, N., Shergill, I.S. and Patel, H.R.H. (2005) Autonomic dysreflexia: the forgotten medical emergency. *Hospital Medicine*, 66 (5): 294–296.

Chikwe, J., Walther, A. and Pepper, J. (2004) The surgical management of mitral valve disease. *British Journal of Cardiology*, 11 (1): 42–47.

Cho, S.-H., Hwang, J.H. and Kim, J. (2008) Nurse staffing and patient mortality in intensive care units. *Nursing Research*, 57 (5): 322–330.

Cholesterol Treatment Triallists (CTT) Collaborators (2008) Efficacy of cholesterol-lowering therapy in 18686 people with diabetes in 14 randomised trials of statins: a meta-analysis. *Lancet*, 371 (9607): 117–125.

Cholley, P., Thouverez, M., Floret, N., Bertrand, X. and Talon, D. (2008) The role of water fittings in intensive care rooms as reservoirs for the colonization of patients with *Pseudomonas aeruginosa*. *Intensive Care Medicine*, 34 (8): 1428–1433.

Chonghaile, M.N., Higgins, B.D., Costello, J. and Laffey, J.G. (2008) Hypercapnic acidosis attenuates lung injury induced by established bacterial pneumonia. *Anesthesiology*, 109 (5): 837–848.

Chowell, G., Bertozzi, S.M., Colchero, M.A., Lopez-Gatell, H., Alpuche-Aranda, C., Hernandez, M. and Miller, M.A. (2009) Severe respiratory disease concurrent with the circulation of H1N1 influenza. *New England Journal of Medicine*, 361 (7): 674–679.

Christensen, M. (2007) Noise levels in a general intensive care unit: a descriptive study. *Nursing in Critical Care*, 12 (4): 188–197.

Chua, D. and Ignaszewski, A. (2009) Clopidogrel in acute coronary syndromes. *British Medical Journal*, 338 (7701): 998–1002.

Chumbley, G. (2011) Use of ketamine in uncontrolled acute and procedural pain. *Nursing Standard*, 25 (15–17): 35–37.

Chummun, H., Tilley, V. and Ibe, J. (2010) 3,4-methylenedioxyamphetamine (ecstasy) use reduces cognition. *British Journal of Nursing*, 19 (2): 94–100.

Chychula, N.M. and Sciamanna, C. (2002) Help substance abusers attain and sustain abstinence. *The Nurse Practitioner*, 27 (11) 30–47.

Ciancio, G. (2006) A randomized long-term trial of tacrolimus/sirolimus versus tacrolimums/mycophenolate versus cyclosporine/sirolimus in renal transplantation: three-year analysis. *Transplantation*, 81 (6): 845–852.

Clarke, C.M. (2000) Children visiting family and friends on adult intensive care units: the nurse's perspective. *Journal of Advanced Nursing*, 31 (2): 330–338.

Clarke, G. (1993) Mouthcare and the hospitalised patient. *British Journal of Nursing*, 2 (4): 225–227.

Clay, A.S., Behina, M. and Brown, K.K. (2001) Mitochondrial disease. *Chest*, 120 (2): 634–648.

Clay, H.D. (2000) Validity and reliability of the SjO2 catheter in neurologically impaired patients: a critical review of the literature. *Journal of Neuroscience Nursing*, 32 (4): 194–203.

Clay, M. (2002) Assessing oral health in older people. *Nursing Older People*, 14 (8): 31–32.

Cocker, C. (2009) Weaning from ventilation – current state of the science and art. *Nursing in Critical Care*, 14 (4): 185–190.

Cockett, A. (2010) Cardiac disease, in Cockett, A. and Day, H (eds) *Children's High Dependency Nursing*. Chichester: Wiley-Blackwell, pp. 93–124.

—— and Day, H. (eds) (2010) *Children's High Dependency Nursing*. Chichester: Wiley-Blackwell.

Coeytaux, R.R., Williams, J.W., Gray, R.N. and Wang, A. (2010) Percutaneous heart-valve replacement for aortic stenosis: state of the evidence. *Annals of Internal Medicine*, 153 (5): 314–324.

Coggan, M. (2008) Arterial blood gas analysis. *Nursing Times*, 104 (18): 28–29, and 104 (19): 24–25.

Cogo, P.E., Poole, D., Codazzi, D., Boniotti, C., Capretta, A., Langer, M., Luciana, D., Rossi, C. and Bertolini, G. (2010) Outcomes of children admitted to adult intensive care units in Italy between 2003–2007. *Intensive Care Medicine*, 36 (8): 1403–1409.

Cohen, A.T., Rapson, V.F., Bergmann, J.-F., Goldhaber, S.Z., Kakkar, A.K., Deslandes, B., Huang, W., Zayaruzny, M., Emery, L. and Anderson, F.A. Jr, ENDORSE Investigators (2008) Venous thromboembolism risk and prophylaxis in the acute hospital care setting (ENDORSE study): a multinational cross-sectional study. *Lancet*, 371 (9610): 387–394.

Cohen, J., Brun-Buisson, C., Torres, A. and Jorgensen J. (2004) Diagnosis of infection in sepsis: an evidence-based review. *Critical Care Medicine*, 32 (11): S466–S494.

Coia, J.E., Duckworth, G.J., Edwards, D.I., Farrington, M., Fry, C., Humphreys, H., Mallaghan, C. and Tucker, D.R., Joint Working Party of the British Society of Antimicrobial Chemotherapy, the Hospital Infection Society, and the Infection Control Nurses Association (2006) Guidelines for the control and prevention of meticillin-resistant *Staphylococcus aureus* (*MRSa*) in healthcare facilities. *Journal of Hospital Infections*, 63S: S1–S44.

Cole, L., Bellomo, R., Baldwin, I., Hayhoe, M. and Ronco, C. (2003) The impact of lactate-buffered high-volume hemofiltration on acid-base balance. *Intensive Care Medicine*, 29 (7): 1113–1120.

Collin, N., Haslam, E., Fay, D., Hardman, J. and Horrocks, M. (2009) A review of endovascular management of abdominal aortic aneurysm. *British Journal of Hospital Medicine*, 70 (3): 146–150

Collins, P., Webb, C.M., Chong, C.F. and Moat, N.E., Radial Artery Versus Saphenous Vein Patency (RSVP) Trial Investigators (2008) Radial artery versus saphenous vein patency randomized trial. *Circulation*, 117 (22): 2859–2864.

Combe, D. (2005) The use of patient diaries in an intensive care unit. *Nursing in Critical Care*, 10 (1): 31–34.

Comfort, A. (1977) *A Good Age*. London: Mitchell Beazley.

Compton, F., Wittrock, M., Schaefer, J.-H., Zidek, W., Tepel, M. and Scholze, A. (2008) Noninvasive cardiac output determination using applanation tonometry-derived radial artery pulse contour analysis in critically ill patients. *Anesthesia & Analgesia*, 106 (1): 171–174.

Conde-Agudelo, A. and Romero, R. (2009) Amniotic fluid embolism: an evidence-based review. *American Journal of Obstetrics & Gynecology*, 201 (5): 445–455.

Cooper, D.J. (2003) Lactic Acidosis, in Bersten, A.D. and Soni, N. (eds) *Intensive Care Manual*, 5th edition. Edinburgh: Butterworth-Heinemann, pp. 107–111.

Cooper, N. (2004) Acute care: arterial blood gases. *Student British Medical Journal*, 12: 89–132.

—— and Cramp, P. (2003) *Essential Guide to Acute Care*. London: BMJ Books.

——, Forrest, K. and Cramp, P. (2006) *Essential Guide to Acute Care*, 2nd edition. Oxford: Blackwell Publishing/BMJ Books.

Cooper, S.J. (2004) Methods to prevent ventilator-associated lung injury: a summary. *Intensive and Critical Care Nursing*, 20 (6): 358–365.

Copson, D. (2003) Topical negative pressure and necrotising fasciitis. *Nursing Standard*, 18 (6): 71–80.

Corne, J. and Pointon, K. (2010) *Chest X-ray Made Easy*, 3rd edition. Edinburgh: Churchill Livingstone/Elsevier.

Cotter, G., Moshkovitz, Y., Kaluski, E., Cohen, A.J., Miller, H., Goor, D. and Vered, Z. (2004) Accurate, noninvasive continuous monitoring of cardiac output by whole-body electrical bioimpedance. *Chest*, 125 (4): 1431–1440.

Couchman, B.A., Wetzig, S.M., Coyer, F.M. and Wheeler, M.K. (2007) Nursing care of the mechanically ventilated patient: what does the literature say? Part 1. *Intensive and Critical Care Nursing*, 23 (2): 4–14.

Cox, C. (2010) Legal responsibility and accountability. *Nursing Management*, 17 (3): 18–20.

Cox, W. (2002) Cardiac transplantation, in Hatchett, R. and Thompson, D. (eds) *Cardiac Nursing: A comprehensive guide*. Edinburgh: Churchill Livingstone, pp. 462–480.

Coyer, F.M., Wheeler, M.K., Wetzig, S.M. and Couchman, B.A. (2007) Nursing care of the mechanically ventilated patient: what does the literature say? Part 2. *Intensive and Critical Care Nursing*, 23 (2): 64–70.

Crandall, C.G., Vongpatanasin, W. and Victor, R.G. (2002) Mechanism of cocaine-induced hyperthermia in humans. *Annals of Internal Medicine*, 136 (11): 785–791.

Crawford, D., Greene, N. and Wentworth, S. (2005) *Thermometer Review: UK market survey*. Medicines and Healthcare products Regulatory Agency Evaluation 04144. London: MHRA.

Creagh-Brown, B.C., James, D.A. and Jackson, S.H. (2005) The use of the Tempa.Dot thermometer in routine clinical practice. *Age & Ageing*, 34 (3): 297–299.

Cree, C. (2003) Acquired brain injury: acute management. *Nursing Standard*, 18 (11): 45–54.

Creteur, J., Sibbald, W. and Vincent, J-L. (2000) Hemoglobin solutions – not just red blood cell substitutes. *Critical Care Medicine*, 28 (8): 3025–3034.

Critical Care Stakeholder Forum (2005) *Quality Critical Care: Beyond 'comprehensive critical care'*. London: Critical Care Stakeholder Forum.

Crocker, C. (2009) Weaning from ventilation – current state of the science and art. *Nursing in Critical Care*, 14 (4): 185–190.

Crunden, E. (2010) A reflection from the other side of the bed – an account of what it is like to be a patient and a relative in an intensive care unit. *Intensive and Critical Care Nursing*, 26 (1): 18–23.

Cullis, B. and Macnaughton, P.O. (2007) Sedation and neuromuscular paralysis in the ICU. *Anaesthesia and Intensive Care Medicine*, 8 (1): 32–39.

Cunningham, R. and Dial, S. (2008) Is over-use of proton pump inhibitors fuelling the current epidemic of *Clostridium difficile*-associated diarrhoea? *Journal of Hospital Infection*, 10 (1): 1–6.

Curtis, R.L. (2009) Catheter-related bloodstream infection in the intensive care unit. *Journal of the Intensive Care Society*, 10 (2): 102–108.

Cuthbertson, B.H., Card, G., Croal, B.L., McNeilly, J. and Hillis, G.S. (2007) The utility of B-type natiuretic peptide in predicting postoperative cardiac events and mortality in patients undergoing major emergency non-cardiac surgery. *Anaesthesia*, 62 (9): 875–881.

——, Rattray, J., Campbell, M.K., Gager, M., Roughton, S., Smith, A., Hull, A., Breeman, S., Jenkinson, D., Hernández, D., Johnston, M., Wilson, C. and Waldmann, C. (2009) The PRaCTICal study of nurse-led intensive care follow-up programmes for improving long-term outcomes from critical illness: a pragmatic randomised controlled trial. *British Medical Journal*, 339 (7728): 106.

Dallmeyer, R. (2000) Pharmacological support in paediatric intensive care, in Williams, C. and Asquith, J. (eds) *Paediatric Intensive Care Nursing*. Edinburgh: Churchill Livingstone, pp. 395–418.

Dandona, P., Chaudhuri, A., Ghanim, H. and Mohanty, P. (2007) Effect of hyperglycaemia and insulin in acute coronary syndromes. *American Journal of Cardiology*, 99 (11a): 12H–18H.

Danter, J.H. (2003) Geriatric assessment. *Nursing2003*, 33 (12): 52–54.

Darouiche, R. (2006) Spinal epidural abscess. *New England Journal of Medicine*, 355 (19): 2012–2020.

Darovic, G.O. (2002a) Physical assessment of the pulmonary system, in Darovic, G.O. (ed.) *Hemodynamic Monitoring: Invasive and noninvasive clinical application*, 3rd edition. Philadelphia, PA: WB Saunders, pp. 43–56.

—— (2002b) Arterial pressure monitoring, in Darovic, G.O. (ed.) *Hemodynamic Monitoring: Invasive and noninvasive clinical application*, 3rd edition. Philadelphia, PA: WB Saunders, pp. 133–160.

Davenport, A. and Stevens, P. (2008) *Clinical Practice Guidelines: Acute kidney injury*, 4th edition. London: UK Renal Association.

Davies, J., Tibby, S.M. and Murdoch, I.A. (2005) Should parents accompany critically ill children during inter-hospital transport? *Archives of Disease in Childhood*, 90 (12): 1270–1273.

Davies, J.H. and Hassell, L.L. (2001) *Children in Intensive Care*. Edinburgh: Churchill Livingstone.

Davis, J.L., Morris, A., Kallet, R.H., Powell, K., Chi, A.S., Bensley, M., Luce, J.M. and Huang, L. (2008) Low tidal volume ventilation is associated with reduced mortality in HIV-infected patients with acute lung injury. *Thorax*, 63 (11): 988–993.

Davoudian, P. and Blunt, M. (2009) Outcome from intensive care and measuring performance. *Surgery*, 27 (5): 212–215.

Davydow, D.S., Desai, S.V., Needham, D.M. and Bienvenu, O.J. (2008) Psychiatric morbidity in survivors of the acute respiratory distress syndrome: a systematic review. *Psychosomatic Medicine*, 70 (4): 512–519.

——, Gifford, J.M., Desai, S.V., Bienvenu, O.J. and Needham, D.M. (2009) Depression in general intensive care unit survivors: a systematic review. *Intensive Care Medicine*, 35 (5): 796–809.

Dawson, D. (2005) Development of a new eye care guideline for critically ill patients. *Intensive and Critical Care Nursing*, 21 (2): 118–122.

Day, A. (2001) The nurse's role in managing constipation. *Nursing Standard*, 16 (8): 41–44.

Dean, B. (1997) Evidence-based suction management in accident and emergency – a vital component of airway care. *Accident and Emergency Nursing*, 5 (2): 92–97.

de Backer, D., Biston, P., Devriendt, J., Madl, C., Chochrad, D., Aldecoa, C., Brasseur, A., Defrance, P., Gottignies, P. and Vincent, J.L. (2010) Comparison of dopamine and norepinephrine in the treatment of shock. *New England Journal of Medicine*, 362 (9): 779–789.

de Barbieri, I., Frigo, A.C. and Zampieron, A. (2009) Quick change versus double pump while changing the infusion of inotropes: an experimental study. *Nursing in Critical Care*, 14 (4): 200–206.

de Beauvoir, S. (1970) *Old Age*. London: Penguin.

Dedhia, J.D. and Mushambi, M.C. (2007) Amniotic fluid embolism. *Continuing Education in Anaesthesia, Critical Care & Pain*, 7 (5): 152–156.

Deeny, P. (2005) Care of older people in critical care: the hidden side of the moon. *Intensive and Critical Care Nursing*, 21 (6): 325–327.

de Keulenaer, B.L., de Waele, J.J., Powell, B. and Malbrain, M.L.N.G. (2009) What is normal intra-abdominal pressure and how is it affected by positioning, body mass and positive end-expiratory pressure? *Intensive Care Medicine*, 35 (6): 969–976.

de Laat, E.H.E., Schoonhoven, L., Picklers, P., Verbeek, A.L.M. and van Achterberg, T. (2006) Epidemiology, risk and prevention of pressure ulcers in critically ill patients: a literature review. *Journal of Wound Care*, 15 (6): 269–275.

de Laet, I.E. and Malbrain, M.L.N.G. (2007) Intra-abdominal hypertension and abdominal compartment syndrome: what do we know today? *Care of the Critically Ill*, 23 (1): 4–14.

Dellinger, R.P., Levy, M.M., Carlet, J.M., Bion, K., Parker, M.M., Jaeschke, R., Reinhart, K., Angus, D.C., Brun-Buisson, C., Beale, R., Calandra, T., Dhainaut, J.-F., Gerlach, H., Harvey, M., Marini, J.J., Marshall, J., Ranieri, M., Ramsay, G., Sevransky, J., Thompson, B.T., Townsend, S., Vender, J.S., Zimerman, J.L. and Vincent, J.-L. (2008) Surviving Sepsis Campaign: international guidelines for management of severe sepsis and septic shock: 2008. *Intensive Care Medicine*, 34 (1): 17–60.

Demaria, R.G., Carrier, M., Fortier, S., Martineau, R., Fortier, A., Cartier, R., Pellerin, M. Hébert, Y., Bouchard, D., Pagé, P. and Perrault, L.P. (2002) Reduced mortality and strokes with off-pump coronary artery bypass grafting surgery in octogenarians. *Circulation*, 106 (12): I5–I10.

Demir, F. and Dramali, A. (2005) Requirement for 100% oxygen before and after closed suction. *Journal of Advanced Nursing*, 51 (3): 245–251.

Deogaonkar, A., Gupta, R., DeGeorgia, M., Sabharwel, V., Gopakumaran, B., Schubert, A. and Provencio, J.J. (2004) Bispectral Index monitoring correlates with sedation scales in brain-injured patients. *Critical Care Medicine*, 32 (12): 2403–2406.

de Oliveira, C., Watt, R. and Hamer, M. (2010) Tooth-brushing, inflammation, and risk of cardiovascular disease: results from Scottish Health Survey. *British Medical Journal*, 340 (7761): 1400.

507

Derak, S., Mehta, S., Stewart, T.E., Smith, T., Rodgers, M., Buchman, T.G., Carlin, B., Lowson, S. and Granton, J., Multicenter Oscillatory Ventilation for Acute Respiratory Distress Syndrome Trial (MOAT) Study Investigators (2002) High-frequency oscillatory ventilation for acute respiratory distress syndrome in adults. *American Journal of Respiratory and Critical Care Medicine*, 166 (6): 801–808.

Dernaika, T.A., Keddissi, J.I. and Kinasewitz, G.T. (2009) Update on ARDS: beyond the low tidal volume. *American Journal of the Medical Sciences*, 337 (5): 360–367.

Deroy, R. (2000) Crystalloids or colloids for fluid resuscitation – is that the question? *Current Anaesthesia and Critical Care*, 11 (1): 20–26.

de Smet, A.M.G.A., Kluytmans, J.A.J.W., Cooper, B.S., Mascini, E.M., Benus, R.F.J., van der Werf, T.S., van der Hoeven, J.G., Picklers, P., Bogaers-Hofman, D., van der Meer, N.J.M., Bernards, A.T., Kuijper, E.J., Joore, J.C.A., Leversetin-van Hall, M.A., Bindels, A.J.G.H., Jansz, A.P., Wesselink, R.M.J., de Jongh, B.M., Dennesen, P.J.W, van Asselt, G.J., te Velde, L.F., Frenay, I.H.M.E., Kaasjager, K., Bosch, F.H., van Iterson, M., Thijsen, S.F.T., Kluge, G.H., Pauw, W., de Vries, J.W., Kaan, J.A., Arends, J.P., Aarts, L.P.H.J., Sturm, P.D.J., Harinck, H.I.J., Voss, A., Uijtendaal, E.V., Blok, H.E.M., Thieme Groen, E.S., Pouw, M.E., Kaalkman, C.J. and Bonten, M.J. (2009) Decontamination of the digestive tract and oropharynx in ICU patients. *New England Journal of Medicine*, 360 (1): 20–31.

Detriche, O., Berre, J., Massaut, J. and Vincent, J.-L. (1999) The Brussels sedation scale: use of a simple clinical sedation scale can avoid excessive sedation in patients undergoing mechanical ventilation in the intensive care unit. *British Journal of Anaesthesia*, 83 (5): 698–701.

Devendra, D., Liu, E. and Eisenbarth, G.S. (2004) Type 1 diabetes: recent developments. *British Medical Journal*, 328 (7442): 750–754.

Devlin, J.W., Fong, J.J., Howard, E.P., Skrobik, Y., McCoy, N., Yasuda, C. and Marshall, J. (2008) Assessment of delirium in the intensive care unit: nursing practices and perceptions. *American Journal of Critical Care*, 17 (6): 555–565.

Devlin, M. (2000) The nutritional needs of the older person. *Professional Nurse*, 16 (3): 951–955.

de Waele, J.J., Hoste, E.A.J., Baert, D., Hendricks, K., Rijckaert, D., Thibo, P., van Biervliet, P., Blot, S.I. and Colardyn, F. (2007) Relative adrenal insufficiency in patients with severe acute pancreatitis. *Intensive Care Medicine*, 33 (10): 1754–1760.

Dewhurst, A. and Rawlins, T. (2009) Percutaneous valve replacement and repair in the adult: techniques and anaesthetic considerations. *Current Anaesthesia & Critical Care*, 20 (4): 155–159.

Dezfulian, C., Shiva, S., Alekseyenko, A., Pendyal, A., Besiser, D.G., Munasinghe, J.P., Anderson, S.A., Chesley, C.F., Hoek, V. and Gladwin, M.T. (2009) Nitrite therapy after cardiac arrest reduces reactive oxygen species generation, improves cardiac and neurological function, and enhances survival via reversible inhibition of mitochondrial complex I. *Circulation*, 120 (10): 897–905.

DH (Department of Health) (1997) *A Bridge to the Future: Nursing standards, education and workforce planning in paediatric intensive care*. London: HMSO.

—— (1998) *Code of Practice for the Diagnosis of Brain Stem Death*. London: HMSO.

—— (2000a) *Comprehensive Critical Care: A review of adult critical care services*. London: Department of Health.

—— (2000b) *An Organisation with a Memory*. London: Department of Health.

—— (2000c) *Health Services Circular HSC 2000/26*. London: Department of Health.

—— (2001) *National Service Framework for Older People*. London: Department of Health.

—— (2002) *National Service Framework for Diabetes*. London: Department of Health.

—— (2005) *A National Framework to Support Local Workforce Strategy Development: A guide for HR directors in the NHS and social care*. London: The Stationery Office.

—— (2006) *Modernising Nursing Careers*. London: Department of Health.

—— (2007a) *Screening for Meticillin-resistant Staphylococcus aureus (MRSa) colonisation (Saving Lives)*. London: Department of Health.

—— (2007b) *High Impact Intervention 1: Central venous care bundle*. London: Department of Health.

—— (2008a) *National Infarct Angioplasty Project*. London: Department of Health.

—— (2008b) *Organs for Transplants*. London: Department of Health.

—— (2008c) *End of Life Care Strategy*. London: Department of Health.

—— (2009a) *NHS 2010–2015: From good to great. Preventative, people-centred, productive*. London: Department of Health.

—— (2009b) New H1N1v influenza: current situation and next steps. Letter, dated 2 July 2009 (Gateway ref: 12167).

—— (2010a) *Midwifery 2010: Delivering expectations*. London: Department of Health.

—— (2010b) *Six Years On: Delivering the Diabetes National Service Framework*. London: Department of Health.

Dhillon, R., Clark, J. (2009) Infection in the intensive care unit (ICU). *Current Anaesthesia & Critical Care*, 20 (4): 175–182.

Dhond, G.R. and Dob, D.P. (2000) Critical care of the obstetric patient. *Current Anaesthesia and Critical Care*, 11 (2): 86–91.

Dickson, S.J., Batson, S., Copas, A.J., Edwards, S.G., Singer, M. and Miller, R.F. (2007) Survival of HIV-infected patients in the intensive care unit in the era of highly active antiretroviral therapy. *Thorax*, 62 (11): 964–968.

Dickstein, K., Cohen-Solal, A., Filippatos, G., McMurray, J.V.C., Ponikowski, P., Poole-Wilson, P.A., Strömberg, A., van Veldhuisen, D.J., Atar, D., Hoes, A.W., Keren, A., Mebazaa, A., Nieminen, M., Priori, S.G. and Swedberg, K., Task Force for the Diagnosis and Treatment of Acute and Chronic Heart Failure of the European Society of Cardiology (2008) ESC Guidelines for the diagnosis and treatment of acute and chronic heart failure 2008. *European Heart Journal*, 29 (19): 2388–2442.

Dimond, B. (2008) *Legal Aspects of Nursing*, 5th edition. Harlow: Pearson Education.

di Giantomasso, D., May, C.N. and Bellomo, R. (2002) Norepinephrine and vital organ blood flow. *Intensive Care Medicine*, 28 (12): 1804–1809.

di Mario, C., Dudek, D., Piscione, F., Mielecki, W., Stefano, S., Murena, E., Dimopoulos, K., Manari, A., Gaspardone, A., Ochala, A., Zmudka, K., Bolognese, L., Steg, P.G. and Flather, M., CARESS-in-AMI Investigators (2008) Immediate angioplasty versus standard therapy with rescue angioplasty after thrombolysis in the Combined Abciximab RE-teplase Stent Study in Acute Myocardial Infection (CARESS-in-AMI): an open, prospective, randomised, multi-centre trial. *Lancet*, 371 (9612): 559–568.

Dive, A., Foret, F., Jamart, J., Bulpa P. and Installe E. (2000) Effects of dopamine on gastro-intestinal motility during critical illness. *Intensive Care Medicine*, 26 (7): 901–907.

Dodek, P., Keenan, S., Cook, D., Heyland, D., Jacka, M., Hand, L., Muscedere, J. and Brun-Buisson, C., Canadian Critical Care Trials Group, Canadian Critical Care Society (2004) Evidence-based clinical practice guideline for the prevention of ventilator-associated pneumonia. *Annals of Internal Medicine*, 141 (4): 305–313.

Doig, G.S., Heighes, P.T., Simpson, F., Sweetman, E.A. and Davies, A.R. (2009) Early enteral nutrition, provided within 24h of injury or intensive care unit admission, significantly reduces mortality in critically ill patients: a meta-analysis of randomised controlled trials. *Intensive Care Medicine*, 35 (12): 2018–2027.

Donaldson, L.J., Rutter, P.D., Ellis, B.M., Mytton, O.T., Pebody, R.G. and Yardley, I.E. (2010) Mortality from pandemic A/H1N1 2009 influenza in England: public health surveillance study. *British Medical Journal*, 340 (7737): 82.

REFERENCES

Dougherty, L. and Lister, S. (eds) (2004) *The Royal Marsden Hospital Manual of Clinical Nursing Procedures*, 6th edition. Oxford: Blackwell Science.

—— (eds) (2008) *The Royal Marsden Hospital Manual of Clinical Nursing Procedures*, 7th edition. Oxford: Wiley-Blackwell.

Douglas, J.M. and Spaniol, S.E. (2009) A multimodal approach to the prevention of postoperative stroke in patients undergoing coronary artery bypass surgery. *American Journal of Surgery*, 197 (5): 587–590.

Dowdy, D.W., Dinglas, V., Mendez-Tellez, P.A, Bienvenu O.J., Sevransky, J., Dennison, C.R., Shanholtz, C. and Needham, D.M. (2008) Intensive care unit hypoglycaemia predicts depression during early recovery from acute lung injury. *Critical Care Medicine*, 36 (10): 2726–2733.

Dowsett, C. and White, R.J. (2010) Delivering quality and high impact actions. *British Journal of Healthcare Management*, 16 (2): 92.

Drakulovic, M.B., Torres, A., Bauer, T.T., Nicholas, J.M., Nogue, S. and Ferrer, M. (1999) Supine body position as a risk factor for nosocomial pneumonia in mechanically ventilated patients: a randomised trial. *Lancet*, 354 (9193): 1851–1858.

Drucker, P.F. (1974) *Management*. London: Butterworth-Heinemann.

Dua, K. and Banerjee, A. (2010) Gullain-Barré syndrome: a review. *British Journal of Hospital Medicine*, 71 (9): 495–498.

Dubé, L. and Granry, J-C. (2003) The therapeutic use of magnesium in anesthesiology, intensive care and emergency medicine: a review. *Canadian Journal of Anesthesia*, 50 (7): 732–746.

Duncan, A.W. (2009) Upper respiratory tract obstruction in children, in Bersten, A.D. and Soni, N. (eds) *Intensive Care Manual*, 6th edition. Edinburgh: Butterworth-Heinemann Elsevier, pp. 1093–1100.

Durairaj, L. and Schmidt, G.A. (2008) Fluid therapy in resuscitated sepsis: less is more. *Chest*, 133 (1): 252–263.

Durward, A. (2002) Chloride and the anion gap: a clinical guide to establishing the cause of metabolic acidosis. *International Journal of Intensive Care*, 9 (1): 26–31.

Dutta, R., Baha, S. and Al-Shaikh, B. (2006) Humidification, humidifiers and nebulizers. *CPD Anaesthesia*, 8 (2): 78–82.

Dyer, B., Barrow, A. and Coakley, J. (2009) Critical care-associated weakness. *Anaesthesia and Intensive Care Medicine*, 10 (3): 141–143.

Easby, D. and Dalrymple, P. (2009) Monitoring arterial, central and pulmonary capillary wedge pressure. *Anaesthesia and Intensive Care Medicine*, 10 (1): 38–44.

Echols, J., Friedman, B., Mullins, R.F. and Still, J.M. Jr (2004) Initial experience with a new system for the control and containment of fecal output for the protection of patients in a large burn centre. *Chest*, 126 (4 supplement): 862S.

Edouard, A.R., Vanhille, E., Le Moigno, S., Benhamou, D. and Mazoit, J.-X. (2005) Non-invasive assessment of cerebral perfusion pressure in brain injured patients with moderate intracranial hypertension. *British Journal of Anaesthesia*, 94 (2): 216–221.

EfCCNa (European federation of Critical Care Nursing associations) (2007) *Position Statement on Workforce Requirements within European Critical Care Nursing*. Blaricum, Netherlands: EfCCNa.

Egerod, I., Schwartz-Nielsen, K.H., Hansen, G.M. and Lörckner, E. (2007) The extent and application of patient diaries in Danish ICUs in 2006. *Nursing in Critical Care*, 12 (3): 159–167.

Eggert, S.M. and Jarwood, C.J. (2003) Percutaneous tracheostomy. *BJA CEPD Reviews*, 3 (5): 139–142.

Egi, M., Bellomo, R., Stachowski, E., French, C.J. and Hart, G. (2006) Variability of blood glucose concentration and short-term mortality in critically ill patients. *Anesthesiology*, 105 (2): 244–252.

510

Ehlenbach, W.J., Hough, C.L., Crane, P.K., Haneuse, S.J.P.A., Carson, S.S., Curtis, J.R. and Larson, E.B. (2010) Association between acute care and critical illness hospitalization and cognitive function in older adults. *JAMA*, 303 (8): 763–770.

Eisenstaedt, R., Penninx, B.W.J.H. and Woodman, R.C. (2006) Anemia in the elderly: current understanding and emerging concepts. *Blood Reviews*, 20 (4): 213–216.

El-Ansary, D., Adams, R., Torns, L. and Elkins M. (2000) Sternal instability following coronary artery bypass grafting. *Physiotherapy Theory and Practice*, 16 (1): 27–33.

Eliopoulos, C. (2001) *Gerontological Nursing*, 5th edition. Philadelphia, PA: Lippincott.

Eliott, P. (2003) Rational use of inotropes. *Anaesthesia and Intensive Care*, 4 (9): 292–296.

Elliott, R., McKinley, S. and Fox, V. (2008) Quality improvement program to reduce the prevalence of pressure ulcers in an intensive care unit. *American Journal of Critical Care*, 17 (4): 328–334.

El-Radhi, A.S. and Patel, S. (2006) An evaluation of tympanic thermometry in a paediatric emergency department. *Emergency Medicine Journal*, 23 (1): 40–41.

El Solh, A.A., Akinnusi, M.E., Alsawalha, L.N. and Pineda, L.A. (2008) Outcome of septic shock in older adults after implementation of the sepsis 'bundle'. *Journal of the American Geriatrics Society*, 56 (2): 272–278.

Ely, E.W., Truman, B., Shintani, A., Thomason, J.W., Wheeler, A.P., Gordon, S., Francis, J., Speroff, T., Gautam, S., Margolin, R., Sessler, C.N., Dittus and R.S., Bernard, G.R. (2003) Monitoring sedation status over time in ICU patients: reliability and validity of the Richmond Agitation-Sedation Scale (RASS). *JAMA*, 289 (22): 2983–2991.

——, Stephens, R.K., Jackson, J.C., Thomason, J.W.W., Truman, B., Gordon, S., Robert, S. and Bernard, G.R. (2004) Current opinions regarding the importance, diagnosis, and management of delirium in the intensive care unit: a survey of 912 healthcare professionals. *Critical Care Medicine*, 32 (1): 106–112.

Endacott, R. (1999) Role of the allocated nurse and shift leader in the intensive care unit: findings of an ethnographic study. *Intensive and Critical Care Nursing*, 15 (1): 10–18.

—— (2007) Caring for relatives in intensive care – an exemplar of advanced practice. *Nursing in Critical Care*, 12 (1): 4–5.

Eriksson, T., Lindahl, B. and Bergbom, I. (2010) Visits in an intensive care unit: an observational hermeneutic study. *Intensive & Critical Care Nursing*, 26 (1): 51–57.

Erlen, J.A. (2004) Wanted – nurses. *Orthopaedic Nursing*, 23 (4): 289–292.

Esteban, A., Frutos-Vivar, F., Ferguson, N.D., Arabi, Y., Apeztegufa, C., González, M., Epstein, S.K., Hill, N.S., Nava, S., Soares, M.-A., D'Empaire, G., Alía, I. and Anzueto, A. (2004) Noninvasive positive pressure ventilation for respiratory failure after extubation. *New England Journal of Medicine*, 350 (24): 2452–2460.

Ethics Committee of the Society of Critical Care Medicine (1997) Consensus statement of the Society of Critical Care Medicine's Ethics Committee regarding futile and other possible inadvisable treatments. *Critical Care Medicine*, 25 (5): 887–891.

Everest, E. and Munford, B. (2009) Transport of the critically ill, in Bersten, A.D. and Soni, N. (eds) *Intensive Care Manual*, 6th edition. Edinburgh: Butterworth-Heinemann Elsevier, pp. 31–42.

Eves, N.D. and Ford, G.T. (2007) Helium-oxygen: a versatile therapy to 'lighten the load' of chronic obstructive pulmonary disease (COPD). *Respiratory Medicine: COPD Update*, 3 (3): 87–94.

Eynon, C.A. and Menon, K.D. (2002) Critical care management of head injury. *Anaesthesia & Critical Care*, 3 (4): 135–139.

Faber, P., Ronald, A. and Millar, W. (2005) Methylthioninium chloride: pharmacology and clinical applications with special emphasis on nitric oxide mediated vasodilatory shock during cardiopulmonary bypass. *Anaesthesia*, 60 (6): 575–587.

511

Fajardo-Dolci, G., Gutierrez-Vega, R., Arboleya-Casanova, H., Villalobos, A., Wilson, K.S., García, S.G., Sotelo, J., Villalobos, J.A.C. and Díaz-Olavarrietta, C. (2010) Clinical characteristics of fatalities due to influenza A (H1N1) virus in Mexico. *Thorax*, 65 (6): 505–509.

Fallis, W.M. (2005) The effect of urine flow rate on urinary bladder temperature in critically ill adults. *Heart & Lung*, 34 (3): 209–216.

Fan, T., Wang, G., Mao, B., Ziong, Z., Zhang, Y., Liu, X., Wang, L. and Yang, S. (2008) Prophylactic administration of paraenteral steroids for preventing airway complications after extubation in adults: meta-analysis of randomised placebo controlled trials. *British Medical Journal*, 337 (7678): 1088–1091.

Farley, A. and McLafferty, E. (2008) Nursing management of the patient with hypothermia. *Nursing Standard*, 22 (17): 43–46.

Farrell, P. and Sittlington, N. (2009) The normal baby, in Fraser, D.M. and Cooper, M.A. (eds) *Myles Textbook for Midwives*, 15th edition. Edinburgh: Churchill Livingstone Elsevier, pp. 763–784.

Fearnhead, N.S. (2007) Acute lower gastrointestinal bleeding. *Medicine*, 35 (3): 164–167.

Feil, N. (1993) *The Validation Breakthrough*. Baltimore, MD: Health Professionals Press.

Feldt, K. (2000) The checklist of non-verbal pain indicators. *Pain Management Nursing*, 1 (1): 13–21.

Ferrara, J.L.M., Levine, J.E., Reddy, P. and Holler, E. (2009) Graft-versus-host disease. *Lancet*, 373 (9674): 1550–1561.

Ferrer, M., Sellarés, J., Valencia, M., Carrillo, A., Gonzalez, G., Badia, J.R., Nicolas, J.M. and Torres, A. (2009) Non-invasive ventilation after extubation in hypercapnic patients with chronic respiratory disorders: randomised controlled trial. *Lancet*, 374 (9695): 1082–1088.

Figg, K.K. and Nemergut, E.C. (2009) Error in central venous pressure measurement. *Anesthesia & Analgesia*, 108 (4): 1209–1211.

Figueroaa-Ramos, M.I., Arroyo-Novoa, C.M., Lee, K.A., Padilla, G. and Puntillo, K.A. (2009) Sleep and delirium in ICU patients: a review of mechanisms and manifestations. *Intensive Care Medicine*, 35 (5): 781–795.

File, T.M. Jr and Tsang, K.W.T. (2005) Severe acute respiratory syndrome. *Treatments in Respiratory Medicine*, 4 (2): 95–106.

Finfer, S., Ranieri, V.M., Thompson, B.T., Barrie, P.S., Dhainaut, J.F., Douglas, I.S., Garlund, B., Marshall, J.C. and Rhodes, A. (2008) Design, conduct analysis and reporting of a multinational placebo-controlled trial of activated protein C for persistent septic shock. *Intensive Care Medicine*, 36 (11): 2973–2979.

Finnell, J.T. and Harris, C.R. (2000) Cardiovascular toxicity of selected drug overdoses. *Topics in Emergency Medicine*, 22 (1): 29–41.

Firmin, R.K. and Killer, H.M. (1999) Extracorporeal membrane oxygenation. *Perfusion*, 14 (4): 291–297.

Firth, M. and Prather, C.M. (2002) Gastrointestinal motility problems in the elderly patient. *Gastroenterology*, 122 (6): 1688–1700.

Firth-Cozens, J. (2001) Cultures for improving patient safety through learning: the role of teamwork. *Quality in Health Care*, 10 (supplement II): ii26–ii31.

—— and Mowbray, D. (2001) Leadership and the quality of care. *Quality in Health Care*, 10 (supplement II): ii3–ii7.

Fisher, L. and Macnaughton, P. (2006) Electrolyte and metabolic disturbances in the critically ill. *Anaesthesia and Intensive Care Medicine*, 7 (5): 151–154.

Fisher, S., Walsh, G. and Cross, N. (2002) Nursing management of the cardiac surgical patient, in Hatchett, R. and Thompson, D. (eds) *Cardiac Nursing: A comprehensive guide*. Edinburgh: Churchill Livingstone, pp. 426–461.

Fogarty, A. and Lingford-Hughes, A. (2004) Addiction and substance misuse. *Medicine*, 32 (7): 29–33.

Fonseca, J.E., Méndez, F., Cataño, C., Arias, F. (2005) Dexamethasone treatment does not improve the outcome of women with HELLP syndrome: a double-blind placebo-controlled, randomized clinical trial. *American Journal of Obstetrics and Gynecology*, 193 (5): 1591–1598.

Fontana, R.J. (2008) Acute liver failure including acetaminophen overdose. *Medical Clinics of North America*, 92 (4): 761–794.

Ford, P.N.R., Thomas, I., Cook, T.M., Whitley, E. and Peden, C.J. (2007) Determinants of outcome in critically ill octogenarians after surgery: an observational study. *British Journal of Anaesthesia*, 99 (6): 824–829.

Forrest, E.H. (2009) The management of alcoholic hepatitis. *British Journal of Hospital Medicine*, 70 (12): 680–684.

Forsythe, S.M. and Schmidt, G.A. (2000) Sodium bicarbonate for the treatment of lactic acidosis. *Chest*, 117 (1): 260–267.

Fortune, P.-M. and Playfor, S. (2009) Transporting critically ill children. *Anaesthesia and Intensive Care Medicine*, 10 (10): 510–513.

Fourcade, O., Simon, M.-F., Litt, L., Samii, K. and Chap, H. (2004) Propofol inhibits human platelet aggregation induced by proinflammatory lipid mediators. *Anesthesia & Analgesia*, 99 (2): 393–398.

Fowler, R.A., Lapinsky, S.E., Hallett, D., Detsky, A.S., Sibbald, W.J., Slutsky, A.S. and Stewart, T.E., Toronto SARS Critical Care Group (2003) Critically ill patients with severe acute respiratory syndrome. *JAMA*, 290 (3): 367–373.

Foxall, F. (2008) *Arterial Blood Gas Analysis*. Keswick: M&K Update.

Freeman, B.D., Isabella, K., Lin, N. and Buchman, T.G. (2000) A meta-analysis of prospective trials comparing percutaneous and surgical tracheostomy in critically ill patients. *Chest*, 118: (5): 1412–1418.

Fried, M.J., Bruce, J., Colquhoun, R. and Smith, G. (2010) Inter-hospital transfers of acutely ill adults in Scotland. *Anaesthesia*, 65 (2): 136–144.

Friese, R.S., Diaz-Arrastia, R., McBride, D., Frankel, H. and Gentilello, L.M. (2007) Quantity and quality of sleep in the surgical intensive care unit: are our patients sleeping? *Journal of Trauma: Injury, Infection, and Critical Care*, 63 (6): 1210–1214.

——, Bruns, B. and Sinton, C.M. (2009) Sleep deprivation after septic insult increases mortality independent of age. *Journal of Trauma*, 66 (1): 50–54.

Fuccio, L., Laterza, L., Zagari, R.M., Cennamo, V., Grilli, D. and Bazzoli, F. (2008) Treatment of *Helicobacter pylori* infection. *British Medical Journal*, 337 (7672): 747–750.

Fuentebella, J. and Kerner, J.A. (2009) Refeeding syndrome. *Pediatric Clinics of North America*, 56 (5): 1201–1210.

Fukuda, S. and Warner, D.S. (2007) Cerebral protection. *British Journal of Anaesthesia*, 99 (1): 10–17.

Fulbrook, P. (1997) Core body temperature measurement: a comparison of axilla, tympanic membrane and pulmonary artery blood temperature. *Intensive and Critical Care Nursing*, 13 (5): 266–272.

Fullwood, D. and Sargent, S. (2010) An overview of sedation for adult patients in hospital. *Nursing Standard*, 24 (39): 48–56.

Furlan, J.C., Urbach, D.R. and Fehlings, M.G. (2007) Optimal treatment for severe neurogenic bowel dysfunction after chronic spinal cord injury: a decision analysis. *British Journal of Surgery*, 94 (9): 1139–1150.

Gaasbeek, A. and Meinders, E. (2005) Hypophosphatemia: an update on its etiology and treatment. *American Journal of Medicine*, 118 (10): 1094–1101.

Gacouin, A., Camus, C., Gros, A., Isslame, S., Marque, S., Lavoué, S., Chimot, L., Donnio, P.-Y. and Le Tulzo, Y. (2010) Constipation in long-term ventilated patients: associated factors and impact on intensive care unit outcomes. *Critical Care Medicine*, 38 (10): 1933–1938.

Gaffney, A.M., Widhurt, S.M., Annich, G.M. and Radomski, M.W. (2010) Extracorporeal life support. *British Medical Journal*, 341 (7780): 982–986.

Gagné, R.M. (1975) *Essentials of Learning for Instruction*. New York: Holt, Reinhart & Winston.

Gagné, R.M. (1985) *The Condition of Learning and Theory Instruction*. London: Holt, Reinhart & Winston.

Gajic, O., Rana, R., Winters, J.L., Yilmaz, M., Mondez, J.L., Rickman, O.B., O'Byrne, M.M., Evenson, L.K., Malinchoc, M., DeGoey, S.R., Afessa, B., Hubmayr, R.D. and Moore, S.B. (2007) Transfusion-related acute lung injury in the critically ill. *American Journal of Respiratory and Critical Care Medicine*, 176 (9): 886–891.

Gallagher, R. and McKinley, S. (2009) Anxiety, depression and perceived control in patients having coronary artery bypass grafts. *Journal of Advanced Nursing*, 65 (11): 2386–2396.

Gallego, P.H., Craig, M.E., Hing, S. and Donaghue, K.C. (2008) Role of blood pressure in development of early retinopathy in adolescents with type 1 diabetes: prospective cohort study. *British Medical Journal*, 337 (7668): 497–499.

Galvin, S., Campbell, M., Marsh, B. and O'Brien, B. (2010) Cocaine-related admissions to an intensive care unit: a five-year study of incidence and outcomes. *Anaesthesia*, 65 (2): 163–166.

Gammon, J., Morgan-Samuel, H. and Gould, D. (2008) A review of the evidence for suboptimal compliance of healthcare practitioners to standard/universal infection control precautions. *Journal of Clinical Nursing*, 17 (2): 157–168.

Gandhi, N.R., Nunn, P., Dheda, K., Schaaf, H.S., Zignol, M., van Soolingen, D., Jensen, P. and Bayona, J. (2010) Multidrug-resistant and extensively drug-resistant tuberculosis: a threat to global control of tuberculosis. *Lancet*, 375 (9728): 1830–1843.

Garner, A. and Sibthorpe, B. (2002) Will he get back to normal? Survival and functional status after intensive care therapy. *Intensive and Critical Care Nursing*, 18 (33): 138–145.

Garretson, S. and Malberti, S. (2007) Understanding hypovolaemic, cardiogenic and septic shock. *Nursing Standard*, 50 (21): 46–55.

Garry, P., Garry, D. and Kapila, A. (2010) Surviving sepsis – the physiology behind why we should intervene early. *Care of the Critically Ill*, 25 (2): 36–39.

Garvey, G. and Belligan, G. (2009) MRSA: isolation could do more harm than good, in Ridley, S. (ed.) *Critical Care Focus 16: Infection*. London: Intensive Care Society, pp. 73–89.

Gastmeier, P. and Geffers, C. (2007) Prevention of ventilator-associated pneumonia: analysis of studies published since 2004. *Journal of Hospital Infection*, 67 (1): 1.

Gattinoni, L., Pesenti, A., Bombino, M., Pelosi, P. and Brazzi, L. (1993) Role of extracorporeal circulation in adult respiratory distress syndrome management. *New Horizons*, 1 (4): 603–612.

Geeraerts, T., Merceron, S., Benhamou, D., Vigué, B. and Duranteau, J. (2008) Non-invasive assessment of intracranial pressure using ocular sonography in neurocritical care patients. *Intensive Care Medicine*, 34 (11): 2062–2067.

Germain, S., Wyncoll, D. and Nelson-Piercy, C. (2006) Management of the critically ill obstetric patient. *Current Obstetrics & Gynaecology*, 16 (3): 125–133.

Ghajar, J. (2000) Traumatic brain injury. *Lancet*, 356 (9233): 923–929.

Ghiassi, S., Sun, Y.-S., Kim, V.B., Scott, C.M., Nifong, W., Rotondo, M.F. and Chitwood, R. Jr (2004) Methylene blue enhancement of resuscitation after refractory hemorrhagic shock. *Journal of Trauma, Injury, Infection and Critical Care*, 57 (3): 515–521.

Ghuran, A. and Nolan, J. (2000) Recreational drug misuse: issues for the cardiologist. *Heart*, 83 (6): 627–633.

Giantin, V., Toffanello, E.D., Enzi, G., Perissinotto, E., Vangelista, S., Simonato, M., Ceccato, C., Mantato, E. and Sergi, G. (2008) Reliability of body temperature measurements in hospitalised older patients. *Journal of Clinical Nursing*, 17 (11): 1518–1525.

514

Giantso, V., Liratzopoulos, N., Efraimidou, M., Alepopoulou, E., Kartali-Ktenidou, S., Minopoulos, G.I., Zakynthinos, S. and Manolas, K.I. (2005) Both early-onset and late-onset ventilator-associated pneumonia are caused mainly by potentially multi-resistant bacteria. *Intensive Care Medicine*, 31 (11): 1488–1494.

Giles, K.A., Pomposelli, F., Hamdan, A., Wyers, M., Jhaveri, A. and Schermerhorn, M.L. (2009) Decrease in total aneurysm-related deaths in the era of endovascular aneurysm repair. *Journal of Vascular Surgery*, 49 (3): 543–551.

Girault, C., Breton, L., Richard, J-C., Tamion, F., Vandelet, P., Aboab, J., Leroy, J. and Bonmarchand, G. (2003) Mechanical effects of airway humidification devices in difficult to wean patients. *Critical Care Medicine*, 31: 1306–1311.

Girou, E. (2003) Prevention of nosocomial infections in acute respiratory failure patients. *European Respiratory Journal*, 22 (supplement 42): 72s–76s.

Glaspole, I.N. and Williams, T.J. (1999) Lung transplantation. *Medicine*, 27 (11): 146–148.

Goffman, E. (1963) *Stigma*. London: Penguin.

Goh, J. and Gupta, A.K. (2002) The management of head injury and intracranial pressure. *Current Anaesthesia & Critical Care*, 13 (3): 129–137.

Goldacre, M.J. and Roberts, S.E. (2004) Hospital admission for acute pancreatitis in an English population, 1963–98: database study of incidence and mortality. *British Medical Journal*, 328 (7454): 1466–1469.

Goldfrad, C. and Rowan, K. (2000) Consequences of discharges from intensive care at night. *Lancet*, 355 (9210): 1138–1142.

Goldhill, D.R., Badacsonyi, A., Goldhill, A.A. and Waldmann, C. (2008) A prospective observational study of ICU patient position and frequency of turning. *Anaesthesia*, 63 (5): 509–515.

González, E.L.M., Johansson, S., Wallander, M.-A. and García Rodríguez, L.A. (2009) Trends in the prevalence and incidence of diabetes in the UK: 1996–2005. *Journal of Epidemiology and Community Health*, 63 (4): 332–336.

Gonzalez, J.C.M. (2008) Gastric residuals – are they important in the management of enteral nutrition? *Clinical Nutrition Highlights*, 4 (1): 2–8.

Gopal, S., Jayakumar, D. and Nelson, P.N. (2009) Meta-analysis on the effect of dopexamine on in-hospital mortality. *Anaesthesia*, 64 (6): 589–594.

Gould, D. (2008) Enterococcal infection. *Nursing Standard*, 22 (27): 40–43.

Grap, M.J., Munro, C.L., Ashtiani, B. and Bryant, S. (2003) Oral care interventions in critical care: frequency and documentation. *American Journal of Critical Care*, 12 (2): 113–118.

Grebenik, C.R. and Sinclair, M.E. (2003) Which inotrope? *Current Paediatrics*, 13 (1): 6–11.

Green, C. (2003) DIC and other coagulopathies in the ICU. *Anaesthesia and Intensive Care*, 4 (5): 147–149.

Greene, S.L., Dargan, P.I. and Jones, A.L. (2005) Acute poisoning: understanding 90% of cases in a nutshell. *Postgraduate Medical Journal*, 81 (954): 204–216.

Greenhalgh, J., Hockenhull, J., Rao, N., Dundar, Y., Dickson, R.C. and Bagust, A. (2010) Drug-eluting stents versus bare metal stents for angina or acute coronary syndromes. *Cochrane Database of Systematic Reviews*, issue 5, art. no. CD004587; doi: 10.1002/14651858.CD004587.pub2.

Greenlee, M., Wingo, C.S., McDonough, A.A., Youn, J.-H. and Kone, B.C. (2009) Narrative review: evolving concepts in potassium homeostasis and hypokalaemia. *Annals of Internal Medicine*, 150 (9): 619–625.

Greenwood, J. (1998) Critical care nurse perceptions of family needs. *Heart & Lung*, 20 (2): 189–201.

Griffiths, R.D. (2003) Nutrition support in critically ill septic patients. *Current Opinion in Nutrition & Metabolic Care*, 6 (2): 203–210.

—— and Bongers, T. (2005) Nutrition support for patients in the intensive care unit. *Postgraduate Medical Journal*, 81 (960): 629–636.

Grimm, M., Rinaldi, M., Yonan, N.A., Arpesella, G., Arizón Del Prado, J.A., Pulpón, L.A., Villemot, J.P., Frigerio, M., Rodriguez Lambert, J.L., Crespo-Leiro, M.G., Almenar, L., Duveau, D., Ordonez-Fernandez, A., Gandjbakhch, J., Maccherini, M. and Laufer, G. (2006) Superior prevention of acute rejection by tacrolimus vs. cyclosporine in heart transplant recipients – a large European trial. *American Journal of Transplantation*, 6 (6) 1387–1397.

Güneş, Ü.Y. and Zaybak, A. (2008) Does the body temperature change in older people? *Journal of Clinical Nursing*, 17 (17): 2284–2287.

Guenter, P.A., Settle, R.G., Perlmutter, S., Marino, P.L., DeSimone, G.A. and Rolandelli, R.H. (1991) Tube feeding-related diarrhoea in acutely ill patients. *Journal of Parenteral and Enteral Nutrition*, 15 (3): 277–280.

Gunn, S.R., Early, B.J., Zenati, M.S. and Ochoa, J.B. (2009) Use of a nasal bridle prevents accidental nasoenteral feeding tube removal. *Journal of Parenteral and Enteral Nutrition*, 33 (1): 50–54.

Gunn, T. (1992) *The Man with Night Sweats*. London: Faber.

Gunning, K. (2009) Hepatic failure. *Anaesthesia and Intensive Care Medicine*, 10 (3): 124–126.

Gupta, R.K., Nikkar-Esfahani, A. and Jamjoom, D.Z.A. (2010) Spontaneous intracerebral haemorrhage: a clinical review. *British Journal of Hospital Medicine*, 71 (9): 499–506.

Gustafsson, C. and Fagerberg, I. (2004) Reflection, the way to professional development? *Journal of Clinical Nursing*, 13 (3): 271–280.

Guyton, A.C. and Hall, J.E. (2005) *Textbook of Medical Physiology*, 11th edition. Philadelphia, PA: Elsevier Saunders.

Habashi, N.M. (2005) Other approaches to open-lung ventilation: airway pressure release ventilation. *Critical Care Medicine*, 33 (3): S228–S240.

Haenggi, M., Ypparila-Wolters, H., Buerki, S., Schlauri, R., Korhonen, I., Takala, J. and Jokob, S.M. (2009) Auditory event-related potentials, bispectral index, and entropy for the discrimination of different levels of sedation in intensive care unit patients. *Anesthesia & Analgesia*, 109 (3): 807–816.

Haider, A.W., Larson, M.G., Franklin, S.S. and Levy, D. (2003) Systolic blood pressure, diastolic blood pressure, and pulse pressure as predictors of risk for congestive heart failure in the Framingham study. *Annals of Internal Medicine*, 138 (1): 10–16.

Haines, L., Wan, K.C., Lynn, R., Barrett, T.G. and Shield, J.P.H. (2007) Rising incidence of type 2 diabetes in children in the U.K. *Diabetes Care*, 30 (5): 1097–1101.

Haitsma, J.J. and Lachmann, B. (2002) Partial liquid ventilation in acute respiratory distress syndrome, in Evans, T.W., Griffiths, M.J.D. and Keogh, B.F. (eds) *ARDS*. Sheffield: European Respiratory Society Journals, pp. 208–219.

Haji-Michael, P.G. (2000) Antioxidant therapy in the critically ill. *Care of the Critically Ill*, 16 (3): 88–92.

Hajjeh, R.A., Sofair, A.N., Harrison, L.H., Lyon, G.M., Arthington-Skaggs, B.A., Mirza, S.A., Phelan, M., Morgan, J., Lee-Yang, W., Ciblak, M.A., Benjamin, L.E., Sanza, L.T., Huie, S., Yeo, S.F., Brandt, M.E. and Warnock, D.W. (2004) Incidence of bloodstream infections due to *Candida* species and in vitro susceptibilities of isolates collected from 1998 to 2000 in a population-based active surveillance program. *Journal of Clinical Microbiology*, 42 (4): 1519–1527.

Hale, A.S., Moseley, M.J. and Warner, S.C. (2000) Treating pancreatitis in the acute care setting. *Dimensions of Critical Care Nursing*, 19 (4): 15–21.

Hall, A.P. and Henry, J.A. (2006) Acute toxic effects of 'Ecstasy' (MDMA) and related compounds: overview of pathophysiology and clinical management. *British Journal of Anaesthesia*, 96 (6): 678–685.

Hall, J. and Horsley, M. (2007) Diagnosis and management of patients with *Clostridium difficile*-associated diarrhoea. *Nursing Standard*, 21 (46): 49–56.

Hallworth, D. and McIntyre, A. (2003) The transport of critically ill children. *Current Paediatrics*, 13 (1): 12–17.

Hambley, H. (1995) Coagulation (II): clinical problems in coagulation disorder. *Care of the Critically Ill*, 11 (5): 203–205.

Hampton, J.R. (2008a) *The ECG Made Easy*, 7th edition. Edinburgh: Churchill Livingstone/ Elsevier.

—— (2008b) *The ECG in Practice*, 5th edition. Edinburgh: Churchill Livingstone/Elsevier.

—— (2008c) *150 ECG Problems*, 3rd edition. Edinburgh: Churchill Livingstone.

Handy, J.M. and Soni, N. (2008) Physiological effects of hyperchloraemia and acidosis. *British Journal of Anaesthesia*, 101 (2): 141–150.

Hans-Geurts, I.J.M., Hop, W.C.J., Kok, N.F.M., Lim, A., Brouwer, K.J. and Jeekel, J. (2007) Randomized clinical trial of the impact of early enteral feeding on postoperative ileus and recovery. *British Journal of Surgery*, 94 (5): 555–561.

Harbath, S., Sax, H. and Gastmeier, P. (2003) The preventable proportion of nosocomial infections: an overview of published reports. *Journal of Hospital Infection*, 54 (4): 258–266.

Harcombe, C. (2004) Nursing patients with ARDS in the prone position. *Nursing Standard*, 18 (19): 33–39.

Harioka, T., Matsukawa, T., Ozaki, M., Nomura, K., Sone, T., Kakuyama, M. and Toda, H. (2000) 'Deep-forehead' temperature correlates well with blood temperature. *Canadian Journal of Anaesthesia*, 47 (10): 980–983.

Harris, A. and Misiewicz, J.J. (2001) Management of *Helicobacter pylori* infection. *British Medical Journal*, 323 (7320): 1047–1050.

Harris, O.A., Colford, J.M. Jr, Good, M.C. and Matz, P.G. (2001) The role of hypothermia in the management of severe brain injury: a meta-analysis. *Archives of Neurology*, 59 (7): 1077–1083.

Harris, P.D. and Barnes, R. (2008) The uses of helium and xenon in current clinical practice. *Anaesthesia*, 63 (3): 284–293.

Harrison, D.A. and Rowan, K.M. (2008) Outcome prediction in critical care: the ICNARC model. *Current Opinion in Critical Care*, 14 (5): 506–512.

Hartog, C., Brunkhorst, F.M. and Reinhart, K. (2009) Old versus new starches: what do we know about their difference?, in Vincent, J.-L. (ed.) *Yearbook of Intensive Care and Emergency Medicine*, pp. 233–242.

Hartung, T.K., Schofield, E., Short, A.I., Parr, M.J.A. and Henry, J.A. (2002) Hyponatraemic states following 3,4-methylenedioxymethamphetamine (MDMA, 'ecstasy') ingestion. *QJM*, 95 (7): 431–437.

Harvey, D. and Thomas, A.N. (2010) Survey of the use of capnography in UK intensive care units. *Journal of the Intensive Care Society*, 11 (1): 34–36.

Harvey, L. (2008) *Management of Spinal Cord Injuries*. Edinburgh: Churchill Livingstone.

Hasham, S., Matteucci, P., Stanley, P.R.W. and Hart, N.B. (2005) Necrotising fasciitis. *British Medical Journal*, 330 (7495): 830–833.

Hassall, I., Latif, I., McGrattan, K. and Pugh, M. (2010) Do noise-cancelling headphones improve sleep quality on the intensive care unit? *Journal of the Intensive Care Society*, 11 (1): 64.

Hausmann, H., Potapov, E.V., Koster, A., Krabatsch, T., Stein, J., Yeter, R., Kukucka, M., Sodian, R., Kuppe, H. and Hetzer, R. (2004) Prognosis after the implantation of an intra-aortic balloon pump in cardiac surgery calculated with a new score. *Circulation*, 106 (12): I-203–I-206.

Hawker, F. (2003) Hepatic failure, in Bersten, A.D. and Soni, N. (eds) *Intensive Care Manual*, 5th edition. Edinburgh: Butterworth-Heinemann, pp. 431–441.

Hawthorne, J. and Redmond, K. (1998) *Pain: Causes and management*. Oxford: Blackwell.

Hawton, K., Townsend, E., Deeks, J., Appleby, L., Gunnell, D., Bennewith, O. and Cooper, J. (2001) Effects of legislation restricting pack size of paracetamol and salicylate on self poisoning in the United Kingdom: before and after study. *British Medical Journal*, 322 (7296): 1203–1207.

Hayashida, K.-I., Obata, H., Nakajima, K. and Eisenach, J.C. (2008) Gabapentin acts within the locus coeruleus to alleviate neuropathic pain. *Anesthesiology*, 109 (6): 1977–1984.

Hayden, P. and Wyncoll, D. (2008) Severe acute pancreatitis. *Current Anaesthesia & Critical Care*, 19 (1) 1–7.

Hayes, J. and Jones, C. (1995) A collaborative approach to oral care during critical illness. *Dental Health*, 34 (3): 6–10.

Hayward, J. (1975) Information: A prescription against pain. London: Royal College of Nursing.

Heals, D. (1993) A key to well-being. *Professional Nurse*, 8 (6): 391–398.

Hebert, P.C., Wells, G., Blajchman, M.A. Marshall, J., Martin, C., Pagliarello, G., Tweeddale, M., Schweitzer, I. and Yetisir, E., Transfusion Requirements Investigators for the Canadian Critical Care Trials Group (1999) A multicenter randomized, controlled clinical trial of transfusion requirements in critical care. *New England Journal of Medicine*, 340 (6): 409–417.

Hedges, C. and Redeker, N.S. (2008) Comparison of sleep and mood in patients after on-pump and off-pump coronary artery bypass surgery. *American Journal of Critical Care*, 17 (2): 133–141.

Heintz, B.H., Halilovic, J. and Christensen, C.L. (2010) Vancomycin-resistant enterococcal urinary tract infections. *Pharmacotherapy*, 30 (11): 1136–1149.

Henderson, C. and Macdonald, S. (eds) (2004) *Mayes' Midwifery: A textbook for midwives*, 13th edition. Edinburgh: Baillière Tindall.

Hendricks-Thomas, J. and Patterson, E. (1995) A sharing in critical thought by nursing faculty. *Journal of Advanced Nursing*, 22 (3): 594–599.

Hennessey, I.A.M. and Japp, A.G. (2007) *Arterial Blood Gases Made Easy*. Edinburgh: Churchill Livingstone.

Henricson, M., Berglund, A.-L., Määttä, S., Ekman, R. and Segesten, K. (2008) The outcome of tactile touch on oxytocin in intensive care patients: a randomised controlled trial. *Journal of Clinical Nursing*, 17 (19): 2624–2633.

——, Segesten, K., Berglund, A.-L. and Määttä, S. (2009) Enjoying tactile touch and gaining hope when being cared for in intensive care: a phenomenological hermeneutical study. *Intensive & Critical Care Nursing*, 25 (6): 323–331.

Herman, G., Wilmer, A., Meersseman, W., Milants, I., Wouters, P.J., Bobbaers, H., Bruyinchx, F. and van den Berghe, G. (2007) Impact of intensive insulin therapy on neuromuscular complications in the medical intensive care unit. *American Journal of Respiratory and Critical Care Medicine*, 175 (5): 480–489.

Herridge, M.S., Cheung, A.M., Tansey, C.M., Matte-Martyn, A., Diaz-Granados, N., Al-Saidi, F., Cooper, A.B., Guest, C.B., Mazer, C.D., Meehta, S., Stewart, T.E., Barr, A., Cook, D. and Slutsky, A.S., Canadian Critical Care Trials Group (2003) One-year outcomes in survivors of the acute respiratory distress syndrome. *New England Journal of Medicine*, 348 (8): 683–693.

Hess, D.R. (2002) Mechanical ventilation strategies: what's new and what's worth keeping? *Respiratory Care*, 47 (9): 1007–1017.

Hewitt, J. and Jordan, S. (2004) Prescription drugs: uses and effects. Opioids. *Nursing Standard*, 19 (6): insert.

Heymann, A., Radtke, F., Schiemann, A., Lütz, A., MacGuill, M., Wernecke, K.D. and Spies, C. (2010) Delayed treatment of delirium increases mortality rate in intensive care unit patients. *International Medical Research*, 38 (5): 1584–1595.

Hickey, J.V. (ed.) (2003a) *The Clinical Practice of Neurological and Neurosurgical Nursing*, 5th edition. Philadelphia, PA: Lippincott.

—— (2003b) Intracranial hypertension: theory and management of increased intracranial pressure, in Hickey, J.V. (ed.) *The Clinical Practice of Neurological and Neurosurgical Nursing*, 5th edition. Philadelphia, PA: Lippincott, pp. 285–318.

—— (2003c) Craniocerebral trauma, in Hickey, J.V. (ed.) *The Clinical Practice of Neurological and Neurosurgical Nursing*, 5th edition. Philadelphia, PA: Lippincott, pp. 373–406.

—— (2003d) Vertebral and spinal cord injuries, in Hickey, J.V. (ed.) *The Clinical Practice of Neurological and Neurosurgical Nursing*, 5th edition. Philadelphia, PA: Lippincott, pp. 407–450.

Higgins, C. (2007) *Understanding Laboratory Investigations*, 2nd edition. London: Blackwell Publishing.

Higgins, J., Estetter, B., Holland, D., Smith, B. and Derdak, S. (2005) High-frequency oscillatory ventilation in adults: respiratory therapy issues. *Critical Care Medicine*, 33 (3 supplement): S196–S203.

Higgs, D. (2009a) Critical Care Outreach, in Smith, S.A., Price, A.M. and Chaliner, A. (eds) *Ward-based Critical Care*. Keswick: M&K Publishing, pp. 1–7.

—— (2009b) Critical Care Outreach and the early detection of acute illness, in Moore, T. and Woodrow, P. (eds) *High Dependency Nursing Care*, 2nd edition. London: Routledge, pp. 391–399.

Hillas, G., Vassilakopoulos, T., Plantza, P., Rasidakis, A. and Barakos, P. (2010) C-reactive protein and procalcitonin as predictors of survival and septic shock in ventilator-associated pneumonia. *European Respiratory Journal*, 35 (4): 805–811.

Hillman, K. and Bishop, G. (2004) *Clinical Intensive Care*, 2nd edition. Cambridge: Cambridge University Press.

Hinds, C.J. and Watson, D. (2008) *Intensive Care: A concise textbook*, 3rd edition. Edinburgh: Saunders Elsevier.

Hine, K. (2007) The use of physical restraint in critical care. *Nursing in Critical Care*, 12 (1): 6–11.

Hinkelbein, J. and Genzwuerker, H.V. (2008) Fingernail polish does not influence pulse oximetry to a clinically relevant dimension. *Intensive & Critical Care Nursing*, 24 (1): 4–5.

——, Floss, F., Denz, C. and Krieter, H. (2008) Accuracy and precision of three different methods to determine PCO_2 (PCO_2 vs. $PetCO_2$ vs. $PtcCO_2$) during interhospital ground transport of critically ill and ventilated adults. *Journal of Trauma-Injury Infection & Critical Care*, 65 (1): 10–18.

Hlatky, M.A., Boothroyd, D.B., Bravata, D.M., Boersma, E., Booth, J., Brooks, M.M., Carrié, D., Clayton, T., Danchin, N., Flather, M., Hamm, C.W., Hueb, W.A., Kähler, J., Kelsey, S.F., King, S.B., Kosinski, A.S., Lopes, N., McDonald, K.M., Rodriguez, A., Serruys, P., Sigwart, U., Stables, R.H., Owens, D.K. and Pocock, S.J. (2009) Coronary artery bypass surgery compared with percutaneous coronary interventions for multivessel disease: a collaborative analysis of individual patient data from ten randomised trials. *Lancet*, 373 (9670): 1190–1197.

Ho, A.M.-H., Lee, A., Karmakar, M.K., Dion, P.W., Chung, D.C. and Contardi, L.H. (2003) Heliox vs air-oxygen mixtures for the treatment of patients with acute asthma. *Chest*, 123 (3): 882–890.

Ho, K.M. and Ng, J.Y. (2008) The use of propofol for medium and long-term sedation in critically ill adult patients: a meta-analysis. *Intensive Care Medicine*, 34 (11): 1969–1979.

—— and Power, B.M. (2010) Benefits and risks of furosemide in acute kidney injury. *Anaesthesia*, 65 (3): 283–293.

—— and Sheridan, D.J. (2006) Meta-analysis of frusemide to prevent or treat acute renal failure. *British Medical Journal*, 333 (7565): 420–423.

Ho, L.W.W., Kam, P.C.A. and Thong, C.L. (2005) Disseminated intravascular coagulation. *Current Anaesthesia & Critical Care*, 16 (3): 151–161.

Hobson, C.E., Yavas, S., Segal, M.S., Schold, J.D., Tribble, C.G., Layon, A.J. and Bihorac, A. (2009) Acute kidney injury is associated with increased long-term mortality after cardiothoracic surgery. *Circulation*, 119 (18): 2444–2453.

Hodd, J., Doyle, A., Carter, J., Albarran, J. and Young, P. (2010) Extubation in intensive care units in the UK: an online survey. *Nursing in Critical Care*, 15 (6): 281–284.

Hofhuis, J.G., Spronk, P.E., van Stel, H.F. Schrijvers, A.J., Rommes, J.H. and Bakker, K. (2008a) Experiences of critically ill patients in the ICU. *Intensive and Critical Care Nursing*, 24(5): 300–313.

——, Spronk, P.E., van Stel, H.F., Schrijvers, G.J.P., Rommes, J.H. and Bakker, J. (2008b) The impact of critical illness of perceived heath-related quality of life during ICU treatment, hospital stay and after hospital discharge. *Chest*, 233 (2): 377–385.

Holden, J., Harrison, L. and Johnson, M. (2002) Families, nurses and intensive care patients. *Journal of Clinical Nursing*, 11 (2): 140–148.

Holloway, T. and Penson, J. (1987) Nursing education as social control. *Nurse Education Today*, 7 (5): 235–241.

Hopkins, P.M. (2008) Malignant hyperthermia. *Current Anaesthesia & Critical Care*, 19 (1): 22–33.

Hopkins, R.O., Weaver, L.K., Collingridge, D., Parkinson, R.B., Chan, K.J. and Orme, J.F. Jr (2005) Two-year cognitive, emotional, and quality-of-life outcomes in acute respiratory distress syndrome. *American Journal of Respiratory and Critical Care Medicine*, 171 (4): 340–347.

Hopson, A.S.M. and Greenstein, A. (2007) Intravenous infusions in hyperbaric chambers: effect of compression on syringe function. *Anaesthesia*, 62 (6): 602–604.

Houghton, A.R. and Gray, D. (2008) *Making Sense of the ECG*, 3rd edition. London: Hodder Education.

Houwing, R., Overgoor, M., Kon, M., Jansen, G., van Asbeck, B.S. and Haalboom, J.R.E. (2000) Pressure-induced skin lesions in pigs: reperfusion injury and the effects of vitamin E. *Journal of Wound Care*, 9 (1): 36–40.

Høvdin, G. (2008) Acute bacterial conjunctivitis. *Acta Ophthalmologica*, 86 (1): 5–17.

Howie, A.J. and Ridley, S.A. (2008) Bed occupancy and incidence of meticillin-resistant *Staphylococcus aureus* in an intensive care unit. *Anaesthesia*, 63 (10): 1070–1073.

Huang, L., Quartin, A., Jones, D. and Havlir, D.V. (2006) Intensive care of patients with HIV infection. *New England Journal of Medicine*, 355 (2):173–181.

Hubbard, R.E., Lyons, R.A., Woodhouse, K.W., Hillier, S.L., Wareham, K., Ferguson, B. and Major, E. (2003) Absence of ageism in access to critical care: a cross-sectional study. *Age & Ageing*, 32 (4): 382–387.

Hughes, E. (2004) Understanding the care of patients with acute pancreatitis. *Nursing Standard*, 18 (18): 45–52.

Hughes, M., MacKirdy, F.N., Norrie, J. and Grant, I.S., Scottish Intensive Care Society (2003) Acute respiratory distress syndrome: an audit of incidence and outcome in Scottish intensive care units. *Anaesthesia*, 58 (9): 838–845.

Hughes, R.A.C. and Cornblath, D.R. (2005) Guillain-Barré syndrome. *Lancet*, 366 (9497): 1653–1666.

——, Wijdicks, E.F.M., Benson, E., Cornblath, D.R., Hahn, A.F., Meythaler, J.M., Sladky, J.T., Barohn, R.J. and Stevens, J.C. (2005) Supportive care for patients with Guillain-Barre syndrome. *Archives of Neurology*, 62 (8):1194–1198.

Hugonnet, S., Chevrolet, J.C. and Pittet, D. (2007) The effect of workload on infection risk in critically ill patients. *Critical Care Medicine*, 35 (1): 76–81.

Hui, D.S., Wong, K.T., Ko, F.W., Tam, L.S., Chan, D.P., Woo, J. and Sung, J.J.Y. (2005) The 1-year impact of severe acute respiratory syndrome on pulmonary function, exercise capacity and quality of life in a cohort of survivors. *Chest*, 128 (4): 2247–2261.

Hunningher, A. and Smith, M. (2006) Update on the management of severe head injury in adults. *Care of the Critically Ill*, 22 (5): 124–129.

Hunter, J.D. and Doddi, M. (2010) Sepsis and the heart. *British Journal of Anaesthesia*, 104 (1): 3–11.

Hunter, J.J. and Chien, K.R. (1999) Signalling pathways for cardiac hypertrophy and failure. *New England Journal of Medicine*, 341 (17): 1276–1283.

Hunter, J.P. (2002) Rhabdomyolysis. *Care of the Critically Ill*, 18 (2): 52–55.

Hussein, A. (2009) Thermal disorders, in Bersten, A.D. and Soni, N. (eds) *Intensive Care Manual*, 6th edition. Edinburgh: Butterworth-Heinemann, pp. 837–850.

Hussein, H.K., Lewington, A.J.P. and Kanagasundaram S. (2009) General management of acute kidney injury. *British Journal of Hospital Medicine*, 70 (7): M104–M107.

Hutchins, A., Durand, M.A., Grieve, R., Harrison, D., Rowan, K., Green, J., Cairns, J. and Black, N. (2009) Evaluation of modernisation of adult critical care services in England: time series and cost effectiveness analysis. *British Medical Journal*, 339 (7730): 1130.

Ichai, C., Armando, G., Orban, J.-C., Berthier, F., Rami, L., Samat-Long, C., Grimand, D. and Leverve, X. (2009) Sodium lactate versus mannitol in the treatment of intracranial hypertensive episodes in severe traumatic brain-injured patients. *Intensive Care Medicine*, 35 (3): 471–479.

ICN (International Council of Nurses) (2006) *The ICN Code of Ethics for Nurses*. Geneva: International Council of Nurses.

ICS (Intensive Care Society) (2002) *Guidelines for the Transport of the Critically Ill Adult*. London: Intensive Care Society.

—— (2006) *Critical Insight*. London: Intensive Care Society.

—— (2007a) *Sedation Guidelines*. London: Intensive Care Society.

—— (2007b) *Investigation of Suspected Infection in Critically Ill Patients*. London: Intensive Care Society.

—— (2008) *Standards for Care of Adult Patients with Temporary Tracheostomies*. London: Intensive Care Society.

—— (2009a) *Statement on the Use of Unlicensed Medicines or Licensed Medicines for Unlicensed Uses in Critically Ill Patients*. London. Intensive Care Society.

—— (2009b) *Standards and Recommendations for the Provision of Renal Replacement Therapy on Intensive Care Units in the United Kingdom*. London: Intensive Care Society.

—— (2010) *Medication Concentrations in Critical Care Areas*. London: Intensive Care Society.

Iggulden, H. (2006) *Care of the Neurological Patient*. Oxford: Blackwell Publishing.

Ikegamin, T., Takeromi, A., Soejima, Y., Yoshizumi, T., Sanefuji, K., Kayashima, H., Shimada, M. and Maehara, Y. (2008) Living donor liver transplantation for acute liver failure: a 10-year experience in a single centre. *Journal of the American College of Surgeons*, 206 (3): 412–418.

Imanaka, H., Taenaka, N., Nakamura, J., Aoyama, K. and Hosotani, H. (1997) Ocular surface disorders in the critically ill. *Anesthesia & Analgesia*, 85 (2): 343–346.

International Carotid Stenting Study Investigators (2010) Carotid artery stenting compared with endarterectomy in patients with symptomatic carotid stenosis (International Carotid Stenting Study): an interim analysis of a randomised controlled trial. *Lancet*, 375 (9719): 985–997.

Inward, C. (2008) Haemolytic uraemic syndrome. *Paediatrics and Child Health*, 18 (8): 364–368.

Iotti, G.A., Polito, A., Belliato, M., Pasero, D., Beduneau, G., Wysocki, M., Brunner, J.X., Braschi, A., Brochard, L., Mancedbo, J., Ranieri, V.M., Richard, J.-C.M. and Slutsky, A.S. (2010) Adaptive support ventilation versus conventional ventilation for total ventilatory support in acute respiratory failure. *Intensive Care Medicine*, 36 (8): 1371–1379.

Irwin, G.H. (2007) How to protect a patient with aortic aneurysm. *Nursing 2007*, 37 (2): 36–42.

Isaac, R. and Taylor, B.L. (2003) Fever in ICU patients. *Anaesthesia and Intensive Care*, 4 (5): 153–155.

Isbister, J.P. (2009) Blood transfusion, in Bersten, A.D. and Soni, N. (eds) *Intensive Care Manual*, 6th edition. Edinburgh: Butterworth-Heinemann Elsevier, pp. 995–1010.

Jacobs, M.J., van Eps, R.G.S., de Jong, D.S., Schurink, G.W.H. and Mochtar, B. (2004) Prevention of renal failure in patients undergoing thoracoabdominal aortic aneurysm repair. *Journal of Vascular Surgery*, 40 (6): 1067–1073.

Jain, S. and Belligan, G. (2007) Basic science of acute lung injury. *Surgery*, 25 (3): 112–116.

Jalan, R. and Damink, S.W. (2001) Hypothermia for the management of intracranial hypertension in acute liver failure. *Current Opinion in Critical Care*, 7 (4): 257–262.

Jallali, N. (2003) Necrotising fasciitis: its aetiology, diagnosis and management. *Journal of Wound Care*, 12 (8): 297–300.

James, S.K., Stenestrand, U., Lindbåck, J., Carlsson, J., Scherstén, F., Nilsson, T., Wallentin, L. and Lagerqvist, B., SCARR Study Group (2009) Long-term safety and efficacy of drug-eluding versus bare-metal stents in Sweden. *New England Journal of Medicine*, 360 (19): 1933–1945.

Jeerakathil, T., Johnson, J.A., Simpson, S.H. and Majumdar, S.R. (2007) Short-term risk for stroke is doubled in persons with newly treated type 2 diabetes compared with persons without diabetes. *Stroke*, 38 (6): 1739–1743.

Jeffacote, W.J. and Harding, K.G. (2003) Diabetic foot ulcers. *Lancet*, 361 (9368): 1545–1551.

Jefrey, A. (2003) Insulin resistance. *Nursing Standard*, 17 (32): 47–53.

Jenkins, D.A. (1989) Oral care in the ICU: an important nursing role. *Nursing Standard*, 4 (7): 24–28.

Jenkins, I.A., Playfor, S.D., Bevan, C., Davies, G. and Wolf, A.R. (2007) Current United Kingdom sedation practice in pediatric intensive care. *Pediatric Anesthesia*, 17 (1): 675–683.

Jermitsky, E., Omert, L.A., Dunham, M., Wilberger, J. and Rodriguez, A. (2005) The impact of hyperglycemia on patients with severe brain injury. *Journal of Trauma, Injury, Infection and Critical Care*, 58 (1): 47–50.

Jerreat, L. (2010) Managing diabetic ketoacidosis. *Nursing Standard*, 24 (34): 49–55.

Jevon, P. (2007) Measuring capillary refill time. *Nursing Times*, 103 (12): 26–27.

Jevon, P. (2009) *ECGs for Nurses*, 2nd edition. Oxford: Wiley-Blackwell.

Jiggins, M. and Talbot, J. (1999) Mouth care in PICU. *Paediatric Nursing*, 11 (10): 23–26.

Joanna Briggs Institute (2002) Eye care for intensive care patients. *Best Practice*, 6 (1): 1–6.

Johns, C. (2005) Reflection on the relationship between technology and caring. *Nursing in Critical Care*, 10 (3): 150–155.

Joint British Diabetes Societies Inpatient Care Group (2010) *The Management of Diabetic Ketoacidosis in Adults*. London: NHS Diabetes.

Jolly, S., Newton, G., Horlick, E., Seidelin, P.H., Ross, H.J., Husain, M. and Dzavik, V. (2005) Effect of vasopressin on hemodynamics in patients with refractory cardiogenic shock complicating acute myocardial infarction. *American Journal of Cardiology*, 96 (12): 1617–1620.

Jones, C. (2007) Aftermath of intensive care: the scale of the problem. *British Journal of Hospital Medicine*, 68 (9): 464–466.

——, Skirrow, P., Griffiths, R.D., Humphris, G., Ingleby, S., Eddleston, J., Waldmann, C. and Gager, M. (2004) Post traumatic stress disorder-related symptoms in relatives of patients following intensive care. *Intensive Care Medicine*, 30 (3): 456–460.

Jones, C.V. (2004) The importance of oral hygiene in nutritional support, in White, R. (ed.) *Trends in Oral Health Care*. Dinton: Quay Books, pp. 72–83.

Joshua-Amadi, M. (2002) Recruitment and retention. *Journal of Nursing Management*, 9 (8): 17–21.

Jowett, N.I. and Thompson, D.R. (2007) *Comprehensive Coronary Care*, 4th edition. Edinburgh: Baillière Tindall.

Jung, S., Kim, H. and Yang, H. (2008) The effects of temperature monitoring methods and thermal management methods during spinal surgery. *Anesthesiology*, 109: A1133.

Juurlink, D.N., Buckley, N.A, Stanbrook, M.B., Isbister, G.K., Bennett, M. and McGuigan, M.A. (2005) Hyperbaric oxygen for carbon monoxide poisoning. *Cochrane Database Systematic Reviews*, issue 1, art. no. CD002041.

Kacmarek, R.M., Wiedemann, H.P., Lavin, P.T., Wedel, M.K., Tutuncu, A.S. and Slutsky, A.S. (2006) Partial liquid ventilation in adult patients with acute respiratory distress syndrome. *American Journal of Respiratory & Critical Care Medicine*, 173 (8): 882–889.

Kahil, A.C. and Sun, J. (2008) How many patients with severe sepsis are needed to confirm the efficacy of drotrecogin alfa activated? A Bayesian design. *Intensive Care Medicine*, 4 (10): 1804–1811.

Kahn, R. (2007) Is the metabolic syndrome a real syndrome? *Circulation*, 115 (13): 1806–1811.

Kam, P.C.A. and Ferch, N.I. (2000) Apoptosis: mechanisms and clinical implications. *Anaesthesia*, 55 (11): 1081–1093.

Kanagasundaram, S. (2007) Renal replacement therapy in acute kidney injury: an overview. *British Journal of Hospital Medicine*, 68 (6): 292–297.

Kannan, A. (2008) Heparinised saline or normal saline? *Journal of Perioperative Practice*, 18 (10): 440–441.

Karali, V., Massa, E., Vassiliadou, G., Chouris, I., Rodin, I. and Bitzani, M. (2008) Evaluation of development of diabetes insipidus in the early phase following traumatic brain injury in critically ill patients. *Critical Care*, 12 (supplement 2): P130.

Kass, J.E. (2003) Heliox redux. *Chest*, 123 (3): 673–676.

Kaye, P. and O'Sullivan, I. (2002) The role of magnesium in the emergency department. *Emergency Medical Journal*, 19 (4): 288–291.

Keays, R.T. (2009) Diabetic emergencies, in Bersten, A.D. and Soni, N. (eds) *Intensive Care Manual*, 6th edition. Edinburgh: Butterworth-Heinemann, pp. 613–620.

Keely, B.R. (1998) Preventing complications: recognition and treatment of autonomic dysreflexia. *Dimensions in Critical Care Nursing*, 17 (4): 170–176.

Kellum, J. and Pinsky, M. (2002) Use of vasopressor agents in critically ill patients. *Current Opinion in Critical Care*, 8 (3): 236–241.

Kelly, C.P. and LaMont, J.T. (2008) *Clostridium difficile* – more difficult than ever. *New England Journal of Medicine*, 359 (18): 1932–1940.

Kelly, H., Grant, K., Williams, S. and Smith, D. (2009) H1N1 swine origin influenza infection in the United States and Europe in 2009 may be similar to H1N1 seasonal influenza infection in two Australian states in 2007 and 2008. *Influenza and Other Respiratory Viruses*, 3 (4): 183–188.

Kelly, T., Timmis, S. and Twelvetree, T. (2010) Review of the evidence to support oral hygiene in stroke patients. *Nursing Standard*, 24 (37): 35–38.

Kemper, M.J., Harps, E. and Muller-Wiefel, D.E. (1996) Hyperkalaemia: therapeutic options in acute and chronic renal failure. *Clinical Nephrology*, 46 (1): 67–69.

Kennedy, D.D., Coakley, J. and Griffiths, R.D. (2002) Neuromuscular problems and physical weakness, in Griffiths, R.D. and Jones, C. (eds) *Intensive Care Aftercare*. Oxford: Butterworth-Heinemann, pp. 7–18.

Kennedy, M.S. (2004) Kinetic therapy: in search of the evidence: it may prevent some pulmonary complications. *American Journal of Nursing*, 104 (12): 22.

Keogh, B.F. and Cordingley, J.J. (2002) Current invasive ventilatory strategies in acute respiratory distress syndrome, in Evans, T.W., Griffiths, M.J.D. and Keogh, B.F. (eds) *ARDS*. Sheffield: European Respiratory Society Journals, pp. 161–180.

Kern, L.S. (2004) Postoperative atrial fibrillation: new directions in prevention and treatment. *Journal of Cardiovascular Nursing*, 19 (2): 103–115.

Kerr, K.G. and Snelling, A.M. (2009) *Pseudomonas aeruginosa:* a formidable and ever-present adversary. *Journal of Hospital Infection*, 72 (4): 338–344.

Kessler, C. (2009) Gylcaemic control in hospital: how tight should it be? *Nursing2009*, 39 (11): 38–43.

Khwannimit, B. and Bhurayanontachai, R. (2009) The performance of customised APAXCHE II and SAPS II in predicting mortality of mixed critically ill patients in a Thai medical intensive care unit. *Anaesthesia and Intensive Care*, 37 (5): 784–790.

Kiekkas, P., Sakellaropoulos, G., Brokalaki, H., Manolis, E., Samios, A., Skartsani, C. and Baltopoulos, G.I. (2008) Nursing workload associated with fever in the general intensive care unit. *American Journal of Critical Care*, 17 (6): 522–533.

Kiening, K.L., Unterberg, A.W., Bardt, T.F., Schneider, G.H. and Lanksch, W.R. (1996) Monitoring of cerebral oxygenation in patients with severe head injuries. Brain tissue pO$_2$ versus jugular vein oxygen saturation. *Journal of Neurosurgery*, 85 (5): 751–757.

Kimberger, O., Cohen, D., Illievich, U. and Lenhardt, R. (2007) Temporal artery versus bladder thermometry during perioperative and intensive care monitoring. *Anesthesia & Analgesia*, 105 (4): 1042–1047.

Kingston, D., Sykes, S. and Raper, S. (2002) Protocol for the administration of haemofiltration fluids and electrolytes using a patient group direction. *Nursing in Critical Care*, 7 (4): 193–197.

Kistemaker, J.A., den Hartog, E.A. and Daanen, H.A. (2006) Reliability of an infrared forehead skin thermometer for core temperature measurements. *Journal of Medical Engineering & Technology*, 30 (4): 252–261.

Kite, K. and Pearson, L. (1995) A rationale for mouth care: the integration of theory with practice. *Intensive and Critical Care Nursing*, 11 (2): 71–76.

Knaus, W.A., Draper, E.A., Wagner, D.P. and Zimmerman, J.E. (1985) APACHE II: a severity of disease classification system. *Critical Care Medicine*, 13 (10): 818–829.

Knoll, G.A. (1999) Tacrolimus versus cyclosporin for immunosuppression in renal transplantation: meta-analysis of randomised trials. *British Medical Journal*, 318 (7191): 1104–1107.

Knoll, M., Lautenschlaeger, C. and Borneff-Lipp, M. (2010) The impact of workload on hygiene compliance in nursing. *British Journal of Nursing*, 19 (16): S18–S22.

Koesters, S.C., Rogers, P.D. and Rajasingham, C.R. (2002) MDMA ('ecstasy') and other 'club drugs': the new epidemic. *Pediatric Clinics of North America*, 49 (2): 415–433.

Kogos, S.C. Jr, Richards, J.S., Banos, J., Schmitt, M.M., Brunner, R.C., Meythaler, J.M., Salisbury, D.B., Renfroe, S.G. and White, A.J. (2005) A descriptive study of pain and quality of life following Guillain-Barre syndrome: one year later. *Journal of Clinical Psychology in Medical Settings*, 12 (2):111–116.

Kokozides, G.E. (2006) Implementation of hemostatic techniques in the treatment of upper gastrointestinal hemorrhage. *Annals of Gastroenterology*, 19(4): 325–334.

Koksal, G.M., Sayilgan, C., Sen, O. and Oz, H. (2004) The effects of different weaning modes on the endocrine stress response. *Critical Care*, 8 (1): R31–R34.

Kollef, M.H., Afessa, B., Anzueto, A., Veremakis, C., Kerr, K.M., Margolis, B.D., Craven, D.E., Roberts, P.R., Arroliga, A.C., Hubmayr, R.D., Restrepo, M.I., Auger, W.R. and Schinner, R., NASCENT Investigation Group (2008) Silver-coated endotracheal tubes and incidence of ventilator-associated pneumonia: the NASCENT randomised trial. *JAMA*, 300 (7): 805–813.

Konstantinides, S.V. (2008) Acute pulmonary embolism revistited. *Postgraduate Medical Journal*, 84 (998): 651–658.

Kozek-Langenecker, S.A. and Sibylle, A. (2005) Effects of hydroxyethyl starch solutions on hemostasis. *Anesthesiology*, 103 (3): 654–660.

Krieg, T., Liu, Y., Rütz, T., Methner, C., Yang, X.-M., Dost, T., Felix, S.B., Stasch, J.-P., Cohen, M.V. and Diowney, J.M. (2009) BAY 58–2667, a nitric oxide-independent guanylyl cyclise activator, pharmacologically post-conditions rabbit and rat hearts. *European Heart Journal*, 30 (13): 1607–1613.

Krishnan, J.A. and Brower, R.G. (2000) High-frequency ventilation for acute lung injury and ARDS. *Chest*, 118 (3): 795–807.

——, Moore, D., Robeson, C., Rand, C.S. and Fessler, H.E. (2004) A prospective, controlled trial of a protocol-based strategy to discontinue mechanical ventilation. *American Journal of Respiratory and Critical care Medicine*, 169 (6): 673–678.

Krumberger, J. (2002) When the liver fails. *RN*, 65 (2): 26–29.

Ksouri, H., Balanant, P.-Y., Tadié, J.-M., Heraud, G., Abboud, I., Lerolle, N., Novara, A., Fagon, J.-Y. and Faisy, C. (2010) Impact of morbidity and mortality conferences on analysis of mortality and critical events in intensive care practice. *American Journal of Critical Care*, 19 (2): 135–145.

Kudst, K.A. (2003) Effect of route and type of nutrition on intestine-derived inflammatory responses. *American Journal of Surgery*, 185 (1): 16–21.

Kulungowski, A.M., Kashuk, J.L., Moore, E.E., Hutting, H.G., Sadaria, M.R, Cothren, C.C., Johnson, J.L. and Sauaia, A. (2009) Hemolysis, elevated liver enzymes, and low platelets syndrome: when is surgical help needed? *American Journal of Surgery*, 198 (6): 916–920.

Kumar, A., Ellis, P., Arabi, Y., Roberts, D., Light, B., Parrillo, J.E., Dodek, P., Wood, G., Kumar, A., Simon, D., Peters, C., Ahsan, M. and Chateau, D., Cooperative Antimicrobial Therapy of Septic Shock Database Research Group (2009) Initiation of inappropriate antimicrobial therapy results in a fivefold reduction of survival in human septic shock. *Chest*, 136 (5): 1237–1248.

——, Roberts, D., Wood, K.E., Light, B., Parrillo, J.E., Sharma, S., Suppes, R., Feinstein, D., Zanotti, S., Taiberg, L., Gurka, D., Mular, A. and Cheang, M. (2006) Duration of hypotension before initiation of effective antimicrobial therapy is the critical determinant of survival in human septic shock. *Critical Care Medicine*, 34 (6): 1589–1596.

Kuo, J. and Butchart, E.G. (1995) Sternal wound dehiscence. *Care of the Critically Ill*, 11 (6): 244–248.

Kuwabara, S., Ogawara, K., Sing, J.-Y., Mori, M., Kanai, K., Hattori, T., Yuki, N., Lin, C. S.-Y., Burke, D. and Bostock, H. (2002) Differences in membrane properties of axonal and demyelinating Guillain-Barré syndromes. *Annals of Neurology*, 52 (2): 180–187.

Lacherade, J.-C., de Jonghe, B., Guezennec, P., Debbat, K., Hayon, J., Monsel, A., Fangio, P., de Vecchi, C.A., Ramaut, C., Outin, H. and Bastuji-Garin, S. (2010) Intermittent subglottic secretion drainage and ventilator-associated pneumonia. *American Journal of Respiratory and Critical Care Medicine*, 182 (7): 910–917.

Lamerton, M. and Albarran, J.W. (1997) Percutaneous balloon mitral valvuloplasty: advancing the nursing perspective. *Nursing in Critical Care*, 2 (2): 88–92.

Lamia, B., Kim, H.K., Hefner, A., Severyn, D., Gomez, H., Puyana, J.C. and Pinsky, M.R. (2008) How accurate are different arterial pressure-derived estimates of cardiac output and stroke volume variation measures in critically ill patients? *Critical Care*, 12 (supplement 2): P100.

Lanfear, J. (2002) The individual with epilepsy. *Nursing Standard*, 16 (4): 43–53.

Lange, N.R., Kozlowski, J.K., Gust, R., Shapiro, S.D. and Schuster, D.P. (2000) Effect of partial liquid ventilation on pulmonary vascular permeability and edema after experimental acute lung injury. *American Journal of Respiratory and Critical Care Medicine*, 162 (1): 271–277.

Langley, J. and Adams, G. (2007) Insulin-based regimens decrease mortality rates in critically ill patients: a systematic review. *Diabetes/Metabolism Research & Reviews*, 23 (3): 184–192.

Lanone, S., Taillé, C., Boczkowski, J. and Aubier, M. (2005) Diaphragmatic fatigue during sepsis and septic shock. *Intensive Care Medicine*, 31 (12): 1611–1617.

Lapinsky, S.E. and Granton, J.I. (2004) Critical care lessons from severe acute respiratory syndrome. *Current Opinion in Critical Care*, 10 (1): 53–58.

Larson, E.L., Cohen, B., Ross, B. and Behta, M. (2010) Isolation precautions for methicillin-resistant *Staphylo-coccus aureus*: electronic surveillance to monitor adherence. *American Journal of Critical Care*, 19 (1): 16–26.

Larvin, M. (1999) Acute pancreatitis. *Surgery*, 17 (11): 261–265.

Laskou, M., Katsiari, M., Mainas, E., Kotsaimani, A., Karampela, I. and Magina, A. (2008) ICU patients: does age make any difference? *Critical Care*, 12 (supplement 2): P496.

Latessa, V. (2002) Endovascular stent-graft repair of descending thoracic aortic aneurysms: the nursing implications for care. *Journal of Vascular Nursing*, 20 (3): 86–93.

Latman, N. (2003) Clinical thermometry: possible causes and potential solutions to electronic, digital thermometer inaccuracies. *Biomedical Instrumentation & Technology*, 37 (3): 190–196.

Laupland, K.B., Kirkpatrick, A.W., Kortbeek, J.B. and Zuege, D.J. (2006) Long-term mortality outcome associated with prolonged admission to the ICU. *Chest*, 129 (4): 954–959.

Lawes, E.G. (2003) Hidden hazards and dangers associated with the use of HME/filters in breathing circuits: their effect on toxic metabolite production, pulse oximetry and airway resistance. *British Journal of Anaesthesia*, 91 (2): 249–264.

Lawson, L., Bridges, E.J., Ballou, I., Eraker, R., Greco, S., Shively, J. and Sochulak, V. (2007) Accuracy and precision of noninvasive temperature measurement in adult intensive care patients. *American Journal of Critical Care*, 16 (5): 485–496.

Lawson, N., Thompson, K., Saunders, G., Saiz, J., Richardson, J., Brown, D., Ince, N., Caldwell, M. and Pope, D. (2010) Sound intensity and noise evaluation in a critical care unit. *American Journal of Critical Care*, 19 (6): e88–e98; doi: 10.4037/ajcc2010180. Available online at http://ajcc.aacnjournals.org/content/19/6.toc (accessed 2 January 2011).

Lee Char, S.J., Evans, L.R., Malvar, G.L. and White, D.B. (2010) A randomised trial of two methods to disclose prognosis to surrogate decision makers in intensive care units. *American Journal of Respiratory and Critical Care Medicine*, 182 (7): 905–909.

Lefkou, E. and Hunt, B.J. (2008) Bleeding disorders in pregnancy. *Obstetrics, Gynaecology and Reproductive Medicine*, 18 (8): 217–223.

Leigh Brown, A.J. (1999) Viral evolution and variation in the HIV pandemic, in Dalgleish, A.G. and Weiss, R.A. (eds) *HIV and the New Viruses*, 2nd edition. San Diego, CA: Academic Press, pp. 29–42.

Lermitte, J. and Garfield, M.J. (2005) Weaning from mechanical ventilation. *Continuing Education in Anaesthesia, Critical Care & Pain*, 5 (4): 113–117.

Lettinga-van de Poll, T., Schurink, G.W.H., de Haan, M.W., Verbruggen, J.P.A.M. and Jacobs, M.J. (2007) Endovascular treatment of traumatic rupture of the thoracic aorta. *British Journal of Surgery*, 94 (5): 525–533.

Levi, M. and ten Cate, H. (1999) Current concepts: disseminated intravascular coagulation. *New England Journal of Medicine*, 341 (8): 586–592.

——, Toh, C.H., Thachil, J. and Watson, H.G. (2009) Guidelines for the diagnosis and management of disseminated intravascular coagulation. *British Journal of Haematology*, 145 (1): 24–33.

Levine, E. (1997) Jewish views and customs on death, in Parkes, C.M. (ed.) *Death and Bereavement across Cultures*. London: Routledge, pp. 98–130.

Lewis, G. (ed.) (2007) *The Confidential Enquiry into Maternal and Child Health (CEMACH). Saving Mothers' Lives: Reviewing maternal deaths to make motherhood safer – 2003–2005. The Seventh Report on Confidential Enquiries into Maternal Deaths in the United Kingdom.* London: CEMACH.

Lewis, S.J. and Heaton, K.W. (1997) Stool form scale as a useful guide to intestinal transit time. *Scandinavian Journal of Gastroenterology*, 32 (9): 920–924.

Lian, J.X. (2010) Interpreting and using the arterial blood gas analysis. *Nursing2010*, 5 (3): 26–36.

Light, R.W., Rogers, J.T., Moyers, J.P., Lee, Y.C.G., Rodriguez, R.M., Alford, W.C. Jr, Ball, S.K., Burrus, G.R., Colthorp, W.H., Glassford, D.M. Jr, Hoff, S.J., Lea, J.W.I.V., Nesbitt, J.C., Petracek, M.R., Starkey, T.D., Stoney, W.S. and Tedder, M. (2002) Prevalence and clinical course of pleural effusions at 30 days after coronary artery and cardiac surgery *American Journal of Respiratory and Critical Care Medicine*, 166 (12): 1567–1571.

Ligtenberg, J.J.M., Meijering, S., Stienstra, Y., van der Horst, I.C.C., Vogelzang, M., Nijsten, M.W.N., Tulleken, J.E. and Zijlstra, J.G. (2006) Mean glucose level is not an independent risk factor for mortality in mixed ICU patients. *Intensive Care Medicine*, 31 (3): 435–438.

Lim, S.-M. and Webb, S.A. (2005) Nosocomial bacterial infections in intensive care units. I: Organisms and mechanisms of antibiotic resistance. *Anaesthesia*, 60 (9): 887–902.

Lim, W., Qushmag, I., Devereaux, P.J., Heels-Ansdell, D., Lauzier, F., Ismaila, A.S., Crowther, M.A. and Cook, D.J. (2006) Elevated cardiac troponin measurements in critically ill patients. *Archives of Internal Medicine*, 166 (22): 2446–2454.

Lindsay, P. (2004) Complications of the third stage of labour, in Henderson, C. and Macdonald, S. (eds) *Mayes' Midwifery: A textbook for midwives*, 13th edition. Edinburgh: Baillière Tindall, pp. 987–1002.

Liwu, A. (1990) Oral hygiene in intubated patients. *Australian Journal of Advanced Nursing*, 7 (2): 4–7.

Llewellyn, L. (2007) Changing inotrope infusions: which technique is best? *Nursing Times*, 103 (8): 30–31.

Long, D.A. and Coulthard, M.G. (2006) Effect of heparin-bonded central venous catheters on the incidence of catheter-related thrombosis and infection in children and adults. *Anaesthesia and Intensive Care*, 34 (4): 481–484.

Long, T. and Sque, M. (2007) An update on initiatives to increase organ donation: a UK perspective. *British Journal of Transplantation*, 2 (2): 10–15.

Lorente, L., Lecuona, M., Jiménez, A., Mora, M.L. and Sierra, A. (2007) Influence of an endo-tracheal tube with polyurethane cuff and subglottic secretion drainage on pneumonia. *American Journal of Respiratory and Critical Care Medicine*, 176 (11): 1079–1083.

Lorgeril, M. de, Salen, P., Marin, J.-L., Boucher, F., Paillard, F. and Leiris, J. de. (2002) Wine drinking and risks of cardiovascular complications after recent acute myocardial infarction. *Circulation*, 106 (12): 1465–1469.

Lough, M.E. (2008) Sedation, agitation, and delirium management, in Urden, L.D., Stacy, K.M. and Lough, M.E. (eds) *Priorities in Critical Care Nursing*, 5th edition. St Louis, MO: Mosby, pp. 99–108.

Low, D. and Milne, M. (2007) Crystalloids, colloids, blood, blood products and blood substitutes. *Anaesthesia and Intensive Care Medicine*, 8 (2): 56–59.

Lower, J. (2003) Using pain to assess neurologic response. *Nursing2003*, 33 (6): 56–57.

Lowthian, P. (1997) Notes on the pathogenesis of serious pressure sores. *British Journal of Nursing*, 6 (16): 907–912.

Lucey, M.R., Mathurin, P. and Morgan, T.R. (2009) Alcoholic hepatitis. *New England Journal of Medicine*, 360 (26): 2758–2769.

Lumb, A. (2005) *Nunn's Applied Respiratory Physiology*, 6th edition. Oxford: Butterworth-Heinemann.

Maben, J. (2009) Splendid isolation? The pros and cons of single rooms for the NHS. *Nursing Management*, 16 (2): 18–19.

McCaffery, M. and Pasero, C. (1999) *Pain Clinical Manual*, 2nd edition. St Louis, MO: Mosby.

McClave, S.A., Martindale, R.G., Vanek, V.W., McCarthy, M., Roberts, P., Taylor, B., Ochoa, J.B., Napolitano, L. and Cresci, G., ASPEN Board of Directors and the American College of Critical Care Medicine (2009) Guidelines for the provision and assessment of nutrition support therapy in the adult critically ill patient. *Critical Care Medicine*, 37 (5): 277–316.

McColl, K.E.L. (2010) *Helicobacter pylori* infection. *New England Journal of Medicine*, 362 (17): 1597–1604.

MacConnachie, A.M. (1997) Ecstasy poisoning. *Intensive and Critical Care Nursing*, 13 (6): 365–366.

McConnell, H. and Cressey, D. (2008) Acute liver failure: focussing on pre-tertiary-transfer care. *Care of the Critically Ill*, 24 (5): 127–133.

McCormack, B. and Manley, K. (eds) (2004) *Practice Development in Nursing*. Oxford: Blackwell.

McGrath, M. (2008) The challenges of caring in a technological environment: critical care nurses' experiences. *Journal of Clinical Nursing*, 17 (8): 1096–1004.

McGuire, P.K., Cope, H. and Fahy, T.A. (1994) Diversity of psychopathy associated with use of 3,4-methylenedioxymethamphetamine ('Ecstasy'). *British Journal of Psychiatry*, 165 (3): 391–395.

Mach, W.J., Knight, A.R., Orr, J.A. and Pierce, J.D. (2009) Apoptosis and haemorrhagic shock. *Journal of Research in Nursing*, 14 (1): 77–88.

Machin, D. and Allsager, C. (2006) Principles of cardiopulmonary bypass. *Continuing Education in Anaesthesia, Critical Care & Pain*, 6 (5): 176–181.

Macias, C.A., Rosengart, M.R., Puyana, J.-C., Linde-Zwirble, W.T., Smith, W., Peitzman, A.B. and Angus, D.C. (2009) The effects of trauma centre care, admission volume, and surgical volume on paralysis after traumatic spinal cord injury. *Annals of Surgery*, 249 (1): 10–17.

Macintosh, I. and Britto, J. (2000) How to Guide: high frequency oscillatory ventilation. *Care of the Critically Ill*, 16 (4): centre insert.

Macintyre, P. and Schug, S.A. (2007) *Acute Pain Management: A practical guide*, 3rd edition. Edinburgh: Saunders Elsevier.

——, Schug, S.A., Scott, D.A., Visser, E.J. and Walker, S.M., Acute Pain Management Scientific Evidence Working Group of the Australian and New Zealand College of Anaesthetists and Faculty of Pain Medicine (2010) *Acute Pain Management: Scientific evidence*, 3rd edition. Melbourne: Australian and New Zealand College of Anaesthetists, Faculty of Pain Medicine.

Mackenzie, A.F. (2005) Activated protein C: do more survive? *Intensive Care Medicine*, 31 (12): 1624–1626.

McKinley, M. (2009) Acute liver failure. *Nursing2009*, 39 (3): 38–44.

McKinley, S., Coote, K. and Stein-Parbury, J. (2003) Development and testing of a Faces Scale for the assessment of anxiety in critically ill patients. *Journal of Advanced Nursing*, 41 (1): 73–79.

McKinnell, J. and Holt, S. (2007) Liver disease and renal dysfunction. *Medicine*, 35 (9): 521–523.

Mackintosh, C. (2007) Assessment and management of patients with post-operative pain. *Nursing Standard*, 22 (5): 49–55.

McLaughlin, N., Leslie, G.D., Williams, T.A. and Dobb, G.J. (2007) Examining the occurrence of adverse events within 72 hours of discharge from the intensive care unit. *Anaesthesia & Intensive Care*, 35 (4): 486–493.

McLean, B. (2001) Rotational kinetic therapy for ventilation/perfusion mismatch. *Connect*, 1 (4): 113–118.

McLellan, S.A., McClelland, D.B.L. and Walsh, T.S. (2003) Anaemia and red blood cell transfusion in the critically ill patient. *Blood Reviews*, 17 (4): 195–208.

Maclennan, J. (2001) Meningococcal group C conjugate vaccines. *Archives of Disease in Childhood*, 84 (5): 383–386.

McLeod, G.A., Davies, H.T.O., Munnoch, N., Bannister, J. and Macrae, W. (2001) Postoperative pain relief using thoracic epidural analgesia: outstanding success and disappointing failures. *Anaesthesia*, 56 (1): 75–81.

McNabb, M. (2004) Maternal and fetal physiological responses to pregnancy, in Henderson, C. and Macdonald, S. (eds) *Mayes' Midwifery: A textbook for midwives*, 13th edition. Edinburgh: Baillière Tindall, pp. 288–311.

Macnaughton, P. (2004) Weaning ventilatory support. *Anaesthesia and Intensive Care Medicine*, 5 (1): 11.

—— (2006) New ventilators for the ICU – usefulness of lung performance reporting. *British Journal of Anaesthesia*, 97 (1): 57–63.

McPhee, J., Eslami, M.H., Arous, E.J., Messina, L.M. and Schanzer, A. (2009) Endovascular treatment of ruptured abdominal aortic aneurysms in the United States (2001–2006): a significant survival benefit over open repair is independently associated with increased institutional volume. *Journal of Vascular Surgery*, 49 (4): 817–826.

McWilliam, S. and Riordan, A. (2010) How to use: C-reactive protein. *Archives of Disease in Childhood – Education & Practice*, 95 (2): 55–58.

Maggiore, S.M., Lelloche, F., Pigeot, J., Taille, S., Deye, N., Durrmeyer, X., Richard, J.-C., Mancebo, J., Lemaire, F. and Brochard, L. (2003) Prevention of endotracheal suctioning-induced alveolar derecruitment in acute lung injury. *American Journal of Respiratory and Critical Care Medicine*, 167 (9): 1215–1224.

Mak, S. and Newton, G.E. (2001) The oxidative stress hypothesis of congestive heart failure. *Chest*, 120 (6): 2035–2046.

Malangoni, M.A. and Martin, A.S. (2005) Outcome of severe acute pancreatitis. *American Journal of Surgery*, 189 (3): 273–277.

Malbrain, M.L.N.G., Chiumello, D., Pelosi, P., Bihari, D., Innes, R., Ranieri, V.M., del Turco, M., Wilmer, A., Brienza, N., Malcangi, V., Cohen, J., Japiassu, A., de Keulenaer, B.L., Daelemans, R., Jacquet, L., Laterre, P.-F., Frank, G., de Souza, P., Cesana, B. and Gattinoni, L. (2005) Incidence and prognosis of intraabdominal hypertension in a mixed population of critically ill patients: a multiple-center epidemiological study. *Critical Care Medicine*, 33 (2): 315–332.

Malfertheiner, P., Chan, F.K.L. and McColl, K.E.L. (2009) Peptic ulcer disease. *Lancet*, 374 (9699): 1449–1461.

Malik, S., Wong, N.D., Franklin, S.S., Kamath, T.V., L'Italien, G.J., Pio, J.R. and Williams, R. (2004) Impact of the metabolic syndrome on mortality from coronary heart disease, cardiovascular disease, and all causes in United States adults. *Circulation*, 110 (10): 1245–1250.

Mallick, A., Elliot, S.C. and Bodenham, A.R. (2008) Early experiences with interventional lung assist. *Care of the Critically Ill*, 24 (6): 145–146.

Maloney, D.G., Appadurai, R. and Vaughan, R.S. (2002) Anions and the anaesthetist. *Anaesthesia*, 57 (2): 140–154.

Mandelstam, M. (2007) *Betraying the NHS*. London: Jessica Kingsley.

Manias, E. and Street, A. (2001) Nurse-doctor interactions during critical care ward rounds. *Journal of Clinical Nursing*, 10 (4): 442–450.

Manley, K. (2004) Transformational culture, in McCormack, B. and Manley, K. (eds) *Practice Development in Nursing*. Oxford: Blackwell Publishing.

—— and McCormac, B. (2008) Person-centred care. *Nursing Management*, 15 (8): 12–13.

Manocha, S., Walley, K.R. and Russell, J.A. (2003) Severe acute respiratory distress syndrome (SARS): a critical care perspective. *Critical Care Medicine*, 31 (11): 2684–2692.

Manojilovich, M. (2005) Predictors of professional nursing practice behaviors in hospital settings. *Nursing Research*, 54 (1): 41–47.

Manson, J.E., Greenland, P., LaCroix, A.Z., Stefanik, M.L., Mouton, C.P., Oberman, A., Perri, M.G., Sheps, D.S., Pettinger, M.B. and Siscovick, D.S. (2002) Walking compared with vigorous exercise for the prevention of cardiovascular events in women. *New England Journal of Medicine*, 347 (10): 716–725.

Mar, G.J., Barrington, M.J. and McGuirk, B.R. (2009) Acute compartment syndrome of the lower limb and the effect of postoperative analgesia on diagnosis. *British Journal of Anaesthesia*, 102 (1): 3–11.

March, A. (2005) A review of respiratory management in spinal cord injury. *Journal of Orthopaedic Nursing*, 9 (1): 19–26.

Margarey, J.M. and McCutcheon, H.H. (2005) 'Fishing with the dead' – recall of memories from ICI. *Intensive & Critical Care Nursing*, 21 (6): 344–354.

Marieb, E.N. and Hoehn, K. (2007) *Human Anatomy and Physiology*, 7th edition. San Francisco, CA: Pearson/Benjamin/Cummings.

Marik, P.E. (2000) Fever in the ICU. *Chest*, 117 (3): 855–869.

—— (2002) Low-dose dopamine: a systematic review. *Intensive Care Medicine*, 28 (7): 877–883.

—— (2010) *Handbook of Evidence-based Critical Care*. New York: Springer-Verlag.

—— and Raghaven, M. (2004) Stress-hyperglycaemia, insulin and immunodulation in sepsis. *Intensive Care Medicine*, 30 (5): 748–756.

—— and Zaloga, G.P. (2002) Adrenal insufficiency in the critically ill: a new look at an old problem. *Chest*, 122 (4): 1784–1796.

——, Baram, M. and Vahid, B. (2008) Does central venous pressure predict fluid responsiveness? *Chest*, 134 (1): 172–178.

Marret, E., Remy, C. and Bonnet, F., Postoperative Pain Forum Group (2007) Meta-analysis of epidural analgesia *versus* parenteral opioid analgesia after colorectal surgery. *British Journal of Surgery*, 94 (6): 665–673.

Marsh, M. (2000) Respiratory anatomy and physiology in infants and children, in Williams, C. and Asquith, J. (eds) *Paediatric Intensive Care Nursing*. Edinburgh: Churchill Livingstone, pp. 61–79.

Marshall, A.P. and West, S.H. (2003) Gastric tonometry and enteral nutrition: a possible conflict in critical care nursing practice. *American Journal of Critical Care*, 12 (4): 349–356.

Martin, C., Viviand, X., Leone, M. and Thirion, X. (2000) Effects of norephinephrine on the outcome of septic shock. *Critical Care Medicine*, 28 (8): 2758–2765.

Martin, S.R. and Foley, M.R. (2006) Intensive care in obstetrics: an evidence-based review. *American Journal of Obstetrics and Gynaecology*, 195 (3): 673–689.

Maslow, A.H. (1954/1987) *Motivation and Personality*, 3rd edition. New York: Harper & Row.

—— (1971) *The Farthest Reaches of Human Nature*. London: Penguin.

Matull, W.R., Pereira, S.P. and O'Donohue, J.W. (2006) Biochemical markers of acute pancreatitis. *Clinical Pathology*, 59 (4): 340–344.

Maunder, T. (1997) Principles and practice of managing difficult behaviour situations in intensive care. *Intensive and Critical Care Nursing*, 13 (2): 108–110.

May, K. (2009) The pathophysiology and causes if raised intracranial pressure. *British Journal of Nursing*, 18 (15): 911–914.

Maybauer, D.M., Talke, P.O., Westphal, M., Maybauer, M.O., Traber, L.D., Enkhbaatar, P., Morita, N. and Traber, D.L. (2006) Positive-end expiratory pressure ventilation increases extravascular lung water due to a decrease in lung lymph flow. *Anaesthesia and Intensive Care*, 34 (3): 329–333.

MDA (Medical Devices Agency) (2001) Tissue necrosis caused by pulse oximeter probes. Medical Devices Agency safety notice, MDA SN 2001 (08), March 2001. London: Medical Devices Agency.

Mebazaa, A., Nieminen, M.S., Packer, M., Cohen-Solal, A., Kleber, F.X., Pocock, S.J., Thakker, R., Padley, R.J., Põder, P. and Kivikko, M., SURVIVE Investigators (2007) Levosimendan vs dobutamine for patients with acute decompensated heart failure. *JAMA*, 297 (17): 1883–1891.

Meek, S. and Morris, F. (2008a) Introduction II – basic terminology, in Morris, F., Brady, W.J. and Camm, J. (eds) *ABC of Clinical Electrocardiography*, 2nd edition. London: BMJ Books, pp. 5–8.

—— (2008b) Introduction I – leads, rate, rhythm, and cardiac axis, in Morris, F., Brady, W.J. and Camm, J. (eds) *ABC of Clinical Electrocardiography*. London: BMJ Books, pp. 1–4.

Mehanna, H.M., Moledina, J. and Travis, J. (2008) Refeeding syndrome: what it is, and how to prevent and treat it. *British Medical Journal*, 336 (7659): 1495–1498.

Mehta, R.L., Paascual, M.T., Soroko, S. and Chertow, G.M., PICARD Study Group (2002) Diuretics, mortality, and nonrecovery of renal function in acute renal failure. *JAMA*, 188 (19): 2547–2553.

Meier, P., Knapp, G., Tamhane, U., Chaturvedi, S. and Gurm, H.S. (2010) Short term and intermediate term comparison of endarterectomy versus stenting for carotid artery stenosis: systematic review and meta-analysis of randomised controlled clinical trials. *British Medical Journal*, 340 (7744): 459.

Meier, R., Ockenga, J., Pertkiewicz, M., Pap, A., Milinic, N., MacFie, J., Löser, C. and Keim, V. (2006) ESPEN guidelines on enteral nutrition: pancreas. *Clinical Nutrition*, 25 (2): 275–284.

Meierkord, H., Boon, P., Engelsen, B., Göcke, K., Shorvon, S., Tinuper, P. and Holtkamp, M. (2010) EFNS guideline on the management of status epilepticus in adults. *European Journal of Neurology*, 17: 348–355.

Meissner, A., Genga, K.R., Studart, F.S., Settmacher, U., Hofmann, G., Reinhart, K. and Sakr, Y. (2010) Epidemiology of and factors associated with end-of-life decisions in a surgical intensive care unit. *Critical Care Medicine*, 38 (4): 1060–1068.

Meister, J. and Reddy, K. (2002) Rhabdomyolysis: an overview. *American Journal of Nursing*, 102 (2): 75–79.

Melzack, R. and Wall, P. (1988) *The Challenge of Pain*, 2nd edition. London: Penguin.

Metheny, N. (1993) Minimising respiratory complications of nasoenteric tube feedings: state of the service. *Heart & Lung*, 22 (3): 213–222.

Meyer, B., Bergmann, A., Wexberg, P., Struck, J., Morgenthaler, N.G., Heinz, G., Pacher, R. and Huelsmann, M. (2008) Copeptin and acute renal failure in critically ill patients. *Critical Care*, 12 (supplement 2): P439.

Meyer, J. and Sturdy, D. (2004) Exploring the future of gerontological nursing outcomes. *International Journal of Older People Nursing* in association with *Journal of Clinical Nursing*, 13 (6b): 128–134.

MHRA (Medicines and Healthcare products Regulatory Agency) (2004) *Medical Device Alert, MDA/2004/020*. London: MHRA.

Michelet, P., Guervilly, C., Hélaine, A., Avaro, J.P., Blayac, D., Gaillat, F., Dantin, T., Thomas, P. and Kerbaul, F. (2007) Adding ketamine to morphine for patient-controlled analgesia after thoracic surgery: influence on morphine consumption, respiratory function, and nocturnal desaturation. *British Journal of Anaesthesia*, 99 (3): 396–403.

Mick, D.J. and Ackerman, M.H. (2004) Critical care nursing for older adults: pathophysiological and functional considerations. *Nursing Clinics of North America*, 39 (3): 473–493.

Mihatsch, M.J., Kyo, M., Morozumi, K. Yamaguchi, Y., Nickeleit, V. and Ryffel, B. (1998) The side-effects of cyclosporin-A and tacrolimus. *Clinical Nephrology*, 49 (6): 356–363.

Miller, E., Hoschler, K., Stanford, E., Andrews, N. and Zambon, M. (2010) Incidence of 2009 pandemic influenza A H1N1 infection in England: a cross-sectional serological study. *Lancet*, 375 (9720): 1100–1108.

Miller, R.F., Allen, E., Copas, A., Singer, M. and Edwards, S.G. (2006) Improved survival for HIV infected patients with severe *Pneumocystis jirovecii* pneumonia is independent of highly active antiviral therapy. *Thorax*, 61 (8): 716–721.

Millson, C. (2009) Update on liver transplantation. *British Journal of Hospital Medicine*, 70 (12): 692–697.

Mitchell, M.D., Anderson, B.J., Williams, K. and Umscheid, C.A. (2009) Heparin flushing and other interventions to maintain patency of central venous catheters: a systematic review. *Journal of Advanced Nursing*, 65 (10): 2007–2021.

Mokhlesi, B., Garimella, P.S., Joffe, A. and Velho, V. (2004) Street drug abuse leading to critical illness. *Intensive Care Medicine*, 30 (8): 1526–1536.

Møller, C.H., Penninga, L., Wetterslev, J., Steinbrüchel, D.A. and Gluud, C. (2008) Clinical outcomes in randomized trials of off- vs. on-pump coronary artery bypass surgery: systematic review with meta-analyses and trial sequential analyses. *European Heart Journal*, 29 (21): 2601–2616.

Möller, M.G., Slaikeu, J.D., Bonelli, P., Davis, A.T., Hoogeboom, J.E. and Bonnell, B.W. (2005) Early tracheostomy versus late tracheostomy in the surgical intensive care unit. *American Journal of Surgery*, 189 (3): 293–296.

Molnar, Z., Shearer, E. and Lowe, D. (1999) N-acetylcysteine treatment to prevent the progression of multisystem organ failure: a prospective, randomised, placebo-controlled study. *Critical Care Medicine*, 27 (6): 1100–1104.

Molyneux, A.J., Kerr, R.S.C., Yu, L.-M., Clarke, M., Sneade, M., Yarnold, J.A. and Sandercock, P., International Subarachnoid Aneurysm Trial (ISAT) Collaborative Group (2005) International Subarachnoid Aneurysm Trial (ISAT) of neurosurgical clipping versus endovascular coiling in 2143 patients with ruptured intracranial aneurysms: a randomised comparison of effects on survival, dependency, seizures, rebleeding, subgroups, and aneurysm occlusion. *Lancet*, 366 (9488): 809–817.

Monaco, F., Drummond, G.B., Ramsay, P., Servillo, G. and Walsh, T.S. (2010) Do simple ventilation and gas exchange measurements predict early successful weaning from respiratory support in unselected general intensive care patients? *British Journal of Anaesthesia*, 105 (3): 326–333.

Monchi, M., Berghmans, D., Ledoux, D., Canivet, J.-L., Dubois, B. and Damas, P. (2004) Citrate vs heparin for anticoagulation in continuous venovenous hemofiltration: a prospective randomized study. *Intensive Care Medicine*, 30 (2): 260–265.

Moniotte, S., Kobzik, L., Feron, O., Trochu, J.N., Gauthier, C. and Balligand, J.L. (2001) Upregulation of β_3-adonoreceptors and altered contractile response to inotropic amines in human failing myocardium. *Circulation*, 103 (12): 1649–1655.

Montejo, J.C., Miñambres, E., Bordejé, L., Masejo, A., Acosta, J., Heras, A., Ferré, M., Fernandez-Ortega, F., Vasquizo, C.I. and Manzanedo, R. (2009) Gastric residual volume during enteral nutrition in ICU patients: the REGANE study. *Intensive Care Medicine*, 36 (8): 1386–1393.

Moore, I., Bhat, R., Hoenich, N., Kilner, A.J., Prabhu, M., Orr, K.E. and Kanagasundaram, N.S. (2009) A microbiological survey of bicarbonate-based replacement circuits in continuous venovenous haemofiltration. *Critical Care Medicine*, 37 (2): 496–500.

Moore, T. and Woodrow, P. (eds) (2009) *High Dependency Nursing: Observation, intervention and support*, 2nd edition. London: Routledge.

Moppett, I.K. (2007) Traumatic brain injury: assessment, resuscitation and early management. *British Journal of Anaesthesia*, 99 (1): 18–31.

Morán, I., Bellapart, J., Vari, A. and Mancebo, J. (2006) Heat and moisture exchangers and heated humidifiers in acute lung injury/acute respiratory distress syndrome patients: effects on respiratory mechanics and gas exchange. *Intensive Care Medicine*, 31 (4): 524–531.

Morgan, R.M.J., Williams, F. and Wright, M.M. (1997) An early warning scoring system for detecting developing critical illness. *Clinical Intensive Care*, 8 (2): 100–101.

Morgan, W.M. III and O'Neill, J.A. Jr (1998) Hemorrhagic and obstructive shock in pediatric patients. *New Horizons*, 6 (2): 150–154.

Mori, H., Hirasawa, H., Oda, S., Shiga, H., Matsuda, K. and Nakamura, M. (2006) Oral care reduces incidence of ventilator-associated pneumonia in ICU populations. *Intensive Care Medicine*, 31 (2): 230–236.

Morrell, N. (2010) Prone positioning in patients with acute respiratory distress syndrome. *Nursing Standard*, 24 (21): 42–45.

Mudawi, T.O., Albouaini, K. and Kaye, D.C. (2009) Sudden cardiac death: history, aetiology and management. *British Journal of Hospital Medicine*, 70 (2): 89–94.

Muecke, S.N. (2005) Effects of rotating night shifts. *Journal of Advanced Nursing*, 50 (4): 433–439.

Mullally, S. (2001) Future clinical role of nurses in the United Kingdom. *Postgraduate Medical Journal*, 77 (907): 337–339.

Munoz-Price, L.S. and Weinstein, R.A. (2008) Acinetobacter infection. *New England Journal of Medicine*, 358 (12): 1271–1281.

Munro, C.L., Grap, M.J., Jones, D.J., McClish, D.K. and Sessler, C.N. (2009) Chlorhexidine, toothbrushing, and preventing ventilator-associated pneumonia in critically ill adults. *American Journal of Critical Care*, 18 (5): 428–437.

Murdoch, J. and Larsen, D. (2004) Assessing pain in cognitively impaired older adults. *Nursing Standard*, 18 (38): 33–39.

Murdoch, S. and Cohen, A. (2000) Intensive care sedation: a review of current British practice. *Intensive Care Medicine*, 26 (6): 922–928.

Murphy, J., Mehigan, B.J. and Keane, F.B.V. (2002) Acute pancreatitis. *Hospital Medicine*, 6 (8): 487–492.

Murphy, N. (2006) An update in acute liver failure: when to transplant and the role of liver support devices. *Clinical Medicine*, 6 (1): 40–46.

Murphy, P.J., Marriage, S.C. and Davis, P.J. (eds) (2009) *Case Studies in Pediatric Critical Care*. Cambridge: Cambridge University Press.

Murphy, T. and Robinson, S. (2006) Renal failure and its treatment. *Anaesthesia and Intensive Care Medicine*, 7 (7): 247–252.

Murray, P.R., Rosenthal, K.S. and Pfaller, M.A. (2009) *Medical Microbiology*, 6th edition. St Louis, MO: Mosby.

Musco, S., Conway, E.L. and Kowey, P.R. (2008) Drug therapy for atrial fibrillation. *Medical Clinics of America*, 92 (1): 121–141.

Musters, C. (2010) Managing patients without their consent: a guide to recent legislation. *British Journal of Hospital Medicine*, 71 (2): 87–90.

Myburgh, J.A., Higgins, A., Jovanovska, A., Lipman, J., Ramakrishnan, N. and Santamaria, J., CAT Study Investigators (2008) A comparison of epinephrine and norepinephrine in critically ill patients. *Intensive Care Medicine*, 34 (12): 2226–2234.

Nachamkin, I., Shadomy, S.V., Moran, A.P., Cox, N., Fitzgerald, C., Ung, H., Corcoran, A.T., Iskander, J.K., Schonberger, L.B. and Chen, R.T. (2008) Anti-ganglioside antibody induction by swine (A/NJ/1976/H1N1) and other influenza vaccines: insights into vaccine-associated Guillain-Barré syndrome. *Journal of Infectious Diseases*, 198 (15 July): 226–233.

Nair, M., Alabi, C. and Hirsch, P.I. (2006) Toxic shock syndrome: a silent killer. *Journal of Obstetrics and Gynaecology*, 26 (8): 825–835.

Nanas, S., Gerovasil, V., Renieris, P., Angelopoulos, E., Poriazi, M., Kritikos, K., Siafaka, A., Baraboutis, I., Zervakis, D., Markakis, V., Rousti, C. and Roussos, C. (2009) Non-invasive assessment of the microcirculation in critically ill patients. *Anaesthesia and Intensive Care*, 37 (5): 733–739.

Nathan, A.T. and Singer, M. (1999) The oxygen trail: tissue oxygenation. *British Medical Bulletin*, 55 (1): 96–108.

Nathens, A.B., Curtis, J.R., Beale, R.J., Cook, D.J., Moreno, R.P., Romand, J.-A., Skerrett, S.J., Stapleton, R.D., Ware, L.B. and Waldmann, C.S. (2004) Management of the critically ill patient with severe acute pancreatitis. *Critical Care Medicine*, 32 (12): 2524–2536.

National Heart, Lung, and Blood Institute Acute Respiratory Distress Syndrome (ARDS) Clinical Trials Network (2006) Comparison of two fluid-management strategies in acute lung injury. *New England Journal of Medicine*, 354 (24): 2564–2575.

Nava, S. and Hill, N. (2009) Non-invasive ventilation in acute respiratory failure. *Lancet*, 374 (9685): 250–259.

NCEPOD (National Confidential Enquiry into Patient Outcome and Death) (2005) *Abdominal Aortic Aneurysm: A service in need of surgery?* London: NCEPOD.

—— (2009) *An Acute Problem*. London: NCEPOD.

—— (2010a) *A Mixed Bag*. London: NCEPOD.

—— (2010b) *An Age Old Problem*. London: NCEPOD.

Netzer, G., Shah, C.V., Iwashyma, T.J., Lanken, P.N., Finkel, B., Fuchs, B., Guo, W. and Christie, J.D. (2007) Association of RCB transfusion with mortality in patients with acute lung injury. *Chest*, 132 (4): 1116–1123.

Nguyen, N.Q., Chapman, M.J., Fraser, R.J., Bryant, L.K. and Holloway, R.H. (2007) Erythromycin is more effective than metoclopramide in the treatment of feed intolerance in critical illness. *Critical Care Medicine*, 35 (2): 483–489.

NHS Estates (2003) *Facilities for Critical Care*. HBN 57. Norwich: The Stationery Office.

NICE (National Institute for Health and Clinical Excellence) (2006) *Nutrition Support in Adults*. London: NICE.

—— (2007a) *Venous Thromboembolism*. Clinical Guideline 46. London: NICE.

—— (2007b) *Head Injury: Triage, assessment, investigation and early management of head injury in infants, children and adults*. London: NICE.

—— (2008) *Laparoscopic Repair of Abdominal Aortic Aneurysm*. London: NICE.

—— (2009a) *Rehabilitation after Critical Illness*. London: NICE.

—— (2009b) *Continuous Subcutaneous Insulin Infusion for the Treatment of Diabetes Mellitus*. London: NICE.

—— (2010a) *Delirium: Diagnosis, prevention and management*. London: NICE.

—— (2010b) *Neuropathic Pain*. Clinical Guideline 96. London: NICE.

—— (2010c) *Chest Pain of Recent Onset*. Clinical Guideline 95. London: NICE.

—— (2010d) *Organ Donation for Transplants Draft Scope for Consultation*. London: NICE.

NICE-SUGAR Study Investigators (2009) Intensive versus conventional glucose control in critically ill patients. *New England Journal of Medicine*, 360 (130): 1283–1297.

Nicholls, S.J., Wang, Z., Koeth, R., Levison, B., DelFraino, B., Dzavik, V., Griffith, O.W., Hathaway, D., Panza, J.A., Nisen, S.E., Hochman, J.S. and Hazen, S.L. (2007) Metabolic profiling of arginine and nitric oxide pathways predicts hemodynamic abnormalities and mortality in patients with cardiogenic shock after acute myocardial infarction. *Circulation*, 116 (20): 2315–2324.

Nightingale, F. (1859/1980) *Notes on Nursing: What it is, and what it is not*. Edinburgh: Churchill Livingstone.

NMC (Nursing and Midwifery Council) (2008a) *The Code: Standards of conduct, performance and ethics for nurses and midwives*. London: NMC.

—— (2008b) *Standards for Medicines Management*. London: NMC.

—— (2009) Position statement: working during a surge in the swine flu pandemic. Available online at www.nmc-uk.org/aarticleprint.aspx?ArticleID=3897 (accessed 19 October 2009).

Nobre, V., Harbarth, S., Graf, J.D., Rohner, P. and Pugin, J. (2008) Use of procalcitonin to shorten antibiotic treatment duration in septic patients: a randomized trial. *American Journal of Respiratory & Critical Care Medicine*, 177 (5): 498–505.

Nolan, J.J. (2002) What is type 2 diabetes? *Medicine*, 30 (1): 6–10.

Norberg, A., Brauer, K.I., Prough, D.S., Gabrielsson, J., Hahn, R.G., Uchida, T., Traber, D.L. and Svensén, C.H. (2005) Volume turnover kinetics of fluid shifts after hemorrhage, fluid infusion, and the combination of hemorrhage and fluid infusion in sheep. *Anesthesiology*, 109 (5): 985–994.

Norwood, M.G.A., Bown, M. J., Lloyd, G. Bell, P.R.F. and Sayers, R.D. (2004) The clinical value of the systemic inflammatory response syndrome in abdominal aortic aneurysm repair. *British Journal of Surgery*, 91 (supplement 1): 112.

Novitzky, N., Jacobs, P. and Rosenstrauch, W. (2008) The treatment of thrombotic thrombo-cytopenic purpura: plasma infusion or exchange? *British Journal of Haematology*, 87 (2): 317–320.

NPSA (National Patient Safety Agency) (2002) *Patient Safety Alert*. Ref. PSA 01. London. NPSA.

—— (2004a) *Achieving Our Aims: Evaluating the results of the pilot CleanyourHands campaign*. London: NPSA.

—— (2004b) *Bowel Care for Patients with Established Spinal Cord Lesions*. London: NPSA.

—— (2005) *Safety Alert: Reducing the harm caused by misplaced nasogastric feeding tubes*. Ref. 0180Jan05. London: NPSA.

—— (2008a) *Problems with Infusions and Sampling from Arterial Lines*. London: NPSA.

—— (2008b) *A Compendium of Patient Safety in Practice*. London: NPSA.

Ntoumenopoulos, G., Presneill, J.J., McElholum, M. and Cade, J.F. (2002) Chest physio-therapy for the prevention of ventilator-associated pneumonia. *Intensive Care Medicine*, 28 (7): 850–856.

Nunn, J.F. (1996) Oxygen consumption and delivery, in Prys-Roberts, C. and Brown, B.R. Jr (eds) *International Practice of Anaesthesia*. Oxford: Butterworth-Heinemann, pp. 1/61/1–10.

Nydegger, A., Heine, R.G., Ranuh, R., Gegati-Levy, R., Crameri, J. and Oliver, M.R. (2007) Changing incidence of acute pancreatitis: 10-year experience at the Royal Children's Hospital, Melbourne. *Journal of Gastroenterology and Hepatology*, 22 (8): 1313–1316.

Nyirenda, M., Tang, J.I., Padfield, P.L. and Seckl, J.R. (2009) Hyperkalaemia. *British Medical Journal*, 339 (7728): 1019–1024.

O'Brien, J.M. Jr, Lu, B., Ali, N.A., Martin, G.S., Aberegg, S.K., Marsh, C.B., Lemeshow, S. and Douglas, I.S. (2007) Alcohol dependence is independently associated with sepsis, septic shock, and hospital mortality among adult intensive care unit patients. *Critical Care Medicine*, 35 (2) 345–350.

Ochola, J. and Venkatesh, B. (2009) Rational approach to fluid therapy in acute diabetic ketoacidosis, in Vincent, J.-L. (ed.) *Yearbook of Intensive Care and Emergency Medicine*, pp. 254–262.

O'Connor, M., Bucknall, T. and Manias, E. (2009) A critical review of daily sedation interruption in the intensive care unit. *Journal of Clinical Nursing*, 18 (9): 1239–1249.

—— (2010) International variations in outcomes from sedation protocol research: where are we at and where do we go from here? *Intensive & Critical Care Nursing*, 26 (4): 189–195.

O'Connor, T.M., O'Halloran, D.J. and Shanahan, F. (2000) The stress response and the hypothalamic-pituitary-adrenal axis: from molecule to melancholia. *QJM*, 93 (6): 323–333.

Oddo, M., Feihl, F., Schaller, M.-D. and Perret, C. (2006) Management of mechanical ventilation in acute severe asthma: practical aspects. *Intensive Care Medicine*, 31 (4): 501–510.

Odell, M. (1996) Intracranial pressure monitoring, nursing in a district general hospital. *Nursing in Critical Care*, 1 (5): 245–247.

O'Donoghue, S.D., Dulhunty, J.M., Bandeshe, H.K., Senthuran, S. and Gowardman, J.R. (2009) Acquired hypernatraemia is an independent predictor of mortality in critically ill patients. *Anaesthesia*, 64 (5): 514–520.

O'Grady, N.P., Barie, P.S., Bartlett, J., Bleck, T., Garvey, G., Jacobi, J., Linden, P., Maki, D.G., Nam, M., Pasculle, W., Pasquale, M.D., Tribett, D.L. and Masur, H. (1998) Practice parameters for evaluating new fever in critically ill patients. *Critical Care Medicine*, 26 (2): 392–408.

Oh, E.G., Lee, W.H., Yoo, J.S., Kim, S.S., Ko, I.S., Chu, S.H., Song, E.K. and Kang, S.W. (2009) Factors related to incidence of eye disorders in Korean patients at intensive care units. *Journal of Clinical Nursing*, 18 (1): 29–35.

Ojiako, K., Shingala, H., Schorr, C. and Gerber, D.R. (2008) Comparison of famotidine and pantoprazole for preventing bleeding in the upper gastrointestinal tract of critically ill patients receiving mechanical ventilation. *American Journal of Critical Care*, 17 (2): 142–147.

O'Neill, L.J. and Carter, D.E. (1998) Adult/elderly care nursing: the implications of head injury for family relationships. *British Journal of Nursing*, 7 (14): 842–846.

Oostdijk, E.A.N., de Smet, A.M.G.A., Blok, H.E.M., Groen, E.S.T., van Asselt, G.J., Benus, R.F.J., Bernards, S.A.T., Frénay, I.H.M.E., Jansz, A.R., de Jongh, B.M., Kaan, J.A., Hall, L.-V., Mascini, E.M., Pauw, W., Sturm, P.D.J., Thijsen, S.F.T., Kluytmans, J.A.J.W. and Bonten, M.J.M. (2010) Ecological effects of selective decontamination on resistant gram-negative bacterial colonization. *American Journal of Respiratory and Critical Care Medicine*, 181 (5): 452–457.

O'Reilly, M. (2003) Oral care of the critically ill: a review of the literature and guidelines for practice. *Australian Critical Care*, 16 (3): 101–109.

Orme, J., Romney, J.S., Hopkins, R.O., Pope, D., Chan, K.J., Thomsen, G., Crapo, R.O. and Weaver, L.K. (2003) Pulmonary function and health-related quality of life in survivors of acute respiratory distress syndrome. *American Journal of Respiratory and Critical Care Medicine*, 167 (5): 690–694.

Ormrod, J.A., Ryder, T., Chadwick, R.J. and Bonner, S.M. (2005) Experiences of families when a relative is diagnosed brain stem dead: understanding of death, observation of brain stem death testing and attitudes to organ donation. *Anaesthesia*, 60 (10): 1002–1008.

O'Shea, P. (1997) Altered consciousness and stroke, in Goldhill, D.R. and Withington, P.S. (eds) *Textbook of Intensive Care*. London: Chapman & Hall, pp. 495–502.

O'Toole, S. (1997) Alternatives to mercury thermometers. *Professional Nurse*, 12 (11): 783–786.

Oudemans-van Straaten, H.M., Wester, J.P.J., de Pont, A.C. and Schetz, M.R.C. (2006) Anticoagulation strategies in continuous renal replacement therapy: can the choice be evidence based? *Intensive Care Medicine*, 32 (2): 188–202.

Page, V. (2008) Sedation and delirium assessment in the ICU. *Care of the Critically Ill*, 24 (6): 153–158.

—— (2010) Management of delirium in the intensive care unit. *British Journal of Hospital Medicine*, 71 (7): 372–376.

Palevsky, E.M. (2009) Intensity of continuous renal replacement therapy in acute kidney injury. *Seminars in Dialysis*, 22 (2): 151–154.

Palma, S., Cosano, A., Mariscal, M., Martinez-Gallego, G., Medina-Cuadros, M. and Delgado-Rodriguez, M. (2007) Cholesterol and serum albumin as risk factors for death in patients undergoing general surgery. *British Journal of Surgery*, 94 (3): 369–375.

Palsson, R., Niles, J. (1999) Regional citrate anticoagulation in continuous venovenous hemofiltration in critically ill patients with a high risk of bleeding. *Kidney International*, 55 (5): 1991–1997.

Pamba, A. and Maitland, K. (2004) Capillary refill: prognostic value in Kenyan children. *Archives of Disease in Childhood*, 89 (10): 950–955.

Pandharipande, P.P., Shintani, A., Peterson, J. and Ely, W. (2004) Sedative and analgesic medications are independent risk factors in ICU patients for transitioning into delirium. *Critical Care Medicine*, 32 (12 supplement): A19.

Pareek, M. and Stephenson, I. (2007) Clinical evaluation of vaccines for pandemic influenza H5N1. *British Journal of Hospital Medicine*, 68 (2): 80–84.

Park, C. (2007) Diabetic ketoacidosis. *Journal of the Royal College of Physicians of Edinburgh*, 37 (1): 40–43.

Park, W.G., Yeh, R.W, Triadafilopoulos, G. (2008) Injection therapies for variceal bleeding disorders of the GI tract. *Gastrointestinal Endoscopy*, 67 (2): 313–332.

Parnaby, C. (2004) A new anti-embolism stocking. *British Journal of Perioperative Nursing*, 14 (7): 302–307.

Parnell, A.D. and Massey, N.J. (2009) Postoperative care of the adult cardiac surgical patient. *Anaesthesia and Intensive Care Medicine*, 10 (9): 430–436.

Parrott, A.C., Lees, A., Garnham, N.J., Jones, M. and Wesnes, K. (1998) Cognitive performance in recreational users of MDMA or 'ecstasy': evidence for memory deficits. *Journal of Psychopharmacology*, 12 (1): 79–83.

Parry, N., Evans, I. and Southall, P. (2010) What's the potassium? *Journal of the Intensive Care Society*, 11 (2): 146.

Pastor, C.M., Maatthay, M.A. and Frossard, J.-L. (2003) Pancreatitis-associated acute lung injury. *Chest*, 124 (6): 2341–2351.

Patel, B.M., Chittock, D.R., Russell, J.A. and Walley, K.R. (2002) Beneficial effects of short-term vasopressin infusion during severe septic shock. *Anaesthesia*, 96 (3): 576–582.

Patel, D. and Meakin, G.H. (2000) Paediatric airway management. *Current Anaesthesia & Critical Care*, 11 (5): 262–268.

Patil, B.B. and Dowd, T.C. (2000) Physiological functions of the eye. *Current Anaesthesia & Critical Care*, 11 (6): 291–298.

Patti, S., Goodfellow, J.A., Iyadurai, S. and Hilton-Jones, D. (2008) Approach to critical illness polyneuropathy and myopathy. *Postgraduate Medical Journal*, 84 (993): 354–360.

Patton, G.C., Coffey, C., Carlin, J.B., Degenhardt, L., Lynskey, M. and Hall, W. (2002) Cannabis use and mental health in young people: cohort study. *British Medical Journal*, 325 (7374): 1195–1198.

Payen, J.-F., Bru, O., Bosson, J.-L., Lagrasta, A., Novel, E., Deschaux, I., Lavagne, P. and Jacquot, C. (2001) Assessing pain in critically ill sedated patients by using a behavioral pain scale. *Critical Care Medicine*, 29 (12): 2258–2263.

Peake, J., Peiffer, J.J., Abbiss, C.R., Nosaka, K., Okutsu, M., Laursen, P.B. and Suzuki, K. (2008) Body temperature and its effect on leukocyte mobilization, cytokines and markers of neutrophil activation during and after exercise. *European Journal of Applied Physiology*, 102 (4): 391–401.

Peate, I. (2004) An overview of meningitis: signs, symptoms, treatment and support. *British Journal of Nursing*, 13 (3): 796–801.

Peek, G., Mugford, M., Tiruvoipati, R., Wilson, A., Allen, E., Thalanany, M., Hibbert, C., Trueside, A., Clemens, F., Cooper, N., Firmin, R.K. and Elbourne, D., CESAR trial collaboration (2009) Efficacy and economic assessment of conventional ventilator support versus extracorporeal membrane oxygenation for severe adult respiratory failure (CESAR): a multicentre randomised controlled trial. *Lancet*, 374 (9698): 1351–1363.

Pender, L.R. and Frazier, S.K. (2005) The relationship between dermal pressure ulcers, oxygenation and perfusion in mechanically ventilated patients. *Intensive and Critical Care Nursing*, 21 (1): 29–38.

Pépin, J., Valiquette, L. and Cossette, B. (2005) Mortality attributable to nosocomial *Clostridium difficile*-associated disease during an epidemic caused by a hypervirulent strain in Quebec. *Canadian Medical Association Journal*, 173 (9): 1037–1042.

Peppelenbosch, N., Cuypers, P.W.M., Vahl, A.C., Vermassen, F. and Buth, J. (2005) Emergency endovascular treatment for the ruptured aortic aneurysm and the risk of spinal cord ischaemia. *Journal of Vascular Surgery*, 42 (4): 608–614.

Perez-Padilla, R., de la Rosa-Zamboni, D., de Leon, S.P., Hernandez, M., Quiñones-Falconi, F., Bautista, E., Ramirez-Venegas, A., Rojas-Serrano, J., Ormsby, C.E., Corrales, A., Higuera, A., Mondragon, E. and Cordova-Villalobos, J.A., INER Working Group on Influenza (2009) Pneumonia and respiratory failure from swine-origin influenza A (H1N1) in Mexico. *New England Journal of Medicine*, 361 (7): 680–680.

Perlino, C.A. (2001) Postoperative fever. *Medical Clinics of North America*, 85 (5): 1141–1149.

Peters, R.J.G., Mehta, S. and Yusuf, S. (2007) Acute coronary syndromes without ST segment elevation. *British Medical Journal*, 334 (16 June): 1265–1269.

Petrov, M.S., Correia, M.I. and Windsor, J.A. (2008) Nasogastric tube feeding in predicted severe acute pancreatitis. A systemic review of the literature to determine safety and tolerance. *Journal of the Pancreas*, 9 (4): 440–448.

Petter, A.H., Chiolero, R.L., Cassina, T., Chassot, P.-G., Muller, X.M. and Revelly, J.-P. (2003) Automatic 'respirator/weaning' with adaptive support ventilation: the effect on duration of endotracheal intubation and patient management. *Anesthesia & Analgesia*, 97 (6): 1743–1750.

Phoenix, S.I., Paravastu, S., Columb, M., Vincent, J.-L. and Nirmalan, M. (2009) Does a higher positive end expiratory pressure decrease mortality in acute respiratory distress syndrome? A systematic review and meta-analysis. *Anesthesiology*, 110 (5): 1098–1105.

Pickworth, T. (2003) Acute pancreatitis. *Anaesthesia and Intensive Care*, 4 (4): 106–107.

Pierce, J.D., Cackler, A.B. and Arnett, M.G. (2004) Why should you care about free radicals? *American Journal of Nursing*, 67 (1): 38–42.

Pilcher, D.V., Duke, G.J., George, C., Bailey, M.J. and Hart, G. (2007) After-hours discharge from intensive care increases the risk of readmission and death. *Anaesthesia & Intensive Care*, 35 (4): 477–485.

Pinhu, L., Whitehead, T., Evans, T. and Griffiths, M. (2003) Ventilator-associated lung injury. *Lancet*, 361 (9354): 332–340.

Pipbeam, S.P. (2006) Ventilator graphics, in Pilbeam, S.P. and Cairo, J.M. (eds) *Mechanical Ventilation: Physiological and clinical applications*, 4th edition. St Louis, MO: Mosby Elsevier, pp. 177–204.

Pisani, M.A. (2009) Considerations in caring for the critically ill older patient. *Intensive Care Medicine*, 24 (2), 83–95.

——, King, S.Y.-J., Kasl, S.V., Murphy, T.E. and Araujo, K.L.-B. (2009) Days of delirium are associated with 1-year mortality in an older intensive care unit population. *American Journal of Respiratory and Critical Care Medicine*, 180 (11): 1092–1097.

Pitkin, A., Scott, R. and Salmon, J. (1997) Hyperbaric oxygen therapy in intensive care. *British Journal of Intensive Care*, 7 (3): 107–113.

Pitt, T. (2007) Management of antimicrobial-resistant *Acinitobacter* in hospitals. *Nursing Standard*, 21 (35): 51–56.

Pittet, D. and Boyce, J.M. (2001) Hand hygiene and patient care: pursuing the Semmelweis legacy. *Lancet Infectious Diseases* (April): 9–20.

Pleym, H., Wahba, A., Videm, V., Asberg, A., Lydersen, S., Bjella, L., Dale, O. and Stenseth, R. (2006) Increased fibrinolysis and platelet activation in elderly patients undergoing coronary bypass surgery. *Anesthesia & Analgesia*, 102 (3): 660–667.

Pneumatikos, I.A., Dragoumanis, C.K. and Bouros, D.E. (2009) Ventilator-associated pneumonia of endotracheal tube-associated pneumonia? *Anesthesiology*, 10 (3): 673–680.

Polderman, K.H. and Girbes, A.R.J. (2002) Central venous catheter use. Part 1: mechanical complications. *Intensive Care Medicine*, 28 (1): 1–17.

Pollard, B.J. (2005) Neuromuscular agents and reversal agents. *Anaesthesia and Intensive Care Medicine*, 6 (6): 189–192.

Porter, J.B. (2009) Optimizing iron chelation strategies in β-thalassaemia major. *Blood Reviews*, 23 (supplement 1): S3–S7.

Pottle, A. (2007) Measuring cholesterol levels. *Nursing Standard*, 21 (46): 42–47.

Pouwer, F., Geelhoed-Duijvestijn, P.H.L.M., Tack, C.J., Bazelmans, E., Beekman, A.-J., Heine, R.J. and Snoek, F.J. (2010) Education and psychological aspects: prevalence of comorbid depression is high in out-patients with type 1 or type 2 diabetes mellitus: results from three out-patient clinics in the Netherlands. *Diabetic Medicine*, 27: 217–224.

Póvoa, P. (2002) C-reactive protein: a valuable marker of sepsis. *Intensive Care Medicine*, 28 (3): 235–243.

Powell, K., Davis, L., Morris, A.M., Chi, A., Bensley, M.R. and Huang, L. (2009) Survival for patients with HIV admitted to the ICU continues to improve in the current era of combination antiretroviral therapy. *Chest*, 135 (1): 11–17.

Powell, T. (2004) *Head Injury: A practical guide*, 2nd edition. Bicester: Speechmark.

Powell-Tuck, J., Gosling, P., Lobo, D.N., Allison, S.P., Carlson, G.L., Gore, M., Lewington, A.J., Pearse, R.M. and Mythen, M.G. (2008) *British Consensus Guidelines on Intravenous Fluid Therapy for Adult Surgical Patients. GIFTASUP.* London: BAPEN, Association for Clinical Biochemistry, Association of Surgeons of Great Britain and Ireland, Society of Academic and Research Surgery, Renal Association, Intensive Care Society.

Power, B. (2009) Acute cardiac syndromes, investigations and interventions, in Bersten, A.D. and Soni, N. (eds) *Intensive Care Manual*, 6th edition. Edinburgh: Butterworth-Heinemann, pp. 155–177.

Powner, D.J. and Bernstein, I.M. (2003) Extended somatic support for pregnant women after brain death. *Critical Care Medicine*, 31(4): 1241–1249.

Pratt, L.W., Ferlito, A. and Rinaldo, A. (2008) Tracheostomy: historical review. *Laryngoscope*, 118 (9): 1597–1606.

Pratt, R.J., Pellowe, C.M., Wilson, J.A., Loveday, H.P., Harper, P.J., Jones, S.R.L.J., McDougall, C. and Wilcox, M.H. (2007) Epic 2: national evidence-based guidelines for preventing healthcare-associated infections in NHS hospitals in England. *Journal of Hospital Infection*, 65 (supplement 1): S1–S64.

Preise, J.-C., Devos, P., Ruiz-Santana, S., Mélot, C., Annane, D., Groeneveld, J., Iapichino, G., Leverve, X., Nitenberg, G., Singer, P., Wernerman, J., Joannidis, M., Stecher, A. and Chioléro, R. (2009) A prospective randomised multi-centre controlled trial on tight glycaemic control by intensive insulin therapy in adult intensive care units: the Glucontrol study. *Intensive Care Medicine*, 35 (10): 1738–1748.

Preller, J. and Wilson, P. (2009) Multi-resistant Gram negative organisms in ICU, in Ridley, S. (ed.) *Critical Care Focus 16: Infection.* London: Intensive Care Society, pp. 28–45.

Preston, S.D., Southall, A.R., Neil, M. and Das, S.K. (2008) Geriatric surgery is about diseases not age. *Journal of the Royal Society of Medicine*, 101: 409–415.

Price, L.C., Germain, S., Wuncoll, D. and Nelson-Piercy, C. (2009) Management of the critically ill obstetric patient. *Obstetrics, Gynaecology and Reproductive Medicine*, 19 (12): 350–358.

Prinha, S. and Rowan, K. (2008) Patients' and relatives' experiences of intensive care. *Journal of the Intensive Care Society*, 9 (1): 91.

Prinssen, M., Verhoeven, E.L.G., Buth, J. Cuypers, P.W.M., van Sambeek, M.R.H.M., Balm, R., Buskens, E., Grobbee, D.E. and Blankensteijn, J.D. (2004) A randomised trial comparing conventional and endovascular repair of abdominal aortic aneurysms. *New England Journal of Medicine*, 351 (16): 1607–1618.

Pritchard, J. (2008) What's new in Guillain-Barré syndrome? *Postgraduate Medical Journal*, 84 (996): 522–538.

Puchakayala, M.R. (2006) Descending thoracic aortic aneurysms. *Continuing Education in Anaesthesia, Critical Care & Pain*, 6 (2): 54–59.

Pun, B.T. and Ely, E.W. (2007) The importance of diagnosing and managing ICU delirium. *Chest*, 132 (2): 624–626.

Putensen, C., Theuerkauf, N., Zinserling, J., Wrigge, H. and Pelosi, P. (2009) Meta-analysis: ventilation strategies and outcomes of the acute respiratory distress syndrome and acute lung injury. *Annals of Internal Medicine*, 151 (8): 566–576.

Quenot, J.-P., Thiery, N. and Barbar, S. (2009)When should stress ulcer prophylaxis be used in the ICU? *Current Opinion in Critical Care*, 15 (2): 139–143.

Raeburn, C.D, Sheppard, F., Barsness, K.A., Ayra, J. and Harken, A.H. (2002) Cytokines for surgeons. *American Journal of Surgery*, 183 (3): 268–273

Rakel, B. and Herr, K. (2004) Assessment and treatment of postoperative pain in older adults. *Journal of PeriAnesthesia Nursing*, 19 (3): 194–208.

Ramnarayan, P., Thiru, K., Paslow, R.C., Harrison, D.A., Draper, E.S. and Rowan, K.M. (2010) Effect of specialist retrieval teams on outcomes in children admitted to paediatric intensive care units in England and Wales: a retrospective cohort study. *Lancet*, 376 (9742): 698–704.

Ramsay, M.A., Savege, T.M., Simpson, B.R. and Goodwin, R. (1974) Controlled sedation with alphaxolone-alphadolone. *British Medical Journal*, 1974–2 (920): 656–659.

Ramsay, P., Huby, G., Thompson, A. and Walsh, T. (2008) Quality of life among survivors of prolonged critical illness: a mixed methods study. *Critical Care*, 12 (supplement 2): P508.

Ranasinghe, A.M. and Bonser, R.S. (2004) Interventions for thoracic aortic disease, in Treasure, T., Hunt, I., Keogh, B. and Pagano, D. (eds) *The Evidence for Cardiothoracic Surgery*. Shrewsbury: tfm Publishing, pp. 253–272.

Rance, M. (2005) Kinetic therapy positively influences oxygenation in patients. *Nursing in Critical Care*, 10 (1): 35–41.

Randhawa, G. (1997) Enhancing the health professional's role in requesting transplant organs. *British Journal of Nursing*, 6 (8): 429–434.

Rang, H.P., Dale, M.M., Ritter, J.M. and Flower, R.J. (2007) *Pharmacology*, 6th edition. Edinburgh: Churchill Livingstone Elsevier.

Rankin, J. (2006) Godzilla in the corridor: the Ontario SARS crisis in historical perspective. *Intensive & Critical Care Nursing*, 22 (3): 130–137.

Rashid, M., Goldin, R. and Wright, M. (2004) Drugs and the liver. *Hospital Medicine*, 65 (8): 456–461.

Rathbun, S.W., Whitsett, T.L., Vesely, S.K. and Raskob, G.E. (2004) Clinical utility of D-dimer in patients with suspected pulmonary embolism and nondiagnostic lung scans or negative CT findings. *Chest*, 125 (3): 851–855.

Rattenbury, N., Mooney and G., Bowen, J. (1999) Oral assessment and care for inpatients. *Nursing Times*, 95 (49): 52–53.

RCN (Royal College of Nursing) (2003a) *Guidance for Nurse Staffing in Critical Care*. London: RCN.

—— (2003b) *Standards for Infusion Therapy*. London: RCN.

—— (2005) *Meticillin-resistant Staphylococcus aureas (MRSa)*. London: RCN.

—— (2008) *Bowel Care, including Digital Rectal Examination and Manual Removal of Faeces*. London: RCN.

RCOG (Royal College of Obstetricians and Gynaecologists) (2007) *Green Top Guide 28: Thromboembolic Disease in Pregnancy and the Puerperium: Acute management*. London: RCOG.

—— (2009) *Green Top Guide 52: Prevention and Management of Postpartum Haemorrhage*. London: RCOG.

RCP (Royal College of Physicians) (2008) *Non-invasive Ventilation in Chronic Obstructive Pulmonary Disease: Management of acute type 2 respiratory failure*. London: RCP.

—— (2010) Unstable Angina and NSTEMI: The early management of unstable angina and non-ST-segment elevation myocardial infarction. London: The National Clinical Guideline Centre for Acute and Chronic Conditions/RCP.

Redfern, S.J. and Ross, F.M. (eds) (2006) *Nursing Older People*, 4th edition. Edinburgh: Churchill Livingstone.

Rees, D.C., Williams, T.N. and Gladwin, M.T. (2010) Sickle-dell disease. *Lancet*, 376 (9757): 2018–2031.

Regan, E.N. (2009) How to care for a patient with a tracheostomy. *Nursing2009*, 39 (8): 34–39.

Reid, C.L. and Campbell, I.T. (2004) Metabolic physiology. *Current Anaesthesia & Critical Care*, 15 (3): 209–217.

Reid, M.B. and Cottrell. D. (2005) Nursing care of patients receiving intra-aortic balloon pump counterpulsation. *Critical Care Nurse*, 25 (5): 40–49.

Reilly, D.E. (1980) *Behavioural Objectives: Evaluation in nursing*. New York: Appleton Century Crofts.

Reilly, M.P. and Rader, D.J. (2003) The metabolic syndrome: more than the sum of its parts. *Circulation*, 108: 1546–1551.

Rello, J., Koulenti, D., Blot, S., Sierra, R., Diaz, E., de Waele, J.J., Macor, A., Agbaht, K. and Rodriguez, A. (2007) Oral care practices in intensive care units: a survey of 59 European ICUs. *Intensive Care Medicine*, 33 (6): 1066–1070.

Remy, B., Deby-Dupont, G. and Lamy, M. (1999) Red blood cell substitutes: fluorocarbon emulsions and haemoglobin solutions. *British Medical Bulletin*, 55 (1): 277–298.

Renal Replacement Therapy Investigators (2009) High intensity continuous renal replacement therapy does not improve mortality in critically ill patients. *New England Journal of Medicine*, 361 (17): 1627–1638.

Reneman, L., Booij, J., de Bruin, K., Reitsma, J.B., de Wolff, F.A., Gunning, W.B., den Heeten, G.J. and van den Brink, W. (2001) Effects of dose, sex and long-term abstention from use on toxic effects of MDMA (ecstasy) on brain serotonin levels. *Lancet*, 358 (9296): 1864–1869.

Renton, M.C. and Snowden, C.P. (2005) Dopexamine and its role in the protection of hepatospanchnic and renal perfusion in high-risk surgical and critically ill patients. *British Journal of Anaesthesia*, 94 (4): 459–467.

Resuscitation Council (UK) (2010) *Resuscitation Guidelines*. London: Resuscitation Council.

Reynolds, R.M., Padfield, P.L. and Seckl, J.R. (2006) Disorders of sodium balance. *British Medical Journal*, 332 (7543): 702–705.

Ricard, J-D., Dreyfus, D. and Saumon, G. (2003) Ventilator-induced lung injury. *European Respiratory Journal*, 22 (supplement 42): 2s–9s.

Ricaurte, G.A. and McCann, U.D. (2005) Recognition and management of complications of new recreational drug use. *Lancet*, 365 (9477): 2137–2145.

Richardson, A., Allsop, M., Coghill, E. and Turnock, C. (2007) Earplugs and eye masks: do they improve critical care patients' sleep? *Nursing in Critical Care*, 12 (6): 278–286.

Richardson, J.D., Cocanour, C.S., Kern, J.A., Garrison, R.N., Kirton, O.C., Cofer, J.B., Spain, D.A. and Thomason, M.H. (2004) Perioperative risk assessment in elderly and high-risk patients. *Journal of the American College of Surgeons*, 199 (1): 133–146.

Rickes, S. and Uhle, C. (2009) Advances in the diagnosis of acute pancreatitis. *Postgraduate Medical Journal*, 85 (1002): 208–212.

Ricks, E. (2007) Critical illness polyneuropathy and myopathy: a review of evidence and the implications for weaning from mechanical ventilation. *Physiotherapy*, 93 (2): 151–156.

Ridley, S. (2005) Critical care needs of the elderly. *Geriatric Medicine*, 35 (2): 11–16.

—— (2009) *Critical Care Focus 16: Infection*. London: Intensive Care Society.

—— and Morris, S. (2006) The cost-effectiveness of intensive care in the UK. *Journal of the Intensive Care Society*, 7 (3): 58.

—— (2007) Cost effectiveness of adult intensive care in the UK. *Anaesthesia*, 62 (6): 547–554.

Riker, R.R., Fraser, G.L., Simmons, L.E., Wilkins and M.L. (2001) Validating the Sedation-Agitation Scale with the Bispectral Index and Visual Analog Scale in adult ICU patients after cardiac surgery. *Intensive Care Medicine*, 27 (5): 853–858.

Riley, B. (2009) Acute cerebrovascular complications, in Bersten, A.D. and Soni, N. (eds) *Intensive Care Manual*, 6th edition. Edinburgh: Butterworth-Heinemann Elsevier, pp. 551–561.

Roberts, I., Yates, D., Sandercock, P., Farrell, B., Wasserberg, J., Lomas, G., Cottingham, R., Svoboda, P., Brayley, N., Mazairac, G., Laloe, V., Munoz-Sanchez, A., Arango, M., Hartzenberg, B., Khamis, H., Yutthakasemsunt, S., Komolafe, E., Olldashi, F., Yadav, Y., Murillo-Cabezas, F., Shakur, H. and Edwards, P. (2004) Effect of intravenous corticosteroids on death within 14 days in 10008 adults with clinically significant head injury (MRC CRASH trial): randomised placebo-controlled trial. *Lancet*, 364: 1321–1328.

Robertson, C.S. (2001) Management of cerebral perfusion pressure after traumatic brain injury. *Anesthesiology*, 95 (6): 1513–1517.

Rodden, A.M., Spicer, L., Diaz, V.A. and Steyer, T.E. (2007) Does fingernail polish affect pulse oximeter readings? *Intensive and Critical Care Nursing*, 23 (1): 51–55.

Rodseth, R.N. (2009) B type natriuretic peptide – a diagnostic breakthrough in peri-operative cardiac risk assessment? *Anaesthesia*, 64 (2): 165–178.

Rogers, C.R. (1951) *Client-centred Therapy*. London: Constable.

—— (1967) *On Becoming a Person*. London: Constable.

—— (1983) *Freedom to Learn for the 80s*. New York: Merrill.

Romyn, D.M. (2001) Disavowal of the Behaviorist Paradigm in nursing education: what makes it so difficult to unseat? *Advances in Nursing Science*, 23 (3): 1–10.

Roper, N., Logan, W. and Tierney, A. (1996) *The Elements of Nursing*, 4th edition. Edinburgh: Churchill Livingstone.

Ros, C., McNeill, L. and Bennett, P. (2009) Review: nurses can improve patient nutrition in intensive care. *Journal of Clinical Nursing*, 18 (17): 2406–2415.

Rosenberg, J. and Eisen, L.A. (2008) Eye care in the intensive care unit: narrative review and meta-analysis. *Critical Care Medicine*, 36 (12): 3151–3155.

Rosendale, J.D., Kauffman, H.M., McBride, M.A. Chabalewski, F.L., Zaroff, J.G., Garrity, E.R., Delmonico, F.L. and Rosengard, B.R. (2003) Aggressive pharmacologic donor management results in more transplanted organs. *Transplantation*, 75 (4): 482–487.

Ross, A. and Crumpler, J. (2007) The impact of an evidence-based practice education program on the role of oral care in the prevention of ventilator-associated pneumonia. *Intensive and Critical Care Nursing*, 23 (3): 132–136.

Ross, N. and Eynon, C.A. (2005) Intracranial pressure monitoring. *Current Anaesthesia & Critical Care*, 16 (5): 255–261.

Rossi, S., Zanier, E.R., Mauri, I., Columbo, A. and Stocchetti, N. (2001) Brain temperature, body core temperature, and intracranial pressure in acute cerebral damage. *Journal of Neurology, Neurosurgery and Psychiatry*, 71 (4): 448–454.

Rousseau, A., Bak, Z., Janerot-Sjoberg, B. and Sjoberg, F. (2005) Acute hyperoxemia-induced effects on regional blood flow, oxygen consumption and central circulation in man. *Acta Physiologica Scandinavica*, 183 (3): 231–240.

Rudge, C. (2010) Organ donation: we can solve the shortage. *Nursing in Critical Care*, 15 (3): 229–233.

Russell, J.A., Walley, K.R., Singer, J., Gordon, A.C., Hébert, P.C., Cooper, D.J., Holmes, C.L., Mehta, S., Granton, J.T., Storms, M.M., Cook, D.J., Presneill, J.J. and Ayers, D., VASST Investigators (2008) Vasopressin versus norepinephrine infusion in patients with septic shock. *New England Journal of Medicine*, 358 (9): 877–887.

Russell, K. (2008) Personal hygiene: eye care, in Dougherty, L. and Lister, S. (eds) *The Royal Marsden Hospital Manual of Clinical Nursing Procedures*, 7th edition. Oxford: Wiley-Blackwell, pp. 629–646.

Russell, R.R. and McAuley, D. (2009) Management of non-accidental injury on the pediatric intensive care unit, in Murphy, P.J., Marriage, S.C. and Davis, P.J. (eds) *Case Studies in Pediatric Critical Care*. Cambridge: Cambridge University Press, pp. 155–161.

Ryan, J. (2004) Aesthetic physical caring – valuing the visible. *Nursing in Critical Care*, 9 (4): 181–187.

Rylah, B. and Vercueil, A. (2010) Intensive therapy of the patient with liver disease. *British Journal of Hospital Medicine*, 71 (7): 377–381.

Sacks, O. (1990) *Awakenings*, revised edition. London: Picador.

Saenger, A.K. and Jaffe, A.S. (2007) The use of biomarkers for the evaluation and treatment of patients with acute coronary syndromes. *Medical Clinics of North America*, 91 (4): 657–681.

Safar, M.E., Levy, B.I. and Struijker-Boudier, H. (2003) Current perspectives on arterial stiffness and pulse pressure in hypertension and cardiovascular diseases. *Circulation*, 107 (22): 2864–2869.

Safdar, N. and Maki, D.G. (2004) The pathogenesis of catheter-related bloodstream infection with noncuffed short-term central venous catheters. *Intensive Care Medicine*, 30 (1): 62–67.

Saggs, P. (2000) Liver failure in the critically ill. *Nursing in Critical Care*, 5 (1): 40–48.

Saidi, M. and Brett, S. (2009) Pandemic influenza: clinical epidemiology, in Ridley, S. (ed.) *Critical Care Focus 16: Infection.* London: Intensive Care Society, pp. 117–134.

Sakka, S.G., Klein, M., Reinhart, K. and Meier-Hellmann, A. (2002) Prognostic value of extravascular lung water in critically ill patients. *Chest*, 122 (6): 2080–2086.

Salukhe, T.V. and Wyncoll, D.L.A. (2002) Volumetric haemodynamic monitoring and continuous pulse contour analysis – an untapped resource for coronary and high dependency care units? *British Journal of Cardiology*, 9 (1 AIC): 20–25.

Samanta, A. and Samanta, J. (2004) NICE guideline and law: clinical governance implications for trusts. *Clinical Governance*, 9 (4): 212–215.

Samuelson, K.A.M., Lundberg, D. and Fridlund, B. (2007) Stressful experiences in relation to depth of sedation in mechanically ventilated patients. *Nursing in Critical Care*, 12 (2): 93–104.

Saranto, K. and Kinnunen, U.-M. (2009) Evaluating nursing documentation – research designs and methods: systematic review. *Journal of Advanced Nursing*, 65 (3): 464–476.

Sargent, S. (2006) Pathophysiology, diagnosis and management of acute pancreatitis. *British Journal of Nursing*, 15 (18): 999–1005.

Sarvimaki, A. and Sanderlin Benko, S. (2001) Values and evaluation in health care. *Journal of Nursing Management*, 9 (3): 129–137.

Sasso, F.C., Carbonara, O., Nasti, R., Campana, B., Marfalla, R., Torella, M., Nappi, G., Torella, R. and Cozzolino, D. (2004) Glucose metabolism and coronary heart disease in patients with normal glucose tolerance. *JAMA*, 291 (15): 1857–1863.

Sayar, S., Turget, S., Dogan, H., Rkici, A., Yurtsever, S., Demirkan, F., Doruk, N. and Taşdelen, B. (2009) Incidence of pressure ulcers in intensive care unit patients at risk according to the Waterlow scale and factors influencing the development of pressure sores. *Journal of Clinical Nursing*, 18 (5): 765–774.

Scalea, T.M., Bochicchio, G.V., Bochicchio, K.M., Johnson, S.B., Joshi, M. and Pyle, A. (2007) Tight glycemic control in critically injured trauma patients. *Annals of Surgery*, 246 (4): 605–612.

Scales, K. and Pilsworth, J. (2007) A practical guide to extubation. *Nursing Standard*, 22 (2): 44–48.

Scannapieco, F.A., Stewart, E.M. and Mylotte, J.M. (1992) Colonization of dental plaque by respiratory pathogens in medical intensive care patients. *Critical Care Medicine*, 20 (6): 740–745.

Schalk, B.W.M., Deeg, D.J.H., Penninx, B.W.J.H., Bouter, L.M. and Visser, M. (2005) Serum albumin and muscle strength: a longitudinal study in older men and women. *Journal of the American Geriatrics Society*, 53 (8): 1331–1338.

Scheinkestel, C.D., Bailey, M., Myles, P.S., Jones, K., Cooper, D.J., Millar, I.L. and Tuxen, D.V. (1999) Hyperbaric or normobaric oxygen for acute carbon monoxide poisoning: a randomised controlled clinical trial. *Medical Journal of Australia*, 170 (5): 203–210.

Schifano, F., Corkery, J., Deluca, P., Oyefeso, A. and Ghodse, A.H. (2006) Ecstasy (MDMA, MDA, MDEA, MBDB) consumption, seizures, related offences, prices, dosage levels and deaths in the UK (1994–2003). *Journal of Psychopharmacology*, 20 (3): 456–463.

Schlösser, F.J.V., Vaartjes, I., van der Heijden, G., Moll, F.L., Verhagen, H.J.M., Muhs, B.E., de Borst, G.J., Tiel Groenestege, A.T.T., Kardaun, J.W.P.F., de Bruin, A., Reitsma, J.B., van der Graaf, Y. and Bots, M.L. (2010) Mortality after elective abdominal aortic aneurysm repair. *Annals of Surgery*, 261 (1): 158–164.

Schneemilch, C.E., Bachmann, H., Ulrich, A., Elwert, R., Halloul, Z. and Hachenberg, T. (2006) Clonidine decreases stress response in patients undergoing carotid endartrectomy under regional anesthesia: a prospective, randomized, double-blinded, placebo-controlled study. *Anesthesia & Analgesia*, 103 (2): 297–302.

Schofield, E., Lawman, S., Volans, G. and Henry, J. (1997) Drugs of abuse: clinical features and management. *Emergency Nurse*, 5 (6): 17–22.

Schramko, A., Suojaranta-Ylinen, R., Kuitunen, A., Raivio, P., Kukkonen, S. and Niemi, T. (2010) Hydroxyethylstarch and gelatine solutions impair blood coagulation after cardiac surgery: a prospective randomized trial. *British Journal of Anaesthesia*, 104 (6): 691–697.

Schuerer, D.J.E., Kolovos, N.S., Kayla, B.V. and Coopersmith, C.M. (2008) Extracorporeal membrane oxygenation. *Chest*, 134 (1): 179–184.

Schuetz, P., Christ-Crain, M., Thomann, R., Falconnier, C., Wolbers, M., Widmer, I., Neidert, S., Fricker, T., Blum, C., Schild, U., Regez, K., Schoenenberger, R., Henzen, C., Bregenzer, T., Hoess, C., Krause, M., Bucher, H.C., Zimmerli, W. and Mueller, B., ProHOSP Study Group (2009) Effects of procalcitonin-based guidelines vs standard guidelines on antibiotic use in lower respiratory tract infections: the ProHOSP randomized controlled trial. *JAMA*, 302 (10): 1059–1066.

Schutte, J.M., Steegers, E.A.P., Schuitemaker, N.W.E., Santema, J.G., Boer, K. de, Pel, M., Vermeulen, G., Visser, W. and Roosmalen, J. van, The Netherlands Maternal Mortality Committee (2010) Rise in maternal mortality in the Netherlands. *British Journal of Obstetrics and Gynaecology*, 117 (4): 399–406.

Schwacha, M.G. and Chaudry, I.H. (2000) Sex hormone-mediated modulation of the immune response after trauma, haemorrhage or sepsis, in Galley, H.F. (ed.) *Critical Care Focus 4: Endocrine disturbance*. London: BMJ Books, pp. 36–56.

Schweickert, W.D., Gehlbach, B.K., Pohlman, A.S., Hall, J.B. and Kress, J.P. (2004) Daily interruption of sedative infusions and complications of critical illness in mechanically ventilated patients. *Critical Care Medicine*, 32 (6): 1272–1276.

——, Pohlman, M.C., Pohlman, A.S., Nigos, C., Pawlik, A.J., Esbrook, C.L., Spears, L., Miller, M., Franczyk, M., Deprizio, D., Schmidt, G.A., Bowman, A., Barr, R., McAllister, K.E., Hall, J.B. and Kress, J.P. (2009) Early physical and occupational therapy in mechanically ventilated, critically ill patients: a randomised controlled trial. *Lancet*, 373 (9678): 1874–1882.

Scott, E.M., Leaper, D.J. and Clark, M. (2001) Effects of warming therapy on pressure ulcers: a randomised trial. *AORN Journal*, 73 (5): 921–938.

Scottish National Blood Transfusion Service (2007) *Better Blood Transfusion Level 1: Safe transfusion practice*. Self-directed Learning Pack. Edinburgh: Effective Use of Blood Group, Scottish National Blood Transfusion Service.

Seaton-Mills, D. (2000) Prone positioning in ARDS: a nursing perspective. *Clinical Intensive Care*, 11 (4): 203–208.

Selby, I.R. and James, M.R. (1995) Severe metabolic and respiratory acidosis. *British Journal of Intensive Care*, 5 (7): 222–225.

Seligman, M.E.P. (1975) *Helplessness: On depression, development and death*. New York: W H Freeman.

Semple, D.N., Ebmeier, K.P., Glabus, M.F., O'Carroll, R.E. and Johnstone, E.C. (1999) Reducing *in vivo* binding to the serotonin transporter in the cerebral cortex of MDMA ('ecstasy') users. *British Journal of Psychiatry*, 175 (July): 63–69.

Serruys, P.W., Morice, M.-C., Kappetein, A.P., Colombo, A., Holmes, D.R., Mack, M.J., Ståhle, E., Feldman, T.E., van den Brand, M., Bass, E.J., Dyck, N.V., Leadley, K., Dawkins, K.D. and Mohr, F.W., SYNTAX Investigators (2009) Percutaneous coronary intervention versus coronary-artery bypass grafting for severe coronary artery disease. *New England Journal of Medicine*, 360 (10): 961–972.

Sessler, C.N. and Varney, K. (2008) Patient-focused sedation and analgesia in the ICU. *Chest*, 133 (2): 552–565.

Sessler, D.I. (2008) Temperature monitoring and perioperative thermoregulation. *Anesthesiology*, 109 (2): 318–338.

Sever, M.S., Vanholder, R. and Lameire, N. (2006) Management of crush related injuries after disasters. *New England Journal of Medicine*, 354 (10): 1052–1063.

Shangraw, R.E. (2000) Acid-base balance, in Miller, R.D. (ed.) *Anesthesia*, 5th edition. Philadelphia, PA: Churchill Livingstone, pp. 1383–1401.

Shannon-Lowe, J., Matheson, N.J., Cooke, F.J. and Aliyu, S.H. (2010) Prevention and medical management of *Clostridium difficile* infection. *British Medical Journal*, 340 (7747): 605–662.

Sharma, R. and Kaddoura, S. (2005) The definition and management of acute coronary syndromes. *Current Anaesthesia & Critical Care*, 16 (5): 305–312.

Sharman, A., Gardiner, D. and Girling, K. (2010) Anticoagulant use in renal replacement therapy in the Mid Trent Critical Care Network: a survey of practice. *Journal of the Intensive Care Society*, 11 (2): 138–143.

Sharp, L.S., Rozycki, G.S. and Feliciano, D.V. (2004) Rhabdomyolysis and secondary renal failure in critically ill surgical patients. *American Journal of Surgery*, 188 (6): 801–806.

Shehabi, Y. and Innes, R. (2002) Sedation and analgesia in the 21st century. *Egyptian Journal of Anaesthesia*, 18: 143–155.

Sherry, K.M. and Barham, N.J. (1997) Cardiovascular pharmacology, in Goldhill, D.R. and Withington, P.S. (eds) *Textbook of Intensive Care*, London: Chapman & Hall, pp. 245–253.

Shiao, J., Koh, D., Lo, L.-H., Lim, M.-K. and Guo, Y. (2007) Factors predicting nurses' consideration of leaving their job during the SARS outbreak. *Nursing Ethics*, 14 (1): 5–17.

Short, A.F., McVeigh, S.K., Flynn, J.M. and Moores, L.K. (2001) Intensive care unit outcomes for patients with thrombotic thrombocytopenic purpura. *Clinical Intensive Care*, 12 (2): 73–79.

Shortgen, F., Girou, E., Deye, N. and Brochard, L. (2008) The risk associated with hyperoncotic colloids in patients with shock. *Intensive Care Medicine*, 4 (12): 2157–2168.

Shroyer, A.L., Grover, F.L., Hattler, B., Collins, J.F., McDonald, G.O., Kozora, E., Lucke, J.C., Baltz, J.H. and Novitzky, D., Veterans Affairs Randomized On/Off Bypass (ROOBY) Study Group (2009) On-pump versus off-pump coronary-artery bypass surgery. *New England Journal of Medicine*, 361 (19): 1827–1837.

Shuhaiber, J.H., Hur, K. and Gibbons, R. (2010) The influence of preoperative use of ventricular assist devices on survival after heart transplantation: propensity score matched analysis. *British Medical Journal*, 340 (7742): 354.

Shuster, M.H., Haines, T., Sekula, L.K., Kern, J. and Vazquez, J.A. (2010) Reliability of intra-bladder pressure measurement in intensive care. *American Journal of Critical Care*, 19 (1): 29–39.

Sillender, M. (2002) The liver and pregnancy. *Care of the Critically Ill*, 18 (6): 181–186.

Simon, V. (2006) HIV/AIDS epidemiology, athogenesis, prevention, and treatment. *Lancet*, 368 (9534): 489–504.

Simons, K.J. and Simons, E.R. (2010) Epinephrine and its use in anaphylaxis: current issues. *Current Opinion in Allergy and Clinical Immunology*, 10 (4): 354–361.

Singer, M. and Webb, A.R. (1997) *Oxford Handbook of Critical Care*. Oxford: Oxford University Press.

Singer, P., Berger, M., van den Berghe, G., Biolo, G., Calder, P., Forbes, A., Griffiths, R., Kreyman, G., Levere, X. and Pichard, C. (2009) ESPEN guidelines on parenteral nutrition: intensive care. *Clinical Nutrition*, 28 (4): 387–400.

Sisodiya, S.M. and Duncan, J. (2004) Epilepsy, epidemiology, clinical assessment and natural history. *Medicine*, 32 (10): 47–51.

Siva, S. and Pereira, S.P. (2007) Acute pancreatitis. *Medicine*, 35 (3): 171–177.

Sjauw, K.D., Engström, A.E., Vis, M.M., van der Schaaf, R.J., Baan, J. Jr, Koch, K.T., de Winter, R.J., Piek, J.J., Tijssen, J.G.P. and Henriques, J.P.S. (2009) A systematic review and meta-analysis of intra aortic balloon pump therapy in ST-elevation myocardial infarction: should we change the guidelines? *European Heart Journal.* Available online at http://eurheartj.oxford journals.org/content/early/2009/01/23/eurheartj.ehn602.full.pdf+html (accessed 29 December 2010).

Skeie, G.O., Apostolski, S., Evoli, A., Gilhus, N.E., Illa, I., Harms, L., Hilton-Jones, D., Melms, A., Verschuuren, J. and Horge, H.W. (2010) Guidelines for treatment of autoimmune neuromuscular transmission disorders. *European Journal of Neurology*, 17: 893–902.

Skinner, B.F. (1971) *Beyond Freedom and Dignity*. London: Penguin.

Skinner, R. and Watson, D. (1997) Renal failure, in Goldhill, D.R. and Withington, P.S. (eds) *Textbook of Intensive Care*. London: Chapman & Hall, pp. 435–440.

Skipworth, R.J.E., Stewart, G.D., Ross, J.A., Guttridge, D.C. and Fearon, K.C.H. (2006) The molecular mechanisms of skeletal muscle wasting: implications for therapy. *The Surgeon*, 4 (5): 273–283.

Smith, A. and Taylor, C. (2005) Analysis of blood gases and acid-base balance. *Surgery*, 23 (6): 194–198.

Smith, D.H. (2007) Managing acute acetaminophen toxicity. *Nursing2007*, 37 (1): 58–63.

Smith, M. (2007) A care bundle for management of central venous catheters. *Paediatric Nursing*, 19 (4): 41–45.

Smith, P.M. (2000) Portal hypertension. *Surgery*, 18 (7): 153–156.

Smith, R., Hay, A., Hilditch, G. and Wallace, P. (2004) Transfer of adults between intensive care units in the United Kingdom: demographics. *Journal of the Intensive Care Society*, 5 (3): 125–128.

Smith-Blair, N., Pierce, J.D. and Clancy, R.L. (2003) The effect of dobutamine infusion on fractional diaphragm thickening and diaphragm blood flow during fatigue. *Heart & Lung*, 32 (2): 111–120.

Soni, N. and Wagstaff A. (2005) Fungal infection. *Current Anaesthesia & Critical Care*, 16 (5): 231–241.

Sontag, S. (1989) *AIDS and its Metaphors*. London: Penguin.

Soo, L.H., Gray, D., Young, T. and Hampton, J.R. (2000) Circadian variation in witnessed out of hospital cardiac arrest. *Heart*, 84 (4): 370–376.

Soydemir, F. and Kenny, L. (2006) Hypertension in pregnancy. *Current Opinion in Obstetrics & Gynaecology*, 16 (6): 315–320.

Spahn, D.R., Waschke, K.F., Standl, T., Motsch, J., van Huynegem, L., Welte, M., Gombotz, H., Coriat, P., Verkh, L., Faithfull, S. and Keipert, P., European Perflubron Emulsion in Non-Cardiac Surgery Study Group (2002) Use of perflubron emulsion to decrease allogeneic blood transfusion in high-blood-loss non-cardiac surgery: results of a European phase 3 study. *Anesthesiology*, 97 (6): 1338–1349.

Spirt, M.J. and Stanley, S. (2006) Update on stress ulcer prophylaxis in critically ill patients. *Critical Care Nurse*, 26 (1): 18–28.

Spodick, D.H. (2003) Acute cardiac tamponade. *New England Journal of Medicine*, 349 (7): 684–690.

Spragg, R.G., Lewis, J.F, Wurst, W., Häfner, D., Baughman, R.P., Wewers, M.D. and Marsh, J.J. (2003) Treatment of acute respiratory distress syndrome with recombinant surfactant protein C surfactant. *American Journal of Respiratory and Critical Care Medicine*, 167 (11): 1562–1566.

Sprung, C.L., Annane, D., Keh, D., Moreno, B., Singer, M., Freivogel, K., Weiss, Y.G., Benbenishty, J., Kalenka, A., Forst, H., Laterre, P.-F., Reinhart, K., Cuthbertson, B.H., Payen, D. and Briegel, J., CORTICUS Study Group (2008) Hydrocortisone therapy for patients with septic shock. *New England Journal of Medicine*, 358 (2): 111–124.

——, Cohen, R., Adini, B. (2010) Recommendations and standard operating procedures for intensive care unit and hospital preparations for an influenza epidemic or mass disaster. *Intensive Care Medicine*, supplement 1.

Sprung, J., Kindscher, J.D., Wahr, J.A. Levy, J.H., Monk, T.G., Moritz, M.W. and O'Hara, P.J. (2002) The use of bovine hemoglobin glutamer-250 (Hemopure®) in surgical patients: results of a multicenter, randomized, single-blinded trial. *Anesthesia & Analgesia*, 94 (4): 799–808.

Sque, M., Long, T., Payne, S. and Allardyce, D. (2008) Why relatives do not donate organs for transplants: 'sacrifice' or 'gift of life'? *Journal of Advanced Nursing*, 61 (2): 134–144.

Stanhope, N. (2006) Temperature measurement in the phase 1 PACU. *Journal of PeriAnesthesia Nursing*, 21 9(1): 27–36.

Stanisstreet, D., Walden, E., Jones, C. and Graveling, A. (2010) *The Hospital Management of Hypoglycaemia in Adults with Diabetes Mellitus*. London: NHS Diabetes.

Stanley, A.J. and Hayes, P.C. (1997) Portal hypertension and variceal haemorrhage. *Lancet*, 350 (9036): 1235–1239.

Stansfeld, S.A. and Matheson, M.P. (2003) Noise pollution: non-auditory effects on health. *British Medical Bulletin*, 68: 243–257.

Stasseno, P., di Tommaso, L., Monaco, M., Iorio, F., Pepino, P., Spampinato, N. and Vosa, C. (2009) Aortic valve replacement. *Journal of the American College of Cardiology*, 54 (20): 1862–1868.

Steegers, E.A.P., van Dadelszen, P., Duvekot, J.J. and Pijnenborg, R. (2010) Pre-eclampsia. *Lancet*, 376 (9741): 631–644.

Steele, A.G. and Sabol, V. (2005) Common gastrointestinal disorders, in Morton, P.G., Fontaine, D.K., Hudak, C.M. and Gallo, B.M. (eds) *Critical Care Nursing: A holistic approach*, 8th edition. Philadelphia, PA: Lippincott Williams & Wilkins, pp. 953–992.

Steggall, M.J. (2007) Urine samples and urinalysis. *Nursing Standard*, 22 (14–16): 42–45.

Stein, R.A. (2009) Lessons from outbreaks of H1N1 influenza. *Annals of Internal Medicine*, 151 (1): 59–62.

Steinhubl, S.R., Bhaat, D.L., Brennan, D.M., Montalescot, G., Hankey, G.J., Eikelboom, J.W., Berger, P.B. and Topol, E.J., CHARISMA Investigators (2009) Aspirin to prevent cardiovascular disease: the association of aspirin dose and clopidogrel with thrombosis and bleeding. *Annals of Internal Medicine*, 150 (6): 379–386.

Stokes, T., Shaw, E.J., Juarez-Garcia, A., Camosso-Stefinovic, J. and Baker, R. (2004) *Clinical Guidelines and Evidence Review for the Epilepsies: Diagnosis and management in adults and children in primary and secondary care*. London: Royal College of General Practitioners.

Stolz, D., Smyrnios, N., Eggimann, P., Pargger, H., Thakkar, N., Siegemund, M., Marsch, S., Azzola, A., Rakic, J., Mueller, B. and Tamm, M. (2009) Procalcitonin for reduced antibiotic exposure in ventilator-associated pneumonia: a randomised study. *European Respiratory Journal*, 34 (6): 1364–1375.

Storey, M. and Jordan, S. (2008) An overview of the immune system. *Nursing Standard*, 23 (15–17): 47–56.

Strahan, E.H.E. and Brown, R.J. (2005) A qualitative study of the experience of patients following transfer from intensive care. *Intensive and Critical Care Nursing*, 21 (3): 160–171.

Strandvik, G., Shoukrey, K. and Al-Shaikh, B. (2006) A review of medical gas provision for critical care – an intensivist's perspective. *CPD Anaesthesia*, 8 (2): 54–61.

Strøm, T., Martinussen, T. and Toft, P. (2010) A protocol of no sedation for critically ill patients receiving mechanical ventilation: a randomised trial. *Lancet*, 375 (9713): 475–480.

Suarez, J.I., Tarr, R.W. and Selman, W.R. (2006) Aneurysmal subarachnoid haemorrhage. *New England Journal of Medicine*, 354 (4):387–396.

Sud, S., Friedrich, J.O., Taccone, P., Polli, F., Adhikari, N.K.J., Latini, R., Pesenti, A., Guérin, C., Mancebo, J., Curley, M.A.Q., Fernandez, R., Chan, M.-C., Beuret, P., Voggenreiter, G., Sud, M., Tognoni, G. and Gattinoni, L. (2010a) Prone ventilation reduces mortality in patients with acute respiratory failure and severe hypoxaemia: systematic review and meta-analysis. *Intensive Care Medicine*, 36 (4): 585–599.

——, Sud, M., Friedrich, J.O., Meade, M.O., Ferguson, N.D., Wunsch, H. and Adhikari, N.K.J. (2010b) High frequency oscillation in patients with acute lung injury and acute respiratory distress syndrome (ARDS): systematic review and meta-analysis. *British Medical Journal*, 340 (7759): 1290.

Sullivan, J. (2000) Positioning of patients with severe traumatic brain injury: research-based practice. *Journal of Neuroscience Nursing*, 32 (4): 204–209.

Sung, J.J.Y. (2009) Acute gastrointestinal bleeding, in Bersten, A.D. and Soni, N. (eds) *Intensive Care Manual*, 6th edition. Edinburgh: Butterworth-Heinemann, pp. 471–478.

—— (2010) Peptic ulcer bleeding: an expedition of 20 years from 1989–2009. *Journal of Gastroenterology and Hepatology*, 25 (2): 229–233.

Suresh, P., Mercieca, F., Morton, A. and Tullo, A.B. (2000) Eye care for the critically ill. *Intensive Care Medicine*, 26 (2): 162–166.

Suriadi, Sanada, H., Sugama, J., Thigpen, B., Kitagawa, A., Kinosita, S. and Murayama, S. (2006) A new instrument for predicting pressure ulcer risk in an intensive care unit. *Journal of Tissue Viability*, 16 (3): 21–26.

Surviving Sepsis Campaign (2007) *Survive Sepsis: The official training programme of the Surviving Sepsis Campaign.* Sutton Coldfield: Good Hope Hospital.

Sykes, E. and Cosgrove, J.F. (2007) Acute renal failure and the critically ill surgical patient. *Annals of the Royal College of Surgeons of England*, 89 (1): 22–29.

Szaflarski, N.L. (1996) Preanalytic error associated with blood gas/pH measurement. *Critical Care Nurse*, 16 (3): 89–100.

Tabata, M., Grab, J.D., Khalpey, Z., Edwards, F.H., O'Brien, S.M., Cohn, L.H. and Bolman, M. III (2009) Prevalence and variability of internal mammary artery graft use in contemporary multivessel coronary artery bypass graft surgery. *Circulation*, 120 (11): 935–940.

Taccone, P., Pesenti, A., Latini, R., Polli, F., Vagginelli, F., Mietto, C., Caspani, L., Raimondi, F., Bordone, G., Iapichino, G., Mancebo, J., Guérin, C., Ayzac, L., Blanch, L., Fumagalli, R., Tognoni, G. and Gattinoni, L., Prone-Supine II Study Group (2009) Prone positioning in patients with moderate and severe acute respiratory distress syndrome: a randomized controlled trial. *JAMA*, 302 (18): 1977–1984.

Tambyraja, A.L. and Chamlers, R.T.A. (2009) Aortic aneurysms. *Surgery*, 27 (8): 342–345.

Tan, R., Knowles, D., Streater, C. and Johnston, A.J. (2009) The use of peripherally inserted central catheters in intensive care: should you pick the PICC? *Journal of the Intensive Care Society*, 10 (2): 95–98.

Task Force (2007) Task Force for the Diagnosis and Treatment of Non-ST-segment Elevation Acute Coronary Syndromes of the European Society of Cardiology (2007) Guidelines for the diagnosis and treatment of non-ST-elevation acute coronary syndromes. *European Heart Journal*, 28 (13): 1598–1660.

—— (2008a) Task Force on the Diagnosis and Management of Acute Pulmonary Embolism of the European Society of Cardiology (2008) Guidelines on the diagnosis and management of acute pulmonary embolism. *European Heart Journal*, 29 (18): 2276–2315.

——(2008b) Task Force on the Management of ST-segment Elevation Acute Myocardial Infarction of the European Society of Cardiology (2008) Management of acute myocardial infarction in patients presenting with persistent ST-segment elevation. *European Heart Journal*, 29 (23): 2909–2945.

—— (2010a) Task Force for the Management of Atrial Fibrillation of the European Society of Cardiology (2010) Guidelines for the management of atrial fibrillation. *European Heart Journal*, 31: 2369–2429.

—— (2010b)Task Force on Myocardial Revascularization of the European Society of Cardiology and the European Association for Cardio-Thoracic Surgery (2010) Guidelines on myocardial revascularization. *European Heart Journal*, 31 (20): 2501–2555.

Tassaux, D., Gainnier, M., Battisti, A. and Jolliet, P. (2005) Helium-oxygen decreases inspiratory effort and work of breathing during pressure support in intubated patients with chronic obstructive pulmonary disease. *Intensive Care Medicine*, 31 (11): 1501–1507.

Teare, J. and Smith, J. (2004) Using focus groups to explore the views of parents whose children are in hospital. *Paediatric Nursing*, 16 (5): 30–34.

Tembo, A.C. and Parker, V. (2009) Factors that impact on sleep in intensive care. *Intensive & Critical Care Nursing*, 25 (6): 314–322.

Teoh, L.S.G., Gowardman, J.R., Larsen, P.D., Green, R. and Galletly, D.C. (2000) Glasgow Coma Scale: variation in mortality among permutations of specific total scores. *Intensive Care Medicine*, 26 (2): 157–161.

Terragni, P.P., del Sorbo, L., Mascia, L., Urbino, R., Martin, E.L., Birocco, A., Faggiano, C., Quintel, M., Gattinoni, L. and Ranieri, V.M. (2009) Tidal volume lower than 6 ml/kg enhances lung protection. *Anesthesiology*, 111 (4): 826–835.

Therapondos, G. and Hayes, O.C. (2002) Management of gastro-oesophageal varices. *Clinical Medicine*, 2 (4): 297–302.

Thomas, B. and Bishop, J. (2007) *Manual of Dietetic Practice*. Oxford: Blackwell.

Thomas, N.J. and Carcillo, J.A. (1998) Hypovolemic shock in pediatric patients. *New Horizons*, 6 (2): 120–129.

Thorpe, D. and Harrison, L. (2002) Bowel management: development of guidelines. *Connect*, 2 (2): 61–66.

Thumbikat, P., Hussain, N. and McClelland, M.R. (2009) Acute spinal cord injury. *Surgery*, 27 (7): 280–286.

Thygesen, K., Alpert, J.S. and White, H.D., Joint ESC/ACCF/AHA/WHF Task Force for the Redefinition of Myocardial Infarction (2007) Universal definition of myocardial infarction. *European Heart Journal*, 28 (13): 2525–2538.

Tibballs, J. (2003) Equipment for paediatric intensive care, in Bersten, A.D. and Soni, N. (eds) *Intensive Care Manual*, 5th edition. Edinburgh: Butterworth-Heinemann, pp. 1075–1086.

Tidswell, M. (2001) Prone ventilation. *Clinical Intensive Care*, 12 (5–6): 193–201.

Tillyard, A., Keays, R. and Soni, N. (2005) The diagnosis of acute renal failure in intensive care: mongrel or pedigree? *Anaesthesia*, 60 (9): 903–914.

Tingle, J. (2007) Recurring themes in NHS complaints. *British Journal of Nursing*, 16 (5): 265.

Tobin, M.J., Laghi, F. and Jurban, A. (2010) Ventilator-induced respiratory muscle weakness. *Annals of Internal Medicine*, 153 (4): 240–245.

Todaro, J.F., Shen, B.J., Niaura, R., Spiro, A. III and Ward, K.D. (2003) Effect of negative emotions on frequency of coronary heart disease (The Normative Aging Study). *American Journal of Cardiology*, 92 (8): 901–906.

Tonkin, A. (2004) The metabolic syndrome – a growing problem. *European Heart Journal*, 6 (supplement A): A37–A42.

Torres, A., Ewig, S., Lode, H. and Carlet, J., European HAP Working Group (2009) Defining, treating and preventing hospital acquired pneumonia: European perspective. *Intensive Care Medicine*, 35 (1): 9–29.

Toubia, N. and Sanyal, A.J. (2008) Portal hypertension and variceal hemorrhage. *Medical Clinics of North America*, 92 (3): 551–574.

Trachsel, D., McCrindle, B.W., Nakagawa, S. and Bohn, D. (2005) Oxygenation index predicts outcome in children with acute hypoxemic respiratory failure. *American Journal of Respiratory and Critical Care Medicine*, 172 (2) 206–211.

Traynor, M. (2009) Humanism and its critiques in nursing research literature. *Journal of Advanced Nursing*, 65 (7): 1560–1567.

Treadwell, S.D. and Robinson, T.G. (2007) Cocaine use and stroke. *Postgraduate Medical Journal*, 83 (980): 389–394.

Treloar, D.M. (1995) Use of a clinical assessment tool for orally intubated patients. *American Journal of Critical Care*, 4 (5): 355–360.

Tremper, K.K. (2002) Perfluorochemical 'red blood cell substitutes': the continued search for an indication. *Anesthesiology*, 97 (6): 1333–1334.

Trost, J.C. and Hills, L.D. (2006) Intra-aortic balloon counterpulsation. *American Journal of Cardiology*, 97 (9): 1391–1398.

Trouiller, P., Fangio, P., Paugam-Burtz, C., Appéré-de-Vecchi, C., Merckx, P., Louvet, N., Pease, S., Outin, H., Mantz, J. and de Jonghe, B. (2009) Frequency and clinical impact of preserved bispectral index activity during deep sedation in mechanically ventilated ICU patients. *Intensive Care Medicine*, 35 (12): 2096–2104.

Trzeciak, S., Dellinger, R.P., Chansky, M.E., Arnold, R.C., Schorr, C., Milcarek, B., Hollenberg, S.M. and Parrillo, J.E. (2007) Serum lactate as a predictor of mortality in patients with infection. *Intensive Care Medicine*, 33 (6): 970–977.

Tufnell, D.J. and Hamilton, S. (2008) Amniotic fluid embolism. *Obstetrics, Gynaecology and Reproductive Medicine*, 18 (8): 213–216.

Turnbull, B. (2008) High-flow humidified oxygen therapy used to alleviate respiratory distress. *British Journal of Nursing*, 17 (19): 1226–1230.

Turvill, J.L., Burroughs, A.K. and Moore, K.P. (2000) Change in occurrence of paracetamol overdose in UK after introduction of blister packs. *Lancet*, 355 (9220): 2048–2049.

Uchino, S., Bellomo, R., Morimatsu, H., Morgera, S., Schetz, M., Tan, I., Bouman, C., Macedo, E., Gibney, N., Tolwani, A., Oudemans-van Straaten, H., Ronco, C. and Kellum, J.A. (2007) Continuous renal replacement therapy: a worldwide practice survey. *Intensive Care Medicine*, 33 (9): 1563–1570.

Uhl, W., Isenmann, R. and Buchler, M.W. (1998) Infections complicating pancreatitis: diagnosing, treating, preventing. *New Horizons*, 6 (supplement 2): S72–S79.

——, Buchler, M.W., Malfertheiner, P., Beger, H.G., Adler, G. and Gaus, W., German Pancreatitis Study Group (1999) A randomised, double-blind, multicentre trial of octreotide in moderate to severe acute pancreatitis. *Gut*, 45 (1): 97–104.

UK EVAR Trial Investigators (2010) Endovascular versus open repair of abdominal aortic aneurysm. *New England Journal of Medicine*, 362 (20): 1863–1871.

UK Working Party on Acute Pancreatitis (2005) UK guidelines for the management of acute pancreatitis. *Gut*, 54: supplement III.

Unroe, M., Mahn, J.M., Carson, S.S., Govert, J.A., Martinu, T., Sathy, S.J., Clay, A.S., Chia, J., Gray, A., Tulsky, J.A. and Cox, C.E. (2010) One-year trajectories of care and resource utilization for recipients of prolonged mechanical ventilation. *Annals of Internal Medicine*, 153 (3): 167–175.

Uyar, M., Demirag, K., Olgun, E., Cankayali, I. and Moral, A.R. (2005) Comparison of oxygen cost of breathing between pressure-support ventilation and airway pressure release ventilation. *Anaesthesia and Intensive Care*, 33 (2): 218–222.

Valencia, E. (2000) Pancreatitis: slowly improving the approach. *Care of the Critically Ill*, 16 (3): 98–102.

van den Berghe, G. and de Zegher, F. (1996) Anterior pituitary function during critical illness and dopamine treatment. *Critical Care Medicine*, 24 (9): 1580–1590.

——, Wouters, P., Weekers, F. Verwaest, C., Bruyninckx, F., Schetz, M., Vlasslelaers, D., Ferdinande, P., Lauwers, P. and Bouillon, R. (2001) Intensive insulin therapy in critically ill patients. *New England Journal of Medicine*, 345 (19): 1359–1367.

van de Werf, F., Ardissino, D., Betriu, A., Cokkinos, D.V., Falk, E., Fox, K.A., Julian, D., Lengyel, M., Neumann, F.J., Ruzyllo, W., Thygesen, C., Underwood, S.R., Vahanian, A., Verheugt, F.W. and Wijns, W. (2003) Management of acute myocardial infarction in patients presenting with ST-segment elevation. *European Heart Journal*, 24 (1): 28–66.

van Doorn PA. (2005) Treatment of Guillain-Barre syndrome and CIDP. *Journal of the Peripheral Nervous System*, 10 (2):113–127.

Vandromme, M.J., Griffin, R.L., Weinberg, J.A. and Rue, L.W. III (2010) Lactate is a better predictor than systolic blood pressure for determining blood requirement and mortality: could prehospital measures improve trauma triage? *Journal of the American College of Surgeons*, 210 (5): 861–869.

van Horn, E. and Tesh, A. (2000) The effect of critical care hospitalization on family members: stress and responses. *Dimensions of Critical Care Nursing*, 19 (4): 40–49.

Vanhoutte, P.M. (2002) Ageing and endothelial dysfunction. *European Heart Journal*, 4 (supplement A): A8–A17.

VA/NIH Acute Kidney Injury Trial Network (2008) Intensity of renal support in critically ill patients with acute kidney injury. *New England Journal of Medicine*, 359 (1): 7–20.

van Melle, J.P., de Jonge, P., Honig, A., Schene, A.H., Kuyper, A.M.G., Crijns, H.J.G.M., Schins, A., Tulner, D., van den Berg, M. and Ormel, J., MIND-IT Investigators (2007) Effects of antidepressant treatment following myocardial infarction. *British Journal of Psychiatry*, 190 (6): 460–466.

van Santvoort, H., Besselink, M.G., de Vries, A.C., Boermeester, M.A., Fischer, K., Bollen, T.L., Cirkel, G., Schaapherder, A.F., Nieuwenhuijs, V.B., van Goor, H., Dejong, C.H., van Eijck, C.H., Witteman, B.J., Weusten, B.L., van Laarhoven, C.J., Wahab, P.J., Tan, A.C., Schwartz, M.P., van der Harst, E., Cuesta, M.A., Siersema, P.D., Gooszen, H.G. and van Erpecum, K.J., Dutch Acute Pancreatitis Study Group (2009) Early endoscopic retrograde cholangiopan-creatography in predicted severe acute biliary pancreatitis: a prospective multicenter study. *Annals of Surgery*, 250 (1): 68–75.

van Welzen, M. and Carey, T. (2002) Autonomic dysreflexia: guidelines for practice. *Connect*, 2 (1): 13–21.

Varon, J. and Acosta, P. (2008) Therapeutic hypothermia. *Chest*, 133 (5): 1267–1274.

Vaughan, B. and Pillmoor, M. (1989) *Managing Nursing Work*. London: Scutari.

Vedio, A.B., Chinn, S., Warburton, F.G., Griffiths, M.P., Leach, R.M. and Treacher, D.F. (2000) Assessment of survival and quality of life after discharge from a teaching hospital general intensive care unit. *Clinical Intensive Care*, 11 (1): 39–46.

Veith, F.J., Baum, R.A., Ohki, T., Amor, M., Adiseshiah, M., Blankensteijn, J.D., Buth, J., Chuter, T.A.M., Fairman, R.M., Gilling-Smith, G., Harris, P.L., Hodgson, K.J., Hopkinson, B.R., Ivancev, K., Katzen, B.T., Lawrence-Brown, M., Meier, G.H., Malina, M., Makaroun, M.S., Parori, J.C., Richter, G.M., Rubin, G.D., Stelter, W.J., White, G.H., White, R.A., Wisselink, W. and Zarins, C.K. (2002) Nature and significance of endoleaks and endotension: summary of opinions expressed at an international conference. *Journal of Vascular Surgery*, 35 (5): 1029–1035.

Vincent, J.-L., Rello, J., Marshall, J., Silva, E., Anzueto, A., Martin, C.D., Moreno, R., Lipman, J., Gomersall, C., Sakr, Y. and Reinhart, K., EPIC II Group of Investigators (2009) International study of the prevalence and outcomes of infection in intensive care units. *JAMA*, 203 (21): 2323–2329.

Viscusi, E.R., Siccardi, M., Damaraju, C.V., Hewitt, D.J. and Kershaw, P. (2007) The safety and efficacy of fentanyl iontrophoretic transdermal system compared with morphine intravenous patient-controlled analgesia for postoperative pain management: an analysis of pooled data from three randomized, active-controlled clinical studies. *Anesthesia & Analgesia*, 105 (5): 1428–1436.

Vizcaychipi, M., Keays, R. and Soni, N. (2007) Anaesthesia and intensive care for HIV patients. *Anaesthesia and Intensive Care Medicine*, 8 (2): 44–47.

Vlahakes, G.J. (2001) Haemoglobin solutions in surgery. *British Journal of Surgery*, 88 (12): 1553–1555.

Voelker, R. (2000) Movement after brain death. *JAMA*, 283 (6): 734.

Wagih, M.I. and Arthurs, G. (2008) Central venous pressure. *Care of the Critically Ill*, 24 (3): 53–57.

Wagstaff, A.T.J. (2009) Oxygen therapy, in Bersten, A.D. and Soni, N. (eds) *Intensive Care Manual*, 6th edition. Edinburgh: Butterworth-Heinemann Elsevier, pp. 316–326.

Wahr, J.A. and Tremper, K.K. (1996) Oxygen measurement and monitoring techniques, in Prys-Roberts and C., Brown, B.R. Jr (eds) *International Practice of Anaesthesia*. Oxford: Butterworth-Heinemann, pp. 2/159/1–19.

Wainberg, M.A. (1999) HIV resistance to antagonists of viral reverse transcriptase, in Dalgleish, A.G. and Weiss, R.A. (eds) *HIV and the New Viruses*, 2nd edition. San Diego, CA: Academic Press, pp. 223–250.

Wake, D. (1995) Ecstasy overdose: a case study. *Intensive and Critical Care Nursing*, 11 (1): 6–9.

Wald, R., Quinn, R.R., Luo, J., Li, P., Scales, D.C., Mamdani, M.M. and Ray, J.G., University of Toronto Acute Kidney Injury Research Group (2009) Chronic dialysis and death among survivors of acute kidney injury requiring dialysis. *JAMA*, 302 (11): 1179–1185.

——, Waiker, S.S., Liangos, O., Pereira, B.J.G., Chertow, G.M. and Jaber, B.L. (2006) Acute renal failure after endovascular vs open repair of abdominal aortic aneurysm. *Journal of Vascular Surgery*, 43 (3): 460–466.

Waldmann, C. and Barnes, R. (2004) Cannulation of central veins. *Anaesthesia and Intensive Care Medicine*, 5 (1): 6–9.

Walker, J. (2009) Spinal cord injuries: acute care management and rehabilitation. *Nursing Standard*, 23 (42): 47–56.

Wall, P.D. and Melzack, R.W. (eds) (1999) *Textbook of Pain*, 4th edition. Edinburgh: Churchill Livingstone.

Wallace, C.I., Dargan, P.I. and Jones, A.L. (2003) Paracetamol overdose: an evidence based flowchart to guide management. *Emergency Medicine Journal*, 19 (3): 202–205.

Wallace, T.W., Abdullah, S.M., Drazner, M.H., Das, S.R., Khera, A., McGuire, D.K., Wians, F., Sabatine, M.S., Morrow, D.A. and de Lemos, J.A. (2006) Prevalence and determinants of troponin T elevation in the general population. *Circulation*, 113 (16): 1958–1965.

Wallen, K., Chaboyer, W., Thalib, L. and Creedy, D.K. (2008) Symptoms of acute posttraumatic stress disorder after intensive care. *American Journal of Critical Care*, 17 (5): 534–543.

Walltmahmed, M. (2006) Insulin therapy in the management of type 1 and type 2 diabetes. *Nursing Standard*, 21 (6): 50–56.

Walsh, S.B., Tang, T., Wijewardena, C., Yarham, S.I., Boyle, J.R. and Gaunt, M.E. (2007) Postoperative arrhythmias in general surgical patients. *Annals of the Royal College of Surgeons of England*, 89 (2): 91–95.

Walter, T. (1997) Secularization, in Parkes, C.M., Laungani, P. and Young, B. (eds) *Death and Bereavement Across Cultures*, London: Routledge, pp. 166–187.

Walunj, A., Thomson, G., Hent, N., Dunning, J. and Brett, S. (2010) Global networking and pandemic influenza. *Journal of the Intensive Care Society*, 11 (3): 165–170.

Wang, P., Gong, G., Li, Y. and Li, J. (2010) Hydroxyethyl starch 130/0.4 augments healing of colonic anastamosis in a rat model of peritonitis. *American Journal of Surgery*, 199 (2): 232–239.

Ward, B. and Park, G.R. (2000) Humidification of inspired gases in the critically ill. *Clinical Intensive Care*, 11 (4): 169–176.

Warkentin, T.E. (2003) Heparin-induced thrombocytopenia: pathogenesis and management. *British Journal of Haematology*, 121 (4): 535–555.

Warren, H.S., Suffredini, A.F., Eichacker, P.Q. and Munford, R.S. (2002) Risks and benefits of activated protein C treatment for severe sepsis. *New England Journal of Medicine*, 347 (13): 1027–1030.

Washington, G.T. and Matney, J.L. (2008) Comparison of temperature measurement devices in post anesthesia patients. *Journal of PeriAnesthesia Nursing*, 23 (1): 36–48.

Waterhouse, C. (2005) The Glasgow Coma Scale and other neurological observations. *Nursing Standard*, 19 (33): 56–64.

Waterlow, J. (1985) A risk assessment card. *Nursing Times*, 81 (48): 49–55.

—— (1995) Pressure sores and their management. *Care of the Critically Ill*, 11 (3): 121–125.

—— (2005) *Pressure Sore Prevention Manual*. Taunton: Waterlow.

Waters, C. (2008) Delirium in the intensive care unit: a narrative review of published assessment tools and their relationship between ICU delirium and clinical outcomes. *Journal of the Intensive Care Society*, 9 (1): 46–50.

Watkins, L.D. (2000) Head injuries: general principles and management. *Surgery*, 18 (9): 219–224.

Watson, C., Wilkinson, J.N. and Ali, N. (2010) Critical care management of obstetric patients. *British Journal of Hospital Medicine*, 71 (7): 382–387.

Watson, J.B. (1924/1998) *Behaviourism*. New Brunswick, NJ: Transaction Publishers.

Watson, R. (2001) Assessing gastrointestinal (GI) tract functioning in older people. *Nursing Older People*, 12 (10): 27–28.

Weaver, L.K. (2009) Carbon monoxide poisoning. *New England Journal of Medicine*, 360 (12): 1217–1225.

Weetman, C. and Allison, W. (2006) Use of epidural analgesia in post-operative pain management. *Nursing Standard*, 20 (44): 54–64.

Weinert, C. and McFarland, L. (2004) The state of intubated patients. *Chest*, 126 (6): 1883–1890.

Weiss, M., Dullenkopf, A., Fischer, J.E., Keller, C., Gerber, A.C. and the European Paediatric Endotracheal Intubation Study Group (2009) Prospective randomized controlled multi-centre trial of cuffed or uncuffed endotracheal tubes in small children. *British Journal of Anaesthesia*, 103 (6): 867–873.

Welch, C., Harrison, D., Short, A. and Rowan, K. (2008) The increasing burden of alcoholic liver disease on United Kingdom critical care units: secondary analysis of a high quality clinical database. *Journal of Health Services Research & Policy*, 13 (supplement 2): 40–44.

Welch, J. (2002) Kinetic therapy. *Care of the Critically Ill*, 18 (6): centre insert.

Weller, A.S. (2001) Body temperature and its regulation. *Anaesthesia and Intensive Care Medicine*, 2 (5): 195–198.

Wellwnius, G.A, Mukamal, K.J., Kulshreshtha, A., Asonganyi, S. and Mittleman, M.A. (2008) Depressive symptoms and the risk of atherosclerotic progression among patients with coronary artery bypass grafts. *Circulation*, 117 (18): 2312–2319.

Welsch, D., Tilley, R. and Rhodes, A. (2001) Cardiovascular complications of cocaine. *Clinical Intensive Care*, 12 (5–6): 241–244.

Wenham, T. and Pittard, A. (2009) Intensive Care Unit environment. *Continuing Education in Anaesthesia, Critical Care & Pain*, 9 (6): 178–183.

Werner, C. and Engelhard, K. (2000) Cerebral resuscitation: current concepts and perspectives, in Adams, A.P. and Cashman, J.N. (eds) *Recent Advances in Anaesthesia and Analgesia 21*. Edinburgh: Churchill Livingstone, pp. 77–90.

—— (2007) Pathophysiology of traumatic brain injury. *British Journal of Anaesthesia*, 99 (1): 4–9.

West, E., Raffery, A.M. and Lankshear, A. (2004) *The Future Nurse: Evidence of the impact of registered nurses*. London: Royal College of Nursing.

Weston, D. (2008) *Infection Prevention and Control*. Chichester: John Wiley & Sons.

Westphal, M., James, M.F.M., Kozek-Langenecker, S., Stocker, R., Guidet, B. and van Aken, H. (2009) Hydroxyethyl starches. *Anesthesiology*, 111 (1): 187–202.

Wetherell, J.L., Maser, J.D. and van Balkom, A. (2005) Anxiety disorders in the elderly: outdated beliefs and a research agenda. *Acta Psychiatriica Scandinavia*, 111 (6): 401–402.

White, H. and Venkatesh, B. (2008) Cerebral perfusion pressure in neurotrauma: a review. *Analgesia & Anesthesia*, 107 (3): 979–988.

WHO (World Health Organization) (2005) *Clean Care is Safer Care*. Geneva: WHO.

—— (2007) Ethical considerations in developing a public health response to pandemic influenza. Geneva: WHO.

—— (2008) Addressing Ethical Issues in Pandemic Influenza Planning. Geneva: WHO.

—— (2009) *Nurses and Midwives: A force for health*. Copenhagen: WHO.

Whyte, D. and Robb, Y. (1999) Families under stress: how nurses can help. *Nursing Times*, 95 (30): 50–52.

Wiener, R.S. and Welch, H.G. (2007) Trends in the use of the pulmonary artery catheter in the United States, 1993–2004. *JAMA*, 298 (4): 423–429.

——, Wiener, D.C. and Larson, R.J. (2008) Benefits and risks of tight glucose control in critically ill adults: a meta-analysis. *JAMA*, 300: 933–944.

Wilkins, R.L., Hodgekin, J.E. and Lopez, B. (2004) *Fundamentals of Lung and Heart Sounds*, 3rd edition. St Louis, MO: Mosby.

Wilkinson, K. (1997) Paediatric physiology and general considerations, in Goldhill, D.R. and Withington, P.S. (eds) *Textbook of Intensive Care*. London: Chapman & Hall, pp. 345–353.

Williams, A.J. (1998) Assessing and interpreting arterial blood gases. *British Medical Journal*, 317: 1213–1216.

Williams, A.M. and Irurita, V.F. (2004) Therapeutic and non-therapeutic interpersonal interactions: the patient's perspective. *Journal of Clinical Nursing*, 13 (7): 806–815.

Williams, J., Oenning, V. and Tuomaia, B. (2005) Cardiovascular alterations, in Sole, M.L., Klein, D.G. and Moseley, M.J. (eds) *Critical Care Nursing*, 4th edition. St Louis, MO: Elsevier Saunders, pp. 291–350.

Williams, J.M.L. and Williamson, R.C.N. (2010) Alcohol and the pancreas. *British Journal of Hospital Medicine*, 71 (10): 556–561.

Williams, T.A. and Leslie, G.D. (2004) A review of the nursing care of enteral feeding tubes in critically ill adults: part I. *Intensive and Critical Care Nursing*, 20 (6): 330–343.

—— (2005) A review of the nursing care of enteral feeding tubes in critically ill adults: part II. *Intensive and Critical Care Nursing*, 21 (1): 5–15.

——, Martin, S., Thomas, L., Leen, T., Tamaliunas, S., Lee, K.Y. and Dobb, G. (2008) Duration of mechanical ventilation in an adult intensive care unit after introduction of sedation and pain scales. *American Journal of Critical Care*, 17 (4): 349–356.

Wilson, J., Woods, I., Fawcettt, J., Whall, R., Dibb, W., Morris, C. and McManus, E. (1999) Reducing the risk of major elective surgery: randomised controlled trial of preoperative optimisation of oxygen delivery. *British Medical Journal*, 318 (7191): 1099–1103.

Wilson, L.A. (2005) Urinalysis. *Nursing Standard*, 19 (35): 51–54.

Wilson, P.W.F. and Grundy, S.M. (2003) The metabolic syndrome: practical guide to origins and treatment: part 1. *Circulation*, 108 (12): 1422–1425.

Wilson, S.R., Hirsch, N.P. and Appleby, I. (2005) Management of subarachnoid haemorrhage in a non-neurosurgical centre. *Anaesthesia*, 60 (5): 470–485.

Winer, J.B. (2008) Gullain-Barré syndrome. *British Medical Journal*, 337 (7663): 227–230.

Winser, H. (2001) An evidence base for adult resuscitation. *Professional Nurse*, 16 (7): 1210–1213.

Winslow, E.H. and Jacobson, A.F. (1998) Dispelling the petroleum jelly myth. *American Journal of Nursing*, 98 (11): 16.

Wittenberg, M.D., Kaur, N. and Walker, D.A. (2010) The challenge of HIV disease in the intensive care unit. *Journal of the Intensive Care Society*, 11 (1): 26–30.

Wittlinger, M., Schläpfer, M., de Conno, E., Z'graggen, B.R., Reyes, L., Booy, C., Schimmer, R.C., Seifert, B., Burmeister, M.-A., Spahn, D.R. and Beck-Schimmer, B. (2010) The effects of hydroxyethyl starches (HES 130/0.42 and HES 200/0.5) on activated renal tubular epithelial cells. *Anesthesia & Analgesia*, 110 (2): 531–540.

Wong, H.R. (1998) Potential protective role of the heat shock response in sepsis. *New Horizons*, 6 (2): 194–200.

Woodrow, P. (2009) End-of-life care, in Moore, T. and Woodrow, P. (eds) *High Dependency Nursing: Observation, intervention and support*, 2nd edition. London: Routledge, pp. 400–408.

Woods, S. and Gray, S.J. (2009) Cardiopulmonary bypass. *Anaesthesia and Intensive Care Medicine*, 10 (9): 416–420.

Wren, M. (2009) *Clostridium difficile*: How big? How bad?, in Ridley, S. (ed.) *Critical Care Focus 16: Infection*. London: Intensive Care Society, pp. 46–55.

Wright, B. (2007) *Loss and Grief*. Keswick: M&K Update.

Writing Committee of the Second World Health Organization Consultation on Clinical Aspects of Human Infection with Avian Influenza A (H5N1) Virus (2008) Update on Avian Influenza A (H5N1) virus infection in humans. *New England Journal of Medicine*, 358 (3): 261–273.

Wu, Y.-K., Tsai, Y.-H., Lan, C.-C., Huang, C.-Y., Lee, C.-H., Kao, K.-C. and Fu, J.-Y. (2010) Prolonged mechanical ventilation in a respiratory-care setting: a comparison of outcome between tracheostomized and translaryngeal intubated patients. *Critical Care*, 14 (2): R26.

Wunsch, H. and Mapstone, J. (2005) High-frequency ventilation versus conventional ventilation for the treatment of acute lung injury and acute respiratory distress syndrome: a systematic review and Cochrane analysis. *Anesthesia & Analgesia*, 100 (6): 1765–1772.

Wyffels, P.A.H., Sergeant, P. and Wouters, P.F. (2010) The value of pulse pressure and stroke volume variation as predictors of fluid responsiveness during open chest surgery. *Anaesthesia*, 65 (7): 704–709.

Wyncoll, D.L.A. (2009) Management of acute poisoning, in Bersten, A.D. and Soni, N. (eds) *Intensive Care Manual*, 6th edition. Edinburgh: Butterworth-Heinemann Elsevier, pp. 903–912.

Xavier, G. (2000) The importance of mouth care in preventing infection. *Nursing Standard*, 14 (18): 47–51.

Yassin, J. and Wyncoll, D. (2005) Management of intractable diarrhoea in the critically ill. *Care of the Critically Ill*, 21 (1): 20–24.

Yellon, D.M. and Hausenloy, D.J. (2007) Myocardial reperfusion injury. *New England Journal of Medicine*, 357 (11): 1121–1135.

Ympa, Y.P., Sakr, Y., Reinhart, K. and Vincent, J.-L. (2005) Has mortality from acute renal failure decreased? A systematic review of the literature. *American Journal of Medicine*, 118 (8): 827–32.

Yoshida, T., Rinka, H., Kaji, A., Yoshimoto, A., Arimoto, H., Miyaichi, T. and Kan, M. (2009) The impact of spontaneous ventilation on distribution of lung aeration in patients with acute respiratory distress syndrome: airway pressure release ventilation versus pressure support ventilation. *Anesthesia & Analgesia*, 106 (6): 892–900.

Young, J., Stiffleet, J., Nikoletti, S. and Shaw, T. (2006) Use of a Behavioral Pain Scale to assess pain in ventilated, unconscious and/or sedated patients. *Intensive & Critical Care Nursing*, 22 (1): 32–39.

Young, J.B. and Sturdy, D. (2007) Improving care for older people in general hospitals. *Geriatric Medicine*, 37 (4): 39–41.

Yu, M., Nardella, A. and Pechet, L. (2000) Screen tests of disseminated intravascular coagulation: guidelines for rapid and specific laboratory diagnosis. *Critical Care Medicine*, 28 (6): 1777–1780.

Zaar, M., Lauritzen, B., Secher, N.H., Krantz, T., Nielsen, H.B., Madsen, P.L. and Johansson, P.I. (2009) Initial administration of hydroxyethyl starch vs lactated Ringer after liver trauma in the pig. *British Journal of Anaesthesia*, 102 (2): 221–226.

Zeeleder, S., Hack, E. and Wuillemin, W.A. (2005) Disseminated intravascular coagulation in sepsis. *Chest*, 128 (4): 2864–2875.

Zeeman, G.G., Fleckenstein, J.L., Twicker, D.M. and Cunningham, F.G. (2004) Cerebral infarction in eclampsia. *American Journal of Obstetrics & Gynecology*, 190 (3): 714–720.

Zimetbaum, P. (2007) Amiodarone for atrial fibrillation. *New England Journal of Medicine*, 356 (9): 935–941.

Zimmer, S.M. and Burke, D.S. (2009) Historical perspective – emergence of influenza A (H1N1) viruses. *New England Journal of Medicine*, 361 (3): 279–285.

Zimmerman, J.E., Kramer, A.A., McNair, D.S. and Malila, F.M. (2006) Acute Physiology and Chronic Health Evaluation (APACHE) IV: hospital mortality assessment for today's critically ill patients. *Critical Care Medicine*, 34 (5): 1297–1310.

Zirakzadeh, A. and Patel, R. (2006) Vancomycin-resistant *Enterococci*: colonization, infection, detection, and treatment. *Mayo Clinical Proceedings*, 81 (4): 529–536.

Index

Page numbers in italic type indicate figures and tables.

ABCDE approach
  children 116–119
  CNS injury 356–359
  DIC 262
  drug overdose 450–452
  gastrointestinal bleeds 402
  influenza pandemics 143–144
  transfer of patients 465–466
abdominal aortic aneurysm (AAA) repair
    347
abdominal compartment syndrome 411,
    485
abruptio placentae 485
abscesses, pancreatic 436
abuse, reporting 120
accountability 458–461
ACE inhibitors 289
acetylcholine 64–65
acidaemia 176
acid/base balance *see* arterial blood gas
        (ABG) analysis
acidosis 88, 92, 173–175, *174*, 176, 181,
        307–308, 385, 395, 411, 489
  compensation 181–182
  diabetic ketoacidosis 443–444
Acinetobacter 133
action potential 218, *218*

activated protein C 322
acute coronary syndromes (ACS)
        see coronary artery disease
acute fatty liver 418
acute kidney injury (AKI) 126, 141, 380,
        386–388, 411
  effects on body systems 384–385
  management
    diuretics 385–386
    fluid challenges 385
  rhabdomyolysis 386
  types
    intrinsic 380–381
    postrenal 381–382
    volume-responsive 380
  see also haemofiltration; kidneys
acute lung injury (ALI)
  transfusion-related (TRALI) 330
  see also acute respiratory distress
        syndrome (ARDS)
acute phase proteins 251
acute respiratory distress syndrome
        (ARDS) 34, 37, 38, 39, 270,
        272–274
  conventional ventilation 270–272
  rescue therapies 276–281
acute tubular necrosis (ATN) 380, 381

adaptive pressure ventilation (APV) *see* pressure-regulated volume control (PRVC)

adaptive support ventilation (ASV) 35–36

adenosine triphosphate (ATP) 87, 166, 249, 307

adrenaline (epinephrine) 8, 337, *339*, 341

adrenergic agonists *see* inotrope/vasopressor therapy

adrenocorticotrophic hormone (ACTH) 8, 305

aerolised viruses 144

ageing *see* older people, ageing

ageism 127

agranulocytes 201, 202, *202*
  lymphocytes 255–256, 311

AIDS-related complex (ARC) 256–257, 258–259

airborne infection 135

air emboli, central lines 191

air-trapping (auto-PEEP) 156

airway management 48, 57–58, 143
  children 116–117
  CNS injury 357
  drug overdose 450–451
  endotracheal suction 55–57, 278
  extubation 43, 49–50
    stridor 50
  humidification 53–55, *54*
  intubation 48–49
    problems 52–53, *53*
  pandemics 143
  positioning 271–272
  tracheostomy 50–52
  during transfer 465
  see also ventilation; ventilators

airway pressure release ventilation (APRV) 36

albumin 175, 203, 409
  for infusion *328*, 331

alcohol-induced illness 407, 434

alcohol rubs 136

alfentanil 61, 73

alkaline phosphatase 409

alkalosis 173, 175, 176

alpha receptors 337–339, *339*

alpha 2 antagonists 61

alveoli *see* lungs

ambulance transfer *see* transfer of patients

amitriptyline 76

ammonia 87

amniotic fluid embolus 419

amphetamine sulphate ('speed') 450

amylase 435

anabolism 87, 485
  see also metabolism

anacrotic notch 187, 485

anaemia 158, 201
  sickle cell disease 168

anaesthetics 61, 74

analgesia *see* pain management

anaphylactic shock 311, 485

anaphylactoid syndrome, pregnancy 419

aneurysms *see* vascular surgery

angina, unstable (UA) 286–291, *287*

angioplasty 294–295

angiotensinogen 410

anion gap 180–181

antibiotics 91, 135, 320–321
  see also infection

antibodies 255–256, 311

anticoagulants 392–393
  see also clotting

antidepressants, overdose 447–448

antidiuretic hormone (ADH; vasopressin) 343, 361, 400, 441

anti-emetics 76

antioxidants 251

antipsychotic drugs 62

antipyretic drugs 83

antispasmodic drugs 92

anxiolysis *see* sedation

aorta
  aneurysms 347–348
  aortic stenosis 295–296
  aortic valve 187
  IABPs 312–313, *312*
  see also arteries

APACHE scoring system 127, 480

apnoea backup, ventilators 34, 35

apoptosis, cells 249

arrhythmias *see* heart, dysrhythmias

arterial blood gas (ABG) analysis 172, 182–183
  acid/base balance 172, 173–176, *174*, 298, 383
    acidosis/alkalosis 88, 92, 173–175, *174*, 176, 181, 307–308, 385, 395, 411, 489

buffering 172, 175
    citric acid cycle 87–88, *88*, 249
    compensation 181–182
    pH measurement 172–173
  interpreting results 177–181, *178*
  sampling methods/errors 176–177
'arterial swing' 187
arteries
  blood pressure 185–188, *187*, 242
  carotid 82, 348, 349
  saturation 179
  temperature 82
  see also aorta; arterial blood gas (ABG)
      analysis; coronary artery disease;
      haemodynamic monitoring; vascular
      surgery
artificial ventilation *see* ventilation
ascites 410, 485
aspirate, gastric 89–90
aspiration pneumonia 53
aspirin 83, 289
assault, touch/restraint as 25–26, 62,
    258
assisted spontaneous breathing (ASB)
    43–44
asthma 38, 39, 54, 61
asystole 231
atelectasis 50, *56*, 166, 485
atelectrauma 42
atherosclerosis 186
  aneurysms 347–348
  see also coronary artery disease
atracurium 65
atrial dysrhythmias 222–225, *222–223*,
    225–226, 299
atrial ectopics 221–222, *221*
atrioventricular blocks 226–227, *226–228*
auscultation 151–153
  breath sounds 151–152, *152*
autocycling, ventilators 39
autoimmune disorders 250, 257
  type 1 diabetes 442
autologous transfusion 294, 485
autonomic nervous system 305, 311,
    372–373
  stress responses 19, 72, 290, 311, 361
    autonomic hyper-reflexia 364–365
    sympathetic responses 8, 53, 56, 98,
        305, 311, 341
axillary temperature 82

bacteria 131–133
  commensal 91, 132, 486
    translocation 89, 91
  see also antiobiotics; infection
bacterial pneumonia 257
balloon pumps 312–313, *312*
balloon tamponade 401, *401*, 485
barometric pressure 162
barotrauma 35, 42, 43, 154, 485
barrier nursing 22
basal skull fracture 359
base excess (BE) 180
Behavioral Pain Scale (BPS) 73
Behaviourism 12–14
benzodiazepines 20, 60–61
'best interests' 25–26
beta-blockers 289, 401
beta receptors 337–339, *339*
bicarbonate 166, 175, 176, 180,
    395
bigeminy 229, *229*
bilevel positive airway pressure 36
bilirubin 383, 408, 411
bioimpedance 193
biomarkers
  cardiac 286, 288
  creatinine *209*, 210, 382
  cytokines 80, 249–250, *250*, 319,
      487
  for pancreatitis 435
  procalcitonin 321, *321*
biotrauma 42
'bird flu' 140–141
bispectral index (BIS) 63, 65
bladder 82, 364
  urinary catheters 82, 386, 412
  see also kidneys
bleeding/haemorrhage 262, 264, 277
  cardiac surgery 297–298
  gastrointestinal 399–404, *401*
  haematuria 382–383
  haemorrhage shock 310
  intra-abdominal 437
  intracranial 365
  liver failure 410
  pregnancy 418
  vascular surgery 349
blepharitis 105, 485
blink reflexes 104–105
block, sensory 74

blocks, heart
  atrioventricular 226–227, *226–228*
  bundle branch 228, *228*
blood 199–200, 210–212
  biochemistry 204–208, *209*, 210
  erythrocytes *200*, 201
  leucocytes 201–202, *202*, 250,
    255–256
  plasma 163, 166, 201
    plasma proteins 175, 203
  platelets 202–203
  see also bleeding/haemorrhage; clotting;
    gas carriage; haemodynamic
    monitoring; haemofiltration;
    haemoglobin (Hb)
blood–brain barrier 61, 64, 238, 342,
    409
blood cultures 134–135
blood gases *see* arterial blood gas (ABG)
    analysis
blood pressure
  arterial 185–188, *187–188*, 237
  central venous 188–191, *190*, 337
  see also haemodynamic monitoring;
    inotrope/vasopressor therapy
blood sugar *see* glucose
blood transfusion 80, 294, *328*,
    330–331
  alternative fluids *328*, 333–334
Böhr effect 485
Bolam test 459, 486
bone marrow 200
bowel care 91, 94–95
  bowel sounds 89
  Bristol Stool Form Chart 92
  constipation 93
  diarrhoea 91–93
  and spinal cord injury 364, *364–365*
  see also nutrition
Braden Scale 111–112
bradycardia 53, 220, 223, 486
brain
  atrophy 125
  oedema 238, 358
  perfusion pressure 237–238
  rotation 359
  see also central nervous system (CNS);
    central nervous system (CNS)
    injury; cranium; neurological
    monitoring

brainstem death 424–425, *425*
  brain death incubation 420
breathing *see* respiration; respiratory
    monitoring
Bristol Stool Form Chart 92
brittle bones 126
bronchoconstriction 34, 56
bronchodilators 55
bronchospasm 50, 152
  asthma 38, 39, 54, 61
B-type natiuretic peptide 288
buccal cavity 98
  see also mouthcare
buffering 172, 175
bundle branch block 228, *228*
Bundle of Kent 225
bypass *see* cardiac surgery

cachectin *see* tumour necrosis factor
    (TNF)
calcitonin 321, *321*
calcium *178*, 208–210, *209*
  brittle bones 126
  hyper-/hypocalcaemia 436, 488
calcium channels 81, 218, *218*, 248–249
  calcium channel blockers 289
calories 486
Candida 134, 318
candidiasis 99
cannulae *see* catheters/cannulae
capillaries 326, 327
capillary leak 250, 311, 318, 321
capillary occlusion pressure 52, 110,
    486
capillary refill 185
capnography 158, 193
carbaminoglobin 166
carbon dioxide 33–34, 163
  dissociation 167, *167*
  end-tidal (capnography) 158, 193
  hypercapnia 88, 105, 167, 173–174,
    488
    permissive 37, 270–271, 490
  hypocapnia 238, 488
  partial carbon dioxide rebreathing
    193
  removal 34, 37, 278
  see also arterial blood gas (ABG)
    analysis; gas carriage; gas
    exchange

carbon monoxide poisoning 168, 279, 280
cardiac arrhythmias/dysrhythmias *see* heart, dysrhythmias
cardiac markers 286, 288
cardiac oedema 225, 226
cardiac output/index (CO/CI) 193, 337
cardiac output studies *see* flow monitoring
cardiac surgery 293, 301–303
   bypass grafts 293, 295, 296
   IABPs and VADs 312–314, *312–314*
   open-heart surgery 293–294
   PCI/pPCI 294–295
   post-operative nursing 296–301
   pump oxygenators 276–277, 293, 294
   valve surgery 295–296
   see also transplants
cardiac tamponade 41, 298, 309–310, 491
cardiogenic shock 309
cardioplegia 294
cardiopulmonary bypass (CPB) *see* pump oxygenators
cardiovascular system 326
   ageing 125
   children 117–118, *118*
   CNS injury 357–358
   drug overdose 451
   effects of AKI 384
   epidemic influenza 144
   instability, pancreatitis 436–437
   pregnancy 417
   and shock 308
   during transfer 466
   ventilation complications 41–42
   see also blood pressure; coronary artery disease; haemodynamic monitoring; heart; perfusion; vascular surgery
cardioversion, chemical/electrical 220
carina 48, *49*, 54
carotid arteries 82, 348, 349
catabolism 87, 360, 486
   see also metabolism
catecholamine 24
catheters/cannulae 135, 187
   central venous 135, 188, *188*
      insertion/removal 190–191
      PICCs 191
   haemofilters 392

   intraventricular 241–242
   jugular vein 241
   PCI/pPCI 294–295
   pulmonary artery 192
   suction 56–57, 99
   TIPSS 402
   urinary 82, 386, 412
cations 180–181
C. difficile 92, 133
cell metabolism *see* metabolism
cellular pathology 248, 252–253
   cell membranes 248–249, *248*
   free radicals 166, 249, 251–252, 487
   mitochondria 87, 164, 249
   necrosis and apoptosis 249
   see also responses, inflammatory
central lines *see* central venous catheters (CVCs)
central nervous system (CNS) 235
   ageing 125
   see also autonomic nervous system; neurological disability; neurological monitoring; nervous system; sympathetic nervous system
central nervous system (CNS) injury 257, 356–357, 366–369
   ABCDE approach 356–359
   epilepsy 361–362, *362*, 366
   pituitary damage 361
   positioning 361
   prognosis/psychological problems 365–366
   spinal cord injury 357–358, 362–364
      autonomic hyper-reflexia (dysreflexia) 364–365
      positioning/moving 363
   traumatic brain injury 358, 359
      haemorrhage 365
      nursing care 359–361, *360*
central venous catheters (CVCs) 135, 188, 190–191, 318
central venous pressure (CVP) 188–191, *190*, 337
   see also haemodynamic monitoring
cerebral atrophy 125
cerebral oedema 238, 358, 409
cerebral perfusion pressure (CPP) 237–238
cerebrospinal fluid (CSF) 120, 235–236, 359

chemical cardioversion *see* drugs, cardiology
chest lead placement, ECG 216, *216*
chest shape/movement 150, 151, 278
children *see* paediatrics
chloral hydrate 119
chloramphenicol eye-drops 106, *107*
chlordiazepoxide 20
chlorhexadine 100
chloride *178*, 205, *209*
　hyper-/hypochloraemia 174–175, 205, 329, 488
cholesterol 289
chronic obstructive pulmonary disease (COPD) 34, 54, 153, 167
chronotropic effects 338, 486
circadian rhythm 24, 486
circulation *see* cardiovascular system
circus movement 225
citrate 393
citric acid (Krebs') cycle 87–88, *88*, 249, 489
clinical scoring 127, 480
　APACHE 127, 480
　delirium 19–20
　GCS 238–241, 359
　pain 73
　pressure sores 111–112
　sedation 62, *62–63*, *63*
　stool forms *92*
clonidine 61, 144, 349
clopidogrel 289
closed-circuit suction 56
Clostridium difficile 92, 133
clotting 202–203, 204, 277
　clot breakdown (fibrinolysis) 204, 261, 262
　DIC 261–264, 265–266, 410
　DVT (thromboembolism; VTE) 203, 261, 264–265, 363, 372, 418–419
　and haemofilters 392–393
　and IABPs 313
　pulmonary embolism 203, 261
　thrombolytics (clot busters) 289
coagulation *see* clotting
cocaine 449, 449–450
colloid osmotic pressure (COP) 326–327, 486
colloids *328*, 330–333

colostomy care 94
commensal bacteria 91, 132, 486
communication 23
　with older people 125, 127
　and oral hygiene 97
　with relatives 6
　and the senses 21–22
compensation, metabolic/respiratory 181–182
complaints about care 461
complements 486
compliance
　cranium 235–236
　lungs 154, *154–155*, 156
compound sodium lactate 329
computerised tomography (CT) 358
concentration gradients 173
confidentiality 8, 258, 367
confusion 150
　see also delirium
'coning' (tentorial herniation) 120, 491
consciousness, GCS 238–241, 359
constipation 93
consumption of oxygen/index (VO2/I) 195
consumptive coagulopathy 262
contact lenses 105
continuous positive airway pressure (CPAP) 36, 278
continuous renal replacement therapies (CRRTs) *see* haemofiltration
contre-coup 359
controlled mandatory ventilation (CMV) 35
convection, kidneys 390–391, *391*, 491
'Cooley's anaemia' 168
cooling 83
core temperature 81
Cori cycle 486
cornea 104–105
coronary artery bypass grafts (CABGs) *295*, 296
coronary artery disease 290–291
　cardiac markers 286, 288
　myocardial infarction 24, 226, 228, 251–252, 287, 299, 309
　　ECG lead changes 218, *219*
　　STEMI (STE-ACS)/NSTEMI (NSTE-ACS) 286–291, *287*, 293

treatment/drugs 287–288, 289–290
see also cardiac surgery; heart
cortisol 24
costs *see* professional issues, costs
coughing, intubation 52
'crackle' 152
cranium 235–236, *236–237*
   basal skull fracture 359
C-reactive protein (CRP) 205, *209*
creatine kinase (CK) 288
creatinine *209*, 210, 382
crepitations (rales/crackle) 152
crichothyroidotomies 52
cricoid pressure 48
Critical Care Outreach 7–8
critical illness neuropathy/myopathy
   371
crystalloids *328*, 329
cuff pressures
   blood pressure 186
   intubation 52, *53*
Cullen's sign 486
culture
   and pain 71
   and organ donation 427
CVVH/CVVHD *see* haemofiltration
cyanosis 150
cytokines 80, 249–250, *250*, 319, 487

Daltons/kiloDaltons 489
dantrolene sodium 81
D-dimers 204, 261, 262, 487
dead space 49, 50, 52, 54, 158, 163, 308,
   487
death 424–425, *425*
   brain death incubation 420
decompensation, liver 409–411
deep forehead temperature 82
deep vein thrombosis (DVT;
   thromboembolism; VTE) 203,
   261, 264–265, 363, 372,
   418–419
dehiscence 487
deliberate self-harm (DSH) *see* self-
   poisoning
delirium 19–20, 125
delivery of oxygen/index (DO2/I) 194
dentures 101
depolarising/non-depolarising drugs 64–65,
   487

depression 447–448
dermatomes 74, *75*
dextrans *328*, 332
diabetes insipidus 361, 426, 441
diabetes mellitus 441–442
   HHS/HONKS 444
   ketones 384, 442
      ketoacidosis 443–444
   metabolic syndrome 442–443
   see also glucose; urinalysis
dialysis 391, 487
   see also haemofiltration
diamorphine (heroin) 73
diarrhoea 91–93, 111, 133
diastolic pressure 185–186
diazepam 60–61
dicrotic notch 187, 487
diffuse axonal injury 487
diffusion 33, 39, 487
disability, ABCDE approach *see*
   neurological disability
disseminated intravascular coagulation
   (DIC) 261–263, 265–266, 410
   nursing care 264
   related pathologies 263
dissociation, oxygen/carbon dioxide
   157, 158, 164, *165*, 167, *167*
distributive shock 310–311
   see also sepsis
diuretics 385–386
dobutamine *339*, 340, 341–342
documentation 136, 461
dopamine *339*, 342
dopexamine (hydrochloride) 342, 386
Doppler assessment 349, 490
double pumping 339
down regulation, receptors 338
dressings, tracheostomies 52
drug abuse/misuse *see* self-poisoning
drug clearance, haemofiltration 395
drug-eluting stents (DESs) 295
drugs
   analgesics 73–76, *75*
   anticoagulants 392–393
   antipsychotics 62
   antipyretics 83
   antispasmodics 92
   cardiology 220, 289
   children 118, 119
   diuretics 385–386

half-life 60, 488
inotropes/vasopressors 337–345, *339*
neuromuscular blockade (chemical paralysis) 62, 64–65, 81, 357
pregnancy 420
sedation 60–62
steroids 321–322
see also self-poisoning
duty of care 8, 459
dysreflexia 364–365
dysrhythmias *see* heart, dysrhythmias

ears
hearing 21–22
ototoxicity 490
tympanic temperature 82
eclampsia 418
E. coli 174, 487
'Ecstasy' (MDMA) 449, 450
ectopics 220–222, *221–222*
bigeminy/trigeminy 229, *229*
ejection fraction 195, 487
elderly, the *see* older people
electrocardiography (ECG) 215–219, *215–219*, 286
electroencephalography (EEG) 63
electrolytes 92, *178*, 360, 428, 436, 451
emphysema 34
encephalopathy, hepatic 406, 409
endarterectomy 349
endogenous infection 131
'endoleak' 348, 487
endoscopy 400
endotracheal tubes (ETTs) 22, 48–50, *49*
children 116–117
problems 52–53, *53*, 101
suction 55–57, 278
endovascular aneurysm repair (EVAR) 347, 349–350
end-tidal carbon dioxide (capnography) 158, 193
energy 87–88, *88*, 249
enteral nutrition 89–90
Enterococci 133
epicardial wires 299
epidemics *see* pandemics
epidural opioids 74, *75*
epilepsy 61
CNS injury 361–362, *362*, 366

epinephrine *see* adrenaline
erythrocytes 163, *200*, 201
Escherichia coli 174, 487
estimated glomerular filtration rate (eGFR) 382
ethics
ageism 127
HIV/ARC 258
organ donation 427
rationing in pandemics 142–143
stereotyping 71, 124
exogenous infection 131
expired positive airway pressure (EPAP) 36
exposure, ABCDE approach
children 118–119
during transfer 466
exposure keratopathy 21, 104, 105, 489
extracorporeal membrane oxygenation (ECMO) *see* pump oxygenators
extravasation 487
extravascular lung water (EVLW) 195, 273
extubation *see* airway management; ventilators, weaning
eyes
damage/infection 104–108, *107*
eye muscle paralysis 65
pupil size/response, GCS 239–240
vision distortion/absence 21

faeces
and skincare 111
see also bowel care
fat metabolism 87, *88*, 126
fatty acids 490
fentanyl 61, 73
fibrillation
atrial 192, 195, 214, 221, 223, 224, 299
ventricular 230, *230*
fibrin degradation products (FDPs) 204, 261, 262
fibrin meshes 262
fibrinolysis (clot breakdown) 204, 261, 262
'fight or flight' responses 8, 98, 305, 341
filtration
glomerular filtration rate (GFR) 210, 382, 418
see also haemofiltration

finger clubbing 150
fitting
 children 118
 CNS injury 359
 eclampsia 418
 see also epilepsy
flow graphs 154, *155*
flow monitoring 191–195, *192*, 487
flow:volume loops 156, *157*
fluconazole 134
fluid management 326–327, 334–335
 ARDS 273
 CNS injury 358
 fluid challenges 385
 intravenous fluids 328–335, *328*
  colloids *328*, 330–333
  crystalloids 329
 oxygen-carrying fluids *328*, 333–334
 water distribution 326, *326*
 see also blood; perfusion
fluids, excessive
 acute fluid collections 435
 ascites 410, 485
 bowels 91
 cardiac tamponade 41, 298, 309–310
 pleural effusions 297
 see also oedema
fluids, physiological
 cerebrospinal fluid 120, 235–236, 359
 fluid loss 189
flumazenil 61
flutter, atrial 224, *225*
foetal haemoglobin (HbF) 168
follow-up clinics 25
fraction of inspired oxygen 37, 162, 164, 166, 278
free oxygen radicals 166, 249, 251–252, 487
fresh frozen plasma (FFP) 331
fungal infection 134, 318
furosemide 385–386

gabapentin 76
gallstones 434, 437
gamma-aminobutyric acid (GABA) 60
gas analysis *see* arterial blood gas (ABG) analysis
gas carriage 162, 169–170
 of carbon dioxide 166–167
 cell respiration 164–165

dissociation, oxygen/carbon dioxide 157, 158, 164, *165*, 167, *167*
 gas pressures 162–163, *162*
 Heliox 167–168
 hyperbaric oxygenation 113, 279–280
 of oxygen 163, 200–201, 238
 oxygen debt/toxicity 166, 321
gas exchange 33, 34, 37, 39, 153, 278
gastric irrigation 402
gastric motility 76
gastric residual volume (aspirate) 89–90
gastric tonometry 176
gastric tubes 89
gastrointestinal system
 ageing 126
 bleeding 399–404, *401*
 effects of AKI 384
 and HIV 257
 pancreas 308, 434–435
 and pregnancy 417
 see also bowel care; liver; pancreatitis
gelatins *328*, 331–332
gingivitis 98
Glasgow Coma Scale (GCS) 238–241, 359
glomerular filtration rate (GFR) 210, 382, 418
glucose *178*, 206–207, *209*, 329, 442, 444
 hyper-/hypoglycaemia 118, 207, 360, 384, 411, 417, 436, 441, 443, 488
 HHS/HONKS 444
glycaemic control *see* glucose
glyceryl trinitrate 289
glycosides 488
glycosuria 384, 488
graft versus host disease (GvHD) 428–429
gram positive/negative organisms 132–133, 318
granulocytes 201, 202, *202*
Grey Turner's sign 488
Guillain-Barré syndrome (GBS) 34, 141, 372–375

haematocrit (Hct) 201
haematology *see* blood
haemodynamic monitoring 185, 195–197, 349
 arterial pressure 185–186, *187–188*

central venous pressure 189–190, *190*, 337
  CVC use/removal 135, 188, 190–191
  PICCs 191
  flow monitoring 191–195, *192*
  ultrasound 195
haemofiltration 208, 322, 390–391, *390–391*, 395–397
  anticoagulation, filters 392–393
  monitoring/problems 393–395
haemoglobin (Hb) 163, 163–164, 164, 166, 200–201, 330
  derivatives 333–334
  foetal Hb 168
  haemoglobinopathies 168
   anaemia 158, 168, 201
haemolysis 206, 262
haemolytic uraemic syndrome (HUS) 263
haemorrhage *see* bleeding/haemorrhage
Haldane effect 167, 488
half-life 488
hallucinations 23
haloperidol 20, 62
hand hygiene 136
Hartmann's 329
head injury *see* central nervous system (CNS) injury; neurological monitoring
health and safety *see* safety
healthcare-associated infections (HAIs) 131, 133, 135
health promotion 290
 drug misuse 452–453
heart
  dysrhythmias 53, 191, 214, 232–233
   asystole 231
   atrial 222–226, 222–226, 299
   blocks 226–228, 226–228, 299
   ectopics 220–222, 221–222
   post-operative 298–299
   pulseless electrical activity 231
   and reperfusion injury 251–252
   treatments 219–220
   ventricular 228–230, *229–230*
  electrocardiography 215–219, *215–219*, 286
  oedema 225, 226
  tamponade 41, 298, 309–310
  see also cardiovascular system; coronary artery disease

heart–lung machines *see* pump oxygenators
heat/moisture exchangers (HMEs) 54, 55
heatstroke 81
Helicobacter pylori 399
Heliox 167–168
helium 167, 313
HELLP syndrome 419–420
heparin 392–393
  HITTS 263
hepatic encephalopathy 406, 409
hepatitis 408
heroin (diamorphine) 73
herpes simplex 99
hertz (Hz) 488
hierarchy of needs, Maslow 14
high-dependency units (HDUs) 8
high-flow haemofiltration 322
high-flow humidified nasal oxygen 36
high-frequency ventilation (HFV/HFOV/HFJV) 277–279
highly active antiretroviral therapy (HAART) 256
HIV/ARC 256–257, 258–259
holistic care 6, 14
HONKS 444
hot-water humidifiers 54–55
HRQL scoring system 480
Humanism 12, 14, 15
humidification, airways 53–55, *54*
hydrogen ions 172–173, 175
hydrogen peroxide 251
hygiene 136
  oral *see* mouthcare
hyperalderostonism 488
hyperbaric oxygenation 113, 279–280
hypercalcaemia 488
hypercapnia 88, 105, 167, 173–174, 488
  permissive 37, 270–271, 490
hyperchloraemia 174–175, 205, 329, 488
hyperglycaemia 207, 360, 384, 417, 436, 441, 443, 488
  HHS/HONKS 444
hyperkalaemia 206, 308, 385, 488
hypermagnesaemia 208
hypernatraemia 205, 488
hyperosmolar hyperglycaemic state (HHS) 444
hyperoxia 166

hyperphosphataemia 207–208
hyperpyrexia 81
hypersalivation 53, 372
hypertension
  cardiac surgery 297
  GBS 372
  intra-abdominal 411–412, 437
  intracranial 235–236, 236–237, 358,
    359–360
  intraocular 105
  pregnancy 417, 418
  pulmonary 194, 272
  vasogenic 238
hypertonic saline dextran (HSD) 332
hyperventilation 173, 357
hypervolaemia 294, 333, 488
hypoalbuminaemia 175, 203
hypocalcaemia 436, 488
hypocapnia 238, 488
hypochloraemia 488
hypoglycaemia 118, 207, 360, 411, 443,
  488
hypokalaemia 92, 206, 299, 331, 385,
  488
hypomagnesaemia 208, 436
hyponatraemia 205, 488
hypoperfusion *see* shock
hypophosphataemia 207–208
hypotension 83, 195, 262, 305
  cardiac surgery 297
  GBS 372
  haemofiltration 395
  liver failure 410
  pulmonary 194
  see also acute kidney injury (AKI)
hypothalamic-pituitary-adrenal (HPA)
  axis 8, 305
hypothermia 83–84, 294
  children 118–119
hypothalamus 80
hypoventilation 173
hypovolaemia 83, 126, 186, 187, 488
  hypovolaemic shock 310
hypoxia 33, 37, 50, 56, 117, 164, 238,
  249, 250, 251
  myocardial 220
  oxygen debt 166, 321

ibuprofen 76
ICU Outreach *see* Critical Care Outreach

immune system 249–251, 255–256
  immunocompromise 53, 80, 131, 373,
    410, 488
  immunodeficiency 201, 256, 257
    HIV/ARC 256–257, 258–259
  transplants 428–429
    immunosuppression 429
immunoglobins 89
independent lung ventilation 39–40
infection 80, 131, 137–138, 428
  bacteria 131–133
    necrotising fasciitis 112–113
  from CVCs 135, 190–191
  fungi 134, 318
  healthcare-associated/nosocomial 131,
    133, 134, 135, 490
  meningitis 120–121
  oral 98–99
  pancreatitis 436
  screening and control 134–136
    signs and symptoms of infection
     319
  and white cells 201, 255–256
  see also immune system; pneumonia;
    responses, inflammatory; sepsis
influenza *see* pandemics
information
  and pain 71
  and relatives 6, 8
inotrope/vasopressor therapy 337,
  343–345
  adrenaline (epinephrine) 8, 337, *339*,
    341
  alpha/beta receptors 337–339, *339*
  calculations 340
  dobutamine *339*, 340, 341–342
  dopamine *339*, 342
  dopexamine (hydrochloride) 342
  noradrenaline (norepinephrine) 8, *339*,
    340, 341
  phosphodiesterase inhibitors 342–343
  safety 339–340
inspiratory:expiratory (I:E) ratio 38–39
insulin 206–207
  see also diabetes mellitus
interleukins 80, 249–250, 250, 319, 488
interventional lung assist (iLA) 277
intra-abdominal haemorrhage 437
intra-abdominal pressure (IAP) 411–412,
  437

intra-aortic balloon pumps (IABPs) 312–313, *312*
intracellular oedema 249
intracranial haemorrhage 365
intracranial pressure (ICP) 235–236, *236–237*
  measurement 241–242, *241*, 359–360
intraocular pressure 105
intrathoracic pressure 38, 41, 42, 195
intravenous fluids 328–335, *328*
intrinsic AKI 380–381
intubation *see* airway management
inverse ratio ventilation (IRV) 39, 271
ionised calcium 488
irrigation
  bladder 364
  gastric 402
ischaemia 24, 226, 380, 489
isoenzymes 288
isolation 22
isosorbide mono-/dinitrate 289
isothermic saturation boundary 53, 54, 489
itching (pruritis) 411

jaundice 411
jejunal tubes 89
jet ventilation 278–279
joules 489
jugular venous bulb saturation 241
junctional (nodal) ectopics 221
junctional (nodal) rhythm 225, *226*

keratitis 104, 105, 489
keratopathy 21, 104, 105, 489
ketamine 61, 73, 74, 119
  recreational use 450
ketoacids 174
ketones 384, 442
  diabetic ketoacidosis 443–444
kidneys 299
  acid/base balance 175
  ageing 126
  diuretics 385–386
  glomerular filtration rate 210, 382, 418
  and midazolam 60
  renin-angiotensin-aldosterone cascade 305, 348, 381, 410
  and shock 308

urinalysis 382–385
urine output 206, 208, 380, 381, 382, 395, 418
  see also acute kidney injury (AKI); haemofiltration
kilocalories 489
kiloDaltons 489
kilopascals (kPa) 172
kinetic therapy 272
Krebs' (citric acid) cycle 87–88, *88*, 249, 489
Kussmaul respiration 489

laboratory screening 134–135
labour 417
lactate *178*, 181, 329
laryngeal oedema 50
laxatives 93
'Lazarus' signs 425
left cardiac work/index (LCW/I) 194
left ventricular stroke work/index (LVSW/I) 194
legal issues/litigation 120, 367, 459, 460, 461
leucopaenia 201
leucocytes 201–202, *202*, 250, 255–256, 382–383
leukotrines 250, 319, 489
lifelong learning 14–15
limb assessment, GCS 240–241
limb electrodes, ECG 216
lipase 435
lips 101
liquid ventilation 279
liver
  acute fatty liver 418
  ageing 126
  artificial livers 412
  chemical buffers 175
  liver failure 405–408, *408*, 412–414
    decompensation signs 409–411
    intra-abdominal pressure 411–412
    liver function tests 408–409, *408*
  pregnancy 417
  and shock 308
  and ventilation 42
logarithms 172–173
loop of Henle 489
lorazepam 60–61
lumbar puncture 120

lungs
    acid/base balance 173–174, *174*, 181–182
    alveolar arterial gradient 179
    compliance 154, *154–155*, 156
    gas exchange 33, 34, 37, 39, 153, 278
    lung rest, ARDS 271
    oedema 33, 36, 189, 195, 273, 320
    pulmonary arteries 82, 192, 194
    pulmonary embolism 203, 261
    pulmonary hyper-/hypotension 194, 272
    see also acute lung injury (ALI); airway management; gas carriage; respiration; respiratory failure; respiratory monitoring; ventilation
lymphocytes 255–256, 311
lyposis 442

macula densa 489
magnesium 208, *209*, 436
malignant hyperpyrexia 81
malnutrition *see* nutrition
management of ICUs 470–473, 475–477
    morale 473–475
        break relief 474
mannitol 358, 386
manometers 190
Marfan's syndrome 348, 489
Maslow, Abraham 12, 14
maternal mortalities 416
MDMA ('Ecstasy') 449, 450
mean arterial pressure (MAP) 185–186, 237
meningitis 120–121
Mental Capacity Act 2005 25–26
metabolism 33–34, 80, 83, 173, 249, 307, 384
    acid/base balance 174–175
        acidosis 88, 92, 174–175, 176, 181, 307–308, 385, 395, 411, 489
        citric acid cycle 87–88, *88*, 249
        compensation 181–182
    blood 330–331
    energy 87–88, *88*, 249
    lactate *178*, 181
    metabolic syndrome 442–443
metabolites *178*
methaemoglobin (MetHb) 168
metoclopramide 76

microcirculation 185
microvascular obstruction/necrosis 262
midazolam 60–61, 118
millimoles 489
'Minnesota' tubes 401, *401*
minute volume 37
mitochondria 87, 164, 249, 307, 489
mitral valve disease/stenosis 295–296
Molecular Adsorbent Recirculating System (MARS) 412
Monro-Kellie hypothesis 235, 489
morale, staff 473–475
    break relief 474
morbidity/mortality 481–482
    maternal 416
    older people 126
morphine 61, 73, 74, 118, 119
mouthcare 97, 99–100, 101–102
    infection 98–99
    lips 101
    plaque 98, 100
    pressure sores 101
    removal of secretions 56, 99
    saliva 97–98, *98*, 100
    teeth and dentures 100, 101
MRSa/MSSa 132–133, 318
multi-organ dysfunction syndrome (MODS) 112–113, 318, 319–320
myelin 70
myocardium
    beta2 receptors 338
    oxygenation 194, 220, 286, *287*, 308
    stunning 251
myocardial infarction (MI) *see* coronary artery disease
myocyte membranes 218
myoglobin 288
    rhabdomyolysis 386

nasal cavity *54*
nasojejunal tubes 89
nasopharyngeal probes 82
natiuretic peptides 288
nausea, anti-emetics 76
near infrared spectroscopy (NIRS) 195
nebulisation/nebulisers 55
necrosis
    acute tubular 380, 381
    cells 249
    tissues 113

necrotising fasciitis 112–113, 311
negligence 458–459
nervous system 235
    effects of AKI 384
    ICU-acquired weakness 371
        Guillain-Barré syndrome (GBS) 34,
            141, 372–375
    neuropathic pain 76
    see also central nervous system (CNS);
        central nervous system (CNS)
        injury; neurological monitoring
neurogenic shock 311
neurological disability
    children 118
    CNS injury 358–359
    drug overdose 451–452
    during transfer 466
    epidemic influenza 144
neurological monitoring 235, 242–244, 300
    cerebral blood flow 237–238
    cerebral oedema 238
    Glasgow Coma Scale 238–241, 359
    intracranial pressure 235–236, 236–237
        measurement 241–242, 241, 359–360
    jugular venous bulb saturation 241
neuromuscular blockade (chemical
        paralysis) 62, 64–65, 81, 357
neuropathy see peripheral neuropathy
neurotransmitters
    acetylcholine 64–65
    GABA 60
neutrophils 202, 202, 319
nitrates 289
nitric oxide 250, 251, 319, 489
nitrite 383
nitrogen 87, 166
nociceptors 70
nodal (junctional) ectopics 221
nodal (junctional) rhythm 225, 226
noise levels 24
non-invasive ventilation (NIV) 36, 43–44
non-ST elevation (NSTE-ACS/NSTEMI)
        286–291, 287
non-steroidal anti-inflammatory drugs
        (NSAIDs) 76, 83
non-verbal cues, pain 72
noradrenaline (norepinephrine) 8, 339, 340,
        341
nosocomial infections 131, 133, 134, 135,
        490

nurse:patient ratios 7
nursing see professional issues
nutrition 87, 94–95
    CNS injury 360
    energy 87–88, 88, 249
    enteral 89–90
    older people 126
    and pancreatitis 437
    parenteral 90
    refeeding syndrome 90–1
    see also bowel care
nystatin 99

obstetrics see pregnancy
obstructive shock 309
ocular damage see eyes, damage/infection
oedema
    cardiac 225, 226
    cerebral 238, 358, 409
    intracellular 249
    laryngeal 50
    pancreatic 435
    periorbital 21
    pregnancy 417
    pulmonary 33, 36, 189, 195, 273,
        320
    from ventilation 42
oesophageal balloons 401, 401
oesophageal probes 82
'off-pump' coronary artery bypass
        (OPCAB) 294
older people 124, 128–129
    admission criteria 126–127
    ageing 124–125
        physiology 125–126
    ageism 127
    pain 71
    pyrexia 80
oliguria 380, 381, 395
oncotic pressure 490
'one-way weaning' 44
open-heart surgery 293–294
'open lung' strategies, ventilation 36, 38
opioids 61, 73–74
    epidural 74, 75
    patient-controlled analgesia 74–76
oral cavity 98
    removing secretions 56, 99
    see also mouthcare
organ donation see transplants

organ failure *see* multi-organ dysfunction
     syndrome (MODS)
oscillatory ventilation 278
osmolality/osmolarity of fluids *328*, 490
osmosis 490
ototoxicity 490
overdoses *see* self-poisoning
oximetry *see* pulse oximetry
oxygen 54, 117, 162–163, 194–195
    dissociation 157, 158, 164, *165*
    fraction of inspired oxygen 37, 162, 164,
        166, 278
    free radicals 166, 249, 251–252, 487
    high-flow humidified nasal oxygen 36
    hypoxia 33, 37, 50, 56, 117, 164, 238,
        249, 250, 251
       myocardial 220
       oxygen debt 166, 321
    jugular vein saturation 241
    partial pressure of arterial oxygen 37,
        162, 163
    see also arterial blood gas (ABG)
        analysis; gas carriage; gas
        exchange
oxygenation 34, 37, 38, 194
    hyperbaric 113, 279–280
    myocardial 194, 220, 286, *287*, 308
    oxygenation failure 33–34
    preoxygenation, suction 56
    pulse oximetry 157–158
    pump oxygenators 276–277, 293,
        294
oxygen-carrying fluids *328*, 333–334
oxygen debt 166, 321
oxygen index (OI) 157
oxygen toxicity 37, 42, 166

packed cell volume (PCV) 201
paediatrics 116, 121–122
   ABCDE approach 116–119
   extubation 50
   meningitis 120–121
   pyrexia 80
   sedation 118, 119, 144
   transfer 119, 119–120
   ventilation 35
pain management 69, 73, 76–78, 299–300,
      360, 428
   assessment 72–73
   central stimuli, GCS 239

children 118
drugs 73–76
physiology 70, *71*
   neuropathic pain 76, 372
psychology 70–71
pancreas 308
   pancreatic juice 434–435
pancreatitis 434–435, *435*, 438–439
   complications 435–436
   symptoms 436–437
   treatments 437
pancuronium 65
pandemics 140–141, 144–145
   influenza 140, 141–142
      'bird' and 'swine flu' 140–141
      prevention 144
      treatment 143–144
   rationing of resources 142–143
paracetamol 76, 83
   overdose 448
   see also liver, liver failure
paralysis, chemical *see* neuromuscular
      blockade
paralytic ileus 89
parenteral nutrition (PN) 90
paroxysms 490
partial carbon dioxide rebreathing
      193
partial pressure of arterial oxygen (PaO_2)
      37, 162, 163, 165
patient-centred care 5, 14, 15
patient-controlled analgesia (PCA)
      74–76
patient group directions (PGDs) 460–461
peptic ulcers 399
percutaneous coronary intervention (PCI)
      294–295
percutaneous intubation 51
percutaneous vascular repair 347
perfluorocarbons (PFCs) 279
perfusion 33, 83, 150, 158, 167, 327
   abdominal 411
   ageing 126
   cerebral 237–238
   renal 380
   reperfusion injury 166
   and vascular disease 349
   see also cardiovascular system;
      haemodynamic monitoring; shock
      (hypoperfusion)

periodontitis 98
periorbital oedema 21
peripheral cooling 83
peripherally inserted central cannulae
    (PICCs) 191
peripheral neuropathy 76, 371
    Guillain-Barré syndrome 34, 141,
        372–375
peripheral responses, GCS 241
peripheral warmth 185
permissive hypercapnia 37, 270–271,
    490
personal protective equipment (PPE)
    136
pethidine 73
pH *see* arterial blood gas (ABG) analysis
philosophy 15–17
    Behaviourism 12–14
    Humanism 12, 14, 15
phosphate 175, 207–208, *209*
phosphodiesterase inhibitors (PDIs)
    342–343
pituitary gland 8, 305, 361
plaque
    arterial 295, 349
    dental 98, 100
plasma 163, 166, 201
    fresh frozen 331
    plasma substitutes *328*, 331–332
plasma proteins 175, 203, 409
platelet-activating factor (PAF) 202, 319
platelets 202–203, 331
plethysmographs ('pleths') 158, 490
pleural effusions 297
pleural rub 152
Pneumocystis jirovici (PJP) 257
pneumonia 89, 136
    aspiration 53
    bacterial pneumonia 257
    ventilator-associated 48, 97, 133, 134
poisoning
    carbon monoxide 168, 279, 280
    and liver failure 407–408
    see also self-poisoning
polycythaemia 200
polyuria 208
positioning of patients
    CNS injury 358, 361, 363
    IAP measurement 412
    prone positioning 271–272

positive end expiratory pressure (PEEP) 36,
    38, 166, 271
    air-trapping (auto-PEEP) 156
positive pressure technique, extubation
    50
positive pressure, ventilation 42–43
post-operative care
    cardiac surgery 296–301
    transplant surgery 428
    vascular surgery 349–351, *350*
postrenal AKI 381–382
post-traumatic stress disorder (PTSD) 25,
    273, 481
potassium *178, 206, 209, 294*
    hyper-/hypokalaemia 92, 206, 299, 308,
        331, 385, 488
pre-eclampsia 418
pregnancy 416–418
    obstetric emergencies 416, 420–422
        amniotic fluid embolus 419
        haemorrhage 418
        HELLP syndrome 419–420
        hypertension 417, 418
        thromboembolism 418–419
    parity 490
    trimesters 491
pressure, physiological
    barotrauma 35, 42, 43, 154, 485
    capillary occlusion 52, 110, 486
    colloid osmotic 326–327, 486
    gases 162–163, *162*, 165
    intra-abdominal 411–412, 437
    intracranial 235–236, *236–237*,
        241–242, *241*, 359–360
    intraocular 105
    intrathoracic 38, 41, 42, 195
    perfusion gradients 327, *327*
    see also blood pressure
pressure, ventilation *see* ventilation;
    ventilators
pressure control (PC) 35
pressure graphs 154, *154*
pressure-regulated volume control (PRVC)
    35
pressure sores *see* skin and skincare,
    pressure sores
pressure support (PS) 36, 43–44
pressure support ventilation (PSV) 36
pressure:volume loops *155*, 156
primary angioplasty/PCI 295

probes
  nasopharyngeal/oesophageal 82
  pulse oximetry 158
procalcitonin 321, *321*, 435
professional issues 9–10, 458, 462
  accountability and negligence 458–461
  confidentiality 8, 258
  costs 277, 479–480, 482–484
    mortality/morbidity 481–482
    scoring systems 127, 480
  dealing with relatives 5–7, 366–367,
      452
  duty of care 8, 459
  holistic care 6, 14
  legal issues/litigation 120, 367, 459, 460,
      461
  levels of care *4*
  nurse education 12–13, 14
    lifelong learning 14–15
  nursing roles 7–8
  patient-centred care 5, 14, 15
  record keeping 461
  see also ethics; management of ICUs;
      psychological care; safety
prokinetics 90
prone positioning 271–272
propofol 61, 119
  propofol syndrome 118
proportional assist ventilation (PAV) 36
proprioceptors 22
prostacyclin 272, 392–393, 490
proteins
  acute phase 251
  body proteins 87
  plasma proteins 175, 203, 409
  proteinuria 383
pruritis 411
pseudocysts, pancreatic 435–436
Pseudomonas 133
psychedelic drugs 23
psychological care 19
  ARDS 273
  CNS injury 360, 366
  coronary disease 290
  HIV/ARC 257
  liver failure 409–410
  of older people 127
  of relatives 6, 366–367
    organ donation 426, 427
  ventilation 44

psychological problems 19, 26–28
  anxiety, intubation 53
  cardiac surgery 300
  circadian rhythm and sleep 24–25
  CNS injury 366
  delirium 19–20, 125
  GBS 373
  isolation 22
  obstetric emergencies 420
  pain 70–71
  sensory 21–24
  stress 8, 19, 257, 290
    PTSD 25, 273, 481
  see also responses, stress
pulmonary artery catheters (PACs) 192
pulmonary artery pressure (PAP) 194
pulmonary artery temperature 82
pulmonary embolism (PE) 203, 261
pulmonary hyper-/hypotension 194, 272
pulmonary oedema 33, 36, 189, 195,
      273, 320
pulmonary vascular resistance/index
      (PVR/I) 194
pulmonary vasodilators 55
pulseless electrical activity (PEA) 231
pulse oximetry 157
  limitations 158
pulse pressure variation (PPV) 195
pulse waveforms 186–187, *187*, 192,
      242
pump oxygenators 276–277, 293, 294
pyrexia 80, 80–81, 358, 361
  children 118–119
  malignant hyperpyrexia 81
  treatment 83
  see also thermoregulation
pyrogens 80

QALYs scoring system 480

radial pulse applanation tonometry 193
radicals, free oxygen 166, 249, 251–252,
      487
rales 152
Ramsay scale 63, *63*
rapid eye movement (REM) 24
rapid shallow breathing index (RSBI)
      157
reality orientation 23, 125
receptors, alpha/beta 337–339, *339*

recombinant erythropoietin 331
record keeping 136, 461
rectal temperature 82
refeeding syndrome 90–1
reflexes *see* responses
relatives, dealing with 5–7, 366–367,
        452
    organ donation 426, 427
remifentanil 61, 73
renal failure *see* acute kidney injury
        (AKI)
renal function *see* kidneys
renin-angiotensin-aldosterone cascade 305,
        348, 381, 410
reperfusion injury 166, 251–252
repolarisation 490
reserve function 124–125
respiration
    acid/base balance 173–174, *174*
        acidosis 173–174, 176
        compensation 181–182
    'arterial swing' 187
    breathing phases 38–39, 153, *153*
    breath sounds 151–152, *152*
    children 117
    CNS injury 357
    effects of AKI 384
    intrathoracic pressure 38, 41, 42, 195
    older people 125
    pregnancy 417
    'respiratory swing' 189
    shallow breathing 150
        rapid shallow breathing index 157
    during transfer 465–466
    see also gas carriage; gas exchange;
        lungs; ventilation; ventilators
respiratory failure 33–34, 372
    ARDS 34, 37, 38, 39, 270–274
        rescue therapies 276–281
    asthma 38, 39, 54, 61
    bronchoconstriction 34, 56
    children 116–117
    COPD 34, 54, 153, 167
    emphysema 34
    and pancreatitis 436
    pulmonary embolism 203
    pulmonary hyper-/hypotension 194
    pulmonary oedema 33, 36, 189, 195,
        273, 320
    and shock 308

ventilator-associated lung injury 37, 38,
        42–43, 270
    see also pandemics; pneumonia;
        ventilation; ventilators
respiratory monitoring 150, 159–160, 193
    auscultation 151–153
        breath sounds 151–152, *152*
    end-tidal carbon dioxide (capnography)
        158, 193
    oxygen index 157
    pulse oximetry 157–158
    rapid shallow breathing index 157
    visual monitoring 150
        sputum 150, *151*
    waveform analysis 153–157, *153–155*,
        157
respiratory rate, ventilators 37
'respiratory swing' 189
responses 4, 15
    Glasgow Coma Scale 238–241, 359
    inflammatory 249–251
        acute coronary syndromes 286–291,
            287
        ARDS 34, 37, 38, 39, 270–274
        SIRS 112–113, 250, 251, 318, 436
        systemic inflammation 319
    MODS 112–113, 318, 319–320
    sensory 23
    spinal reflex ('Lazarus' signs) 425
    stress 19, 72, 290, 311, 361
        autonomic hyper-reflexia 364–365
        sympathetic responses 8, 53, 56, 98,
            305, 311, 341
    see also pain management; sepsis; shock
restraint, as assault 25–26, 62
    see also sedation
reticular activating system 23
rhabdomyolysis 386
rhonchi (wheeze) 152
right cardiac work/index (RCW/I) 194
right ventricular stroke work/index
        (RVSW/I) 194
rocuronium 65
Rogers, Carl 12, 15
rotation, brain 359

Saccharomyces boulardii 92
safety 25–26, 472
    inotrope/vasopressor therapy 339–340
    ventilation 40–1

saline solutions 329, 332
saliva 97–98, *98*
  hypersalivation 53, 372
  replacement 100
SAPS II scoring system 480
saturated fatty acids 490
saturation, arterial 179
scoring systems *see* clinical scoring
sedation 20, 60, 65–67
  assessment 62
    sedation scales 62, 62–63, *63*
    'train of four' 65
  children 118, 119, 144
  CNS injury 357
  drugs 60–62
    paralysing agents 64–65, 81
  sedation holds 43, 64
selective oral/digestive decontamination
    (SOD/SDD) 136
self-poisoning 447, 453–454
  ABCDE approach 450–452
  drugs 447–450
    'body packing' 449
  health promotion 452–453
  symptoms 450
self-ventilation 35, 39, 150, 189
senna 93
sensory block 74
sensory problems 21–24
sepsis 318–319, *319*, 322–324
  and MODS 319–320
  systemic inflammation 319
  toxic shock syndrome 311
  treatments 320–322, *321*
  see also shock
septicaemia, nosocomial 134, 135
serotonin 70, 451, 491
severe acute respiratory syndrome (SARS)
    140–141
shiftleadership *see* management of ICUs
shock (hypoperfusion) 87, 89, 144, 249,
    305–307, 314–316, 321
  cardiac interventions 312–313, *312–314*
  children 117
  and CNS injury 357–358
  perfusion failure 307–308
  stages 307–308
  system failure 308
  types 309–311
  see also sepsis

shunting 33, 179, 491
shunts 491
  TIPSS 402
sickle cell disease 168
signs and symptoms of infection (SSI)
    319
sinus rhythms *215*, 217
  sinus arrhythmia 222, *222*
  sinus bradycardia/tachycardia 223
skin and skincare 110, 113–114, 158,
    437
  assessing perfusion 185
  burns, oximetry 158
  necrotising fasciitis 112–113
  post-operative care 300–301
  pressure sores 101, 110–111, 126,
    361
    assessment 111–112
    prevention 112–113
sleep 24–25
smell 23
sodium *178*, 205, *209*
  hyper-/hyponatraemia 205, 488
sodium chloride 329
sodium-potassium pump 248–249
solvent drag, kidneys 390–391, *391*,
    491
sorbitol 91
specific gravity, urine 383–384
'speed' 450
spinal cord
  and pain 70
  see also central nervous system
    (CNS)
spinal cord injury (SCI) 357–358,
    362–364
  positioning/moving 363
  see also central nervous system (CNS)
    injury
spinal reflex ('Lazarus') responses 425
spinal shock 311, 357–358
sputum 150, *151*
staff *see* management of ICUs; professional
    issues
standardised bicarbonate (SBC) 180
Staphylococcus aureus 74, 311
  MRSa/MSSa 132–133, 318
starches *328*, 332–333
starvation *see* nutrition
statins 289

ST-elevation (STE-ACS/STEMI) 286–291, 287, 293
stenosis, aortic/mitral 295–296
stents
    aneurysm repair 347
    carotid artery 349
    drug-eluting 295
stereotyping 71, 124
    ageism 127
sterile water 100, 107
sternotomy 293, 294, 297
steroids 321–322
stethoscopes 151
stoma care 94
stool forms 92
stress, psychological 8, 19, 257, 290
    PTSD 25, 273, 481
stress responses *see* responses, stress
stress ulceration 400
stridor 50, 152
stroke volume/index (SV/I) 193
stroke volume variation (SVV) 195
sucralfate 400
suction
    endotracheal 55–57, 278
    oral secretions 99
sufentanil 61
supraventricular tachycardia (SVT) 223, 223
suxamethonium 65
'swine flu' 141
sympathetic nervous system 215, 301, 311, 364
    stimulation 24, 97, 337, 450, 451
        stress responses 8, 53, 56, 98, 305, 311, 341
synchronised intermittent mandatory ventilation (SIMV) 35
syringe drivers 339
systemic inflammatory response syndrome (SIRS) 112–113, 250, 251, 318, 436
systemic vascular resistance/index (SVR/I) 193–194
systolic pressure 185–186

tachycardia 220, 223, 223, 225, 229–230, 229–230, 286, 308, 491
tachyphylaxis 338
tacrolimus 429

tamponades
    balloon 401, *401*, 485
    cardiac 41, 298, 309–310, 491
taste 22
tear production 104–105, *107*
tears, artificial 106
technology 5
    see also ventilators
teeth and dentures 100, 101
    plaque 98, 100
    see also mouthcare
temperature
    and ABG analysis 178
    cardiac surgery 298
    children 118–119
    measurement 81–83
    peripheral warmth 185
    tracheal gas 54
    see also thermoregulation
temporal artery temperature 82
tentorial herniation 120, 491
terminal care 44
thalassaemia 168
thermometers 81–82
thermoregulation 80, 84–85
    temperature measurement 81–83
    see also hypothermia; pyrexia
thoracic electrical bioimpedance (TEB) 193
thrombocytes *see* platelets
thromboelastography (TEG) 261, 491
thromboembolism *see* deep vein thrombosis (DVT)
thrombolytics 289
thrombosis *see* clotting
thrombotic thrombocytopaenia purpura (TTP) 263
tidal ventilation 34
tidal volumes, ventilators 37, 278
tissue necrosis 113
tissue viability nurses 112
tonometry
    gastric 176
    radial pulse applanation 193
torsades de pointes 219, 230, *230*
total protein (TP) 203
touch 22
    as assault 258
toxic shock syndrome 311
tracheal gas temperatures 54

tracheal ulcers 52
tracheostomy 43, 50–52
'train of four' 65
tramadol 76
transaminases 409
transfer of patients 464–465, 466–468
    ABCDE approach 465–466
    children 119, 119–120
transfusion *see* blood transfusion
transfusion-related acute lung injury
    (TRALI) 330
transjugular intrahepatic portosystemic
    shunt (TIPSS) 402
transmembrane pressure (TMP), filters
    394, 491
transplants 424, 429–430
    brainstem death 424–425, *425*
    cardiac 296, 301
    ethical issues 427
    immune system 428–429
    living donors 427
    nursing care 425–426, 428
    rejection 428
traumatic brain injury (TBI) 358, 359–361,
    360
triclofos 119
trigeminy 229, *229*
trigger levels, ventilators 39, 154
trimesters, pregnancy 491
troponin 286, 288
tuberculosis (TB) 257
tumour necrosis factor (TNF) 80, 249–250,
    250, 319
tunica intima 319, 491
tympanic (ear) temperature 82

ulcers
    gastric 399–400
    tracheal 52
ultrafiltrate 491
ultrafiltration, kidneys 390–391, *390*, 394,
    492
unstable angina (UA) 286–291, *287*
urea *209*, 210
urinalysis 382–385
urinary catheters 82, 386, 412
urine output 206, 208, 380, 381, 382, 395,
    418
    diuretics 385–386
urobilinogen 383

vagal nerve stimulation 53
validation therapy 125
valve surgery 295–296
vancomycin-resistant *Enterococci* (VRE)
    133
variceal bleeding 400
vascular surgery 347, 351–352
    aneurysms 347–348
    post-operative care 349–351, *350*
vasoactive mediators 250, 286, 311, 319,
    321
vasogenic hypertension 238
vasopressin (ADH) 343, 361, 400, 441
vasopressors *see* inotrope/vasopressor
    therapy
vecuronium 65
venous blood pressure *see* central venous
    pressure (CVP)
venous thromboembolism (VTE; DVT)
    203, 261, 264–265, 363, 372,
    418–419
ventilation 32–33, *32*, 34, 44–46, 372
    ARDS 270–272
        rescue therapies 276–281, 293
    cardiac surgery 297
    children 117
    CNS injury 357
    influenza pandemics 143–144
    patient care 40, 44
        kinetic therapy 272
        positioning 271–272
        safety 40–1
        system complications 37, 41–43
    self-ventilation 35, 39, 150
    during transfer 465–466
    see also airway management; lungs;
        respiratory failure; respiratory
        monitoring; sedation; ventilators
ventilator-associated lung injury (VALI) 37,
    38, 42–43, 270
ventilator-associated pneumonia (VAP) 48,
    97, 133, 134
'ventilator eye' 104, 105
ventilators
    apnoea backup 34, 35
    modes and cycles 34–36
        independent lung ventilation 39–40
    settings 37
        inspiratory:expiratory (I:E) ratio
        38–39

inverse ratio ventilation 39, 271
PEEP 36, 38, 166, 271
waveform analysis 153–157, *153–155, 157*
weaning 35–36, 37, 43–44, 157
see also airway management; ventilation
ventricular assist devices (VADs) 312, 313, *314*
ventricular dysrhythmias 228–230, 229–230
ventricular ectopics 222, *222*
bigeminy/trigeminy 229, *229*
ventricular standstill (asystole) 231
vicarious liability 461
viruses *see* pandemics
vision 21
volume-controlled ventilation 35
volume graphs 156, *155*
volume-responsive AKI 380
volutrauma 42, 492
vomiting centre 76

water distribution 326, *326*
Waterlow pressure scoring system 112
Watson, John B. 12

waveform analysis
arterial pressure trace 312, *313*
central venous pressure 189–190, *190*
electrocardiography 215–219, *215–219, 286*
intracranial pressure 241–242, *241*
pulse waveforms 186–187, *187, 192*
respiratory monitoring 153–157, *153–155, 157*
weakness *see* peripheral neuropathy
weaning 35–36, 37, 43–44, 157
tracheostomies 52
wheeze (rhonchi) 152
white blood cells *see* leucocytes
white cell count (WCC) 201, *202*
'whoosh test' 89
Wolff-Parkinson-White (WPW) syndrome 225, *225*

xenografts 296
xerostomia (dry mouth) 97

Yankauer catheters 56, 99, 100
yeasts, digestion 91

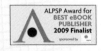
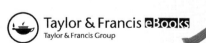